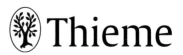

Orthodontic and Dentofacial Orthopedic Treatment

Thomas Rakosi, DDS, MD, MSD, PhD

Professor Emeritus and Former Chairman
Department of Orthodontics
School of Dental Medicine
Albert Ludwigs University
Freiburg, Germany

Thomas M. Graber, DMD, MSD, PhD, Odont Dr hc, DSc, ScD †

Former Clinical Professor of Orthodontics
Department of Orthodontics
College of Dentistry
University of Illinois at Chicago
Chicago, IL, USA

With contributions by

R. G. "Wick" Alexander, William J. Clark, Jason B. Cope, Jack G. Dale, M. Ali Darendeliler, John DeVincenzo, Magdalena Kotova, Andrew Kuhlberg, Michael R. Marcotte, Rainer-Reginald Miethke, C. Brian Preston, John J. Sheridan, Alexander Vardimon, Bjørn Zachrisson

1260 illustrations

Thieme
Stuttgart · New York

Library of Congress Cataloging-in-Publication Data is available from the publisher.

Important note: Medicine is an ever-changing science undergoing continual development. Research and clinical experience are continually expanding our knowledge, in particular our knowledge of proper treatment and drug therapy. Insofar as this book mentions any dosage or application, readers may rest assured that the authors, editors, and publishers have made every effort to ensure that such references are in accordance with **the state of knowledge at the time of production of the book.**

Nevertheless, this does not involve, imply, or express any guarantee or responsibility on the part of the publishers in respect to any dosage instructions and forms of applications stated in the book. **Every user is requested to examine carefully** the manufacturers' leaflets accompanying each drug and to check, if necessary in consultation with a physician or specialist, whether the dosage schedules mentioned therein or the contraindications stated by the manufacturers differ from the statements made in the present book. Such examination is particularly important with drugs that are either rarely used or have been newly released on the market. Every dosage schedule or every form of application used is entirely at the user's own risk and responsibility. The authors and publishers request every user to report to the publishers any discrepancies or inaccuracies noticed. If errors in this work are found after publication, errata will be posted at www.thieme.com on the product description page.

© 2010 Georg Thieme Verlag KG
Rüdigerstraße 14, 70469 Stuttgart,
Germany
http://www.thieme.de
Thieme New York, 333 Seventh Avenue,
New York, NY 10001, USA
http://www.thieme.com

Cover design: Thieme Publishing Group
Design and Typesetting by Ziegler + Müller, Kirchentellinsfurt, Germany
Printed in India by Replika Press LTD, Delhi

ISBN 978-3-13-127761-9

Some of the product names, patents, and registered designs referred to in this book are in fact registered trademarks or proprietary names even though specific reference to this fact is not always made in the text. Therefore, the appearance of a name without designation as proprietary is not to be construed as a representation by the publisher that it is in the public domain.

This book, including all parts thereof, is legally protected by copyright. Any use, exploitation, or commercialization outside the narrow limits set by copyright legislation, without the publisher's consent, is illegal and liable to prosecution. This applies in particular to photostat reproduction, copying, mimeographing, preparation of microfilms, and electronic data processing and storage.

In Memoriam

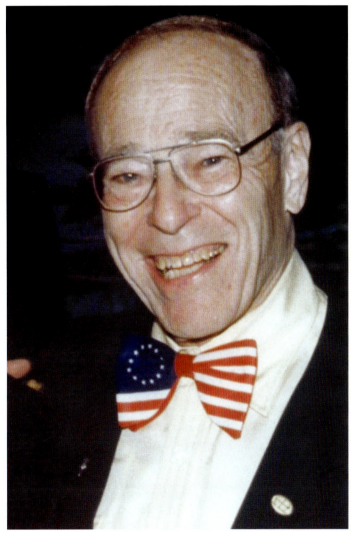

Thomas M. Graber, DMD, MSD, PhD, Odont Dr hc, DSc, ScD, MD, FDSRCS (Eng)
*1917, †2007

Contributors

R. G. "Wick" Alexander, DDS, MSD
Professor of Orthodontics
Baylor College of Dentistry
Texas A & M Health Science Center
Dallas, TX
Private Practice
Arlington, TX, USA

William J. Clark, BDS, DDO
Orthodontist
Fife, Scotland, UK

Jason B. Cope, DDS, PhD
Diplomate, American Board of Orthodontics
Adjunct Associate Professor
Department of Orthodontics
St. Louis University
St. Louis, MI, USA

Jack G. Dale, DDS
Private Practice
Toronto, Ontario, Canada

M. Ali Darendeliler, DDS
Professor and Chair
Discipline of Orthodontics
Faculty of Dentistry
University of Sydney
Head, Department of Orthodontics
Sydney Dental Hospital
Sydney, NSW, Australia

John DeVincenzo, DDS, MS
Clinical Professor
UCSF, Division of Orthodontics
San Luis Obispo, CA, USA

Magdalena Kotova, DDS, PhD
Clinical Department of Stomatology
Third Faculty of Medicine
Charles University
Prague, Czech Republic

Andrew Kuhlberg, DMD, MSD
Private Practice
Avon, CT, USA

Michael R. Marcotte, DDS, MSD
Private Practice
Bristol, CT, USA

Rainer-Reginald Miethke, Dr. med. dent., PhD
Professor and Chair
Department of Orthodontics, Dentofacial Orthopedics
and Pedodontics
Charité, Center for Dental Medicine
Berlin, Germany

C. Brian Preston, BDS, PhD, MS and Certificate in Orthodontics
Department of Orthodontics
School of Dental Medicine
University at Buffalo
The State University of New York
Buffalo, NY, USA

John J. Sheridan, DDS, ABO
Associate Professor
School of Orthodontics
Jacksonville University
Jacksonville, FL, USA

Alexander Vardimon, DDS
Associate Professor and Chairman
Department of Orthodontics
The Maurice and Gabriela Goldschleger School
of Dental Medicine
Head, The International Postgraduate Program in Orthodontics
Tel Aviv University
Tel Aviv, Israel

Bjørn Zachrisson, DDS, MSD, PhD
Professor II
Department of Orthodontics
Faculty of Dentistry
University of Oslo
Oslo, Norway

A Clinical Roadmap for the New Orthodontics

Tom Graber originally prepared this preface but unfortunately he could not finish it. Tom's interest was in international and not national orthodontics—with no dogmatism but looking pragmatically in all directions for methods that help solve various types of treatment problems with selective indication. This was the nature of Tom and his vision.

After Tom's death, it was decided to dedicate this book to his memory. As originally the co-editor of the book, I have completed this preface but maintained the spirit of Tom as well the content of the original.

In what follows, essentially Tom is speaking to us. First-person references convey his own experiences, enthusiasms, and wisdom. My own interpolations will be obvious.

T. Rakosi

Nine volatile years into a millennium we are all acutely aware of many challenges that confront us in diverse fields. Every country in the world faces political, financial, and economic quicksand, and the future is less certain than anyone would wish. In a more professionally parochial survey, the field of orthodontics and dentofacial orthopedics has seen no cataclysmic events, only steady progress based on extensive research around the world. The demand for our services has encouraged the brightest minds to come into our specialty. The financial returns have attracted commercial firms to provide the armamentarium we need, and technical developments have kept pace with scientific progress. Not only are more patients being treated, but "service" is better than ever before. Long-term evidence-based assessment of treatment results is now available. We know pretty well what we can and cannot do in dentofacial orthopedics and orthodontics.

On the other side of the coin, the potential iatrogenic sequelae of our services are common knowledge both within our specialty and in the contingency-fee legal profession. The question "At what price orthodontics?" is answered now in biological, biomechanical, and risk-management arenas. Some of the most comprehensive searches in Medline emanate from law offices, as motivated young legal staff search for all possible untoward effects resulting from our services. No longer are such terms as "crestal bone loss," "dehiscence," "decalcification," "fenestration," "gingival recession," "hypermobility," "interseptal bone loss," "periodontal problems," "root resorption," "TMD," and "traumatic occlusion" exclusive to the professional orthodontic vocabulary!

It is imperative that we practice evidence-based orthodontics. Defensive orthodontics is imperative for both the patient and orthodontist. This, of course, means proper diagnosis and patient selection before anything else. It was to that end that Tom Rakosi, Irmtrud Jonas, and I produced the widely used *Orthodontic Diagnosis* in the Color Atlas of Dental Medicine series (Thieme, 1993), which was printed in more languages than any other orthodontic text. "Dropping the other shoe," so to speak, is this new text *Orthodontic and Dentofacial Orthopedic Treatment*. For this we have assembled an impressive group of world-class clinicians to cover those aspects that we feel are most important for rendering the highest level of service in the safest, most practice-efficient way.

Chapter 1 (Tom Rakosi) recapitulates the fundamentals of orthodontic diagnosis as previously presented in *Orthodontic Diagnosis*, with special emphasis on therapeutic diagnosis. Each patient visit is a diagnostic exercise, assessing what has been accomplished, possible problems, and what remains to be done in the most time- and technique-efficient manner and with the most tissue-conscious approach.

Chapter 2 (Brian Preston) is on preventive orthodontics. Not all orthodontic patients have full-blown malocclusions. Experience has shown that many problems can be intercepted early and fully corrected, thus preventing further damage or smoothing the way for full mechanotherapy later. The experienced diagnostician recognizes these patients and institutes limited procedures that have a definite cost–benefit ratio for all concerned. Some of these problems are covered in *Orthodontic Diagnosis*, but this chapter delineates such instances in more detail—with more of a "how-to" approach. The old saying "An ounce of prevention is worth a pound of cure" is most appropriate here. Such efforts are particularly worthwhile in the area of abnormal perioral habits, with their potential for deforming the developing dentition. The same is true for abnormal respiration. The way to approach each problem is to ask yourself "If this were my child, what would I think was best for the child?"

Chapter 3 (Jack Dale) covers interceptive guidance of occlusion and extraction: the raison d'être, the technique, and long-term results. Jack Dale's magnificent chapters in other books, his lectures around the world, and his dedication to excellence have earned him the preeminent status he now enjoys. His service on the American Board of Orthodontics has provided exemplary guidance to a generation of young orthodontists, stimulating them to become applied biologists, not merely good mechanics, which earned him the prestigious Albert H. Ketcham Award. This chapter, like the others, must be read and re-read to appreciate the full impact of the principles and practice of the best possible combination of diagnostic acumen and therapeutic achievement.

Chapter 4 (Tom Rakosi) discusses the scope and limitations of functional therapy. It emphasizes the principles of differentiation and individualization. We can differentiate between functional orthodontic and functional orthopedic treatment. The principle of the functional orthodontic appliances can be that of force application or force elimination. The precondition for successful treatment is a comprehensive treatment protocol taking into account the individual requirements and peculiarities of the patient.

Chapter 5 (William Clark) takes applied biology a step further, utilizing the Twin Block appliance for posturing the mandible forward and stimulating temporomandibular joint metabolism and optimal growth response. The Bionator has the same mandibular posturing approach, and in addition utilizes a screening effect to prevent deleterious pressures on the dentition by the screening musculature. The Twin Block appliance may have started with occlusal guide planes as recommended by A.M. Schwartz, but it has come a long way and is now capable of treating three-dimensional problems (i.e., sagittal, vertical, and transverse deficiencies). The reader is referred to Dr. Clark's excellent textbooks for a more comprehensive discussion of Twin Block therapy. Like so many of our eminent world-class authors, Dr. Clark is in demand around the world to explain his approach to Class II problems. As with other functional appliances, this does not negate the use of expansion screws or fixed attachments at one or more phases of active treatment. But the approach makes sagittal correction easier, with less potential iatrogenic damage.

Chapter 6 (Alexander Vardimon) employs most of the concepts promulgated by Dr. Clark but adds the use of rare-earth magnets to help in the mandibular propulsion. Having done major NIH-sponsored research with me at the ADA Research Institute, Professor Vardimon was able to show the tissue-conscious nature of these minuscule and powerful coated magnets, in both the attracting and repelling modes, to achieve jaw positioning as well as tooth movement (i.e., bringing down palatally impacted canines). James Moss has done the same.

A full picture of the beneficial effects of the magnets has not been completely determined, but all evidence points to faster, potentially less damaging tooth movement [1]. Use in palatal expansion appliances has proven quite successful, with less potential iatrogenic damage such as root resorption, buccal plate dehiscence, and fenestration [2,3].

Chapter 7 (Ali Darendeliler) on early maxillary expansion is authored by a truly international orthodontist who has worked at renowned universities all over the world; Istanbul, Geneva, North Carolina, and Southern California have been his fields of activity. He is now the head of the leading Orthodontic Department of Australia, in Sydney. Within a very comprehensive research program, research interests include the dental and skeletal effect of orthodontic appliances and the scope and possibilities of maxillary expansion. As well as the diagnostic preconditions of the expansion, the contents of his chapter include timing, types of maxillary expanders, forces produced with maxillary expanders, and their skeletal and dental effects. He stresses the importance of patients' age for the indication of various procedures of expansion and gives important guidelines to the practitioner for successful maxillary expansion.

Chapter 8 (John De Vincenzo) recognizes the use of mandibular propulsion, but uses a fixed inter-arch mechanism, similar to that of Hans Pancherz and the Jasper Jumper, with reciprocal anchorage in the maxillary arch. The idea of combining maxillary molar distalization with mandibular propulsion and potential favorable condylar and glenoid fossa changes with fixed appliances was introduced by Emil Herbst in 1906 and expanded in his book of 1910. His appliances and concepts were amazingly contemporary, as many orthodontists using the Herbst appliance can attest. Whereas Pancherz and his followers (Terry Dischinger et al) feel there is more basal skeletal correction as a result of growth guidance, at least in the short run, since use of the Herbst appliance is limited to 6–7 months DeVincenzo feels that over the long haul the response is essentially dental—i.e., tooth movement. Long-term studies by Pancherz and Ruf show that actual growth of the condyle achieved by adulthood is only 1–2 mm more than normal. But two factors are operative here: One is that these appliances are worn for only a small portion of the growth period—only 6–7 months; but growth occurs over 9–15 years. Predominance of morphological pattern is likely to re-manifest itself in such cases unless subsequent growth guidance through the use of activator/bionator/twin block continues the postural propulsion to some degree. Then too, as Ulrich Paulsen shows in his excellent CAT-scan studies, the modification of the glenoid fossa posterior structure is significant, and most researchers have not measured this important area. Orthopedic surgeons correcting scoliosis or long bone deformities would never limit their guidance to 6 months and still expect a permanent change. We can learn much from medical orthopedics as we resort to growth guidance for longer periods of time, as we have done successfully with Class III malocclusions. As an often-quoted maxim has it: "It is not the tool that you use, but when, why, for how long, with how much force."

Chapter 9 (Michael Marcotte) is essential for anyone seeking to understand the biomechanics of orthodontic therapy for both fixed and removable appliances. Advertisements for new exotic wires and complex brackets may create the impression that they are largely automatic, but that is far from true. Orthodontic biomechanical principles were pretty elementary when I finished my specialty training. Learning by experience was not always pleasant, as so-called anchorage units moved as much as the target teeth. Fundamental concepts stressed appliances that produced so much friction that heavy forces were required to overcome the resistance and, in the process, they produced damage in too many patients. We were handed an edgewise bracket and a series of three or four archwires, leading to a 0.022×0.028 wire that snugly fit the bracket. But even heavy elastics had difficulty moving teeth. The degree of force and length of treatment almost always produced some root resorption and soft-tissue damage.

With leaders in the field such as we have now, our specialty is well founded in biomechanical aspects, with the emphasis on the "bio." Much credit for this revolution goes to the orthodontic department at Indiana University, to sage clinicians like James Baldwin and Charles Burstone, and to their bright young students like Michael Marcotte and Thomas Mulligan, who are teaching generations around the world the basics of moments, couples, and vectors and of control without the severe attendant damage we produced before the Indiana influence on the specialty. Not only has Indiana been the font of biomechanical knowledge (all those mentioned above and many more are outstanding clinicians), but these eminent leaders have made what appears to be a complex aspect of physics very understandable for all. Without this background, no clinician deserves to call himself an orthodontist. Admittedly, reading this chapter for the first time may confuse some novice orthodontic students, but like a sacred text, it must be read again and again! With the information gained, the clinician can understand the raison d'être of all appliances—the advantages and disadvantages of specific problems. Too many orthodontic "pied pipers" who never really understood the underlying principles of the appliances they used, the "set-up" they applied to all patients, or the "rules of use," have tooted their horns to attract willing followers. This is the ugly side of our history.

Unfortunately, this lack of understanding still pervades our specialty. In addition, many nonspecialists read only the advertising claims and learn the hard way by misuse and iatrogenic damage. With those eager-beaver legal vultures circling overhead, we can no longer afford the luxury of learning by trial and error, burying corrected dentitions under permanent retainers. To me, this is the most important chapter in this book for orthodontic students. There are many roads to Rome, many appliances that can accomplish the same result, but only one set of fundamental tissue-conscious principles. Read and understand and don't feel handicapped if it takes three readings to get the full meaning and implications. Try to take short courses given by these leaders if possible. Most graduate orthodontic resident programs have "in-house" teachers of biomechanics: Robert Isaacson, editor of *The Angle Orthodontist* and long-time department head at Minnesota, California, and Virginia; leaders like Ravi Nanda at Connecticut, Rohit Sachdeva of Baylor, Andrew Kuhlberg of Connecticut, Steven Lindauer of Virginia, among others—and I know I have left out some names. Most schools don't have these biomechanical gurus on staff, but if you go to Illinois, for example, you will have all the leaders giving seminars and guiding clinical units, from James Baldwin and Bill Hohlt, through Charles Burstone, Michael Marcotte, Thomas Mulligan, and Bob Isaacson. Learn these principles early, and all appliances will make more sense, or nonsense, to you. No short cuts here!

Chapters 9 through 11 assiduously apply the principles of the biomechanical Bible given in Chapter 9. The early chapters in this book also do, of course, but the guidelines are more important for full fixed mechanotherapy. At least 75% of your practice load will be in this category, perhaps more, as you apply fixed appliances to fine-tune growth guidance cases. As you read the chapters by Marcotte, Kuhlberg, and Alexander, make it a point to return to the profuse illustrations in Chapter 9 to help you understand their implications.

If you need further indoctrination, go to the outstanding chapter by Burstone in the Graber–Vanarsdall graduate orthodontic text [4], to the books by Burstone, Marcotte, and Mulligan, and to the short courses offered by all of them.

Chapter 10 (Andrew Kuhlberg) on the segmented arch technique deals with the culmination of biophysical and biomechanical design developed by Burstone and his staff. It is a popular choice, particularly in the Connecticut area. Marcotte and Kuhlberg were products of this environment and learned the advantages of the segmented arch approach. They will often modify it with continuous arches at various stages of treatment. This chapter gives you a fine description of the technique, its biomechanical justification, and examples of the correction potential if the technique is handled properly. Again compare these cases with those of the other fixed-appliance chapters and judge for yourself whether this is your "cup of tea." The segmented arch technique may be the most biomechanically oriented approach.

Chapter 11 (Wick Alexander) is a good place to turn next. Dr. Alexander is a pioneer in light-wire techniques and has devoted his life to teaching others. He, too, has constantly made changes in his philosophy and appliance units as his experiences and those of his students and disciples point the way to even better control. There is a common thread in the remaining chapters, though: light forces, the lowest possible level that moves teeth. We all have learned the hard way that with too much force we cause hyalinization, stop cellular activity by frontal assault, reduce metabolism, retain catabolic byproducts, and move the tooth or teeth only by undermining resorption mechanotherapy.

Read it in Graber and Vanarsdall [4]. There are other chapters of value, but this is an absolute must for periodontics, etc. Their tissue work is, in my opinion, unexcelled, though European researchers are not far behind. Starting with Sandstedt of Norway in 1904, through Oppenheim of Austria, Noyes of Chicago, Sicher and Weinmann of Austria and the USA, Kaare Reitan, Per Rygh and Birgit Thilander and Annika Isberg of Norway and Sweden, we have a fine heritage of research scientists that matches any field in the world.

The long-term results of Alexander, as well as those of other authors in the light-wire chapters, are bound to be impressive, but standing the test of time is paramount. A balanced occlusion is essential: balanced in contact with the opposing teeth, with the neuromuscular envelope, with function and parafunction, and with facial esthetics. This is not an easy assignment with the myriad of facial types we encounter. Study of the case reports should be afforded concentration and considerable time. Look for criteria of stability, look for tissue health as well as esthetic achievement.

Chapter 12 (Magdalena Kotova), authored by a well-known, leading orthodontist of the Orthodontic Department of the Charles University Prague; deals with implants in orthodontics. Czech orthodontics has had some internationally well-known representatives such as Miroslav Adam, Frantisek Kraus, Ferdinand Skaloud, and Bedrich Neumann. During World War II and the following Iron Curtain period, communication with the West was interrupted and it was difficult to obtain even the scientific literature, let alone equipment or material. As soon as the Iron Curtain dropped, the new generation made up for the lost time. They worked enthusiastically, studying the new literature, visiting famous universities, organizing courses with leading orthodontists and so on, aiming to lift Czech orthodontics to an international level. Two of the exponents of this new generation are Magdalena Kotova and Milan Kaminek. Proof that Czech orthodontics has come abreast of the times is found in Dr. Kotova's research topics. Implants are one of her research priorities and she has many years of experiences in this field, publishing and lecturing on the subject. The quality of her contribution to this book demonstrates her reputation as an expert in the field.

Tom Graber was always building bridges between nations and orthodontists all over the world. He would be happy and proud to have this contribution in his "Memorial Edition."

Chapter 13 (Rainer-Reginald Miethke) describes treatment with the Invisalign system. Professor Miethke holds the chair of the Charité University, Berlin. He was the first in Germany and one of the first in Europe to include the scope and possibilities of treatment with the Invisalign system in his comprehensive research program. He contributed to improvement of the efficacy of the treatment with new ideas such as "led tooth" or ways of using the attachments. He is active across the world, publishing, lecturing, and teaching treatment with Invisalign.

The death of Tom Graber left a gap in the editorship of the *World Journal of Orthodontics* (WJO). Dr. Efthimia K. Basdra, who took on the editorship in the first phase, has since passed the position on to Dr. Miethke, who is now Editor-in-Chief of the WJO. Open-minded, pragmatic, social-minded, and communicative, he is exactly the right successor of Tom. He is an experienced editor, being the Editor-in-Chief of the Quintessenz journal *Kieferorthopädie*. He has widespread connections, for example, in his capacity as a former visiting professor of the Louisiana State University, New Orleans, and the Royal Dental College, Aarhus, or as the Past-President of the 100 Years EOS congress in Berlin. Thanks to his editorship the journal will continue to be managed in the spirit of Tom Graber.

As with any publication or lecture by Rainer-Reginald Miethke, both the content and the didactic quality of his chapter make an excellent contribution for the practitioner on how to manage the Invisalign treatment.

Chapter 14 (Bjørn Zachrisson) is another gem, presented late in the book to make sure you have already been exposed to the various techniques and the ways of solving tooth size discrepancies, morphological variations, re-crowding, particularly in the lower anterior segment, and so on. Bjørn Zachrisson is considered by many to be the top clinician in the world because of his frequent super-courses around the world, his thorough integrity, his open discussion of potential problems, and his masterful way of presenting his material. It is a "must" for all who can do so to attend one of Bjørn Zachrisson's courses. His experiences in retaining treatment results, the steps he takes to prevent or correct re-crowding, and his means of retaining upper and lower arches are described in his many publications. He took on the assignment of "proximal stripping" because of the frequent need to maintain as much of the treatment correction as possible and to ameliorate situations in which adverse post-treatment changes can occur. The care he takes so as not to reduce interproximal bone or cause loss of gingival contour is important, particularly given the current Invisalign advertising, which relies heavily on technicians stripping teeth on laboratory models. This chapter again must be followed carefully. Too much stripping can produce deleterious consequences, as both Drs. Vanarsdall and Boyd, doubly qualified in orthodontics and periodontics, have shown.

Chapter 15 (John Sheridan) is again an essential for all readers. The retention problem is as controversial today as it was 30 years ago. Charles Tweed once quipped "Retention is not only one of the problems, but it is *the* problem." What to do, when to do it, for how long, and in what particular types of cases? Jack Sheridan, a professor of orthodontics at LSU, as well as a developer of the Essix removable plastic appliance, has a broad range of experience and, together with Zachrisson's chapter, offers the reader some essential information on retention. Sheridan also introduced the air-rotor stripping technique, and the reader is referred to his articles in current orthodontic literature. Here, as with Zachrisson's chapter, timing is vital with retention procedures. The game isn't over with the removal of "braces," as more and more lawyers are suing orthodontists for relapsing malocclusions, claiming that it is due to the orthodontist's incompetence. Informed consent forms must be sure to cover the natural consequences of the post-treatment settling phase, predominance of the morphogenetic pattern, lack of patient compliance with wearing of retaining appliances, the need to wear retainers indefinitely in some cases, and so on. The AAO has produced consent forms to be signed by the patient (or parent of a juvenile) to make sure these factors are explained and understood. As with the consent forms in hospitals before surgery, experience has shown that most potential relapse factors are covered even if they may not seem likely.

The final chapter (Jason Cope) could well be the first if being avant garde means anything. It is hard to believe that Ilizarov, an orthopedic surgeon imprisoned in Siberia in 1964, is the father of this amazing ortho-surgical approach to basal skeletal changes in the craniofacial complex! When I look back at my early efforts to correct skeletal malformations like cleft lip and palate problems and the limitations facing me, the indefinite retention, failures, iatrogenic damage, I say, "If only Ilizarov had been around then!" He was working on long bones, of course, and yet the amount of change he produced was quite amazing.

Orthognathic surgery in the form of LeFort I, II, and III has been around for over 30 years, and some striking changes have been produced. But the iatrogenic potential has always been there, even for the best surgeons. I published a number of orthognathic surgery reports when I was editor of the AJO-DO because it truly was and is dentofacial orthopedics that we need to correct many of the malocclusions we see. But looking at some of these patients, immediately postoperatively, with the swelling, black and blue patina, discomfort, and psychological shock, we would sometimes ask whether it was really worth it—whether we would want to undergo the procedure for what many people consider a mostly cosmetic problem. And the contingency-fee lawyers have again been circling around and quite busy: busy enough to make malpractice insurance rise exponentially to levels between $125 000 and $150 000 a year in some areas. What a breath of fresh air distraction osteogenesis has been for patients, oral and maxillofacial surgeons, and orthodontists. Jason Cope was fortunate enough to have been with Mikhail Samukhov and to have produced a book with him, and is admirably qualified to author this chapter. So the biblical saying "The last shall be first" applies in many ways to Chapter 16. Read this chapter several times, attend courses on the technique, which is fairly widespread now, and read the book by Samukhov and Cope. You will truly be "coping," if you'll excuse the pun, with heretofore unsolvable problems and doing so with minimal potential for untoward results.

I am sure my enthusiasm for all the chapters in this treatment book is obvious. With the *Orthodontic Diagnosis* color atlas alongside, the result will be better, faster, safer, and more pain-free care for our patients. After all, isn't that what we all want? And those legal vultures will turn elsewhere to other fields of medicine and dentistry, where the pickings are better for them! Read enjoy, learn, profit with better, evidence-based patient care!

T. M. Graber
T. Rakosi

Vardimon AD, Graber TM, Drescher D, Bourauel C. Rare earth magnets and Impaction AJO-DO 1991; 100: 494–512

Vardimon AD, Graber TM, Voss LR. Stability of magnetic versus mechanical palatal expansion. Eur J Orthod 1989; 11: 107–115

Vardimon AD, Graber TM, Voss LR, Lenke J. Determinants controlling iatrogenic external root resorption and repaid during and after palatal expansion. Angle Orthod 1991; 61: 113–124

Graber TM, Vanarsdall R, Vig KWL. Orthodontics. Current Principles and Practice. 4th ed. St. Louis: Mosby; 2005

Contents

1 Therapeutic Diagnosis 1
Thomas Rakosi

Essential Diagnostic Records	1	Forecasting (Prediction)	11
Indications, Indices, Etiology	2	The Goal of Treatment and Camouflage	13
Soft Tissues and Function	4	Evidence-based Diagnosis	15
Cephalometrics and Periodontal Assessment	7	Social Requirements	16
Computer Analysis and Video Imaging	9		

2 Preventive Orthodontics 18
Brian Preston

Congenitaly Absence and Supernumerary Teeth	19	Oral Habits	23
Dental Impaction	21	Early Use of Orthodontic Appliances	24
Midline Diastema	21	Mouth Breathing	27
Abnormalities in Tooth Size and Shape	22		

3 Early Treatment: Interceptive Guidance of Occlusion including Serial Extraction followed by Mechanotherapy 33
Jack Dale

The Logic of "Serial Extraction"	33	The Tweed–Merrifield Edgewise Appliance Technique	35
Pioneers and Followers	33	The Tweed–Merrifield Edgewise Appliance	35
Serial Extraction	34	Clinical Case Studies	37
The Multibanded-Multibracket Appliance	34	Conclusion	66

4 Functional Orthodontic and Functional Orthopedic Treatment 68
Thomas Rakosi

The Principles of Functional Appliances	68	The Activator	75
Functional Therapy by Force Elimination:		The Bionator	90
Screening Therapy	69	Functional Jaw Orthopedics and Class II Malocclusions	94

5 The Twin Block Technique 101
William Clark

Proprioceptive Stimulus to Growth	101	Twin Block Construction	104
Twin Blocks	101	Stages of Treatment	105
Case Selection	101	Clinical Management	105
Activation	102	Clinical Case Studies	108
Screw Advancement System	103	Conclusion	126
Appliance Design	104		

6 The Functional Magnetic System ... 127
Alexander Vardimon

The Functional Magnetic System	127	FMS Modus Operandi	131
Myth and Reality	127	Mechanism of Functional Correction	132
FMS Design	128	Clinical Case Studies	137
FMS Fabrication	130		

7 Early Maxillary Expansion ... 155
M. Ali Darendeliler

Growth and Anatomy	155	Early or Late Treatment? Surgically Assisted Maxillary Expansion versus Orthopedic Expansion	174
Clinical and Radiological Diagnosis	155		
Timing of Maxillary Expansion	157	Rapid Maxillary Expansion and Obstructive Sleep Apnea (OSA)	174
Types of Maxillary Expanders	160		
Force Produced with Maxillary Expanders	164	Retention and Stability	175
Rate of Expansion and their Dental and Skeletal Effects	166	Side-Effects of Maxillary Expansion	175
Effects in Different Age Groups	167	Discussion and Conclusion	176
Clinical Case Studies	169		

8 The Interarch Compression Spring in Orthodontics ... 179
John DeVincenzo

Force Vectors, Moments, and Analyses	179	Clinical Case Studies	189
Comparison of ICS with Herbst and Jasper Jumper	184	The Use of the ICS with Orthognathic Surgery	202
Description and Comparison of the Various ICS Appliances	184	Disadvantages of the ICS	204
Effects of ICSs on the Dentition	188	Summary	204

9 Anchorage Control in Orthodontic Extraction Therapy ... 205
Michael Marcotte

Closure of Extraction Sites with Group B Anchorage	205	Closure of Extraction Sites with Group C Anchorage	214
Fabrication and Preactivation of the Titanium T-Loop Retraction Spring	207	Asymmetric Space Closure	219
		Finishing Procedures	221
The Trial Activation	208	Conclusion	221
Extraction Site Closure with Group A Anchorage	210		

10 Segmented Arch Mechanics ... 222
Andrew Kuhlberg

Intrusion Arches and Deep Overbite Correction	222	Transpalatal and Lingual Arches	232
Space Closure and Anchorage Control	227	Summary	234
Root Correction	231		

11 The Alexander Discipline ... 235
R. G. Wick Alexander

Unique Bracket Selection and Prescription	235	Clinical Case Studies	240
Unique Arch Form	238	Evidence-Based Studies	260
Treatment Mechanics	239		

12 Implants and Orthodontics ... 261
Magdalena Kotova

Dental Anchorage	261	Dental Implant Used Temporarily as	
Skeletal Anchorage	261	Orthodontic Anchorage	273
Miniscrew Implant	265	Conclusion	275
Palatal Implant	272		

13 Treatment with the Invisalign System ... 276
Rainer-Reginald Miethke

The Principles of the Invisalign System	276	Clinical Aspects of an Invisalign Treatment	283
The Clinical Approach	278	Indications for Treatment with the Invisalign System	285
Attachments	280	Indications for Extraction Therapy in	
Impression-taking for the Invisalign System	283	Combination with Invisalign Treatment	287

14 Stripping ... 289
Bjørn Zachrisson

Risks in Grinding of Teeth	289	How to Regain Lost Gingival Papillae	296
Amount of Enamel Removal in Stripping	290	Stripping versus Extraction of a Single Mandibular Incisor	296
Instruments for Enamel Reduction and Polishing	291	Predisposition to Caries and Risk of Accelerated	
Optimal Stripping Technique	294	Periodontal Tissue Breakdown after Stripping	296
How to Maintain Normal Gingival Papillae during Orthodontic Treatment	295	Clinical Case Studies	297

15 Active Retention Procedures ... 313
John J. Sheridan

Removable Retainers	313	Clear Plastic Corrective Retainers	323
Impression and Cast Standards	314	Clinical Case Examples	326
Thermoforming Plastic to the Cast	316	Spring Retainers	327
Full-Arch Plastic Retainers: Fabrication, Indications, Contraindications	320	Fixed Bonded and Cemented Retainers	328

16 Treatment Planning for Mandibular Distraction Osteogenesis ... 332
Jason B. Cope

Clinical Case Studies: Mandibular Lengthening	333	Mandibular Widening	348
		Summary	356

Index ... 358

1 Therapeutic Diagnosis

Thomas Rakosi

Orthodontists today tend to have a broad perspective on means of correcting malocclusions. No longer is it a "follow the guru" dictum for mechanotherapy. This new orientation requires a strong diagnostic base and an efficiently oriented treatment philosophy. It places high emphasis on dynamic, comprehensive diagnosis as part of every patient visit during treatment. Such on-going assessment is essential for optimal, stable therapeutic achievement. In this highly efficient practice milieu, it is necessary to establish a basis for objectively assessing the quality and utility of our clinical manipulations. We must individualize our efforts to find out which treatment modality is optimal for a particular patient and to know whether we are "on course" for achieving our practice management objectives.

Essential Diagnostic Records

Therapeutic diagnosis includes:
1. Original diagnostic study and prognostic projections
2. Routine assessments of diagnostic time/rate of progress
3. Dynamic, functional prognostic projections
4. Midcourse changes in treatment methods, as needed
5. Epicritical evaluations of the results and possible iatrogenic sequelae (Fig. 1.**1**)

Even after removal of the appliance, it is the responsibility of the orthodontist to maintain a vigilant eye for any retrogressive changes during and after retention.

The questions to be answered in selecting a valid diagnostic procedure are:
1. Is it available, affordable, accurate, and precise?
2. Will it help patients to achieve and maintain treatment goals?

With dynamic diagnosis today, there is no mechanical Procrustean bed appliance satisfying all needs for all patients. Rather, individual, often unique, combinations of skeletal, neuromuscular, and dental characteristics determine the appliance of choice for a particular task. Potential iatrogenic response must always be considered in this litigious world, where root resorption, bone loss, fenestration, dehiscence, and periodontal problems raise a red flag for malpractice lawyers. True diagnosis is like putting together the pieces of a jigsaw puzzle. Each patient visit must be a diagnostic assessment, and both progress and problems should be recorded in the patient's record. This is risk management today.

The superimposed cephalometric tracings before and after orthodontic treatment of two Class II malocclusions shown in Figure 1.**2** emphasize the critical nature of a definitive diagnosis. Both patients were treated with functional appliances. Each appliance was constructed with the unique individual constellation of malocclusion factors in mind and was modified and used accordingly. The patient in Figure 1.**2a** had a horizontal growth pattern; the one in Figure 1.**2b** had a vertical growth pattern. Different appliance construction and modus operandi allowed the optimum to be achieved for both patients. Growth direction and increments

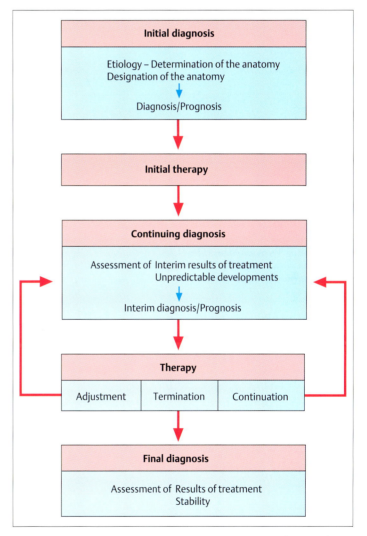

Fig. 1.**1** **Diagram of continuing or therapeutic diagnosis, which is completed only when appliances are removed.** Even then any posttreatment retrogressive changes must be followed and the necessary countermeasures taken.

were critical decisional factors (Fig. 1.**3**). A Class II malocclusion with a horizontal growth pattern can be treated with a conventional activator and anterior positioning of the mandible with simultaneous uprighting of the incisors can be achieved. If we treat a Class II malocclusion with a vertical growth pattern, we must compromise the construction bite with a slight forward position-

2 Therapeutic Diagnosis

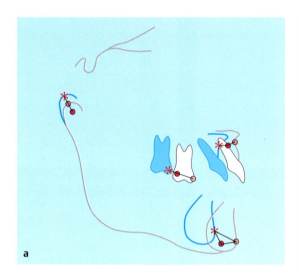
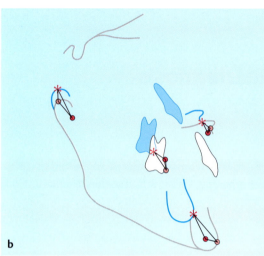

Fig. 1.**2** **Superimposed cephalometric tracings of Class II Division 1 malocclusions, in two different patients, before and after orthodontic treatment.** Note horizontal growth pattern in (**a**) and vertical pattern in (**b**). Different treatment measures are essential.

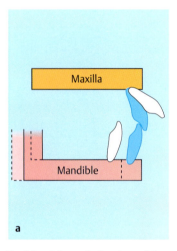
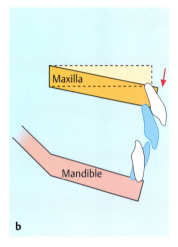

Fig. 1.**3** **Schematic drawings of the appliance design used in treatment of Class II, Division 1 malocclusions in Fig. 1.2.**
a The design for a horizontal growth pattern.
b The design for a vertical growth pattern.

ing and more opening. The mandible will be positioned downward and forward (because of the growth pattern) and a partial camouflage is necessary by retroinclination of the maxillary base and labial tipping of the lower incisors. Depressing the buccal segments can allow upward and forward rotation of the chinpoint, which improves the esthetics of the profile. The vertical dimension must always be considered in planning and executing therapy.

Indications, Indices, Etiology

Before orthodontic treatment is started, the following questions should be answered:
- Why to treat; this refers to the indications and contraindications
- When to treat; the timing of treatment
- Where to treat; in which region or regions of the dentofacial skeleton
- How to treat; which mechanisms and which combination of methods are indicated

It is sometimes difficult to answer the question "Why?" There are many shades of gray between normal occlusion and malocclusion. Despite the current practice-efficiency-inspired brouhaha over one phase versus two phases of treatment, there are no general rules for specific treatment timing. In some cases, it is better to wait until the permanent teeth have erupted; in others, treatment should be initiated during the eruption of permanent teeth or even earlier. Chapter 2 outlines some of the reasons for interceptive treatment; for example, mixed dentition treatment of abnormal habit problems, functional occlusal shifts, and growth guidance problems may well produce a better final result. In other patients, either early or late treatment may produce the same result.

For the patient shown in Figure 1.**4**, for example, a first stage of treatment should have been initiated earlier to prevent the periodontal damage on the labially malposed lower central incisor.

If an orthopedic or growth guidance treatment is indicated, then it is desirable to take advantage of growth increments. The juvenile growth increments can be much greater than those in the peripubertal period, particularly in girls (Fig. 1.**5**).

The cost–benefit–risk ratio should always be considered. To help delineate the indications and treatment effect, various indices have been developed to objectify diagnosis (Peer Assessment Rating (PAR), Index of complexity outcome and treatment (IOTN), etc.). However, indices measure only the normative values before orthodontic treatment, without accounting for the skeletal, functional, or even social aspects. Indices do not make an accurate assessment of the multiple effects of treatment.

Causation is usually multifactorial and is difficult to evaluate because of the compounding and compensating factors. Diagnosis in biological fields is often an initial impression, or probability, subject to later therapeutic response, i.e., therapeutic diagnosis. Hereditary pattern may provide a clue and should be investigated, but environmental factors can also be significant. The environmental influence is often combined with genetic factors (epigenetic), often designated as predisposing causes. The experienced clinician should never be trapped by arbitrary numerical indices. As treatment progresses, therapeutic diagnosis is necessary to intercept any adverse consequences of unexpected treatment responses (Fig. 1.**6**).

Indications, Indices, Etiology 3

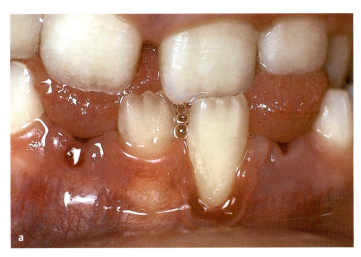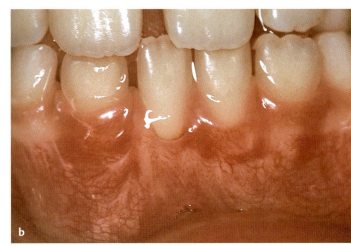

Fig. 1.**4** **Anterior crossbite correction.**
a Before treatment.
b After correction.
Early recognition and interception are important.

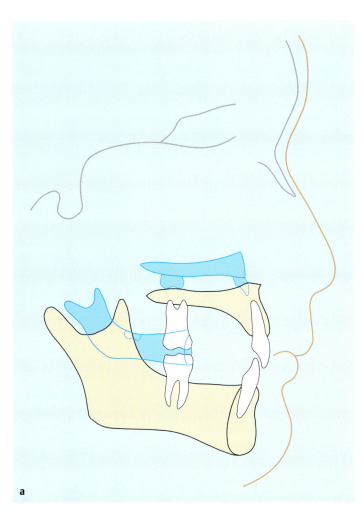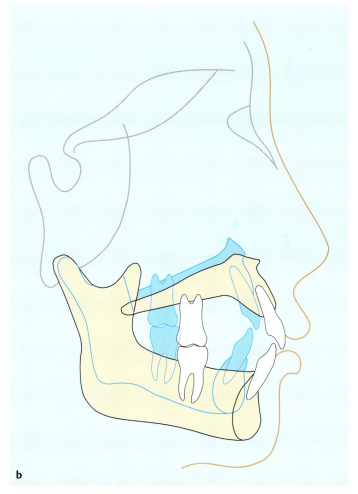

Fig. 1.**5** **Growth changes from birth to adulthood.**
a Between birth and the eighth year of life.
b Between 8 years and the completion of growth.

4 Therapeutic Diagnosis

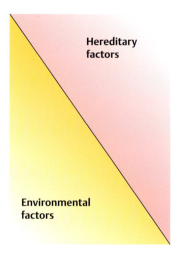

Fig. 1.6 Diagram of the interrelationship between heredity and environment in achieving final pattern. The two are intimately related.

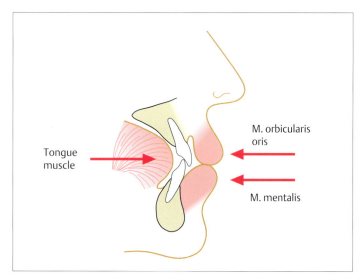

Fig. 1.7 Neuromuscular structures significantly affect tooth position. In normal occlusion, a balance is maintained by soft-tissue structures within and outside the dental arches.

Soft Tissues and Function

Recently, the emphasis in the literature with regard to the role of the neuromuscular environment has changed. Orthodontists are increasingly aware that the position of the teeth is dependent on the equilibrium of the surrounding soft tissues—the "functional matrix" (Fig. 1.**7**). Patients have always been primarily interested in the cosmetic aspects of orthodontics, and the soft tissues are a major component of any attempt at cosmetic improvement. With morphing and video-imaging—discussed later in this chapter—we now have means of enhancing the patient's understanding of the potential and limitations of cosmetic improvement. The spatial relationships of the dentoskeletal components, soft-tissue envelope, and function are becoming more significant in the total diagnostic jigsaw puzzle. The possibilities and limitations of orthodontic treatment are ultimately influenced by the draping soft tissue and muscles, i.e., the functional matrix. By elucidating the limits of soft tissue and functional adaptation, we can differentiate between successful treatment (adapters) and posttreatment relapse (nonadapters). The test of time must be applied.

In patients with malfunction or dysfunction, the first step of treatment is to eliminate the deforming neuromuscular effects. As the great anatomist Harry Sicher said, "Whenever there is a struggle between muscle and bone, muscle wins!" We can then observe an improvement of the malocclusion and prevent further neuromuscular deformation.

The elimination of the dysfunction and reestablishment of a normal lip seal should be the first step of treatment (Fig. 1.**8a, b**). Once this is accomplished, the change is dramatic (Fig. 1.**8c, d**).

Determination of the interocclusal clearance, or freeway space, between upper and lower dentitions at postural resting position (centric relation), as well as any sliding movements on occlusal contact, is often ignored in the diagnostic assessment. Yet this determination is one of the most important because of the dominant role that muscles play in either maintaining the treatment result or causing undesired posttreatment changes. It is vital to remember that the teeth are placed together for only 60–90 minutes in any 24-hour period. The functional matrix suspends the mandible with the teeth 3–4 mm apart the rest of the time, ready for multiple functions such as respiration, deglutition, mastication, and speech. This is the place to begin your diagnostic assessment with a comprehensive functional analysis. This initial assessment should also take temporomandibular joint (TMJ) implications into account. In the new millennium, the orthodontist is responsible for the entire stomatognathic system. The ultimate stability of orthodontic treatment must be a major concern.

Registration of the rest position can be done with a manual functional analysis (Fig. 1.**9**). For illustrative purposes, the kinesiographic 3D registration of the postural rest position provides a graphic record of muscle activity (Fig. 1.**10**). Figure 1.**10** shows the special recording, but it is not really necessary for the functional analysis—only a graphic record. It shows that muscle activity can be recorded graphically, if need be. Alternatively, having a patient swallow and then gently parting the lips without moving the mandible usually gives a good idea of the so-called freeway space between the upper and lower teeth. A functionally balanced relationship between postural rest position and habitual occlusion is shown in Figure 1.**11** (coincidence of centric relation and habitual occlusion).

Tooth interferences and malocclusion can cause sliding movements of the lower jaw into an abnormal position on full occlusal contact. Figure 1.**12a** is a cephalometric tracing that indicates the directional change from initial contact to habitual occlusion (posterior superior displacement of the condyle). Such possible sliding movements must be checked carefully. Less frequently, an anterior or lateral displacement can occur on initial closing contact, particularly in pseudo Class III malocclusions (Fig. 1.**12b**).

Posterior sliding (i.e., displacement) from the physiological rest position can indicate a good prognosis for the correction of the Class II relationship; only the occlusal disturbance need be eliminated.

However, anteriorly directed sliding from rest position can mask a severe Class II malocclusion. Here, both the morphological and functional relationship must be therapeutically influenced.

Soft Tissues and Function 5

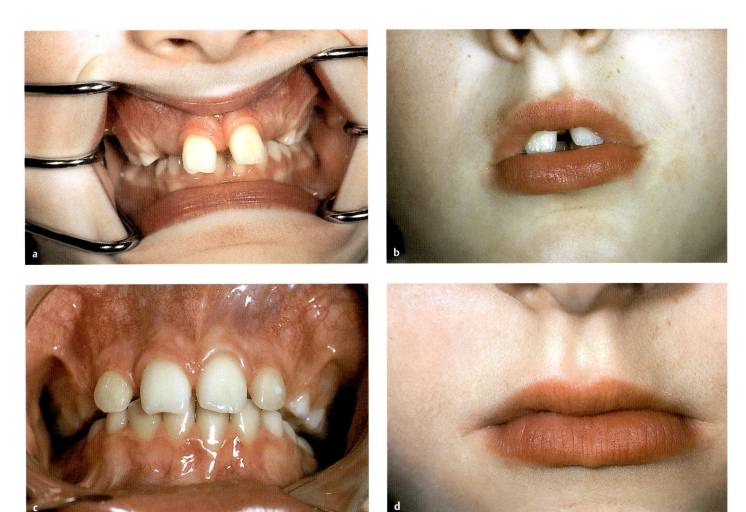

Fig. 1.8 Elimination of oral neuromuscular dysfunction and reestablishment of lip seal.
a, b Before treatment.
c, d After treatment.

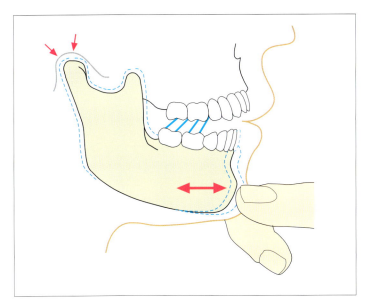

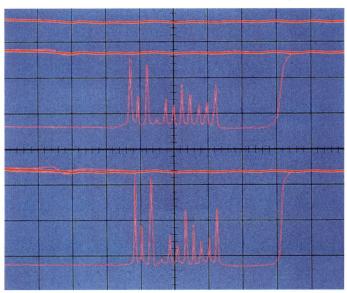

Fig. 1.9 Manipulation of mandible for postural rest and occlusal positions. The rest position is determined by the neuromuscular envelope. Gently guiding the teeth into habitual occlusal position prevents the abnormal protrusive interdental/interarch contact that patients often produce. Forced retrusion can produce deleterious effects.

Fig. 1.10 Kinesiographic recording of rest and habitual occlusion muscle activity.

6 Therapeutic Diagnosis

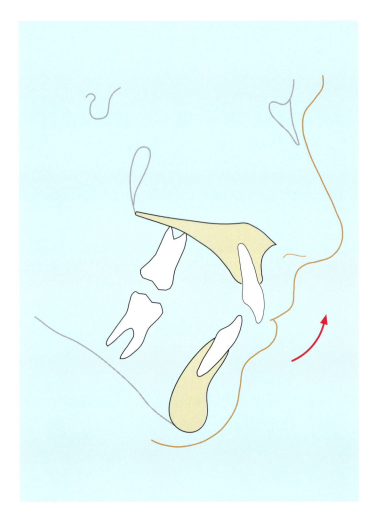

Fig. 1.**11** **The normal path of closure from postural rest position to occlusion as the condyle rotates in the fossa and the mandible closes 3–4 mm into centric occlusion.** Note upward and forward vector.

Fig. 1.**12** **a Posterior superior displacement. b The mandible closes upward and forward from postural rest to initial tooth contact.**
a Final closure, under tooth guidance, is upward and back for both the condyle and the lower dental arch. Such action is often associated with excessive freeway space. This type of displacement exacerbates a Class II relationship and may produce temporomandibular disorder (TMD) sequelae.
b Less frequently, there is anterior tooth guidance and slide from initial tooth contact, as the mandible closes into habitual occlusion, i.e., in a pseudo Class III malocclusion.

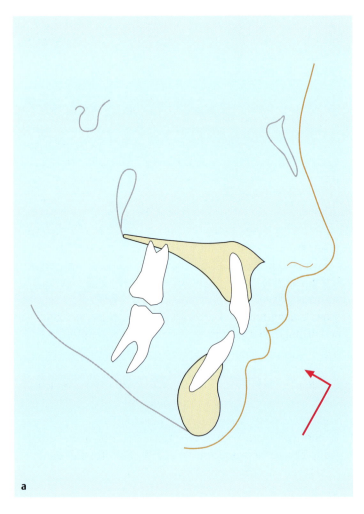

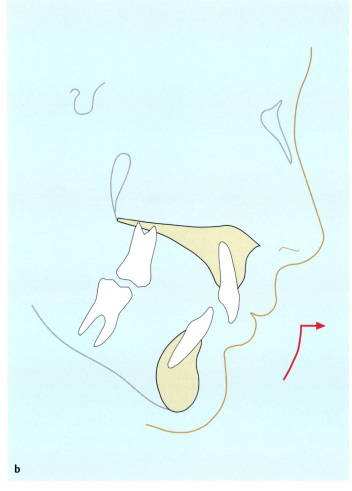

a

b

Cephalometrics and Periodontal Assessment

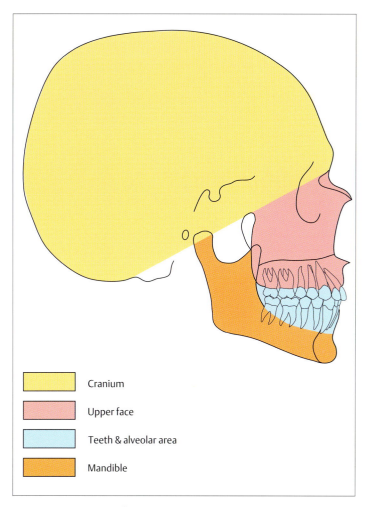

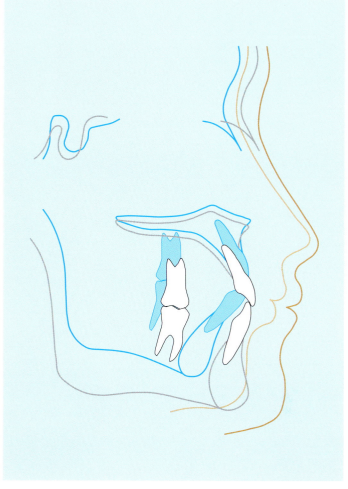

Fig. 1.**13** **Diagnostic analysis recognizes four major structural areas with varying responses to orthopedic and orthodontic treatment.** The least influential is the cranial base (yellow). The most amenable to therapy is the tooth and alveolar bone region (blue). Orthopedic guidance can affect basal maxillary (pink) and mandibular (tan) structures. Diagnostic and prognostic projections must clearly outline the challenges for all areas.

Fig. 1.**14** **Lateral cephalometric tracing illustrates the broad range of normal values for the apical base relationship (ANB angle), ranging from −3° to +8° in a large group of patients with normal occlusion. (Point A in maxilla to nasion to Point B in the mandible.)** Note significant mandibular basal difference with a retrusive − 3 degree reading (blue).

Cephalometrics and Periodontal Assessment

An important goal of the radiographic cephalometric analysis is the localization of the malocclusion features. Four main areas of concern are amenable to cephalometric mensuration. Depending on the area involved, treatment approaches and responses will be different. But measurements alone are totally inadequate: associated periodontal structures are vitally important.

1. At a minimum, at the occlusal level, intervention is possible with selective grinding (equilibration) at any age, including in adults. However, this is the main arena of mechanotherapy and the dental structures are most likely to benefit from orthodontics. Changes needed and produced are easiest to measure with periodic therapeutic diagnosis.
2. At the periodontal level, orthodontic treatment is possible after determination that the status of the periodontal tissues allows movement of teeth, with no deleterious consequences. Before moving teeth, the periodontal status must be critically determined. Any soft-tissue problems must be solved before placement of the appliance. Continuous examination during treatment is imperative, and all measures must be taken to prevent adverse soft-tissue response to orthodontic mechanotherapy.
3. At the level of the maxillary and mandibular basal structures, growth guidance is possible via orthopedic appliances before maturity, particularly in late mixed and early permanent dentition periods. Later, only dentoalveolar camouflage is possible. Treatment timing is important. Cephalometric analysis is a major diagnostic element of treatment timing. With the aid of panoral and periapical radiographs for study of the teeth and associated structures, an initial picture of dentofacial status is obtained. Response—both beneficial and deleterious consequences—then can be determined during treatment.
4. If the abnormality is primarily at the level of the craniofacial sutures and synchondroses (i.e., congenital defects and marked growth abnormalities), usually only combined orthodontics and orthognathic surgery is a viable option for optimal results (Fig. 1.**13**).

The evaluation of the results of radiographic cephalometric analysis requires a comparison with predetermined standards. Several possible standard orientations are possible:

1. To "normal" standards: A norm is a descriptive measure of group behavior meant to serve as a guide, but not designed as a goal for a particular individual.

8   Therapeutic Diagnosis

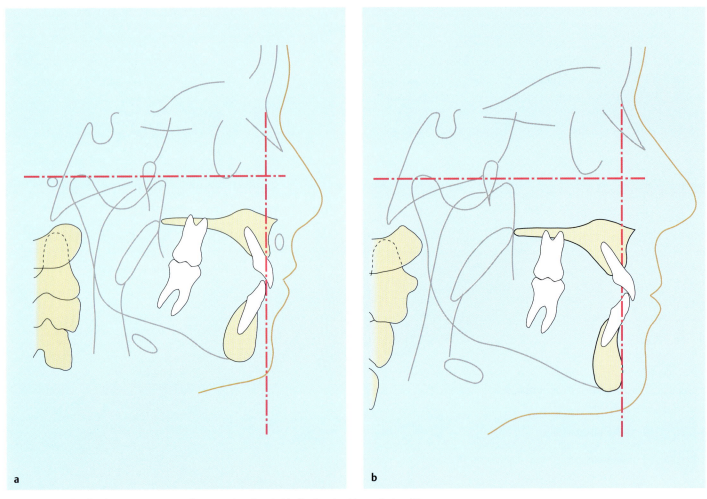

Fig. 1.**15**   **The goals of treatment must reflect initial and probable final sagittal jaw relationship.**

a A mixed dentition patient with a slightly retrognathic profile.

b A cephalometric tracing for the goal of treatment in the permanent dentition.

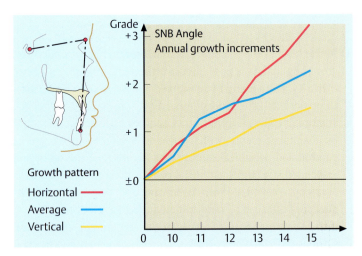

Fig. 1.**16**   **Growth increments vary with different growth patterns.** The chart compares horizontal, average, and vertical growth patterns.

The normative values are clinical assessment standards that serve to orient the clinician in setting goals for planned orthodontic treatment. As Steiner and Graber have both pointed out, they serve as a guide, not a goal for the individual patient (Steiner 1953; Graber 1954). Czasko and Shepard (1984), studying individuals with ideal dental occlusion, found a variation of the ANB apical base measurement between −3° and +8°: a broad range (Fig. 1.**14**). This range of so-called normalcy enhances the possibilities of camouflage treatment for patients.

The goals of orthodontic treatment depend upon the age of the patient. In the mixed dentition, a slight mandibular retrognathism is acceptable because of the forthcoming higher growth increments of the mandible between 9 and 16 years of age (Fig. 1.**15**). This is especially true in the male horizontal pattern, as shown so well by Bjork (1969). Figure 1.**16** shows growth increments of the mandible in the horizontal, average, and vertical growth patterns. The highest increment we can see is in the horizontal pattern.

Little basal skeletal change can be expected in the adult dentition. Orthodontic changes are essentially in the dentoalveolar region. Tooth movement alone is the mechanism for change.

2. To "ideal" standards: Ideals are graphic and mathematical representations of one person's or a group's sense of facial esthetics, not necessarily attainable in any particular patient.
3. To the self: This involves reciprocal comparison of structures, perhaps with earlier records such as previous cephalograms or study models.

Computer Analysis and Video Imaging

Because of the limitations of using mean values in cephalometric criteria, newer, computerized approaches are preferable. These include three-dimensional mesh diagrams, finite element methods (FEM), and tensor analyses. Computers have revolutionized our diagnostic armamentarium. Commercial programs that morph both photographs and cephalograms are no longer a luxury but a necessity for both diagnosis and patient education.

Finite Element Method

The finite element approach (FEM) (Fig. 1.**17**.) describes and quantifies the complex morphological and skeletal changes that occur during craniofacial growth and orthodontic treatment. This method does not require reference frames and is independent of any arbitrary method of registration and superimposition of cephalometric tracings. The technique describes the changes that have taken place; it is not yet sufficiently developed for (routine) orthodontic diagnosis. However, computer software is currently being developed to make finite element analysis easier to use for the clinician, providing an additional approach to assessing the relationship of the various components of the dentofacial complex.

Computerized Procedures

The computer enables rapid and exact evaluation of individual findings, but the well-known acronym GIGO (garbage in, garbage out) applies. The value of any computer-generated result depends on the starting data. However, assuming that proper information is employed, rapid and precise evaluations of individual findings are immediately available for both diagnosis and communication with other professionals via electronic mail. Three-dimensional measurements of dentofacial areas can be made from films, photographs, or plaster study models and can now be sent via e-mail to other professionals, without the need for transmitting original records. This also offers tremendous space saving for patient records. Three-dimensional assessment procedures also offer an exciting new research approach. Individual problems can be correlated and particular problems recognized. But the decisions must still be made by the clinician, who has a greater pool of diagnostic information than that on the monitor screen. The multifactorial and subjective variables are still critical in the final decision making. Diagnosis requires the assembly of multiple bits of information and analysis by the human brain, and weighting and interpreting of results, to arrive at tentative decisions that may well be modified by therapeutic diagnosis during actual treatment.

Various noninvasive computerized procedures are available (see Figs. 1.**18**–1.**20**). MRI (magnetic resonance imaging), for example, provides 3D data directly, with no x-ray exposure. 3D-ultrasound and computerized tomography ("cat-scan," CT) reconstruct information from 2D images. MRI and ultrasound both enable visualization of soft tissue.

The CT scan makes precise images of bone structures, at a precise tissue depth, as chosen by the clinician. This is of particular value in studies of the temporomandibular joint, where conventional 2D radiography obscures the transverse dimension variables. These images will replace the standard and time-honored

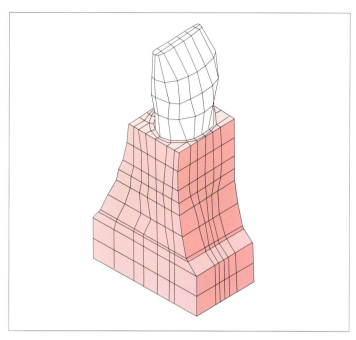

Fig. 1.**17** FEM drawing, modeling the three-dimensional nature of a tooth.

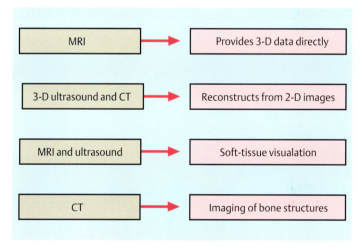

Fig. 1.**18** **Various noninvasive computerized diagnostic procedures.** MRI provides data directly; 3D ultrasound and CT construct images from two-dimensional images. MRI images enhance soft-tissue visualization; CT ("cat scan") images enhance visualization of a structure at a predetermined depth.

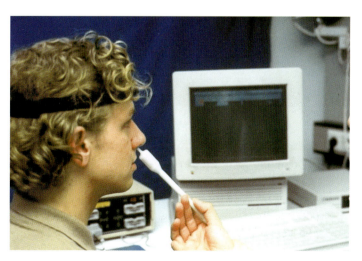

Fig. 1.**19** A noninvasive computer analysis.

10 Therapeutic Diagnosis

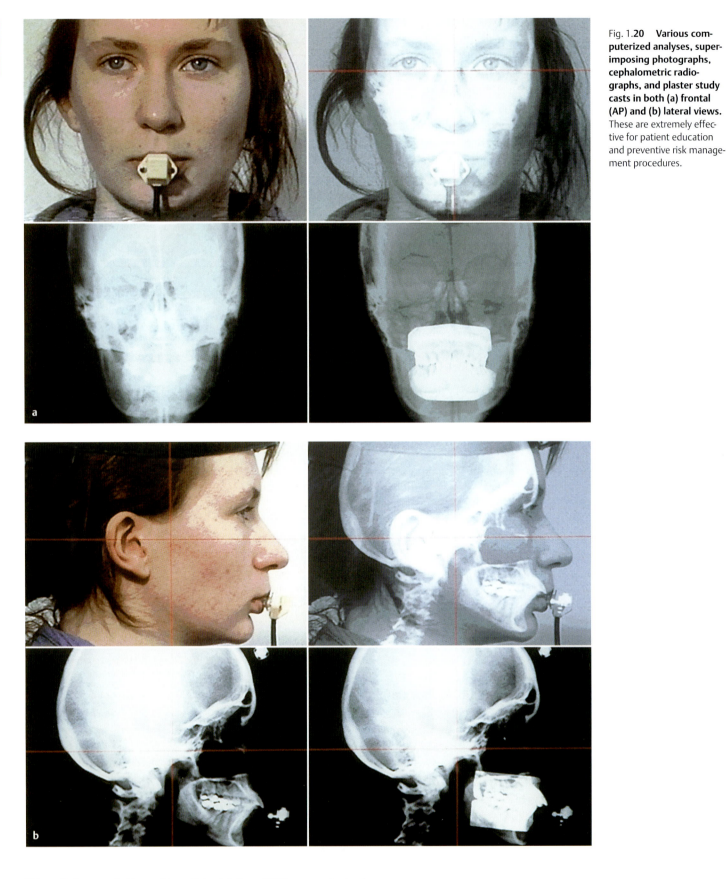

Fig. 1.20 **Various computerized analyses, superimposing photographs, cephalometric radiographs, and plaster study casts in both (a) frontal (AP) and (b) lateral views.** These are extremely effective for patient education and preventive risk management procedures.

2D cephalogram in the not too distant future. With computerized 3D methods and diagnostic tools, we will be able to simultaneously record function or malfunction in three planes of space.

Figure 1.20a,b demonstrates computerized examination with superimposition of cephalograms, casts, and photographs, with a sensor for registration of function.

Video Imaging

Video imaging is not a precise tool for mensuration, but it is suitable for supplying information to patients, to educate and motivate them. It is of value in teaching, helping orthodontic residents to better understand three-dimensional structural relationships and the dynamic role of function. Practice management gurus point up the positive role of patient education and "selling" treatment, but this is coincidental to the diagnostic value (Fig. 1.21).

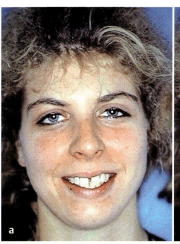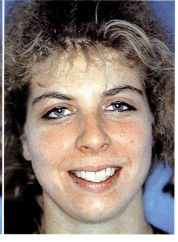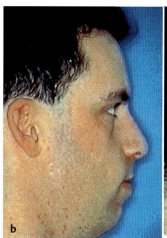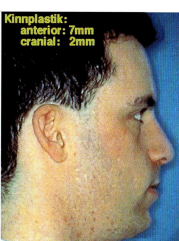

Fig. 1.**21** **Video imaging is an excellent patient education tool.**
a A simple closing of an anterior diastema.
b The changes effected by a simple chin augmentation surgical procedure.
Extensive morphing of facial and dental changes can be done with commercially available programs.

Forecasting (Prediction)

Attempts have been made to predict both biological and therapeutic changes from cephalometric films, and commercial programs have been available for some time (i.e., the Ricketts Rocky Mountain analysis) that project direction and amount of facial and dental changes with specific growth patterns. However, such attempts are largely two-dimensional, allowing for only anteroposterior and vertical projections, and many clinicians feel they are not yet sufficiently accurate. Progress is being made, and newer, 3D bases make this a viable tool, provided soft-tissue assessments, functional analyses, and the like are considered alongside cephalometric measurements.

The goals of these forecasting methods are:
- Localization of the variability or abnormality
- Assessment of potential problems as a result of the variability
- Possible solutions, (i.e., growth guidance, extraction, surgery, or camouflage)
- Timing of control measures (possible autonomous improvement)
- Assessment of probability of success of treatment and potential problems

The major concern with all new diagnostic tools is that we are still making our decisions with a degree of uncertainty because we do not have all the contributing factors in the diagnostic mosaic. The infinite variability of the facial skeleton, even in cases of good occlusion, makes forecasting of the ultimate status less exact than we would like. Outcome predictions are still not sufficiently reliable because of the dynamic, changing milieu of biological problems, too often assessed by only two-dimensional criteria.

To minimize the impact of uncertainty, the consequences and cost of errors (potential iatrogenic sequelae) should constantly be considered. Irreversible commitments must not depend on a cavalier decision process devoid of critical information. This is a sign of professional maturity. Diagnostic tools are improving every day, and it is the responsibility of the clinician to keep abreast of those improvements. Orthodontics is, and is likely to be for some time, the "thinking clinician's" game, but this makes it all more interesting and exciting.

The discrepancy between what we expect and what actually happens during treatment can be considerable. The adage about "The best laid plans of mice and men" applies in orthodontics. Midcourse corrections are often necessary and depend on proper therapeutic diagnosis with each patient visit. There is no Procrustean bed of diagnosis for all malocclusions, any more than for treatment regimens.

It has been emphasized that treatment can be instituted both in the mixed dentition and in the permanent dentition. Each has certain advantages, depending on the problems and morphogenetic pattern associated with the malocclusion. For example, waiting until the early permanent dentition may give a clearer picture of what steps must be taken. While many patients might profit from serial extraction of teeth in an acutely crowded dentition, in borderline cases it might be better to wait until the premolars and canines have erupted and then make the extraction/nonextraction decision. An early treatment decision in a patient with mild crowding (Fig. 1.**22 a–c**) would likely have meant a serial extraction routine for many clinicians. In actuality, the patient was treated with nonextraction, after taking full diagnostic records and periodic observation (Fig. 1.**22 d–f**). The key here was that the crowding was mild. Sometimes there is autonomous improvement in crowding, particularly where the problem is not severe. Watchful waiting and periodic observation paid off for the patient shown in Figure 1.**22**.

The forecast potential for multiple arch length problems, growth increments, and growth direction and growth timing will improve as we increase our knowledge base with diagnostic tools that provide more information prior to placement of the appliance, allowing us to predict with accuracy the consequences of specific interventions for each individual patient. Self-improvement or increasing severity of malocclusions during the pretreatment observation period are decisive concerns for the ultimate success of treatment and the stability of results. Pretreatment observation may increase the load of patients, but the returns in patient service and personal education are gratifying.

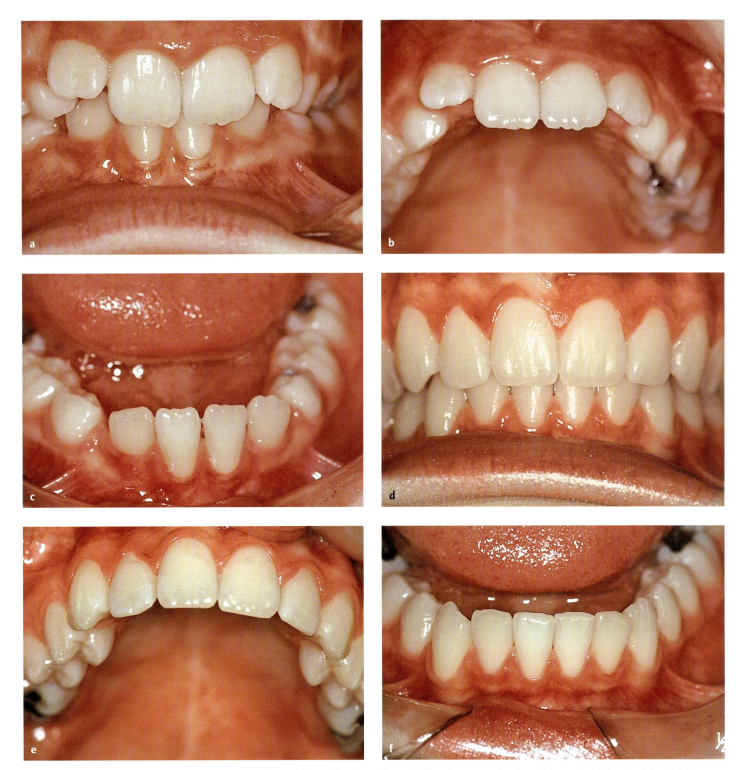

Fig. 1.22 **Treatment timing is important.** In this series of views, the arch length problem could have been treated with serial extraction in the mixed dentition but was not. The results are shown with nonextraction in the permanent dentition.
a–c Initial pretreatment intraoral views.
d–f Posttreatment intraoral views.

In some malocclusions, a trend toward self-improvement can be observed, i.e., a homeostatic reaction. In many Class II and open bite malocclusions, autonomous improvement is seen between the second and sixth years of life (Fig. 1.23).

The Class III malocclusion is more likely to be progressive, with a larger hereditary component. Larger-than-average mandibular growth increments can be seen after the seventh year of life (Fig. 1.24).

An approximate forecast is possible with the help of standards developed through periodic surveys of large numbers of nonorthodontic schoolchildren (Moyers 1973). Again, these values are a guide and not a goal for each individual patient (Fig. 1.25). Moyers differentiates between stable structures (constants) and nonstable areas, which are adaptive to skeletal changes and can be influenced therapeutically.

The Goal of Treatment and Camouflage

Diagnosis has generally been based on an ideal occlusion paradigm. This concept is not evidence-based because the arbitrary ideal occlusion is the exception and not the rule.

The "old glory" skull in the Angle textbook (Angle 1907) (Fig. 1.**26**) is no longer the realistic goal of orthodontic treatment. Achieving a stable, ideal occlusion for all patients is unrealistic. This is an articulator concept that may serve well for artificial dentures, but not for the living, developing, changing human being. Gnathology has been called by Lysle Johnston "the science of how articulators chew." Myriad functional variabilities and responses cannot be sufficiently replicated on a mechanical reproduction of the temporomandibular joint and upper and lower dentitions. It is a fallacy to assume that mandibular opening is a purely rotary action via a hinge axis movement in the glenoid fossa. That is an outmoded mechanical prosthetic concept. The goal must individualized and differentiated. It must be an individualized, achievable optimum, a balance of structural, neuromuscular, and esthetic outcomes that will be stable and will most benefit the individual patient. Careful examination of the patient periodically during active orthodontic treatment provides the best answer for both the patient and the clinician. Altogether too many orthodontists still ignore the role of the draping soft tissue as they expand dental arches off basal bone and into muscle forces.

An important question in assessing the goal for treatment is the three-dimensional status and relationship of the supporting components of the dentofacial complex. Are the skeletal and neuromuscular components balanced before we start? We should try to maintain that balance. If they are unbalanced, it should be our goal to establish a harmonious dentofacial relationship when we have completed mechanotherapy. Figure 1.**27** illustrates a balanced skeletal and neuromuscular frame. Dentoalveolar changes, i.e. tooth movement, should strive to maintain that balance.

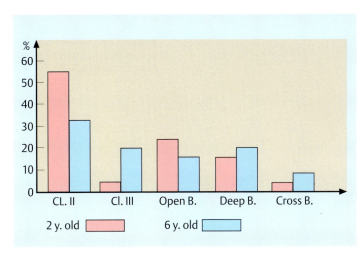

Fig. 1.**23** **The Achilles heel of orthodontics is the lack of an observation period before treatment in young patients.** The applied biological orthodontist of the new millennium, like the pediatrician, does not treat every patient who comes to the practice. For example, studying the frequency of malocclusions between the second and sixth year of life, autonomous improvement often occurs in Class II and open bite malocclusions. The reverse is true for Class III, deep bite, and crossbite problems.

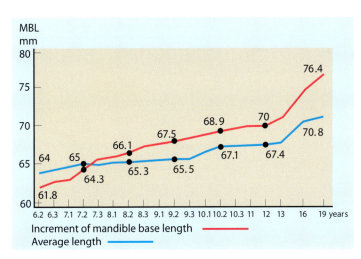

Fig. 1.**24** Class III patients are more likely to become more severe, as this chart from 6.3 to 19 years shows.

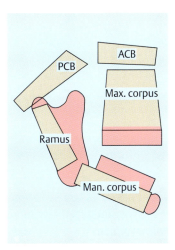

Fig. 1.**25** **The approximate changes in nonstable areas (pink) are compared to the more constant parts of the craniofacial complex (tan) according to Moyers (1973).** Condylar growth is generally more active than growth in the anterior part of the ramus, according to most studies. PCB: posterior cranial base, ACB: anterior cranial base.

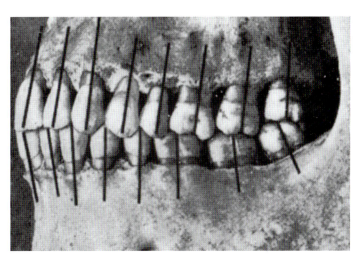

Fig. 1.**26** The alveolodental portion of the classical Angle "Old Glory" skull, demonstrating long axis inclinations.

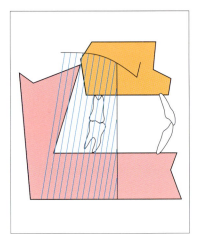

Fig. 1.**27** A diagrammatic representation of a balanced skeletal and neuromuscular relationship in a normal occlusion.

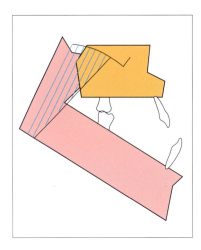

Fig. 1.**28** A dysplastic skeletodental relationship and changed neuromuscular element. Compare with Fig. 1.27.

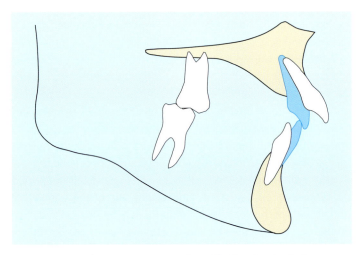

Fig. 1.**29** **Depending on patient age and specific Class II malocclusion characteristics, camouflage treatment may be indicated.** Note lingual tipping of the upper incisors and labial tipping of the lower incisors.

In a dysplastic relationship of skeletal and neuromuscular components, growth guidance, growth enhancement, inhibition, or directional change are usually indicated (Fig. 1.**28**). In some cases, this is not possible, especially in the permanent or adult dentition, and camouflage treatment is necessary. Too often, we have tried to fit a normal occlusion onto an abnormal maxillomandibular relationship. The unstable results and iatrogenic consequences reflect an unrealistic diagnostic study and treatment goal. In severe adult cases, where not even camouflage is possible, a combined orthognathic surgical approach may be necessary. With distraction osteogenesis, this is now an easier and potentially less iatrogenic approach that the traditional sagittal split, LeFort I, and LeFort II orthognathic surgery alternatives (see Chapter 17) Before treatment is started, a thorough diagnostic regimen must be used to decide whether it is possible to attain an achievable optimum via camouflage or whether it is necessary to resort to surgery. Camouflage and presurgical orthodontics require completely different treatment procedures. In camouflage, the compensation consists mostly in tipping of the incisors. Presurgically the incisors must be uprighted by the orthodontist. For camouflage, much depends on the position and inclination of the incisors and jaw bases and the possibility of stable change as we produce an esthetically more acceptable result without surgical assistance.

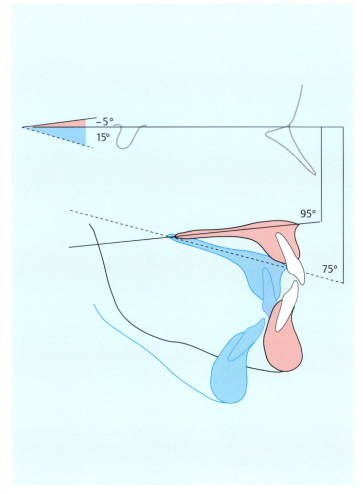

Fig. 1.**30** **An important diagnostic element is the upward (ante) or downward (retro) inclination of the maxillary base.** Just a 5° variation above, with a 15° increase below the sella–nasion plane (a total of 20°) can produce the dramatic changes illustrated.

Figure 1.**29** illustrates possible camouflage of a Class II relationship by lingual tipping of the upper incisors and labial tipping of the lower incisors. The position and inclination of the jaw bases are important considerations, depending on the facial pattern. Besides the inclination of the mandible (mandibular and occlusal planes), the inclination of the maxillary base must also be assessed (Fig. 1.**30**).

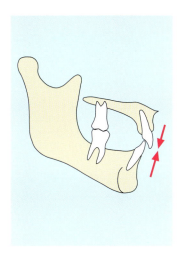

Fig. 1.**31** **Convergent rotation of the upper and lower jaws, which creates and enhances deep bite problems.**

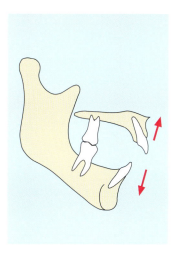

Fig. 1.**32** **Diverging rotation of maxillary and mandibular bases, creating open bite problems (arrows).** Compare with Fig. 1.**31**.

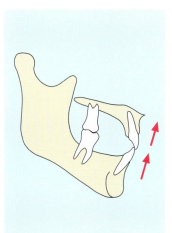

Fig. 1.**33** **Growth rotation of jaws in the same (cranial) direction.**

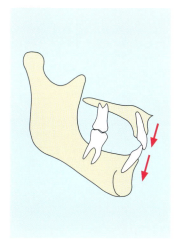

Fig. 1.**34** **Growth rotation of jaws in same (caudal) direction.** Note the arrows showing downward and backward direction of facial growth, which may not be what you want for optimal esthetics.

Depending on the combination of these inclinations, there are various possibilities for treatment: e.g., convergent rotation of the jaw bases (Fig. 1.**31**); horizontal growth pattern, with retroinclination of the maxilla; severe skeletal deep overbite.

Figure 1.**32** illustrates diverging rotation: vertical growth pattern and anteinclination of the maxilla; severe skeletal open bite malocclusion. Prognosis is poor in such patients. The patient must be informed in advance.

Figure 1.**33** illustrates jaw growth rotation in the same cranial direction. For example, a horizontal pattern with anteinclination of the maxilla; compensated skeletal deep overbite; the anteinclination is opening the bite.

Figure 1.**34** shows rotation in the same direction in caudal or downward and backward rotation compensated open bite. The tracing shows a vertical growth pattern with retroinclination of the maxilla; compensated skeletal open bite; the retroinclination is closing the bite.

Study these illustrations carefully and be aware of the challenges to orthodontic, orthopedic, and orthognathic services. If the patient is not informed in advance (i.e., informed consent), the potential for litigation is greatly increased.

Evidence-based Diagnosis

This term is more than semantic euphony. The best treatment regimen for individual malocclusions is the evidence-based decision. A thorough diagnostic study is essential, of course, but the evidence-based decision consists of at least two components:

1. External clinical evidence from systematically updated research
2. Individual clinical expertise; i.e., knowledge plus actual experience by the clinician

The external evidence comes from current randomized, prospective, controlled clinical studies and comprehensive systematic reviews of available literature. The systematic reviews should provide the gold standard for judging whether a particular treatment does more good than harm (Fig. 1.**35 a**). Orthodontic therapy always has the possibility of being a two-edged sword, as the recent increase in malpractice litigation demonstrates. Root resorption, crestal bone loss, periodontal damage, and positional instability are just some of the claims being made in court against orthodontists.

The true gold standard must be a scientifically recognized diagnosis. Anecdotal reports are not enough. Clearly, we still have a way to go before evidence-based results show that we are doing more good than harm in the long run. Orthodontic results need to demonstrate more long-term stability, without indefinite use of posttreatment retaining devices. Figure 1.**35 b** shows the goal

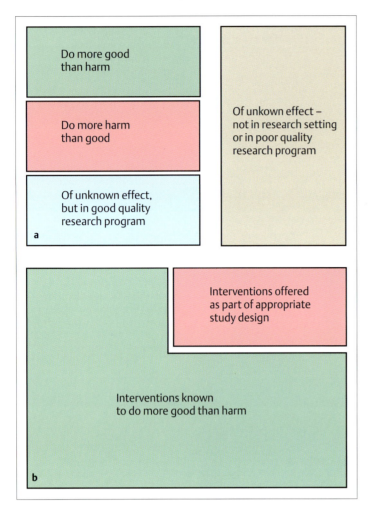

Fig. 1.**35** **Current status of evidence-based orthodontics.** As the diagrams indicate, we must enlarge the green section and reduce the pink iatrogenic and unknown sections (gray) in our total orthodontic therapy results.
a Current situation.
b Goal of evidence-based orthodontics.

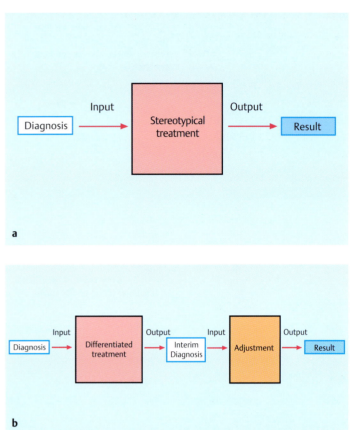

Fig. 1.**36** **The aim of orthodontics in the new millennium.** Not a pragmatic (**a**) but a communicative (**b**) mode of treatment.

of evidence-based orthodontics, relying only on interventions (i.e., treatment) that do maximal good with minimal iatrogenic sequelae.

For a valid research study design, instead of pragmatic evidence, the communicative evidence should be preferred. The pragmatic evidence responds to the same input immutably with the same output; it shapes the patient's problem to suit the intervention; it is an appliance-related therapy (Fig. 1.**36a**).

The communicative evidence responds to a given input with different outputs, corresponding to its internal state, providing information as to whether the clinician's suggestion fits the patient and the individual situation; it is a problem-oriented therapy (Fig. 1.**36b**).

Recently, a major three-university NIH-supported prospective study on mixed dentition treatment received extensive exposure in professional journals, at annual orthodontic meetings, and in the lay press. However, orthodontic residents-in-training had committed major flaws in the execution of the research. They failed, for example, to follow the proper treatment regimen with particular appliances; and several different residents saw patients on successive appointments. The research design was appropriate; the research execution was flawed. It is important that *all* aspects of an evidence-based study be analyzed objectively.

Social Requirements

The social requirements and psychological implications of diagnosis must not be neglected. The practice management efficiency gurus are giving lectures all over the world, telling orthodontists how to see more patients in less time. One management-group norm is 60–80 patients per day. How, then, can adequate time be given to each patient? How can each patient receive meaningful individual attention, therapeutic diagnosis, personal motivation, and psychological support? Patient compliance suffers, and psychological support is hardly possible in this milieu. Treatment decisions and therapeutic improvement require continuing teamwork between the patient and orthodontist. The personal relationship established with each patient can be particularly rewarding, and this is jeopardized by reducing patient contact during treatment.

Orthodontists must respect the personal desires of their patients. This is being jeopardized by the rush to "see" more patients in less time. Evidence-based patient care is a phenomenon that is simply not possible in this superstore environment. Legal entanglements are a reality where personal care of insufficient depth and understanding has been rendered. The increase in litigious involvement by orthodontists cannot all be blamed on the eager-beaver contingency-fee lawyers. The best antidote is a strong personal relationship with each patient. Not only is this more satisfying to the patients, but it makes orthodontic practice more personally rewarding for the clinician over the long haul.

Therapeutic diagnosis is a continuing obligation during and after treatment, as posttreatment "settling" occurs. This euphemism for relapse is too often a tragic consequence that might have been avoided with proper diagnosis, proper control, proper motivation, and a personal relationship. Treat each patient as you would like to be treated or as you would treat your own child.

References

Angle EH. Treatment of Malocclusion of the Teeth and Fractures of the Maxillae. 7th ed. Philadelphia, Pa: SS White Manufacturing Co; 1907.

Bjork A. Prediction of mandibular growth rotation. Am J Orthod. 1969; 55: 585–599.

Casko JS, Shepherd WB. Dental and skeletal variation within the range of normal. Angle Orthod. 1984; 54: 5–17.

Graber TM. A critical review of clinical cephalometric radiography. Am J Orthod. 1954; 40: 1.

Graber TM, Rakosi T, Petrovis AG. Dentofacial Orthodontics with Functional Appliances. 2nd ed. St. Louis, Ma: Mosby; 1997.

Moyers RE. Handbook of Orthodontics. Chicago: Yearbook Medical Publishing; 1973.

Rakosi T, Jonas I, Graber TM. Orthodontic Diagnosis: Color Atlas of Dental Medicine. Stuttgart: Thieme; 1993.

Rakosi T. The relevance of our diagnostic tools to treatment planning. Acta Med Rom. 1994; 32: 217.

Steiner CC. Cephalometrics for you and me. Am J Orthod. 1953; 39: 10.

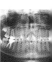

2 Preventive Orthodontics

Brian Preston

Early treatment, preventive (interceptive) orthodontics, and treatment timing are much-debated and still somewhat controversial subjects (Tulloch et al. 1997). A consensus definition of early treatment holds it as treatment started in the primary or mixed dentition to enhance the dental and skeletal development before the eruption of the permanent dentition. But critical to this concept is diagnosis, the recognition of problems that can be prevented or intercepted, allowing the fullest expression of a normal developmental pattern for each child. Different approaches are still applied to various conditions that might require early treatment, although some say early intervention could reduce treatment time or even eliminate the need for treatment at a later stage (Graber 1961). It is a fact that developing malocclusions may be intercepted at any age and at any stage of dental development. If this can be done expeditiously, with minimal time, mechanotherapy investment, and iatrogenic reaction, the efforts are justified.

In a traditional sense, the notion of interceptive orthodontics has referred primarily to occlusal problems that can be treated by pediatric or general dentists and are usually treated by means of removable appliances. This form of treatment is mostly carried out in young patients who are in their deciduous or late mixed-dentition stage of occlusal development. The Achilles heel, however, is comprehensive diagnosis and recognition of skeletal abnormalities and neuromuscular deformation potential. The question is not the appliance, but how, when, and why you use it and the benefits it brings, assessed against waiting until the permanent dentition and comprehensive fixed appliance treatment. In recent years, many dentists have gained a working knowledge of the more elaborate aspects of orthodontic diagnosis and treatment planning, making use, for example, of cephalometric radiographs to identify aberrant craniofacial patterns. With the use of more sensitive diagnostic procedures, the scope of interceptive orthodontics has expanded well beyond its previous boundaries. The standard of care in terms of diagnostic orthodontic records include cephalometric, and dental radiographs, radiographic evidence of skeletal maturation (Turchetta, Fishman, Subtelny 2007), plaster, or digital study casts and extra-, and intra-oral photographs. The amount, direction and timing of growth are important keys in determining a rational, and successful treatment plan. Before commencing orthodontic treatment it would be advantageous if the orthodontist providing the treatment could reliably estimate how future changes in the vertical, or the horizontal relationships of the jaws are related to the incremental skeletal increases and the timing of growth. It is also important to evaluate whether posttreatment growth will affect the long term stability of the treatment results obtained. The initial orthodontic records should also include the results of a comprehensive clinical examination which, in turn should include comments on the patient's primary mode of respiration. While it is possible for general dentists to provide early treatment for skeletal facial abnormalities, the diagnostic process that leads to referral of these patients for appropriate treatment is a very important aspect of interceptive orthodontics. Sound orthodontic diagnosis requires a good understanding of the basics of facial growth, skeletal age, and normal and abnormal facial patterns. Generally, only orthodontists possess this skill to the degree required for optimal therapy. Nevertheless, recognition of developing problems is within the purview of general and pediatric dentists. The knowledge of when to refer for an expert orthodontic consultation parallels the referral by a pediatrician to an ear, nose and throat (ENT) specialist. This chapter gives a broad appraisal of the early treatment potential and various appliances employed, usually by the orthodontist, as part of the total management of the skeletal, neuromuscular, and dental facets of the developing malocclusion. Merely "straightening teeth" is no longer a valid treatment objective in the new millennium (Sarver, Ackerman 2000). It is hoped that the following pages will give all who treat young dental patients a better understanding of the challenges and timing of optimal care, always with what is best for the patient in mind, not for the efficiency of practice management, which might result in longer guidance and fewer income-producing patients but more satisfying results for the orthodontist. Tayer and Burnes (1993) note the writings of Würpel (1931) who cautioned: *The mind of a child is as tender and as lovely as the petals of a full-blown rose. Beware how you touch it! Meet it with all the reverence of your being. Use it with gentle respect and fill it with the honey of love, the perfume of faith and the tenderness of tolerance. Thus shall you fulfill the mission of your life.*

Nonetheless, the push to provide more efficient, and better-individualized orthodontic treatment is likely to gain momentum in the foreseeable future. In undertaking such treatment, we must remember that efficiency greatly impacts our ability to provide a better result in a shorter period of time. Treatment goals must be clearly defined prior to embarking on a sequence of mechanical interventions and, in this respect, timing and degree of interception are the key issues.

There are a number of possibilities with interceptive orthodontics. In some instances, patients present with essentially normal occlusions and interceptive steps are taken to prevent a malocclusion from developing. In other patients, a degree of malocclusion

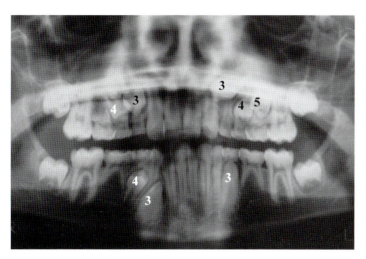
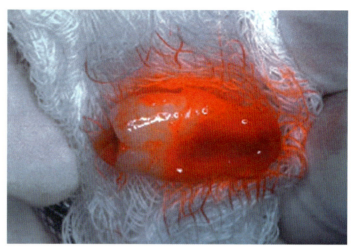

Fig. 2.1 A panoramic radiograph of a 10-year-old boy who presents with both bicuspid teeth congenitally missing in the lower left quadrant and the second bicuspid tooth absent in each of the quadrants on the right side. The orthodontic treatment required the extraction of four bicuspid teeth, and this raised the possibility that one of the bicuspid teeth (upper arrow) in the upper right quadrant can be transplanted to the lower left quadrant (lower arrow) where both bicuspid teeth are absent.

Fig. 2.2 The upper right second bicuspid, with its root approximately one-half to two-thirds completed, has been surgically removed from the patient shown in Figure 2.1 with its root bud intact. The extracted upper bicuspid was placed in a socket prepared in the lower left first bicuspid area. Following orthodontic treatment, the dentition resembled the outcome usually achieved with the extraction of four bicuspid teeth.

is already present and, in these cases, the goal of treatment is to correct the problem and prevent further occlusal deterioration. Examples of occlusal conditions that may require interceptive treatment in young patients include:
- Congenitally missing teeth.
- Supernumerary teeth.
- Ectopic eruption ankylosed teeth.
- Early loss of teeth.
- Midline diastema.
- Habits.
- Crossbites.

Although interceptive treatment is usually associated with young patients, it can be instituted at any age or stage of dental development. For example, mature patients with essentially normal occlusions may need orthodontic treatment to prevent malocclusions from developing as a result of tooth loss, dental attrition, periodontal disease or other etiological factors. The assumption is made that a normal occlusion will be maintained if an incipient malocclusion is diagnosed and treated in a timely manner.

The **congenital absence of a tooth or teeth** results from disturbances that occur during the early stages of odontogenesis. Since the follicles of the primary teeth give rise to the permanent tooth buds, it is not possible to have a permanent tooth if its primary precursor is missing. According to Butler's field theory, the teeth most likely to be congenitally missing would be those furthest from the midline in each series of teeth (Butler 1939). Experience seems to support Butler's theory. If a molar tooth is missing, it is almost always the third molar; if an incisor is missing, it is nearly always the lateral; if a premolar is missing, it is almost always the second rather than the first. The orthodontic problems associated with congenitally absent teeth are complex and they require careful diagnosis and treatment planning. Ultimately, and in the absence of severe crowding of the dental arches the missing tooth or teeth will have to be replaced by prosthetic means that include dental bridges or osseo-integrated implants. No clinician should embark upon a program of planned extractions (serial extractions) prior to obtaining radiographic evidence that all of the permanent teeth are indeed present. Autotransplantation of immature premolars (Figs. 2.1, 2.2) also presents a viable method of restoring edentulous areas for patients whose alveolar growth is not yet complete (Paulsen 2001). The most crucial factors for the survival of transplants and their continued development are ½ to ¾ root development in the transplant, wide open apices and preservation of the periodontal ligament during the surgical procedure (Paulsen, Zachrisson 1992).

The occurrence of **supernumerary teeth** is a less common finding than other dental developmental anomalies (Altug-Atac, Erdem 2007). Moreover, the prevalence of this anomaly differs significantly between races (Zhu at al. 1996). The presence of supernumerary teeth can lead to the abnormal eruption or impaction of the normal series of teeth. The late development of supernumerary teeth can also complicate the post orthodontic retention phase (Fig. 2.3a,b). The occurrence of unerupted supernumerary teeth should be suspected if, during orthodontic treatment, it becomes difficult to move teeth or to correct their abnormal axial inclinations. Supernumerary teeth frequently cause damage to the roots of adjacent teeth. Obviously, panoral radiographs are required at periodic intervals, usually once a year to determine if the developmental status is normal. This is a keystone of interceptive orthodontics.

Supernumerary teeth can also erupt and resemble other teeth in the dental arch (Fig. 2.4) to the extent that it can be difficult to decide which tooth is the anomalous one. Prior to extracting a supernumerary tooth, it is wise under these circumstances to examine all of the teeth involved for vitality and for root integrity.

It is frequently very difficult to determine the exact position of an unerupted, or impacted tooth relative to the roots of its neighbors. In these circumstances, the most important consideration is usually whether the unerupted tooth is located either lingually or buccally to the adjacent teeth. The parallax periapical radiograph technique, introduced by Clark in 1910 for the localization of impacted teeth, is still the preferred method today (Clark 1910; Jacobs 1999). Clark used two periapical radiographs and shifted

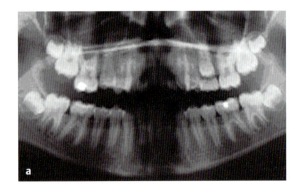
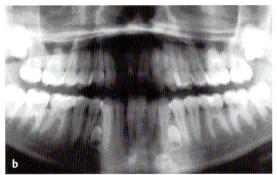

Fig. 2.**3 a** The original radiograph was taken when this female patient was 11 years old. There is no sign of developing teeth in the anterior region of the mandible. **b** Following orthodontic treatment, supernumerary teeth can be seen on the panoramic radiograph taken at age 13 years. The development of a second set of cuspid teeth is a relatively rare phenomenon.

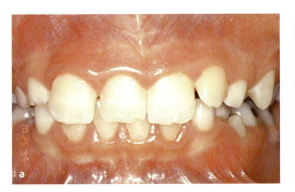
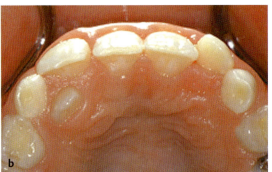

Fig. 2.**4** A patient presents with three maxillary anterior teeth that resemble central incisors. The upper left lateral incisor is in place while the upper right lateral incisor is in the process of erupting in a palatal position. In a situation such as this, care must be taken to distinguish between a malformed, wide upper lateral and a supernumerary central incisor.

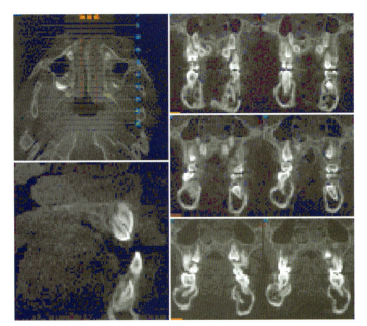

Fig. 2.**5** The CBCT radiograph at top left maps the direction (coronal), as well as the thickness, of the slices of the tissues that will be imaged. The sagittal image at bottom left shows two maxillary central incisors developing in a crowded situation, with one tooth superimposed on the other. The images on the right side are transverse slices of the jaws showing the positions of the developing, and erupted, teeth.

(Mah: Hatcher 2004). Cone-beam computed tomography (CBCT) or cone beam volumetric tomography (CBVT) has followed the trend of computed tomography (CT) in medicine, in which, CT has become one of the most important radiological examinations worldwide. The use of volumetric radiographic techniques is becoming feasible in general dentistry (Fig. 2.**5**), largely because computerized axial tomography (CAT or CT) imaging radiographic machines are being designed specifically for dental use (Mozzo et al. 1998). The images obtained with radiographic machines such as the NewTom 3 G FOV 12 (Quantitative Radiology s.r.l. Verona, Italy) make it possible to determine the positions of unerupted teeth with precision. Radiation doses associated with the latest generation of CBCT machines have been reduced from those resulting from the earlier machines. It should be noted, however, that even conventional radiology potentially contributes significantly to the radiation burden in those less than 19 years old in the United States (Hujoel et al. 2008).

Occasionally, a malpositioned permanent tooth bud, or retained deciduous tooth, can cause the resultant tooth to erupt into an abnormal position. Early loss, or caries, of a deciduous molar may also affect the normal eruption the succedaneous teeth. This condition is called **ectopic eruption,** and it is frequently encountered in the eruption of the maxillary first molars. Ectopic eruption can result in the transposition of teeth, while abnormally erupting teeth can damage the roots of adjacent teeth. For a permanent tooth to erupt, the overlying bone as well as the primary tooth roots must resorb, and the tooth must make its way through the gingiva. **Supernumerary teeth,** pathological entities (Figs. 2.**6**, 2.**7**) and tough fibrous gingival tissue can impede tooth eruption. It becomes abundantly clear that an accurate visualization of developing problems may be the most important interceptive service that can be rendered. For example, the eruption of a tooth from its developmental position within the jaw toward its

the tube in the horizontal plane. In 1952, Richards appreciated that a vertical tube shift could also be carried out. No major changes occurred in the technique until Keur (1986) replaced the periapical radiographs with a combination of a panoramic and an occlusal radiograph (Keur 1986; Stivaros and Mandall 2000; Jacobs 1999). This modification allows a greater tube movement and therefore a greater shift of the image of the impacted tooth.

The clinical application of 3-dimensional craniofacial imaging is one of the most exciting and revolutionary topics in dentistry

Preventive Orthodontics

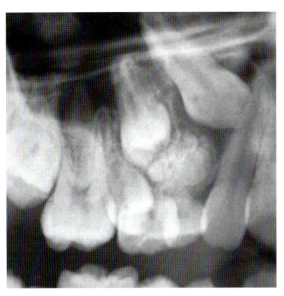

Fig. 2.**6** This figure illustrates how a pathological entity such as an odontome may prevent a tooth from erupting. In this instance the first bicuspid is unable to erupt, while the adjacent cuspid has been pushed into an abnormal eruption path.

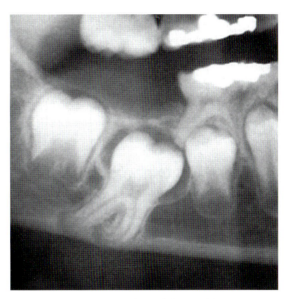

Fig. 2.**8** First permanent molar teeth frequently become impacted due to either the early loss or the prolonged retention of deciduous molars. In this patient, the distal root of the second deciduous molar is impeding the eruption of the first permanent mandibular molar.

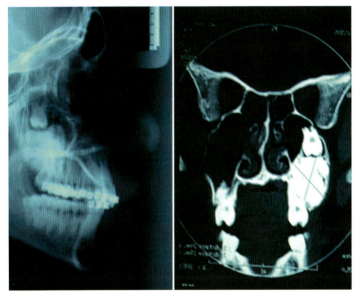

Fig. 2.**7** The radiograph on the left is a cephalometric view of an upper molar displaced into the maxillary antrum by an ossifying lesion. The CT scan on the right taken of the same lesion, shows the exact position of the displaced left maxillary molar.

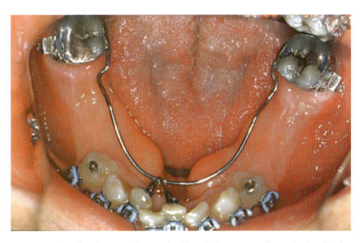

Fig. 2.**9** Lingual arches provide a method by which space can be maintained in the mandibular dental arch. Precision lingual arches can also be used, as in this illustration, to upright or disimpact teeth that have tipped mesially. A passive sectional arch is placed to stabilize the incisor teeth.

functional position in the occlusal plane is a complex process of juggling for space in the growing jaws.

Dental impaction occurs when there is cessation of the eruption of a tooth due to an abnormal eruption path or the presence of an obstacle in its normal eruption path. Factors that may result in the impaction of molar teeth include:
- Dental crowding.
- The early loss of teeth.
- Pathology.
- Dental caries.
- Poor quality restorative work.
- The retention of primary teeth.
- Supernumerary teeth.
- Orthodontic tooth movement.

A number of specific dental anomalies contribute to the observation that mandibular molars are prone to impaction (Fig. 2.**8**). There are a variety of appliances (Fig. 2.**9**) that can be used to de-impact impacted molars but, in a few select cases, the removal of a third molar tooth may be all that is required to allow an impacted second mandibular molar to erupt (Fig. 2.**10**). A always, diagnosis is the name of the interceptive orthodontics game.

A **maxillary midline diastema** is a relatively common occurrence, especially in the mixed-dentition phase of dental development. A maxillary midline space larger than 2 mm rarely closes spontaneously with further development. Care must be taken when closing spaces between the maxillary incisors as these spaces may be part of the "ugly duckling phase" of normal dental development. Space closure during this phase of development

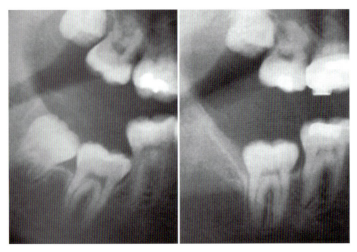

Fig. 2.10   In this patient, the extraction of a wisdom tooth allowed the impacted second lower molar tooth to erupt. The outcome will depend on the crown shapes, as well as the inclinations of the teeth involved.

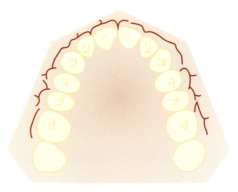

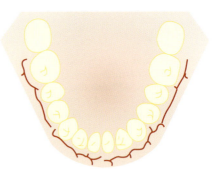

Fig. 2.12   The Bolton formula is used to compare the intermaxillary mesiodistal widths of the permanent teeth up to and including the first permanent molars. If the calculated ratio is greater than 91.3%, the mandibular teeth are too wide and if the ratio is less that 91.3% the maxillary teeth are relatively too large.

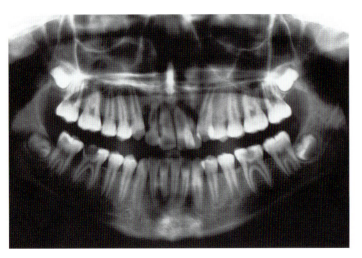

Fig. 2.11   The use of an elastic band, graphically illustrated in this panoramic radiograph, to close spaces between incisor teeth can lead to overeruption of these teeth, or even their exfoliation as is shown here.

may cause the roots of the lateral incisors to push against the crowns of erupting canine teeth. This pressure can result in resorption of the lateral incisor roots or impaction of the erupting canine teeth. The presence of a maxillary midline diastema requires careful investigation, as this occlusal trait can be associated with a wide variety of etiological factors that include:
- A genetic and/or ethnic predisposition.
- The presence of a mesiodens.
- An abnormal maxillary frenum.
- Space occupying lesions.
- A loss of posterior occlusal bite support.
- Class III malocclusion.
- A tooth size discrepancy.
- Normal dental development.
- Habits.

Although some simple solutions have been suggested (Fig. 2.11), the treatment of a midline diastema can present a challenging problem. To quote Dr Graber: *"Do not sit back and wait—Investigate"*.

Abnormalities in **tooth size and shape** result from disturbances that occur during the morphodifferentiation phase of dental development. The most common abnormality is a variation in size, particularly of the maxillary lateral incisors and second premolars. The diagnosis of tooth size discrepancy is based on comparison of the widths of teeth with published tables of expected tooth sizes. The **Bolton analysis** (Fig. 2.12) determines the ratio of the mesiodistal widths of the mandibular versus the maxillary teeth (Bolton 1958; Bolton 1962). In the analysis of the overall Bolton ratio, the relationship of the 12 mandibular teeth to the 12 maxillary teeth is assessed (Stifter 1958). Because of the importance of the canine and incisor relationships, a further analysis is performed to evaluate the ratio between the six lower and the six upper anterior teeth. The normal average for this ratio is 77.2%. Because it is usually easier to reduce than it is to add tooth material, the Bolton analysis assumes that the relatively smaller teeth are of the correct size. In patients with normal occlusal relationships and with good incisor position, tooth size discrepancies may result in spaces, crowding, rotations, and incorrect intercuspations. Tooth size discrepancies may be corrected or improved by extractions or interdental stripping, or by restorative procedures to increase the widths of the teeth that are too narrow. The relevance of the anterior index value is somewhat reduced if the mandibular incisors are severely labioverted and/or if the labiolingual diameters of the incisal edges of the anterior teeth are abnormally large.

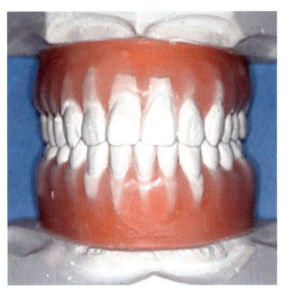

Fig. 2.13 A diagnostic setup, with the lower left lateral extracted and a large upper midline diastema closed. The final orthodontic result obtained for this patient resembled closely the result planned with the diagnostic setup.

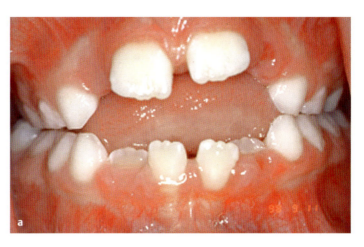
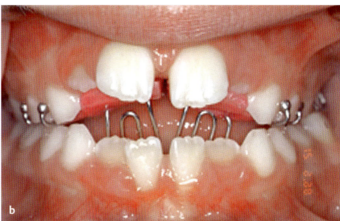
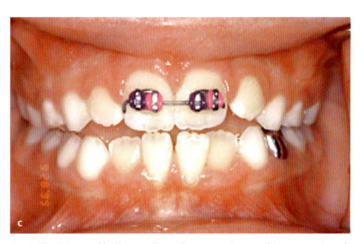

Fig. 2.14 A 9-year-old girl presenting with an **a** anterior open bite was motivated to stop the finger-sucking habit without any orthodontic intervention. **b** Residual open bite closed with tongue crib. **c** Diastema closed with brackets and elastic traction.

Digital technology is having a profound impact on the practice of dentistry and orthodontics. One rapidly growing form of digital technology is the three-dimensional digital dental model, which largely eliminates the use of plaster study models. The electronic dental models usually incorporate an accurate and easy-to-use digital version of the Bolton analysis. Such records may be circulated via e-mail to other dental providers for consultation, an avenue that has not attained its full potential.

Prior to embarking on treatment in patients with tooth size discrepancies, it is useful to perform a diagnostic setup (Fig. 2.13). The diagnostic setup should simulate the extractions, tooth stripping, and the planned orthodontic and restorative work. The diagnostic setup will provide a good indication of the incisor relationships that will be present at the completion of treatment and this, in turn, will give a good indication of the type of retention required for the patient. Such determinations, along with cephalometric and panoral radiographs, provide an excellent prognostic tool for development and treatment timing.

Broadly speaking, the dentition functions within an equilibrium that exists between the pressures exerted by the tongue and by the buccal and labial musculature. Pernicious **oral habits** produce forces that can alter the functional environment in which the dentition operates. Experiments suggest that even very light forces can successfully move teeth, if the force in question is of sufficiently long duration. It seems that for a finger habit to move teeth (Fig. 2.14a–c) the forces created by the finger would have to be applied in a particular direction, at a specific magnitude, and for a length of time that is greater than six hours (Proffit 2000). Carefully taken case histories and patient interviews are time consuming but worth every minute spent with the patient.

Behavioral patterns such as habits are commonly classified as essential or nonessential, innate or learned, and primary or secondary. These terms are largely self-explanatory. Suffice it to say that, if a habit is only one of number of symptoms of an abnormal behavior problem, the psychological aspects of the problem should be the first consideration in treatment. If the emotional development of the child is deemed within normal limits, as is usually the case with most children with finger-sucking habits, and if parental as well as sibling cooperation is reasonably assured, interceptive procedures may be instituted. Habit-breaking appliances are best placed in healthy children who are given other pleasurable activities that can substitute for the finger-sucking habit. Routine diagnostic assessments allow insight into whether a habit is aggravating a malocclusion or whether the problem is transient and self correcting. To remain passive as a malocclusion progresses, and as neuromuscular compensations enhance the malocclusion, could be considered an act of malpractice.

A major challenge in current interceptive orthodontics lies in trying to identify at an early age those patients who could benefit from procedures that may have an orthopedic effect on the developing jaws. Factors that may impact on the **early use of orthodontic appliances** include:

- The type of dental malocclusion
- The craniofacial problem
- The growth pattern of the face.
- The patient's skeletal maturity.
- The patient's growth intensity.
- The dental development of the patient.

It is generally accepted that **extraoral traction appliances** can restrict, or redirect maxillary growth. In patients with midface deficiencies, extraoral forces can be relatively simple to apply, and if used in an appropriate manner, remarkably efficient in protracting retrognathic maxillae.

The question remains: To what extent can **functional orthodontic appliances** enhance mean annual mandibular growth? While some individuals grow more and others less, the answer probably lies in the vicinity of one extra millimeter per year. There is also some support for the belief that, although mandibular growth can be enhanced over the short term, the total predestined mandibular growth will remain the same. This, however, ignores the ability to change the direction of condylar growth and glenoid fossa adaptation. Modern diagnostic techniques such as Cone Beam Computer Tomography may be used with the expectation that they can throw some light on this premise. There is probably considerable advantage for retrogenic (Fig. 2.**15a–c**) patients in obtaining the mandibular growth at an earlier age and in a more favorable direction than would be the case without orthodontic intervention. Regarding the maxilla, there is far less controversy as to the benefits of interceptive treatment instituted to correct retrognathia. In general, it is accepted that interceptive treatment in Class III malocclusions is beneficial, while early treatment for Class II malocclusions requires a good understanding of which patients are most likely to benefit from such intervention.

Commercially available computer programs can be used to digitize lateral skull radiographs and analyze them according to traditional cephalometric analyses. Sometimes these same commercial programs incorporate routines that claim to predict the outcomes of facial growth and/or the effects of orthodontic treatment (Langland 2001). Although **predictions of facial growth** have many real limitations, the concepts are based have a basis in findings that have emerged from research into craniofacial growth

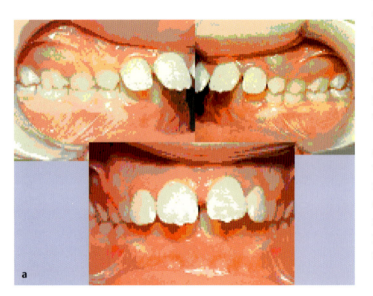

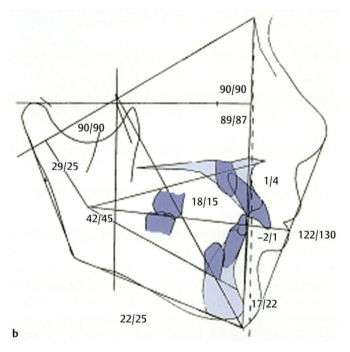

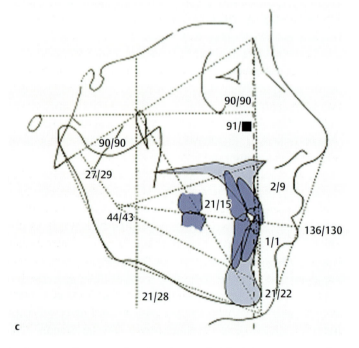

Fig. 2.**15 a** A Class II Division 1 malocclusion observed in a 10-year-old boy. The bite is deep, the overjet is excessive, there is minimal crowding and the arches are in harmony in the transverse dimension. An analysis of the patient's original lateral cephalometric radiograph indicated that he would have above average mandibular growth and that a Herbst functional appliance, to encourage mandibular growth, could be beneficial. The before (**b**) and after (**c**) lateral cephalometric tracings made for the patient shown in **a**. The values shown include both the patient's as well as the age-related mean data for each cephalometric entity. The records indicate that the functional appliance used accomplished mainly dentoalveolar changes, but there is some indication that the patient experienced good mandibular growth during the period of treatment.

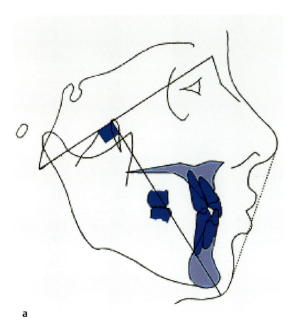
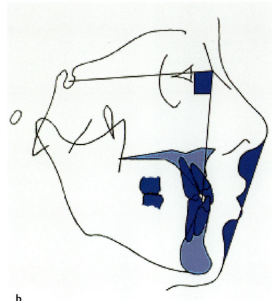

Fig. 2.16 In the short term and without the influence of external factors the angular relationship between the facial axis and the cranial base (**a**) is unlikely to change in a meaningful manner. This is also true for the angular relationship that exists between the maxilla and the cranial base (**b**), measured by the angle sella–nasion–point "A." Without external forces acting on the dentofacial complex, the relationship of the lips to the "E" line will remain essentially constant in the short term.

(Björk and Skeiler 1983). Anatomical features that have been used to predict facial growth on its own, or when combined with orthodontic treatment include:
- Condylar morphology.
- The shapes of the mandibular ramus and body.
- The shape and orientation of the mandibular symphysis.
- The orientation of the buccal, and incisor teeth.
- Specific cephalometric measurements that include assessments of the anterior, and posterior facial heights.

Clinicians who have an interest in orthodontics, and in early orthodontic treatment specifically, should know how to **superimpose** a patient's serial cephalometric radiographs. In this regard, it is important to realize that there are certain, mostly angular, craniofacial relationships that remain relatively constant during growth, and that changes in these relationships can usually be attributed to the effects of orthodontic treatment or to other extraneous factors such as oral habits (Figs. 2.**16 a, b**). It is useful to superimpose serial radiographs on the regions shown in these illustrations even though these superimpositions are more useful in indicating changes in growth direction than they are in showing increases in size due to growth.

Whereas cephalometric superimpositions are used to decide whether and how a patient grew during a specific preceding period, they are equally useful when utilized to determine whether an individual is still experiencing facial growth (Efstratiadis et al. 1999; Ghafari et al. 1998; Palleck et al. 2001). Serial lateral cephalometric radiographs, taken six months apart, can be superimposed to ascertain whether a patient is still growing. This technique is useful in patients who have Class II or Class III malocclusions or in patients who require placement of osseo-integrated implants as part of their comprehensive dental treatment. Craniofacial growth is a complex, three-dimensional process, and it is therefore unlikely that it will be possible in the foreseeable future to predict accurately a patient's facial growth from two-dimensional radiographs. With some experience, however, most dentists should be able to recognize those facial patterns that will remain constant, those that will deteriorate, and those that will improve with time and growth.

Most **Class II malocclusions** appear to result from a mandibular deficiency, rather than from a maxillary excess. While it is not feasible to retract maxillae en masse, **extraoral traction** can be used with some benefit to restrict or guide maxillary growth while allowing the mandible to grow to its full potential. In this regard, mandibular morphology (Figs. 2.**17 a, b**) and skeletal maturity are two of the prime factors that determine whether a deficient mandible will catch up to a larger maxilla. It is probably unrealistic to expect a mandible with a poor growth prognosis to grow vigorously under the influence of an appliance designed to promote mandibular growth. Vertical growth patterns, steep mandibular planes with strong antegonial notching, appear to provide more of a challenge for correction in jaw sagittal discrepancies.

The extremes of facial growth are not found in any one type of malocclusion. It is just as possible for a vertical growth pattern to occur in a Class III craniofacial pattern as in a Class II. The extremes of the vertical and the horizontal facial growth types may require sophisticated orthodontic or combined surgical-orthodontic treatment. It is therefore important to recognize these extremes of facial growth (Fig. 2.**18**) at an early age and, more importantly, to refer them for appropriate consultation and treatment in a timely manner.

The **facial skeleton** develops and operates within a complex soft-tissue environment that supports important life sustaining processes, including such functions as respiration, mastication, and deglutition. The mandible exists in the center of a chain of muscles (Figs. 2.**19**, 2.**20** and Box 2.**1**) that act in close harmony to control the position of the head in space (Bibby and Preston 1981). The center of mass of the human head lies slightly in front of the occipital condyles, which implies that the cranial extensor muscles that insert in the region of the nuccal lines of the occipital bone are usually in tension when the body is in the upright position. This situation leaves the hyoid and facial muscles relatively free to "fine tune" cranial balance while sustaining the other vegetative functions associated with the craniofacial complex. The

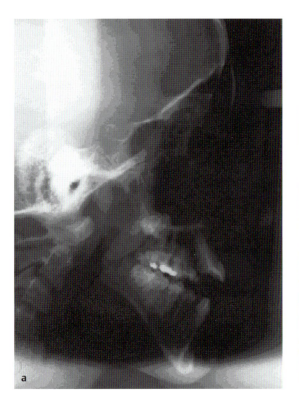
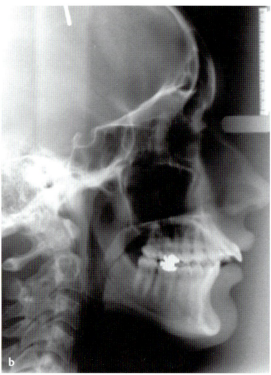

Fig. 2.**17** Malocclusions with the same Angle's classification (Angle 1988) frequently occur in individuals with very different craniofacial developmental patterns. The Class II patient in (a) has a typical vertical, while the Class II patient in (b) has a more horizontal, mandibular growth direction. An important feature of the jaw with the downward growth pattern is the narrow teardrop shaped symphysis while; the mandible with the forward growth has a broader symphysis and a more definite chin button. It is beneficial to develop an understanding of the whole anatomical picture that represents a long (leptoprosopic), or a short and usually broad (euryprosopic) face.

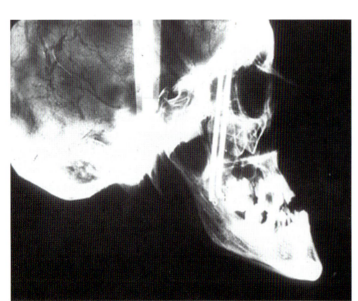

Fig. 2.**18** A lateral cephalometric radiograph of a skull that displays a Class III malocclusion as well as many of the features of an extreme vertical growth pattern. When detected in good time, many Class III malocclusions will benefit from early orthopedic traction that may include a protraction facemask or a chincap (Merwin et al. 1997).

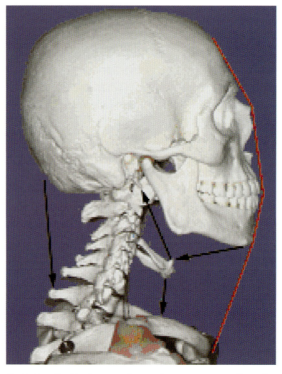

Fig. 2.**19** The black arrows denote the major groups of muscles, the posterior cranial extensors and suprahyoid, and infrahyoid muscles that control the position of the skull on the cervical vertebrae. The red line represents the anterior superficial muscle, and fascial, drape of the face.

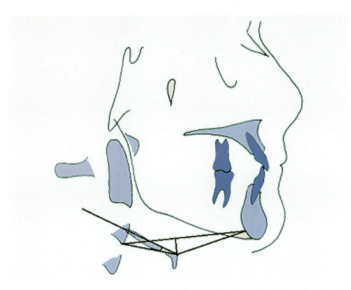

Fig. 2.20 There appears to be a notable degree of order in the dimensions that exist between the structures that constitute the oropharynx as well as the rest of the upper airway. This order is reflected in a triangle, which is formed by the lines that join the anterior inferior border of the third cervical vertebra (C3), to the body of the hyoid bone (H) and to the most posterior, inferior point on the mandibular symphysis (RGn).

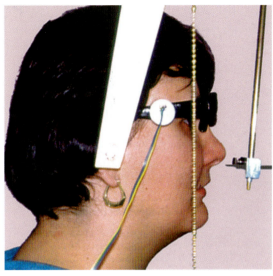

Fig. 2.21 Lateral cephalometric radiographs should be taken with the head in its natural position. Here the patient is wearing a spectacle frame with an electronic inclinometer that is used to find the patient's average natural head position during a ten-minute period of normal daily activity. The patient is subsequently placed in the cephalostat of a cephalographic x-ray machine and the radiograph is exposed while the patient maintains the previously determined average cranial position.

center of mass of a leptocephalic, long narrow, skull lies close to the true vertical plane constructed through the centers of the occipital condyles. When a leptocephalic skull is even slightly extended, its center of mass comes to lie behind the true vertical plane through its supporting occipital condyles. When this happens, the suprahyoid group of muscles, and the muscles that constitute the facial drape, assume greater importance in balancing the skull on the cervical column.

Box 2.1 The Hyoid Triangle.

The distance from "C3", the most inferior-anterior point on the body of the third cervical vertebra, to "H", the most superior-anterior point on the body of the hyoid bone, is remarkably constant (mean = 31.76 mm; SD = 2.9 mm). RGn = the most posterior-inferior point on the mandibular symphysis.

• C3–RGn	• 67.20 mm SD = 6.6 mm
• C3–H	• 31.76 mm SD = 2.9 mm
• H–RGn	• 36.83 mm SD = 5.8 mm

No sexual dimorphism was noted for these measurements.
The distance C3–H represents, in the sagittal plane, the depth of the upper airway in an anatomical region that is subject to cranial and tongue movements. It seems that the suprahyoid muscles can compensate for cervicocranial movements in a manner that keeps the distance C3–H relatively constant.

Cranial posture has been studied in relation to multiple factors that control the position of the skull on the cervical vertebral column (Hanten et al. 2000; Higbie et al. 1999; Huggare 1998; Lee et al. 1995; Linder-Anderson 1979). Current clinical research shows that, in living subjects and while awake, the position of the skull relative to the rest of the body (egocentricity) is controlled with great precision.

Diagnostic photographs as well as cephalometric radiographs should be taken with patients in their natural head position (Fig. 2.21). The exposures made in this manner should also include a true vertical reference line. There is some evidence that cephalometric analyses based on a true vertical reference plane are more reliable than those that rely purely on intracranial reference planes.

Predominant **mouth breathing** is associated with altered cranial posture (Kumar et al. 1995) and this, in turn, is associated with specific facial features that, as a group, constitute adenoidal faces. The nasal mucosa is an erectile tissue that expands and contracts in an almost cyclical fashion. This results in patients breathing alternately through both nostrils or through one or the other. The anterior nasal passages can be obstructed by, among other factors, enlarged turbinates and mucosal engorgement due to perennial allergic rhinitis (Fig. 2.22). Clinicians need to recognize abnormal breathing modes and to refer patients for the appropriate consultation and treatment, should the need arise. The mere fact that some individuals habitually keep their lips apart does not necessarily mean that they are mouth breathers. Routine, periodic diagnostic assessment will provide the best information and timing for optimal interceptive care.

Facial features that have been associated with predominantly oral respiration (reduced nasal breathing) include an increased lower anterior facial height, mandibular retrusion, and increased antegonial notching (Huggare and Laine-Alava 1997; Solow and Tallgren 1976; Solow et al. 1984). The habitual tooth-and-lip-apart posture seen in mouth breathing could facilitate further eruption of the posterior teeth, which, in turn, could lead to an increase in the lower anterior facial height. In mouth breathing, the tongue is postured downward and forward to allow the passage of air through the mouth. The maxillary arch is usually narrower. The clinician does not need sophisticated diagnostic tools to recognize these problems.

Some clinicians believe that it is not possible to evaluate the patency of the upper airway from lateral or, for that matter, fron-

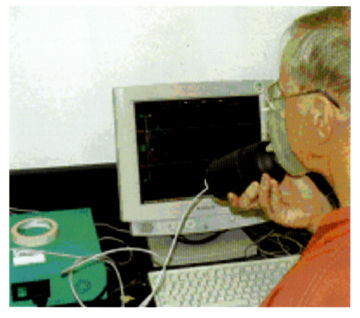

Fig. 2.**22** Rhinomanometry measures the levels of resistance to airflow encountered in the various passages of the upper airway. The rhinomanometer shown here, unlike more expensive units, does not have a steady airflow rate, but it is relatively inexpensive and easy to use. During testing, the resistance to airflow is measured for each nasal passage and also prior to and following the use of nasal decongestants.

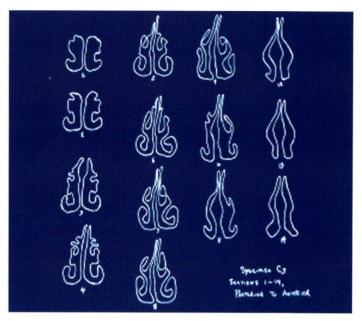

Fig. 2.**23** Tracings of a series of 14 coronal CT sections of the bony nasal air passages. These drawings were published by Vig (1979) to show how difficult it is to judge the patency of the upper airway a from single plane radiograph.

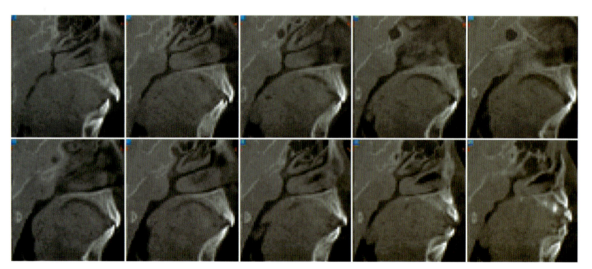

Fig. 2.**24** Sagittal radiographic sections through the nasopharynx of a patient with enlarged adenoidal tissue. On a lateral cephalometric radiograph all of these images would be superimposed and combined into a single picture.

tal cephalometric radiographs. They argue that this process would be similar to guessing what is in a railway tunnel by looking at its entrance. Although it is preferable to study the upper airway with volumetric radiographs (Figs. 2.**23**, 2.**24**), airway analysis performed on cephalometric radiographs (Figs. 2.**25**, 2.**26**) can provide valuable information regarding nasopharyngeal patency.

Despite the obvious problems associated with attempting to diagnose a three dimensional problem from radiographs that reflect only two dimensions, lateral cephalometric radiographs can provide a fairly clear indication of the amount of adenoidal tissue present in the nasopharynx. This area can be enhanced by screens. According to Ricketts, the bony floor of the nasopharynx (Fig. 2.**25**) extends from the anterior of the Atlas vertebra (AA) to the posterior nasal spine (PNS) (Ricketts et al. 1968). The total depth of the bony nasopharynx has also been defined as the distance between PNS and point basion (Ba) located on the anterior margin of the foramen magnum.

Rapid palatal expansion has been proposed as a treatment modality in patients with predominant mouth breathing (Fig. 2.**27**). Usually patients with relatively **narrow upper jaws** present with unilateral or, in severe cases bilateral, buccal crossbites, which are frequently associated with dental midline discrepancies. In these patients, a lateral deviation of the mandible during occlusion may over time result in a permanent facial asymmetry. There are many indications that an early resolution of a posterior crossbite will maintain or restore symmetrical facial growth. A number of indices have been suggested to determine the optimal width of the maxilla (Box 2.**2**).

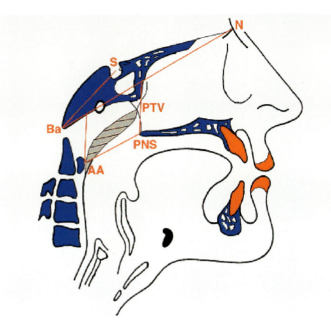

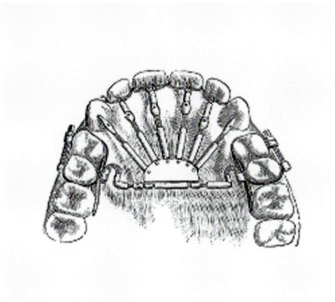

Fig. 2.25 The nasopharynx, as seen on a lateral cephalometric radiograph, is an almost trapezoidal area, enclosed by the line that joins AA and PNS, a section of the line that joins Ba to N as defined by vertical lines through AA and PNS. The percentage of the nasopharynx that is free of soft tissues is available for the passage of respiratory air. In the above diagram the hatched purple area signifies the adenoidal tissue.

Fig. 2.27 A vintage orthodontic appliance that was designed to expand the maxillary dental arch. Because of the relatively heavy forces produced by modern rapid palatal expansion appliances, these appliances are able to separate the midline palatal suture. To accomplish this separation of the palatal suture, the rate of activation of the expansion screws needs careful control.

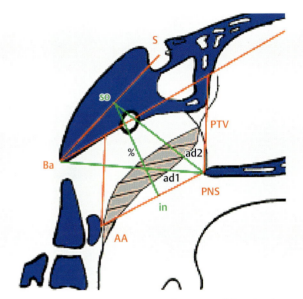

Fig. 2.26 The center of the line joining Ba and S is "so", while "in" is the center of the line joining Ba and PNS. Ricketts suggested that the percentage of the line "so–in" covered by soft tissues corresponded to the relative volume of the adenoidal tissue present in the nasopharynx. The distance to the nearest adenoidal tissue measured along specific lines has also been proposed as a method for determining the patency of the nasopharyngeal airway. Along the line Ba to PNS the nearest adenoidal tissue is signified by the point "ad1" while, point "ad2" signifies the closest adenoidal tissue on the line that joins PNS to "so". In normal children the distance PNS to "ad1" should be in excess of 20 mm, while the distance PNS to "ad2" should be greater than 17 mm. These data represent the combined means for both sexes between the ages of 8 and 16 years of age.

Box 2.2 Pont's Index.

Pont (1909) based his index on a belief that the dental arches should accommodate all of the permanent teeth.

- Upper first bicuspid = $(S \times 100) \div 80$
- Upper first molar = $(S \times 100) \div 64$

S = the combined width of the four upper incisors
Arch widths measured to the center of the occlusal surface of the respective teeth
This belief was closely aligned to the expansionist approach to orthodontic treatment that was popular at the start of the 20th century (see Fig. 2.30). Although Pont's Index did enjoy some popularity in the early 1900, it has fallen out of favor because it does not take account of ethnic variations in tooth size and arch shape. It is better to use the pretreatment mandibular arch form as a guide to the final arch shape than to use Pont's Index for this purpose.

When a patient presents with a relatively narrow maxillary dental arch, there are at least two distinct possibilities. The narrow arch may be due to a constriction of the dentition or to narrowness of the underlying skeletal base. An anteroposterior cephalometric radiograph (Fig. 2.28) may provide clues as to whether a maxillary transverse deficiency has its basis in the dentition, the skeleton, or both.

The original and probably the best-known cephalometric analysis of frontal or AP radiographs is the one devised by Ricketts some forty years ago (Figs. 2.29 and 2.31). The transverse dimension of the maxilla is measured between the left and right Jugal (J) points. The transverse width of the mandible is measured between the left and right Antegonion (Ag) points. As a rough guide, the transverse dimension of the maxilla is normally about 80% of the transverse width of the mandible.

An evaluation of a patient's study models and radiographs will determine whether maxillary expansion, if required, should be dental or skeletal in nature. Skeletal age plays a role in this decision. Once the midline palatal suture has fused, rapid palatal expansion, without surgical augmentation, is probably not a real

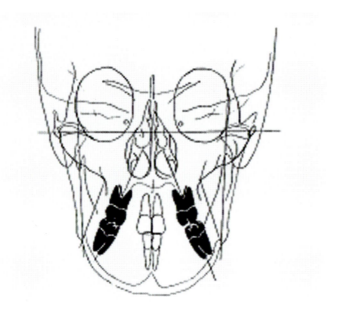

Fig. 2.**28** Frontal radiographs of the craniofacial complex provide metrical data with respect to the widths of the jaws. In the tracing the crowns of the upper molars are inclined buccally (compensated) and this observation provides a good indication that, in this instance, the maxilla is relatively narrow compared to the mandible.

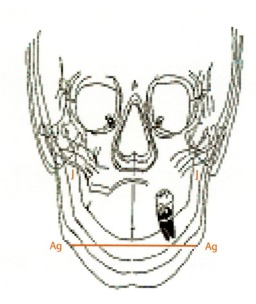

Fig. 2.**29** Data obtained from the Rocky Mountain Diagnostic Services™ indicate that the components of the facial complex, as seen in the frontal view, grow away from a point located on the midline of the face and close to the roof of the nasal cavity. In normal faces the width of the maxillary transverse dimension, measured between the "J" points, is usually close to 80% of the transverse dimension of the mandible, measured between the "Ag" points. A maxillary to mandibular width ratio less than 80% gives a clue to the possibility that the maxilla may require some skeletal expansion.

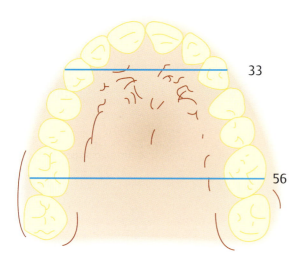

Fig. 2.**30** The mean adult transverse dimensions of the maxillary dentition as presented by the Rocky Mountain Diagnostic Services™. Allowances should be made for differences in arch shape as well as for variations in tooth size.

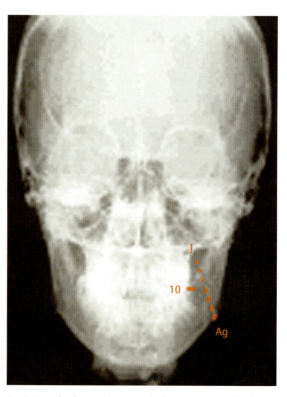

Fig. 2.**31** The distance between the buccal surface of the lower first molar (B6) and the line that joins points "J" and "Ag" measures the transverse linear relationship that exists between the teeth and the denture base. In adults the mean distance between these two entities, on each side of the face, is 10 mm. On a frontal radiograph the upper molars should have a 2 mm positive buccal overjet as compared to the same teeth in the mandible.

option. A number of different maxillary expansion appliances (Fig. 2.**32 a, b**) have been used and they all have their advantages and disadvantages. Rapid palatal expanders are available with designs different from those that are bonded to the teeth. Of these other designs, the hygienic and the Haas palatal expanders are probably the best known.

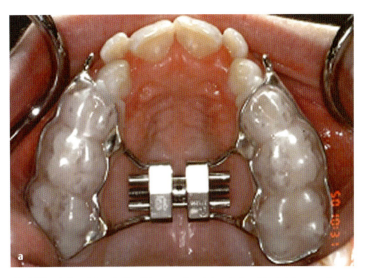
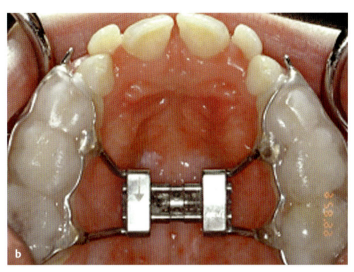

Fig. 2.**32** Before (**a**) and after (**b**) expansion. A bonded rapid palatal expansion appliance is particularly useful in patients who are in their mixed-dentition phase of dental development. In most patients the expansion screw is placed as far distally, and as deep into the vault of the palate, as possible. Bonded expansion appliances are frequently difficult to remove and it is thus prudent to place a debonding screw in each bonded portion of the expander. Hooks for a protraction headgear have been included in this appliance.

Summary

This chapter outlines the many facets of mixed-dentition interceptive orthodontic care. Growth guidance, functional appliances, guided extraction, and palatal expansion are covered in more detail in other chapters of this book and in the extensive bibliography appended to this chapter.

However, the maxim that "an ounce of prevention is worth a pound of cure" is most appropriate for orthodontic guidance of the developing dentition as well as the basal jaw relationships. Applied biology is the name of the game. Mechanotherapy, i.e., "straightening teeth" is most efficient with modern materia technica, but iatrogenic sequelae are always possible. A recent article in the *Angle Orthodontist* by Brezniak and Wasserstein (April 2002) shows the prevalence of OIIRR (orthodontically induced inflammatory root resorption) with conventional "braces." Elimination of abnormal and deforming perioral neuromuscular habits is a valuable service, reducing or eliminating challenges from potential iatrogenic sequelae later. Skeletal apical base dysplasias often respond better during the transitional-dentition period. As Harold Noyes, an eminent pediatrician and orthodontic leader said, "Whenever there is a condition that stands in the way of normal growth and development, it should be eliminated, if possible."

If we emulate the pediatrician who sees his patients routinely, not only when something is wrong, and who gets various tests along the observational highway to make sure the young "rose in bloom" does not deviate from the best possible achievement of development and health, we can render a major service, even though we may never need to place orthodontic appliances. The less we have to mechanically manipulate the teeth, the better it is for all concerned.

References

Altug-Atac AT, Erdem D. Prevalence and distribution of dental anomalies in orthodontic patients. Am J Orthod Dentofacial Orthop 2007; 131: 510–514.

Angle EH. Tweed profile: Dr. Edward Hartley Angle, the Henry Ford of Orthodontics. J Charles H. Tweed Int Found. 1988; 16: 59–76.

Bibby RE, Preston CB. The hyoid triangle. Am J Orthod. 1981; 80(1): 92–97.

Björk A, Skieller V. Normal and abnormal growth of the mandible. A synthesis of longitudinal cephalometric implant studies over a period of 25 years. Eur J Orthod. 1983; 5(1): 1–46.

Bolton WA. Disharmony in tooth size and its relation to analysis and treatment of malocclusion. Angle Orthod. 1958; 28: 113–130.

Bolton WA. The clinical application of a tooth-size analysis. Am J Orthod. 1962; 48: 504–529.

Brezniak N, Wasserstein A. Orthodontically induced inflammatory root resorption. Part 1: the basic science aspects. Angle Orthod. 2002; 72(2): 175–179.

Brezniak N, Wasserstein A. Orthodontically induced inflammatory root resorption. Part 2: the clinical aspects. Angle Orthod. 2002; 72(2): 180–184.

Butler PM. Studies of mammalian dentition. Differentiation of the post-canine dentition. Proc Zool Soc Lond Ser B. 1939; 109: 1–36.

Clark CF. A method of ascertaining the relative position of unerupted teeth by means of film radiographs. Proc R Soc Med Odontol Sectn. 1910; 3: 87–90.

Efstratiadis SS, Cohen G, Ghafari J. Evaluation of differential growth and orthodontic treatment outcome by regional cephalometric superimpositions. Angle Orthod. 1999; 69(3): 225–230.

Turchetta BJ, Fishamn LS, Subtelny JD. Facial growth prediction: A comparison of methodologies. Am J Orthod Dentofacial Orthop 2007; 132: 439–449.

Ghafari J, Baumrind S, Efstratiadis SS. Misinterpreting growth and treatment outcomes from serial cephalographs. Clin Orthod Res. 1998; 1(2): 102–106.

Graber TM. Orthodontics, principles and practice. Philadelphia: WB Saunders; 1961: 550–581.

Hanten WP, Olson SL, Russel JL, Lucio RM, Campbell AH. Total head excursion and resting head posture: normal and patient comparisons. Arch Phys Med Rehabil. 2000; 81(1): 62–66.

Higbie EJ, Seidel-Cobb D, Taylor LF, Cummings GS. Effect of head position on vertical mandibular opening. J Orthop Sports Phys Ther. 1999; 29(2): 127–130.

Hujoel P, Hollender L, Bollen A, Young JD, McGee M, Grosso A. Head-and-neck organ doses from an episode of orthodontic care. Am J Ortho Dentofacial Orthop 20087; 133: 210–217.

Huggare JA, Laine-Alava MT. Nasorespiratory function and head posture. Am J Orthod Dentofac Orthop. 1997; 112(5): 507–511.

Huggare JA. Postural disorders and dentofacial abnormality. Acta Odontol Scand. 1998; 56(6): 383–386.

Jacobs SG. Radiographic localization of unerupted maxillary anterior teeth using the vertical tube shift technique: history and application of the method with some case reports. Am J Orthod Dentofac Orthop. 1999; 116(4): 415–423.

Keur JJ. Radiographic localization techniques. Aust Dent J. 1986; 31: 86–90.

Kumar R, Sidhu SS, Kharbanda OP, Tandon DA. Hyoid bone and Atlas vertebra in established mouth breathers: a cephalometric study. J Clin Pediatr Dent. 1995; 19(3): 191–194.

Langland M. Early treatment and long-range forecasting. Am J Orthod Dentofac Orthop. 2001; 118(3): 247.

Lee WY, Okeson JP, Lindroth J. The relationship between forward head posture and temporomandibular disorders. J Orofac Pain. 1995; 9(2): 161–167.

Linder-Aronson S. Respiratory function in relation to facial morphology and the dentition. Br J Orthod. 1979; 6: 59–71.

Mah J, Hatcher D. Three-dimensional craniofacial imaging. Am J Orthod Dentofacial Orthop 2004; 126: 308–309.

Merwin D, Ngan P, Hagg U, Yiu C, Wei SH. Timing for effective application of anteriorly directed orthopedic force to the maxilla. Am J Orthod Dentofac Orthop. 1997; 112(3): 292–299.

Mozzo P, Procacci C, Tacconi A. A new volumetric CT machine for dental imaging based on the cone-beam technique: preliminary results. Eur Radiol. 1998; 8: 1558–1564.

Palleck S, Foley TF, Hall-Scott J. The reliability of 3 sagittal reference planes in the assessment of Class I and Class III treatment. Am J Orthod Dentofac Orthop. 2001; 119(4): 426–435.

Paulsen HU. Autotransplantation of teeth in orthodontic treatment. Am J Orthod Dentofac Orthop. 2001; 119(4): 336–337.

PaulsenHU, Zachrisson BU. Autotransplantation of teeth and orthodontic treatment planning. In: Andreasen JO, editor. Atlas of replantation and transplantation of teeth. Fibourg: Medi Globe: 1992. pp 258–274.

Pont A. Der Zahn-Index in der Orthodontie. Zahnarzt Orthopadie. 1909; 3: 306–321.

Proffit WR. Contemporary orthodontics. 3rd ed. St. Louis: Mosby; 2000; 118–125.

Ricketts RM, Steele CH, Fairchild RC. Forum on the tonsil and adenoid problem in orthodontics. Am J Orthodont. 1968; 54: 485–514.

Sarver DM, Ackerman JL. Orthodontics about face: The emergence of the esthetic paradigm. Am J. Orthod Dentofacial Orthop 2000; 117: 5: 575–576.

Solow B, Tallgren A. Head posture and craniofacial morphology. Am J Phys Anthrop. 1976; 44: 417–436.

Solow B, Siersbaek-Nielsen S, Greve E. Airway adequacy, head posture, and craniofacial morphology. Am J Orthod Dentofac Orthop. 1984; 86: 214–223.

Stifter J. A study of Pont's, Howes', Neff's and Bolton's analysis on Class I adult dentitions. Angle Orthod. 1958; 28: 215–225.

Stivaros N, Mandall NA. Radiographic factors affecting the management of impacted upper permanent canines. J Orthod. 2000; 27(2): 169–173.

Tayer B, Burnes H. Patient empowerment: the young patient. Am J Orthod Dentofacial Ortop 1993; 103: 365–367.

Tulloch JF, Phillips C, Koch G, Proffit WR. The effect of early intervention on skeletal pattern in Class II malocclusion: a randomized clinical trial. Am J Orthod Dentofacial Orthop 1997; 111: 391–400.

Vig PS. Respiratory mode and morphological types: some thoughts and preliminary conclusions. In: McNamara JA, ed. Naso-respiratory function and craniofacial growth. Michigan: University of Michigan Press; 1979: 233–250.

Würpel EH. Ideals and idealism in orthodontia. Angle Orthod 1993; 1: 14–31.

Zhu JF, Marcushamer M, King DL, Henry RJ. Supernumerary and congenitally absent teeth: a literature review. J Clin Pediatr Dent 1996; 20: 257–258.

3 Early Treatment: Interceptive Guidance of Occlusion including Serial Extraction followed by Mechanotherapy

Jack Dale

The principle of early treatment, associated with the extraction of primary teeth followed by the removal of permanent teeth, was first described by a Frenchman named Robert Bunon in his *Essay on the Diseases of the Teeth* published in 1743, more than 260 years ago.

The Logic of "Serial Extraction"

Kjellgren, a Norwegian, is credited with the introduction of the term "serial extraction," in 1929 (Kjellgren 1947–48). In my opinion, this term is somewhat dangerous because it tends to create a misconception of simplicity, implying that there is nothing more involved than the mere extraction of teeth.

Hotz's term "guidance of eruption," or the term used in the title of this chapter, "guidance of occlusion," are better. These terms are comprehensive; they suggest that a thorough knowledge of growth and development of the dentition and the craniofacial complex is required in making a number of key decisions throughout the developmental period.

The most crucial decision that we, as specialists in orthodontics, are required to make is, "Do we extract teeth or not in the correction of a malocclusion?" Adding the dimension of time, complicating it with growth and development, and carrying out extraction in a serial manner is even more demanding. Serial extraction is not easy, as so many mistakenly believe, and should never be initiated without a comprehensive diagnosis.

In truth, one can extract teeth with the greatest of ease during serial extraction procedures. If the basic principles of diagnosis are ignored, however, the result will be failure and disappointment. It will not only be injurious to the patient but will harm the practitioner's reputation and, ultimately, our specialty of orthodontics. The single most important reason for failure is lack of knowledge and lack of preparation on the part of the clinician.

Serial extraction based on a thorough knowledge and a sound diagnosis and carried out carefully and properly on a select group of patients can be a valuable treatment procedure, and it *is* a treatment procedure. There are those who do not consider interceptive guidance with serial extraction as treatment. But it is this type of treatment that justifies our title "doctor." We are treating a potential major malocclusion utilizing biological principles. Must we be so mechanically oriented that we only consider treatment with appliances? Should we not also be applied biologists?

Serial extraction is an excellent treatment procedure. It can reduce appliance treatment time, the cost of treatment, discomfort to patients, and time lost by both the patients and their parents. It is logical to intercept a malocclusion as early as possible and to reduce or, in rare instances, avoid multibanded-multibracket mechanotherapy at the sensitive teenage period. Why allow an unfavorable dental, skeletal, or soft-tissue relationship to exist for a number of years if it can be wholly or partially corrected early with a minimum of multibanded-multibracket treatment time?

Pioneers and Followers

I consider myself truly fortunate to have learned the basic principles of growth and development of the dentition and the craniofacial complex from a world-renowned educator, research scientist, and authority on this subject, Dr. Coenraad Moorrees at Harvard-Forsyth Orthodontic Program, Harvard University. Dr. Moorrees has been quoted by former students as saying the two things he values most highly are the understanding of craniofacial growth and skill as a diagnostician, and that he believes that the salvation of our specialty lies in nurturing its theoretical foundations (personal communication). When I returned to Toronto from Harvard in 1961, I felt strongly that I must utilize Dr. Moorrees' "theoretical foundations" to become a "skilled diagnostician" in the clinical practice of orthodontics and in the day-to-day caring for my patients.

For 48 years, I have treated many patients utilizing serial extraction with success and satisfaction and have substantiated my use of this procedure with records taken up to 35 years after treatment. The importance of diagnosis cannot be emphasized enough. To differentiate, categorize, and treat serial extraction patients specifically and successfully on a routine basis requires a thorough understanding of the fundamental principles of diagnosis. It is, without question, the key to success.

Several diagnostic analyses related to the teeth and the face, including proportional facial analysis (PFA), craniofacial analysis (CFA), total space analysis (TSA) of the dentition and dental age analysis (DAA) are discussed in the textbook, *Orthodontics, Current Principles and Techniques* (Graber et al., 2005).

The extraction of teeth was performed long before Edward Angle gave his first major paper to the dental profession in 1887. For our purposes, however, the controversy over extraction began with him. In the beginning, it involved such practitioners as Angle himself, Case, Dewey, Grieve, and others. Later, it included Tweed,

Strang, and Brodie. It is still a controversial procedure today, over a century later!

I like to think that the controversy is restricted basically to the borderline problems. It is difficult to believe that there are orthodontists who treat *all* orthodontic problems without the extraction of teeth, or who treat *all* orthodontic problems with extractions. If that is the case, it is tantamount to ignoring morphogenetic pattern and the necessity for diagnosis. I prefer to believe that the majority of practitioners treat patients as individuals and on the basis of a sound diagnosis, extracting teeth in high angle alveolar dental protrusion and tooth-size–jaw-size discrepancies, and treating low-angle, excessive overbite, and spaced dentitions with relatively small teeth on a nonextraction basis.

"Out of the great number of faces that have been formed since the creation of the world, no two have been exactly alike."—William Hogarth.

Serial Extraction

According to the Burlington Growth Study (Burlington Orthodontic Research Project, Report No. 3, 1957), 34% of 3-year-old children enjoy a "normal" occlusion. By the time they reach 12 years of age, only 11% have a "normal" intercuspation, a reduction of 23%. This is attributed to local environmental factors: for example, crowded dentitions resulting from a loss of arch length caused by the premature loss of primary teeth.

Of the remaining 66% of 3-year-old children destined to suffer the ravages of malocclusion, 41% are in a Class I dental relationship, 23% are in a Class II, and only 2% are in Class III. By the time these children reach 12 years of age, 55% have Class I malocclusions, 32% have Class II, and 2% still have Class III, a total increase of 23%. Again, this increase is due primarily to local environmental factors.

Serial extraction is an interceptive procedure designed to assist in the correction of hereditary crowding. Since the malocclusions of the 66% of 3-year-old children are hereditary in nature, with a significant number of tooth-size–jaw-size discrepancies, serial extraction is an invaluable adjunct to interceptive treatment. This is especially true in the 41% Class I malocclusions (**Case Study 3.2**) and, to a lesser extent, the 23% Class II (**Case Study 3.3**).

Class I malocclusions are ideal for serial extraction because the teeth and jaws are in a favorable relationship, and successful treatment is possible with a minimum of mechanotherapy. The ideal conditions for serial extraction are:
- A true, relatively severe, hereditary tooth–size–jaw-size discrepancy
- A mesial step mixed dentition developing into a Class I permanent dentition relationship
- A minimal overjet relationship of the incisor teeth
- A minimal overbite, and
- A craniofacial pattern that is slightly hyperdivergent and orthognathic with a moderate alveolar dental protrusion

My chapter "Interceptive guidance of occlusion with emphasis on diagnosis" in the Graber et al. (2005) textbook outlines and illustrates several signs of a true, hereditary tooth-size–jaw-size discrepancy, which are basic to serial extraction, as well as several signs of environmental crowding, which are not.

In orthodontics we are interested in the ultimate size and the rate of maturation of the jaws, that is, the ultimate size, the rate of maturation, and the emergence of the teeth into the oral cavity and the ultimate treatment result. We are also interested in the adolescent growth spurt of the body and its relation to the accelerated growth in the craniofacial complex. Finally, we must be interested in the relationship between chronological age, skeletal age, and dental age as set out by Moorrees and his associates (see their work between 1961 and 1966, listed in the extensive bibliography at the end of this chapter).

Utilizing information derived from the longitudinal studies of Moorrees and associates, the clinician who is attempting to guide the teeth into a favorable occlusion can more accurately predict important events in the development of the dentition. For instance, we know that the unerupted permanent tooth is literally standing still until half of its root is formed. With this knowledge, we would hesitate to extract the primary first molar if its permanent successor had less than one-half root formation. This would delay rather than accelerate the eruption of the premolar.

We also know that teeth emerge into the oral cavity when three-quarters of their roots are formed. It requires 2½ years for the canine root to go from one-quarter to one-half root length and a 1½ years to go from one-half to three-quarters, when, theoretically, it emerges into the oral cavity. Therefore, if you see a canine root in a radiogram at one-quarter root, you can predict that it will emerge in four years. It requires 1¾ years for the first premolar root to go from one-quarter to one-half root length and 1½ years to go from one-half to three-quarters. Armed with information like this, the clinician, on inspecting the periapical radiogram, can predict the emergence of these teeth and can time their extraction more precisely.

The Multibanded-Multibracket Appliance

When the interceptive guidance of occlusion and serial extraction phase has been completed, the multibanded-multibracket appliance is placed, and active treatment is initiated utilizing, in my case, the modern concepts of The Charles H. Tweed International Foundation for Orthodontic Research and Education developed by Charles H. Tweed, Levern Merrifield, and their colleagues over more than five decades (see work by Tweed, Merrifield et al., from 1946 to 2000 listed in the bibliography).

The treatment objectives after interceptive guidance are:
- Closure of residual extraction spaces
- Improvement of axial inclination of individual teeth
- Correction of rotations
- Correction of the midline discrepancy
- Correction of the residual overbite
- Correction of the residual overjet
- Correction of crossbites
- Refinement of the intercuspation of individual teeth
- Improvement and coordination of arch form, and
- Correction of the class II relationship in some class II patients. (**Case Study 3.3**)
- Charles Tweed's primary objectives in treatment, goals for all orthodontists, include:

- Dental health of the dentition and the supporting and surrounding structures
- Esthetics, including ideal alignment, occlusion and smile
- Balance and harmony within the craniofacial complex, reflected in the facial soft-tissue, especially in the profile
- Function, including canine protected occlusion, incisal guidance and recovery
- Treatment complementing growth and development, including vertical control and a favorable mandibular response
- Stability, respecting the limits of the dentition

These are excellent treatment goals, but they are too general. We must strive for specific treatment goals that are interrelated with one another:
- Counterclockwise (upward and forward) rotation, vertical control with a favorable mandibular response
- FMA reduced, vertical control with a favorable mandibular response
- ANB reduced, skeletal discrepancy reduction by maxillary control with a favorable mandibular response
- Vertical control, high-pull headgear, and serial extraction resulting in a favorable mandibular response
- Alveolar dental correction, uprighting mandibular incisors with anchorage and the extraction of bicuspid teeth
- Crowding corrected, anchorage and extraction
- Anchorage preparation that assists in the retraction of the anterior teeth and the correction of the class II relationship
- Occlusal plane control, vertical control of the posterior teeth, and uprighting of mandibular incisors; flattening of the occlusal plane
- Balance and harmony within the craniofacial complex reflected in the soft-tissue profile, favorable mandibular response, and a reduction of alveolar dental protrusion
- Ideal occlusion in balance and harmony with the supporting and surrounding tissues
- Overtreatment, recovery rather than relapse
- Stability, respecting the limits of the dentition

These specific objectives are illustrated in the comprehensive case reports of G. L. (10 years after treatment (AT)), M. R. (20 years AT) and J. O. (25 years AT), and supported by the results 5–35 years after treatment.

The Tweed–Merrifield Edgewise Appliance Technique

The modern concepts of The Tweed–Merrifield Edgewise Appliance Technique can be summarized as follows.

It was the genius of Dr. Edward Hartley Angle that created the "edgewise appliance." He introduced it in 1928, following intensive experimentation with The "E" arch, the Pin and Tube, and the Ribbon Arch appliances, which he had developed. The world owes to him a debt of gratitude as the real founder and father of modern orthodontics. His work was based on science, developed on dexterity, and consummated in art. He visualized the whole story from beginning to end and he made his vision become a reality.

In 1930, just before he died, he said, "I have finished my work. It is as perfect as I can make it." But we know that this inventive genius, who was always thinking, experimenting, selecting, and discarding, never satisfied with the results at hand, always pondering over possible improvement, would be the last to declare perfection, even if he had attained it. He must have known, even when he made this statement on his deathbed, that his work must go on. He must have been at peace with the knowledge that he had finally found "the right man" to carry out his "beautiful work": Dr. Charles H. Tweed.

The Tweed Foundation has over 100 letters written by Angle to Tweed from 1928 to Angle's death in 1930. During these two years, Angle urged his young disciple to dedicate his life to the development of "the edgewise appliance." Tweed did just that. He concentrated his efforts on the development and advancement of "the edgewise appliance" for 43 years, until his death in 1970, and he established the first pure edgewise practice in the United States.

In 1953, Dr. Levern Merrifield became active in The Tweed Foundation and succeeded Tweed in 1970 as the Director of the Tweed Course. He continued in his leadership role until his death in 2000.

Tweed "diagnosed" a serious problem in orthodontics: facial imbalance and disharmony associated with alveolar dental protrusion and a tooth-size-jaw-size discrepancy. He observed that by creating space with the extraction of teeth and with the correction of the alveolar dental protrusion by uprighting incisors into the space provided, he corrected the facial imbalance and disharmony.

Merrifield devoted his career to the improvement of the "treatment" of this problem to such an extent that the Tweed–Merrifield Edgewise Appliance is one of the most precise instruments for the routine correction of major malocclusions that exists in the world today.

The goal for the future is "prevention," to establish a soft tissue profile in balance and harmony without imbalance and disharmony occurring first.

Thus, it is important to examine potential orthodontic patients by 7 years of age and to determine whether the child could benefit by a "Phase I, Interceptive Guidance," serial extraction period of treatment prior to a "Phase II Tweed–Merrifield Multibanded-Multibracket Edgewise Appliance" treatment when most of the permanent teeth have emerged at 11.5 years of age, prior to the sensitive teenage period.

This chapter discusses the treatment of patients who have benefited from a "Phase I, Interceptive Guidance" serial extraction period of treatment prior to a "Phase II Multibanded-Multibracketed Tweed–Merrifield Edgewise Appliance" period from roughly 11.5 to 13 years of age.

The Tweed–Merrifield Edgewise Appliance

The Tweed–Merrifield edgewise appliance is a neutral bracket appliance with which all the treatment is carried out in wire manipulation for individual situations in individual patients. This contrasts with the straight-wire appliance in which the treatment is primarily in pretorqued, preangulated brackets.

The Tweed–Merrifield edgewise appliance is a series of force systems that include:
- Dentition preparation, including leveling of the brackets and retraction of the canines utilizing an auxiliary high-pull headgear
- Dentition correction, including 10-2 sequential mandibular anchorage preparation and maxillary Class II correction
- Dentition completion, including overtreatment into a super Class I relationship
- Dentition recovery, including a transition from overtreatment occlusion (transitional occlusion) to normal functional occlusion

The results are then retained for 1–2 years depending on the malocclusion being treated.

The modern concepts of the techniques can be summarized as follows:
- Directional force systems
- Sequential 10-2 anchorage
- Readout
- Prescription arches
- Performance testing

The directional force systems technique employs a group of force systems utilizing directional control to position the teeth precisely in both the maxilla and the mandible so that they will be in harmony with their environment.

The sequential 10-2 anchorage concept is a sequential anchorage system wherein the archwire stabilizes 10 teeth while 2 teeth receive the active force. Instead of 12 teeth being simultaneously involved in the anchorage preparation, only two teeth receive active force. The sequence begins with the second molars and is completed with the second premolars. When this type of improved anchorage preparation is used, there is less risk that the mandibular dentition will move unfavorably downward and forward, and patient cooperation is not as crucial.

With readout the objectives of orthodontic treatment can be defined by accurate measurement. Tooth axial inclination and movement can be predetermined, monitored during treatment, and checked for accuracy of final placement.

Prescription arches involve the tabulation of second-order bends (vertical) angulation associated with 10-2 anchorage and readout. They also permit the precise measurement and tabulation of buccolingual axial inclinations of teeth so that third-order bends (torque) can be incorporated in the archwire. Finally, they include first-order bends (horizontal). These prescription arches are designed specifically for individual malocclusions.

Performance testing is a relatively recent development involving the serial measurement of tooth movement and dental relationships so that treatment progress can be evaluated.

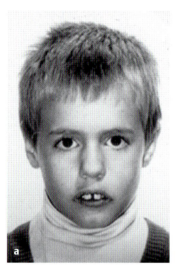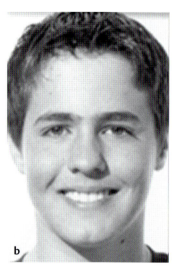

Fig. 3.**1** a **Before treatment:** This young boy, 8 years of age, does not appear to be a particularly happy person with his severely protruding maxillary incisors. b **After early treatment:** At 13 years of age, with orthodontic treatment completed, this handsome young man, with his attractive smile, is enjoying an obvious increase in confidence and self-esteem.

This particular edgewise appliance, originally designed by Tweed and modified by Merrifield and his associates, is the precision instrument utilized in achieving treatment goals. It is characterized by simplicity, efficiency, and comfort; it is hygienic and esthetic and, above all, it has wide range versatility (Vaden et al. 2000).

When all bands and brackets are removed and retainers are placed, a critical stage in the correction of the malocclusion occurs. It is referred to as the "period of recovery." If the corrective procedures only barely achieve the normal relationship of teeth, there will be an inevitable relapse. Any change that occurs will be away from ideal occlusion. If treatment is completed by overcorrection, however, all changes that take place during the recovery period will be toward the ideal relationship.

This treatment protocol provides favorable circumstances for arriving at Tweed's original objectives.

With The Tweed–Merrifield direction force edgewise technology, patients are routinely treated in 18–20 months, primarily because of the efficiency and control of the appliance (see **Case Study 3.1**). When interceptive guidance of occlusion is combined with the edgewise appliance in the correction of specific malocclusions, it reduces mechanotherapy even further (see **Case Studies 3.2** and **3.3**).

To quote Charles Tweed, "When facial deformity has been corrected and mental anguish eliminated, a dull and unhappy facial expression becomes bright and happy. What greater reward could any orthodontist want or expect?" One could add, "The earlier this occurs the better" (Fig. 3.**1**).

Clinical Case Studies

Case Study 3.1 Patient G. L.

- Male
- 14.9 years of age
- Vertical growth
- Hyperdivergent facial pattern (FMA, 30°)
- Skeletal discrepancy: retrognathic mandible (ANB, 9°), (SNB, 71°)
- Maxillary-mandibular alveolar dental protrusion (Z, 55°)
- Class II Division 1 malocclusion
- Tooth-size–jaw-size discrepancy
- Extraction of four first premolar teeth
- Tweed–Merrifield edgewise mechanotherapy

G. L.'s case represents conventional orthodontic treatment, without the advantage of a period of interceptive guidance of occlusion. The treatment was successful and satisfies the general Tweed objectives, but it falls short of the more specific objectives, especially in mandibular response. An earlier and longer period of vertical control could have resulted in a more significant counterclockwise rotation of the mandible. Utilizing serial extraction, a form of vertical control, this has been accomplished many times in our practice as indicated in **Case Study 3.2**, serial extraction Class I, and in **Case Study 3.3**, serial extraction Class II.

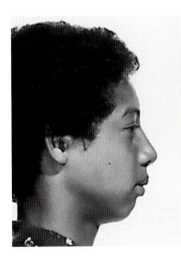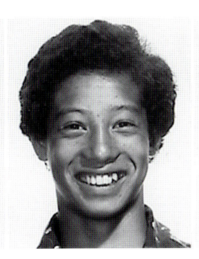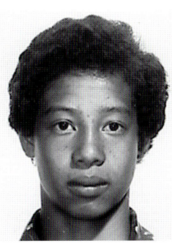

Fig. 3.1.**1** **Face before treatment.** Note retrognathic mandible, with resulting recessive chin, and lack of proportion of the soft-tissue profile. Malalignment of the maxillary anterior teeth is evident when the patient smiles. There is a lack of balance and harmony when the patient's lips are closed.

G. L.—Total Space Analysis

Anterior Arch	
REQUIRED	
Teeth: 1, 2, 3	−40.0
Ceph. correction	−17.0
Soft tissue	−
TOTAL	−57.0
AVAILABLE	+39.0
DEFICIT	−18.0
Mid Arch	
REQUIRED	
Teeth: 4, 5, 6	−59.0
Curve of occlusion	−3.0
TOTAL	−62.0
AVAILABLE	+57.0
DEFICIT	−5.0

Posterior Arch	
REQUIRED	
Teeth: 7, 8	−46.0
AVAILABLE	
Presently available	+32.0
Estimated increase	+3.0
TOTAL	+35.0
DEFICIT	−11.0
TOTAL DEFICIT	**−34.0**

Total space analysis based on research conducted at The Charles H. Tweed Foundation (Merrifield 1978) depicts a significant anterior deficit (**−18.0**) and posterior deficit (**−11.0**), indicating the extraction of four first premolar and four third molar teeth.

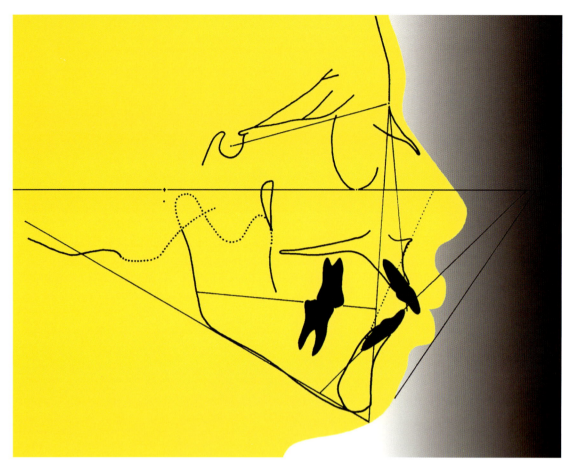

Fig. 3.1.**2 Cephalometric tracing before treatment.** Note skeletal discrepancy (ANB, 9°) resulting from retrognathic mandible (SNB, 71°) and mandible alveolar dental protrusion (IMPA, 107°). Dotted line represents alveolar dental correction objective to a more upright position of the mandibular incisors, which will result in a more balanced soft-tissue profile.

G. L.— Total Space Analysis Difficulty

Anterior arch	Value	Difficulty Factor	Difficulty
Tooth arch discrepancy	1.0	1.5	1.5
Ceph. discrepancy	17.0	1.0	17.0
Soft tissue	0.0	0.5	–
TOTAL	18.0		18.5
Mid arch	**Value**	**Difficulty Factor**	**Difficulty**
Tooth arch discrepancy	2.0	1.0	2.0
Curve of Spee	3.0	1.0	3.0
TOTAL	5.0		5.0
Posterior arch	**Value**	**Difficulty factor**	**Difficulty**
Tooth arch discrepancy	14.0		
Expected increase	+ 3.0		
TOTAL	11.0	0.5	5.5
Horizontal occlusion discrepancy Class II–III	10.0	2.0	20.0
TOTAL DIFFICULTY			**49.0**

Total difficulty **49**, primarily due to cephalometric discrepancy, alveolar dental protrusion (**17.0**), and the Class II relationship (**20.0**).

G.L. CEPH. ANALYSIS

	B.T.	OBJECTIVE
FMA	30	25 (22 - 28)
IMPA	107	87
FMIA	43	68
SNA	80	83
SNB	71	80 (78 - 82)
ANB	9	3 (1 - 5)
OP	6	10 (8 - 12)
Z	55	75 (70 - 80)
PFH/AFH	.61	.70 (.67 - .72)

Fig. 3.1.3 **Cephalometric analysis before treatment**, emphasizing the six measurements that are important in determining success or failure in treatment based on research conducted at The Charles H. Tweed Foundation (Gramling 1987).
FMA indicates a high angle or low angle facial pattern. A favorable response reduces the angle.
SNB indicates mandibular relationship. A favorable response increases the angle.
ANB indicates skeletal discrepancy. A favorable response maintains the angle between 1 and 5°.
OP indicates treatment control. If treatment is controlled and if the posterior teeth are not extruded and the mandibular incisors are not "dumped forward", the occlusal plane will flatten.
Z: A small Z angle indicates a large alveolar dental protrusion. A favorable response would increase the angle.
The posterior face height to anterior face height ratio (**PFH/AFH**) indicates mandibular response. If the ratio increases, the mandible rotates favorably to a lower angle face. If the ratio decreases, the mandible rotates unfavorably in the opposite direction.

G.L.—Cranial Facial Analysis with Difficulty before Treatment (B.T.)

Parameter	Normal range	Patient	Difference
FMA	22–28	30	30 – 28 = 2
ANB	1–5	*9	9 – 5 = 4
Z	70–80	55	70 – 55 = 15
OP	8–12	6	8 – 6 = 2
SNB	78–82	*71	78 – 71 = 7
PFH/AFH	0.62–0.72	0.61 (55/91)	0.67 – 0.61 = 6
Difference	**Difficulty Factor**	**Difficulty**	
		B.T.	
2	5	10	
4	15	*60	
15	2	30	
2	3	6	
7	5	*35	
6	3	18	
TOTAL		**159**	

Total difficulty: **159**.
* Significant difference

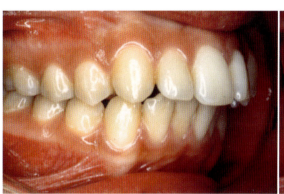 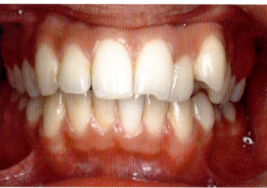

Fig. 3.1.4 **Dentition before treatment.** Note the Class II malocclusion and the protruding and malaligned maxillary anterior teeth. Because of the protrusion, one incisor has been fractured accidentally.

G.L.— Difficulty Summary

TSA difficulty	49.0
CFA difficulty	159.0
TOTAL	208.0
Mild	0–60
Moderate	60–120
*Severe	>120

The patient's orthodontic problem is categorized as severe (**208**, > 120).
It is severe primarily because of the cranial facial factors (**159**, see CFA with Difficulty), and specifically it is severe because of the skeletal discrepancy (ANB, 9°: **60**). More specifically, it is due to the retrognathic mandible (SNB, 71°: **35**), which is also reflected in the soft-tissue profile (Z, 55°: **30**).

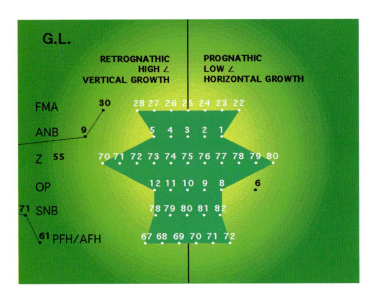

Fig. 3.1.**5** **The wiggle analysis.** The wiggle analysis is based on the normal range of the six Tweed–Merrifield measurements and is designed by Hali and Jack Dale (Dale and Dale 2000). Prior to treatment, except for the OP, the measurements are excessively displaced to the retrognathic, high-angle, vertical growth side of the normal range.

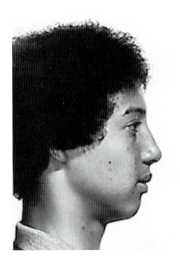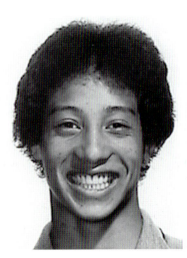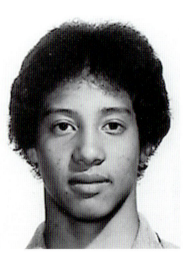

Fig. 3.1.**6** **Face after treatment.** Note that the mandible is still retrognathic, but the face is in balance and harmony and the smile is favorable with ideal alignment.

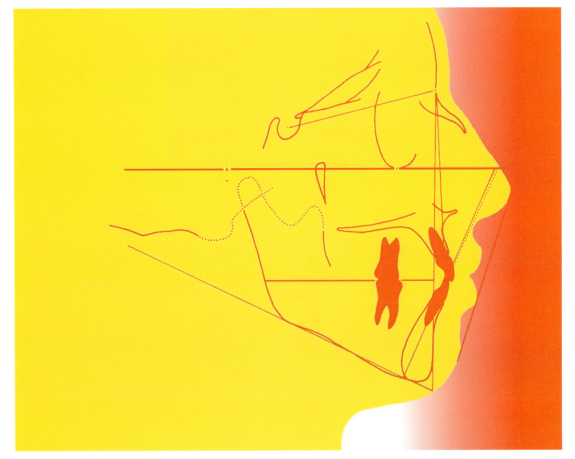

Fig. 3.1.**7** **Cephalometric tracing after treatment.** Note that the alveolar dental correction has been slightly overtreated beyond the dotted objective line. Skeletal discrepancy has been improved (ANB, 9° to 4°), and the alveolar dental protrusion has also been improved (Z, 55° to 71°).

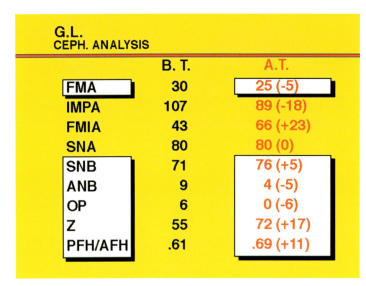

Fig. 3.1.**8** **Cephalometric analysis after treatment with measurements depicting favorable response to treatment according to Tweed objectives:** FMA decreased, SNB increased, ANB decreased, OP flattened (vertical control) Z angle increased and PFH/AFH increased.

G. L.— Cranial Facial Analysis with Difficulty after Treatment (A.T.)

Difference	Difficulty Factor	Difficulty	
		B.T.	A.T.
2	5	10	–
4	15	*60	–
15	2	30	–
2	3	6	+24
7	5	*35	–20
6	3	18	+3
TOTAL		159	+7

The total difficulty has been eradicated and overtreatment has occurred (**159** to **+7**).

There has been a modest improvement in the mandibular response (**35** to **20**). If this patient had been treated by interceptive guidance earlier, the mandibular response would have been more favorable as in Case Study 3.2 and, especially, in Case Study 3.3. Vertical control initiated early provides more time for the mandible to rotate favorably in a counterclockwise direction.

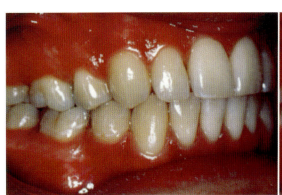 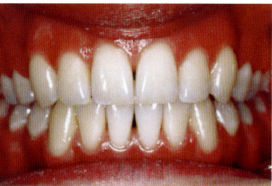

Fig. 3.1.**9** **Dentition after treatment: ideal alignment and occlusion.** The teeth are now in a healthy Class I relationship; the anterior teeth are upright over basal bone; the overjet is corrected, and the incisors are in a favorable overbite relationship.

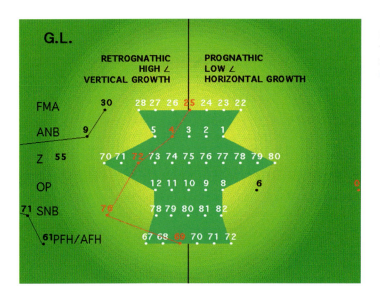

Fig. 3.1.**10** **The wiggle analysis after treatment.** This analysis depicts graphically the significant improvement in all measurements with only the mandibular response falling short of the normal range. All measurements are closer to the normal range.

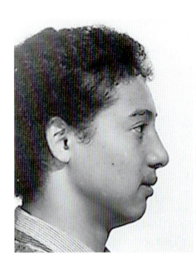
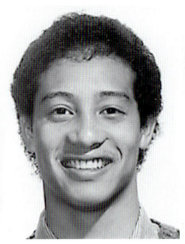
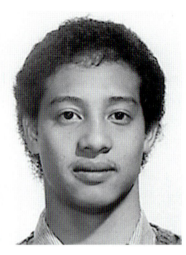

Fig. 3.1.**11 Face 10 years after treatment depicting balance and harmony in the soft tissue.** The soft-tissue profile is still recessive and, because of his maturity, will remain recessive. Nevertheless, he has a beautiful smile exposing a well-aligned dentition.

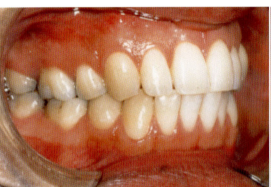
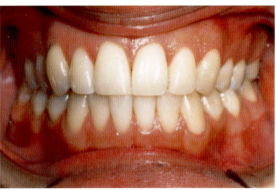

Fig. 3.1.**12 Dentition 10 years after treatment depicting favorable alignment, occlusion, and stability.** This stability indicates that the teeth have been placed in balance with the supporting jaws and the surrounding soft tissue.

Case Study 3.2 Patient M. R.

- Male
- 8.5 years of age
- Vertical growth
- Hyperdivergent facial pattern (FMA, 31°)
- Retrognathic mandible (SNB, 75°) without a skeletal discrepancy (ANB, 3°)
- Maxillary-mandibular alveolar dental protrusion (Z, 57°)
- Class I malocclusion, mixed dentition
- Tooth-size–jaw-size discrepancy
- Serial extraction, including four first premolar teeth
- Tweed–Merrifield edgewise mechanotherapy

M. R.'s case represents the ideal circumstances for interceptive guidance of occlusion, including serial extraction followed by the Tweed–Merrifield edgewise appliance. In this instance, there is a favorable counterclockwise response of the mandible.

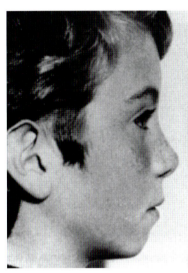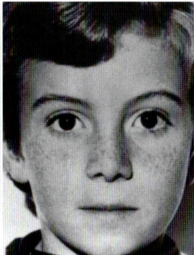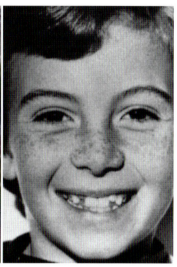

Fig. 3.2.1 **Face before serial extraction reveals a moderate maxillary and mandibular retrognathism resulting in a slightly recessive profile with a moderate prominence of the lips.** The smile reveals a mixed dentition, slightly crowded.

M. R.— Total Space Analysis

Anterior Arch	
REQUIRED	
Teeth: 1, 2, 3	− 39.0
Ceph. correction	− 5.6
Soft tissue	− 6.0
TOTAL	− 50.6
AVAILABLE	+ 33.0
DEFICIT	**− 17.6**
Mid Arch	
REQUIRED	
Teeth: 4, 5, 6	− 54.0
Curve of occlusion	
TOTAL	− 54.0
AVAILABLE	+ 56.0
SURPLUS	+ 2.0

Posterior Arch	
REQUIRED	
Teeth: 7, 8	− 42.0
AVAILABLE	
Presently available	+ 3.0
Estimated increase	+ 24.0
TOTAL	+ 27.0
DEFICIT	**− 15.0**

TSA indicates the extraction of four first premolar and four third molar teeth due to the anterior (**−17.6 mm**) and posterior deficits (**−15 mm**), respectively.

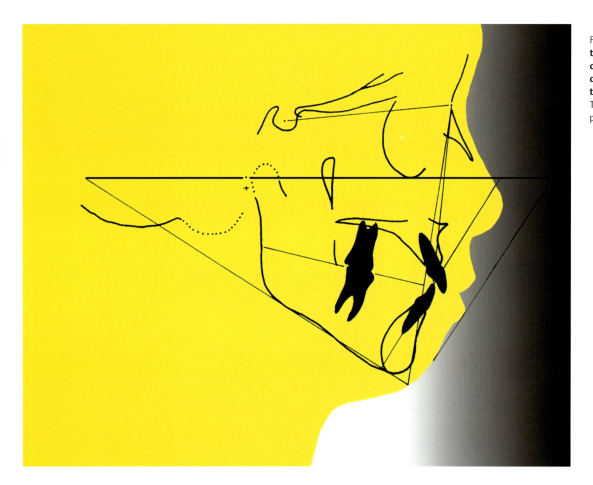

Fig. 3.2.**2** **Cephalometric tracing before serial extraction confirms the maxillary-mandibular retrognathism but with the jaws favorably related.** The profile line confirms the prominent lips.

M. R.— Total Space Analysis Difficulty

Anterior arch	Value	Difficulty Factor	Difficulty
Tooth arch discrepancy	6.0	1.5	9.0
Ceph. discrepancy	5.6	1.0	5.6
Soft tissue	6.0	0.5	3.0
TOTAL	17.6		17.6
Mid arch	**Value**	**Difficulty Factor**	**Difficulty**
Tooth arch discrepancy	2.0	1.0	2.0
Curve of Spee	–	1.0	0.0
TOTAL	2.0		2.0
Posterior arch	**Value**	**Difficulty factor**	**Difficulty**
Tooth arch discrepancy	39.0		
Expected increase	+ 24.0		
TOTAL	15.0	0.5	7.5
Horizontal occlusion discrepancy Class II–III	0.0	2.0	0.0
TOTAL DIFFICULTY			**26.5**

Total difficulty: **26.5**, indicating little difficulty in correcting the dentition.

	B. T.	OBJECTIVE
M.R. CEPH. ANALYSIS		
FMA	31	25 (22 - 28)
IMPA	91	87
FMIA	58	68
SNA	78	83
SNB	75	80 (78 - 82)
ANB	3	3 (1 - 5)
OP	13	10 (8 - 12)
Z	57	75 (70 - 80)
PFH/AFH	.65	.70 (.67 - .72)

Fig. 3.2.**3** **Cephalometric analysis before serial extraction.** The measurements within the boxes are the more significant measurements depicting success or failure in treatment established by The Tweed Foundation (see CS 3.1[3]).
FMA: A favorable response reduces the angle, 31° to 25° in this instance.
SNB: A favorable response increases the angle, 75° to 80° in this instance.
ANB: A favorable response maintains the angle between 1° and 5°, 3° in this instance.
OP: If treatment is controlled and if the posterior teeth are not extruded and the mandibular incisors are not "dumped forward," the occlusal plane will flatten, 13° to 10° in this instance.
Z: A favorable response would increase the angle, 57° to 75° in this instance.
PFH/AFH: If the ratio increases, the mandible rotates favorably to a lower angle face. If the ratio decreases, the mandible rotates unfavorably in the opposite direction. In this instance, the objective is 0.70 from 0.65.

M. R.— Cranial Facial Analysis with Difficulty before Serial Extraction (B.SEXT.)

Parameter	Normal range	Patient	Difference
FMA	22–28	31	31 – 28 = 3
ANB	1–5	3	–
Z	70–80	57	70 – 57 = 13
OP	8–12	13	13 – 12 = 1
SNB	78–82	75	78 – 75 = 3
PFH/AFH	0.62–0.72	0.65	0.67 – 0.65 = 2
Difference	Difficulty Factor	Difficulty B. SEXT.	
3	5	15	
–	15	–	
13	2	26	
1	3	3	
3	5	15	
2	3	6	
TOTAL		65	

Total difficulty **65**, indicating more difficulty in correcting the cranial facial complex.

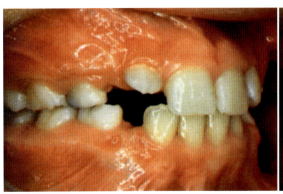
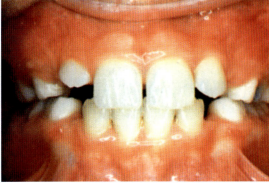

Fig. 3.2.**4 Dentition at initiation of serial extraction with primary canines extracted.** This initiates the correction of the alveolar dental protrusion by uprighting the incisors.

M. R.— Difficulty Summary

TSA difficulty	26.5
CFA difficulty	65.0
TOTAL	**91.5**
Mild	0–60
*Moderate	60–120
Severe	>120

The patient's orthodontic problem (**91.5**) is categorized as moderate (**60–120**), which is suitable for a typical serial extraction treatment. There is an absence of a skeletal discrepancy (ANB, 3°). The difficulty of **65** (see CFA with Difficulty) is due to alveolar dental protrusion (Z, 57°: **26**), a retrognathic mandible (SNB, 75°: **15**), and a high-angle skeletal pattern (FMA, 31°: **15**).

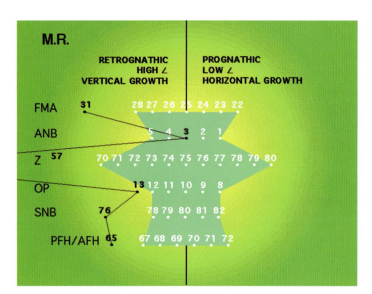

Fig. 3.2.**5** **The wiggle analysis prior to treatment (B.SEXT.).** The measurements are displaced to the retrognathic, high-angle, vertical growth side of the normal range except for the skeletal discrepancy (ANB, 3°). The ANB is within the normal range, confirming that there is not a cranial facial discrepancy and that this is a favorable patient for serial extraction.

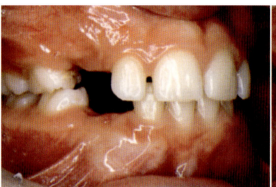
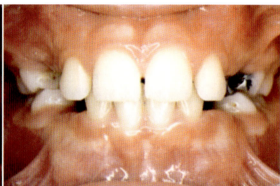

Fig. 3.2.**6** **Dentition during serial extraction.** The primary first molar teeth have been extracted, influencing the permanent first premolar teeth to emerge before the permanent canines.

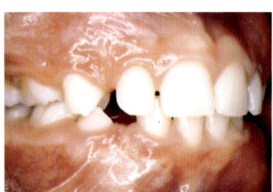
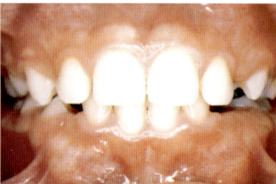

Fig. 3.2.**7** **The first premolar teeth are extracted** to provide space to allow the permanent canines to emerge more favorably.

Clinical Case Studies

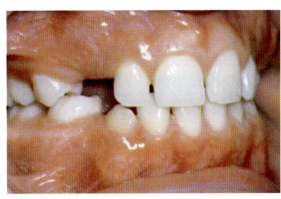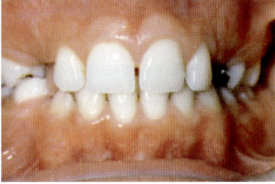

Fig. 3.2.**8** **The permanent mandibular canine teeth are emerging, which are now supporting the mandibular incisors, preventing the increase of the overbite.** The permanent maxillary second premolars have erupted preventing the unfavorable mesial drift of the permanent maxillary first molars into a Class II relationship.

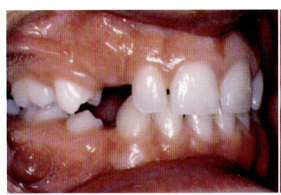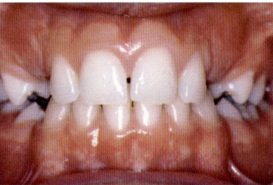

Fig. 3.2.**9** **The permanent mandibular second premolar teeth are emerging.**
It is favorable to have the mandibular premolars emerge after the maxillary to allow the mandibular first molars to drift into a more solid Class I relationship.

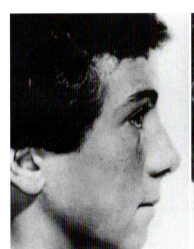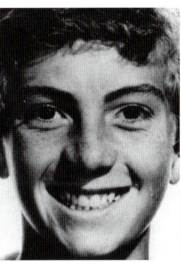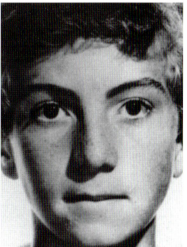

Fig. 3.2.**10** **Face after serial extraction.** Note the quality of the smile at this stage. The smile will be improved by placing the dentition into a more favorable alignment with appliance therapy.

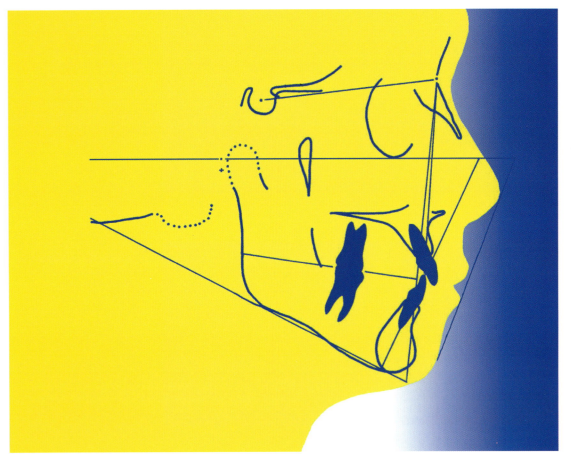

Fig. 3.2.**11 Cephalometric tracing after serial extraction.** The mandible has responded favorably in a counterclockwise rotation (FMA 31° to 27°) (SNB 75° to 78°) (PFH/AFH 0.65 to 0.69). The occlusal plane has flattened (13° to 8°) due to vertical control (molars not extruded, incisors uprighted). Lips are less prominent (Z 57° to 71°). Skeletal relationship remains favorable.

M.R. CEPH. ANALYSIS

	B. T.	A.SEXT.
FMA	31	27 (-4)
IMPA	91	88 (-3)
FMIA	58	65 (+7)
SNA	78	79 (+1)
SNB	75	78 (+3)
ANB	3	2 (-1)
OP	13	8 (-5)
Z	57	71 (+14)
PFH/AFH	.65	.69 (+4)

Fig. 3.2.**12 Cephalometric analysis after serial extraction.** All measurements show a favorable response to serial extraction. Approximately 75% of the patient's response to total treatment occurred during this period without appliance therapy.

M.R.— Cranial Facial Analysis with Difficulty after Serial Extraction (A.SEXT.)

Difference	Difficulty Factor	Difficulty	
		B. SEXT.	A. SEXT.
3	5	15	–
–	15	–	–
13	2	26	–
1	3	3	–
3	5	15	*–
2	3	6	–
TOTAL		65	0

CFA reveals that the total difficulty has been eradicated (**65** to **0**). The mandible has responded favorably (FMA, **15** to **0**). The alveolar dental protrusion has been corrected (Z, **26** to **0**). The retrognathic mandible has been corrected (**15** to **0**) and, with a favorable rotation, the ratio has improved (PFH/AFH, 0.65 to .069: **6** to **0**).

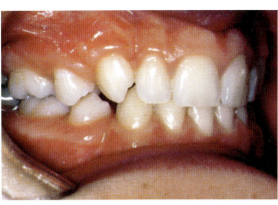 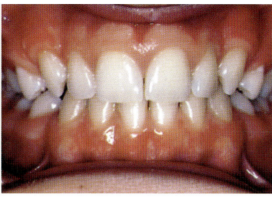

Fig. 3.2.**13 Dentition after serial extraction prior to appliance placement.** Very little mechanotherapy will be required to correct this dentition. Minor corrections remain to be achieved with the edgewise appliance. Only 11 months of edgewise treatment were required to produce an ideal occlusion.

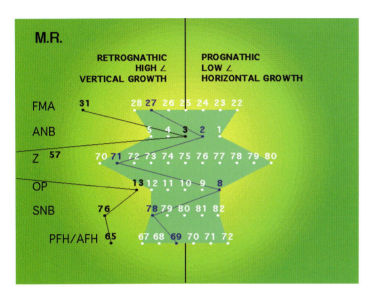

Fig. 3.2.**14 The wiggle analysis after serial extraction.** This analysis graphically depicts the dramatic improvement in all measurements to within the normal range, without the use of any appliance mechanotherapy.

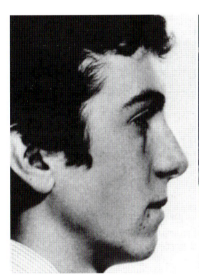 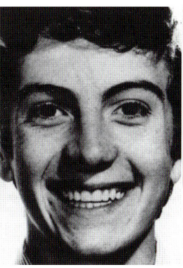 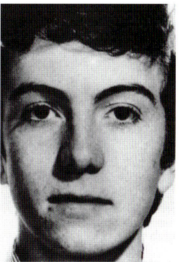

Fig. 3.2.**15 Face after treatment.** Note the improvement in the smile after edgewise treatment. The improvement in the alignment of the teeth significantly improves the smile and the health of the dentition.

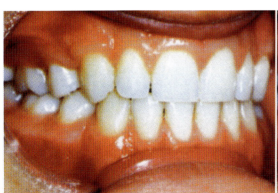 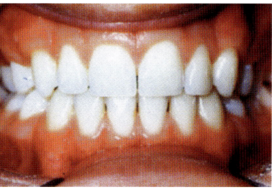

Fig. 3.2.**16 Dentition after treatment depicting a significant improvement after edgewise therapy.** A favorable correction of the alignment also improves function (canine protected occlusion and incisal guidance) and stability. The dentition is in balance with the supporting jaws and the surrounding soft tissues. The teeth have been slightly overcorrected to allow for "recovery".

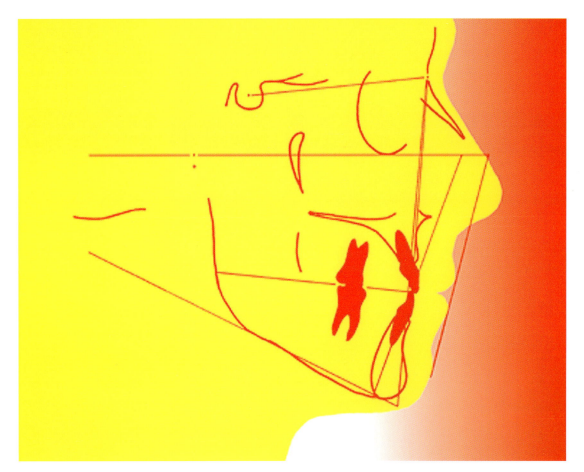

Fig. 3.2.**17** **Cephalometric tracing after treatment depicting balance, harmony, and proportion.** Soft-tissue profile line has improved (see Fig. 3.2.**2** to an ideal relationship with chin, lips, and nose.

M.R. CEPH. ANALYSIS

	B.T.	A.T.
FMA	31	25 (-2)
IMPA	91	85 (-3)
FMIA	58	70 (+5)
SNA	78	79 (0)
SNB	75	79 (+1)
ANB	3	1 (-1)
OP	13	7 (-1)
Z	57	75 (+4)
PFH/AFH	.65	.72 (+3)

Fig. 3.2.**18** **Cephalometric analysis after treatment with measurements depicting further improvement.** The appliance therapy contributed approximately 25% to the total treatment. The mandible continued to rotate favorably (FMA 27° to 25°; SNB 78° to 79°; PFH/AFH 0.69 to 0.72). The occlusal plane continues to flatten with good appliance control (8° to 7°) and the profile result is ideal (Z 71° to 75°).

M.R.— Cranial Facial Analysis with Difficulty after Treatment (A.T.)

Difference	Difficulty Factor	Difficulty		
		B. SEXT.	A. SEXT.	A.T.
3	5	15	–	–
–	15	–	–	–
13	2	26	–	–
1	3	3	–	+3
3	5	15	*–	–
2	3	6	–	–
TOTAL		65	0	+3

The difficulty is totally eradicated, with the occlusal plane slightly overtreated (**0** to **+3**).

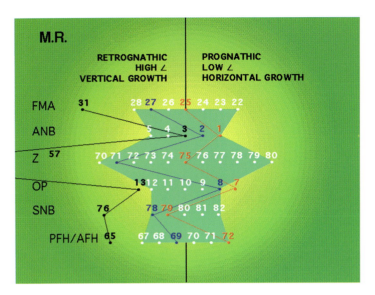

Fig. 3.2.**19** **The wiggle analysis after treatment.** The measurements indicate further progress to the right side within the normal range. Very little change is expected because the posterior, anterior, lateral, and vertical limits of the dentition have not been violated by expansion or extrusion of the teeth.

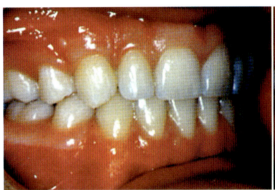
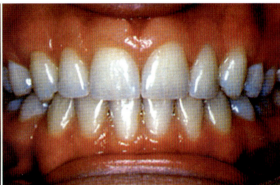

Fig. 3.2.**20** **Dentition 3 years after treatment depicting favorable alignment, occlusion, and stability.** The dentition has recovered into a stable relationship.

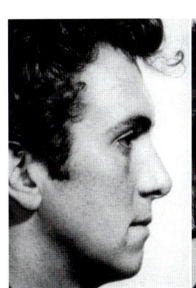
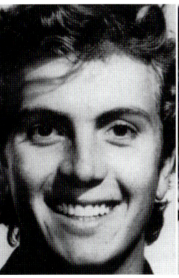
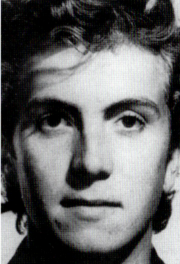

Fig. 3.2.**21** **Face 15 years after treatment depicting favorable proportion, balance, and harmony of the soft tissue and a pleasing smile.** The patient makes his living as a model at this stage.

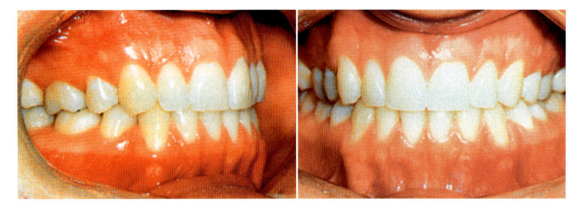

Fig. 3.2.**22** **Dentition 15 years after treatment depicting favorable alignment, occlusion, and stability.** If anything, the dentition and the surrounding structures are more attractive and healthier than they have ever been, in spite of the length of time since treatment.

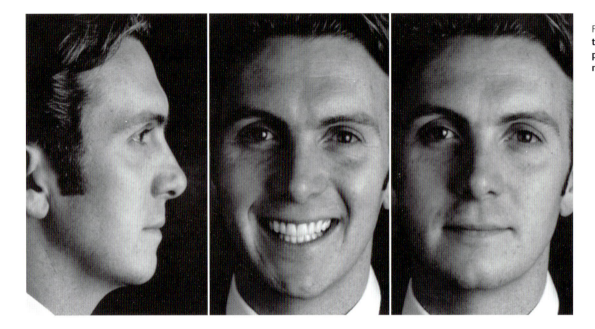

Fig. 3.2.**23** **Face 20 years after treatment depicting favorable proportion, balance, and harmony and a pleasing smile.**

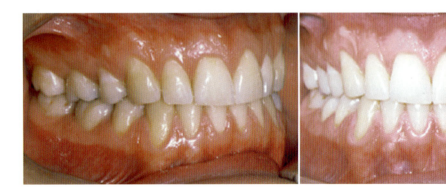

Fig. 3.2.**24** **Dentition 20 years after treatment depicting stability.** We continue to monitor this patient because of his willingness to cooperate and because of his interest in orthodontics.

Case Study 3.3   Patient J. O.

- Male
- 8.5 years of age
- Vertical growth
- Hyperdivergent facial pattern (FMA, 30°)
- Skeletal discrepancy: retrognathic mandible (ANB, 8°) (SNB, 75°)

- Class II Division 1 malocclusion, mixed dentition
- Anterior open bite
- Tooth-size, jaw-size discrepancy
- Serial extraction, including four first premolar teeth
- Tweed–Merrifield edgewise mechanotherapy

J. O.'s case represents Class II interceptive guidance of occlusion including serial extraction followed by the Tweed–Merrifield edgewise appliance treatment. These patients are more difficult to treat and to complete than those with Class I malocclusions because of the skeletal discrepancy and because a thorough knowledge of the edgewise appliance is necessary. A more sophisticated multibanded-multibracket mechanotherapy is required as a result of the more unfavorable growth and development of the craniofacial complex.

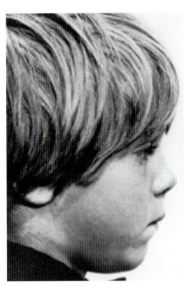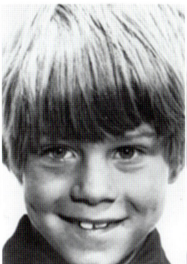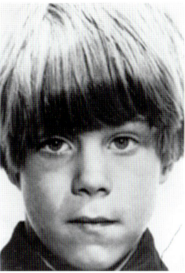

Fig. 3.3.1 **Face before serial extraction.** Note the retrognathic mandible with resulting recessive soft-tissue profile.

J. O.— Total Space Analysis

Anterior Arch	
REQUIRED	
Teeth: 1, 2, 3	− 39.0
Ceph. correction	− 10.4
Soft tissue	−
TOTAL	− 49.4
AVAILABLE	− 34.0
DEFICIT	− 15.4
Mid Arch	
REQUIRED	
Teeth: 4, 5, 6	− 52.0
Curve of occlusion	− 2.5
TOTAL	− 54.5
AVAILABLE	+ 56.0
SURPLUS	+ 1.5

Posterior Arch	
REQUIRED	
Teeth: 7, 8	− 42.0
AVAILABLE	
Presently available	+ 8.0
Estimated increase	+ 21.0
TOTAL	+ 29.0
DEFICIT	− 13.0
TOTAL DEFICIT	**−28.9**

TSA indicates the extraction of four first premolar and four third molar teeth due to the anterior (**−15.4**) and posterior deficits (**−13.0**), respectively.

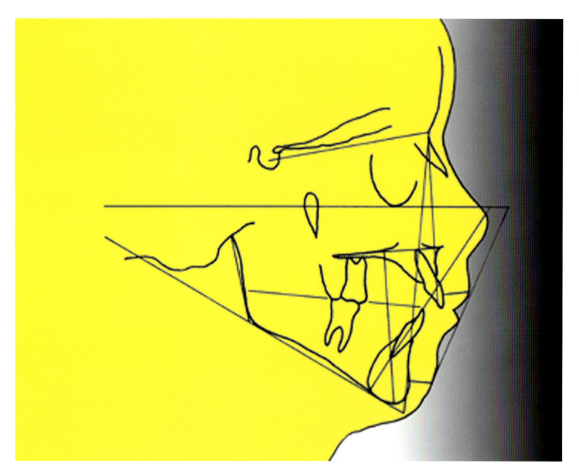

Fig. 3.3.**2 Cephalometric tracing before serial extraction.** Note the recessive profile and the prominent maxillary incisor teeth when he smiles.

J. O.— Total Space Analysis Difficulty

Anterior arch	Value	Difficulty Factor	Difficulty
Tooth arch discrepancy	5.0	1.5	7.5
Ceph. discrepancy	10.4	1.0	10.4
Soft tissue	–	0.5	–
TOTAL	15.4		17.9
Mid arch	**Value**	**Difficulty Factor**	**Difficulty**
Tooth arch discrepancy	+ 4.0	1.0	+ 4.0
Curve of Spee	2.5	1.0	2.5
TOTAL	1.5		1.5
Posterior arch	**Value**	**Difficulty factor**	**Difficulty**
Tooth arch discrepancy	34.0		
Expected increase	+ 21.0		
TOTAL	13.0	0.5	6.5
Horizontal occlusion discrepancy Class II–III	10.0	2.0	20.0
TOTAL DIFFICULTY			**45.9**

Total difficulty **45.9**, more difficult than M. R. (**26.5**). It will therefore be more difficult to correct the dentition in this instance.

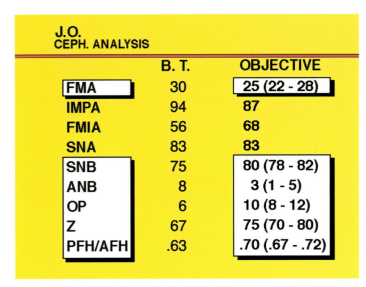

Fig. 3.3.**3** **Cephalometric analysis before serial extraction.** Note the retrognathic mandible (SNB, 75°), the skeletal discrepancy (ANB, 8°), and the high angle facial pattern (FMA, 30°).

J.O.— Cranial Facial Analysis with Difficulty before Serial Extraction (B. SEXT.)

Parameter	Normal range	Patient	Difference
FMA	22–28	30	30 – 28 = 2
ANB	1–5	8	8 – 5 = 3
Z	70–80	67	70 – 67 = 3
OP	8–12	6	8 – 6 = 1
SNB	78–82	75	78 – 75 = 3
PFH/AFH	0.62–0.72	0.63 (39/62)	0.67 – 0.63 = 4
Difference	Difficulty Factor	Difficulty	
		B. SEXT.	
2	5	10	
3	15	*45	
3	2	6	
2	3	6	
3	5	*15	
4	3	12	
TOTAL		94	

Total difficulty **94**, more difficult than M.R. (**65.0**). Skeletal discrepancy (ANB, 8°) is more difficult than M.R. (ANB, 3°) but mandible is the same as M.R. (SNB, 75°); SNA is significantly greater here (SNA 83° vs. 78° for M.R.). To arrive at ANB of 2°, SNB must improve by 8°. To arrive at ANB of 2° for M.R., SNB needed to improve by only 1°.

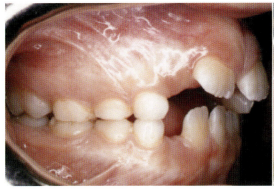
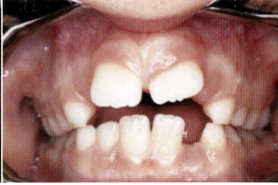

Fig. 3.3.**4** **Dentition before serial extraction depicting open bite and a distal step mixed dentition developing into a Class II permanent relationship.** Vertical control will be absolutely essential during treatment because of the high-angle facial pattern and the anterior open bite.

J.O.— Difficulty Summary

TSA difficulty	45.9
CFA difficulty	94.0
TOTAL	**139.9**
Mild	0–60
Moderate	60–120
*Severe	>120

The patient's orthodontic problem (**139.9**) is categorized as severe (**>120**). It is severe primarily because of the cranial facial discrepancy (**94**). More specifically, there is a skeletal discrepancy (ANB 8°, **45**) due to a relatively retrognathic mandible (SNB 75°, **15**). (see CFA with Difficulty).

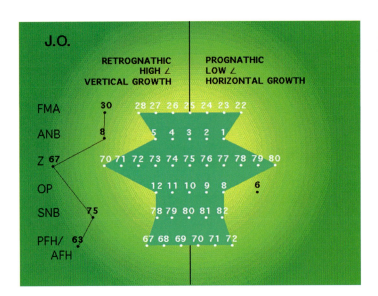

Fig. 3.3.**5** **The wiggle analysis prior to treatment (B.SEXT.).** The measurements are displaced to the retrognathic, high-angle, vertical growth side of the normal range except for the occlusal plane. The significant difference from M.R. here is the skeletal discrepancy (ANB, 8° vs. ANB, 3°).

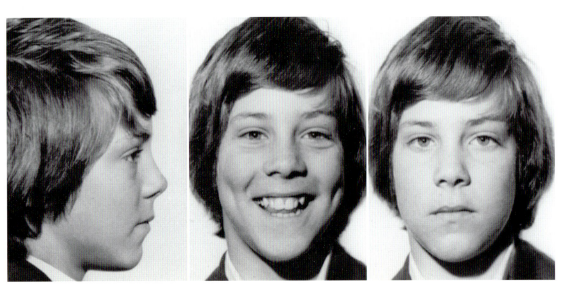

Fig. 3.3.**6** **Face after serial extraction.** Note the quality of the smile at this stage, but also note the improvement in the profile.

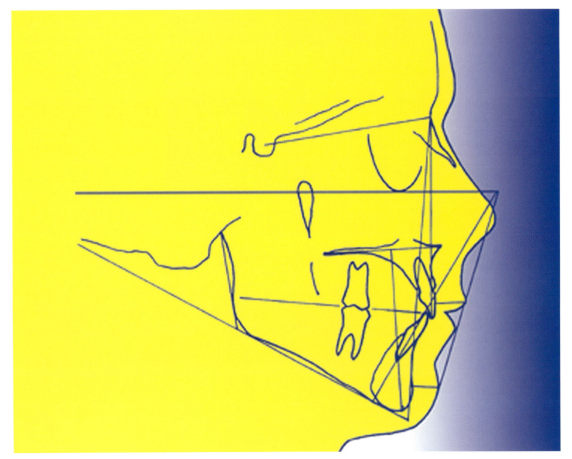

Fig. 3.3.**7** **Cephalometric tracing after serial extraction (A. SEXT.).** Note the improvement in the skeletal discrepancy (ANB 8° to 5°).

Clinical Case Studies

J.O. CEPH. ANALYSIS

	B. T.	A.SEXT.
FMA	30	27 (-3)
IMPA	94	92 (-2)
FMIA	56	61 (+5)
SNA	83	81 (-2)
SNB	75	76 (+1)
ANB	8	5 (-3)
OP	6	6 (0)
Z	67	73 (+6)
PFH/AFH	.63	.65 (+2)

Fig. 3.3.**8 Cephalometric analysis after serial extraction.** Measurements depict favorable response to serial extraction: FMA and ANB decreased and SNB, Z angle, and PFH/AFH increased. The occlusal plane remained the same.

J.O.— Cranial Facial Analysis with Difficulty after Serial Extraction (A. SEXT.)

Difference	Difficulty Factor	Difficulty	
		B. SEXT.	A. SEXT.
2	5	10	–
3	15	*45	–
3	2	6	–
2	3	6	6
3	5	*15	6
4	3	12	6
TOTAL		94	18

CFA reveals that the total difficulty has been reduced from **94** to **18**. The skeletal discrepancy has been reduced and the difficulty eradicated (ANB, 8° to 5°: **45–0**) partly due to the mandibular response (FMA, 30° to 27°: **10–0**; SNB, 75° to 76°: **15–6**). There is still a need for further mandibular response.

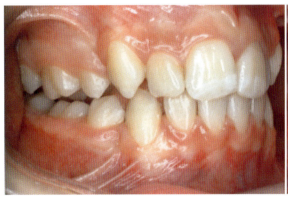 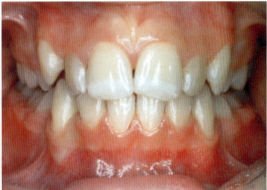

Fig. 3.3.**9 Dentition after serial extraction.** The open bite no longer exists. No appliances were used. With serial extraction the mandibular molars drift forward. This results in a favorable closure of the dentition. The molar relationship depicts this change.

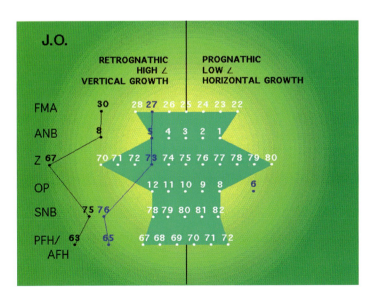

Fig. 3.3.**10 The wiggle analysis after serial extraction.** This analysis graphically depicts the improvement in the five measurements on the left side, with three progressing to the normal range. It also indicates a need for further improvement in the mandibular response, expected in Class II malocclusions.

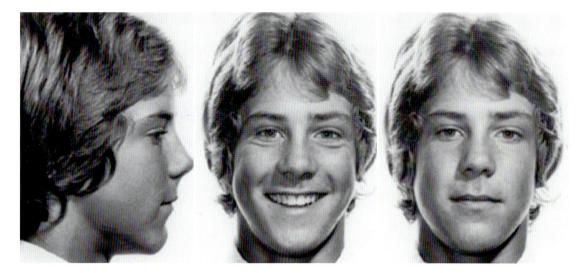

Fig. 3.3.**11** **Face after treatment.** Note the improvement in the smile with the edgewise mechanotherapy. Because the SNA was decreased (83° to 81°) there is an obtuse nasial labial angle. This will improve with further mandibular rotation.

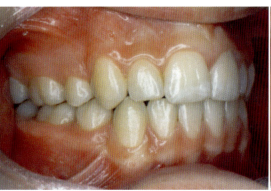 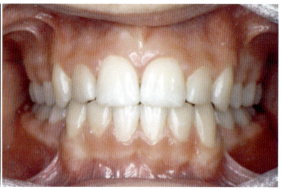

Fig. 3.3.**12** **Dentition after treatment depicting a significant improvement after the edgewise therapy.** The open bite remains closed because posterior teeth were allowed to come forward. If posterior teeth were moved distally to correct the Class II relationship and crowding, the open bite would have remained open or would have become worse.

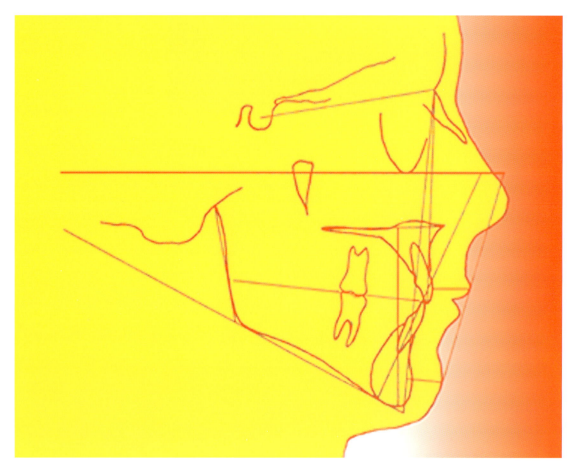

Fig. 3.3.**13** **Cephalometric tracing after treatment, depicting balance and harmony.** The mandible is still relatively retruded. The ANB has been reduced by 5° because SNA has decreased by 4°. That has resulted in an increase in the nasial labial angle. This will improve later.

Clinical Case Studies

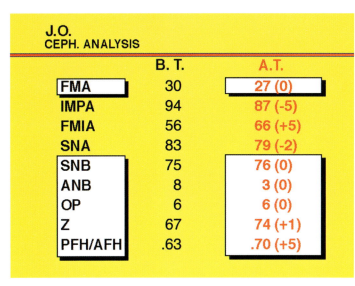

Fig. 3.3.**14 Cephalometric analysis after treatment.** Measurements indicate further improvement. The significant change here is an increase in the PFH/AFH from 0.63 to 0.70.

J. O.— Cranial Facial Analysis with Difficulty after Treatment (A. T.)

Difference	Difficulty Factor	Difficulty		
		B. SEXT.	A. SEXT.	A. T.
2	5	10	–	–
3	15	*45	–	–
3	2	6	–	–
2	3	6	6	6
3	5	*15	6	6
4	3	12	6	–
TOTAL		94	18	12

The difficulty has been further reduced from **18** to **12** and another measurement is within normal range (PFH/AFH, **6–0**).

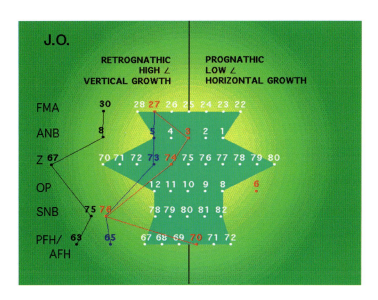

Fig. 3.3.**15 The wiggle analysis after treatment.** Only one measurement remains to the left side of the normal range, (SNB, 76°). This will change dramatically within the next seven years.

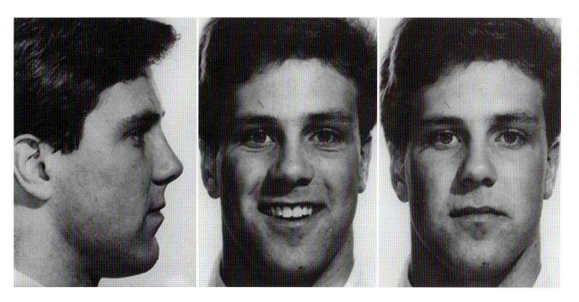

Fig. 3.3.**16 Face 7 years after treatment.** Mandibular growth has significantly strengthened the soft-tissue profile. Note that the nasial labial angle is less obtuse.

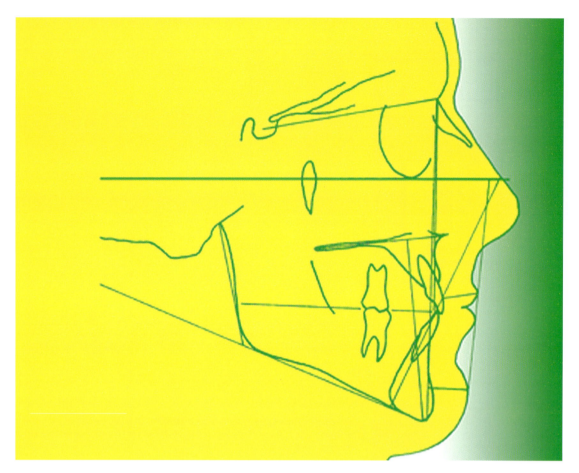

Fig. 3.3.**17 Cephalometric tracing 7 years after treatment with significant mandibular growth.** Also, the profile indicates a significant increase in soft-tissue chin thickness, which helps to strengthen the profile.

J.O. CEPH. ANALYSIS	B. T.	7Y.A.T.
FMA	30	23 (-4)
IMPA	94	91 (+4)
FMIA	56	66 (0)
SNA	83	80 (+1)
SNB	75	79 (+3)
ANB	8	1 (-2)
OP	6	5 (-1)
Z	67	85 (+11)
PFH/AFH	.63	.75 (+5)

Fig. 3.3.**18 Cephalometric analysis 7 years after treatment.** The analysis indicates a further reduction of the FMA by 4° (30° to 23°: 30° to 27°, 27° to 23°), a further decrease of ANB by 7° (8° to 1°: 8° to 5°, 3° to 1°), and an increase in SNB by 3° (75° to 79°: 75° to 76°, 76° to 79°), indicating significant mandibular growth as visualized in the cephalometric tracing.

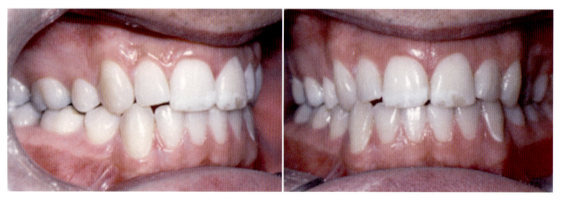

Fig. 3.3.**19 Dentition 7 years after treatment.** The patient, a hockey player at this stage, received a vertical blow to the mandible during a game. He was not wearing a rubber mouth guard. Because there was no protection between his maxillary and mandibular dentition, many cusps were broken and teeth chipped, as indicated by the mesial buccal cusp of the mandibular right first molar tooth and the maxillary left incisor tooth.

J.O.— Cranial Facial Analysis with Difficulty 7 Years after Treatment (7 A.T.)

Difference	Difficulty Factor	Difficulty			
		B.SEXT.	A. SEXT.	A.T.	7A.T.
2	5	10	–	–	–
3	15	*45	–	–	–
3	2	6	–	–	+10
2	3	6	6	6	+9
3	5	*15	6	6	–
4	3	12	6	–	+9
TOTAL		94	18	12	+28

Significant posttreatment growth has the difficulty progressing from **12** to **+28** with the Z angle at **+10°**, indicating a straighter profile, and PFH/AFH at **+9**, indicating rotation of the mandible in a counterclockwise direction.

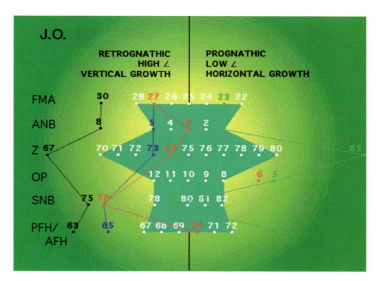

Fig. 3.3.**20** **The wiggle analysis 7 years after treatment.** The mandible is now within the normal range with FMA and ANB. The Z angle, the OP, and the PFH/AFH ratio are well off the right, indicating a stronger profile.

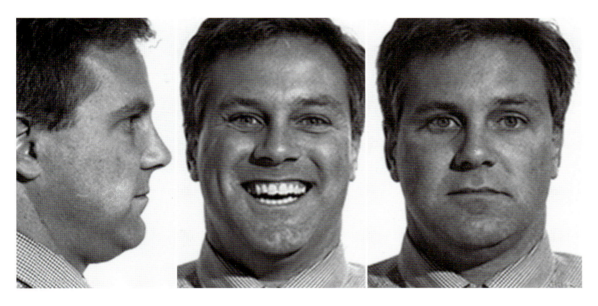

Fig. 3.3.**21** **Face 25 years after treatment indicates favorable balance and harmony.**

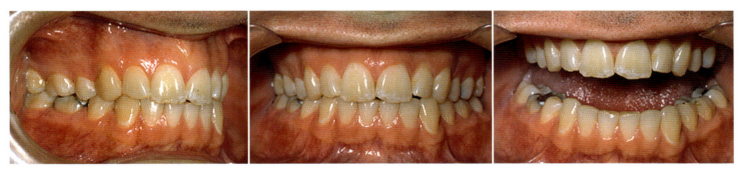

Fig. 3.3.**22** **Dentition 25 years after treatment indicating stability and further chipping of the enamel.** We are now treating his two children. Thus, we will continue to monitor his progress.

Due to space limitations, it is not possible to present comprehensive case reports for more patients. What has been presented is representative of interceptive guidance of occlusion, including serial extraction followed by the Tweed–Merrifield edgewise appliance treatment. In our office, early treatment consists of two periods: (1) Interceptive guidance followed by (2) multibanded-multibracket appliance therapy in class I malocclusions. For a number of class II malocclusions there are three periods: (1) An initial period of interceptive treatment utilizing a high-pull headgear and a partial multibanded-multibracket appliance for one year, followed by (2) a period of interceptive guidance and (3) a final period of active treatment. Figures 3.4.**1**–3.4.**7** provide examples of results achieved by this treatment protocol illustrating stability from 5 to 35 years after treatment is completed.

Recently, I had a patient referred to me for a second opinion. At 8 years of age, with an ANB of 6.5°, the patient was scheduled for surgery at a later date by the first orthodontist. Forty years ago I carried out early treatment on the patient's mother (Fig. 3.**7**), who was the sister of the patient shown in Figure 3.**6**. The mother was one of my ABO patients, and her mandibular response was very similar to that of J.O. Keeping in mind the response of the mother and that of J.O., along with many others, I find it very difficult to predict surgery at 8 years of age.

It has been my experience that early treatment reduces the need for surgery in many patients. I have many adult surgical patients in my practice, but if I have the opportunity to provide early treatment, I will attempt to reduce the necessity for surgery.

The late growth and development that we observed in J.O. could be detrimental to surgical treatment rather than beneficial. The total mandibular response with this Class II patient (J.O.), with a significant skeletal discrepancy (ANB, 8° to 1°) is noticeably better than that of the Class II patient (G.L.), also with a skeletal discrepancy (ANB, 9° to 4°), who did not have the benefit of interceptive guidance over a longer period.

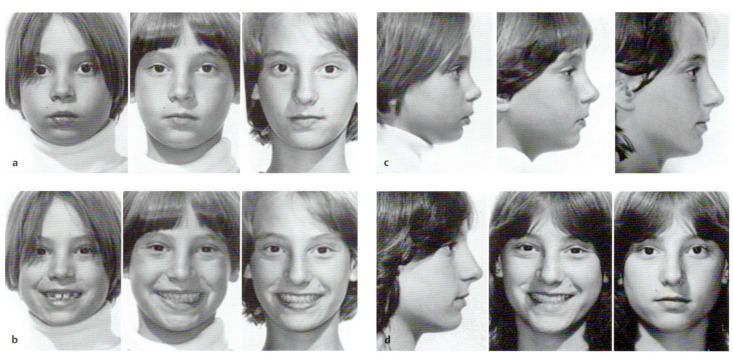

Fig. 3.4.**1 a–d** Sequences before Class II serial extraction (B. SEXT.) (left); after serial extraction (A. SEXT.) (center); after treatment (A. T.) (right).

a Note the improvement in the soft-tissue balance, harmony, and proportion as treatment progresses.
b Note the improvement in the smile as treatment progresses.

c Note the favorable mandibular response in a counterclockwise direction and soft tissue profile as treatment progresses.
d **Five years after treatment:** The patient enjoys beautiful balance, harmony, and proportion in the soft tissue both in the anterior and profile views as well as an attractive smile and a favorable alignment of dentition.

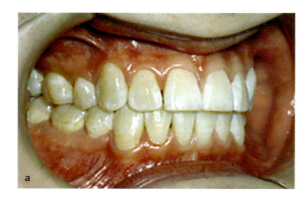
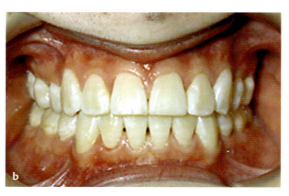

Fig. 3.4.**2** **Six years after treatment:** Ideal alignment and occlusion together with an attractive smile.

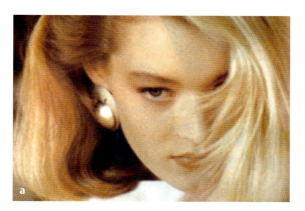
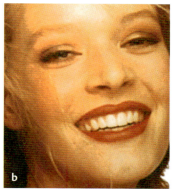

Fig. 3.4.**3** **Eight years after treatment:** A famous model with beautiful facial features and a captivating smile.

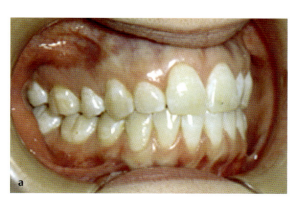
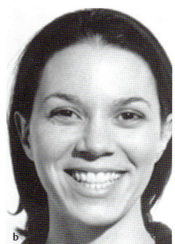

Fig. 3.4.**4** **Ten years after treatment:** The key to a sound occlusion is overtreatment of the maxillary first molars into a super Class I relationship, as seen here in this patient's result.

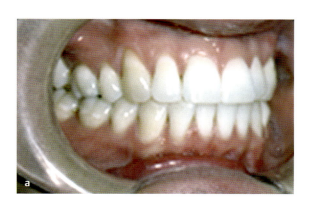
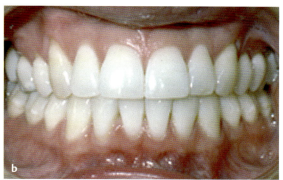

Fig. 3.4.**5** **Fifteen years after treatment:** Probably the most beautiful result that I have achieved during 48 years of practice in orthodontics.

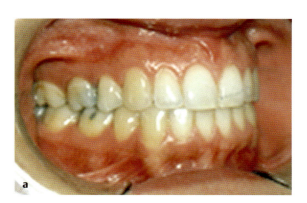
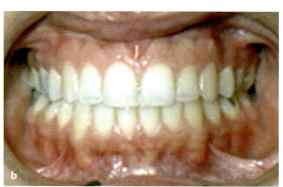

Fig. 3.4.**6** **Eighteen years after treatment:** This patient had minimal retention. If patients are required to wear permanent retainers for the rest of their lives, the teeth are not in balance and harmony with the supporting and surrounding structures.

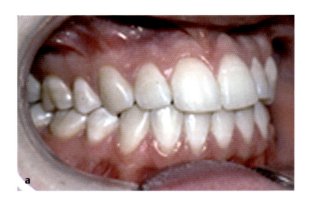
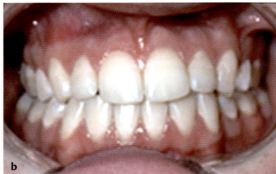

Fig. 3.4.**7** **Twenty-five years after treatment:** Stability is excellent when the dimensions of the dentition are not violated.

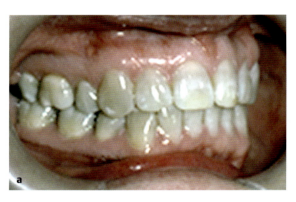
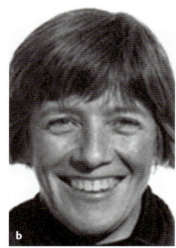

Fig. 3.4.**8** **Thirty-five years after treatment:** This patient still visits our office on a monthly basis with her daughter and I am in a position to observe her results regularly. Soon, I will obtain her records 40 years after treatment.

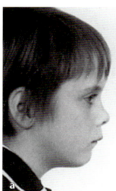
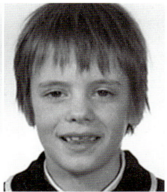
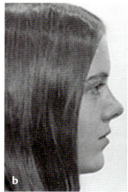
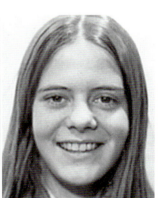
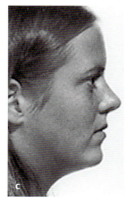
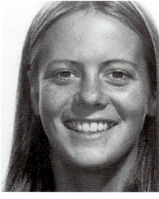

Fig. 3.**5** **An ABO patient treated from age 8 years; this patient had mandibular response similar to that of J.O. [Case Study 3.3].**
- **a** Before serial extraction, 8 years of age, 1962. A recessive profile associated with a retrognathic mandible is evident. An open bite and protrusive maxillary incisors have resulted from a tongue thrust.
- **b** Three years after treatment, 16 years of age, 1970. The mandible has responded favorably in a counterclockwise rotation with early treatment. The profile and smile are both attractive, contributing to the patient's increased self-esteem.
- **c** Nine years after treatment, 22 years of age, 1976. Nothing has changed. Patient displays confidence with attractive facial and dental features.

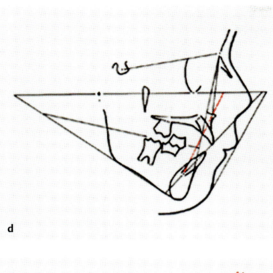
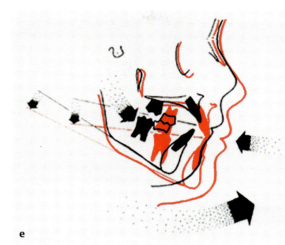
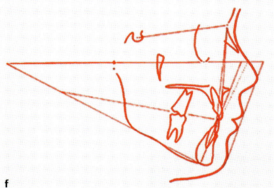
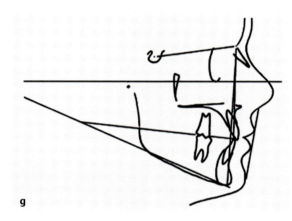
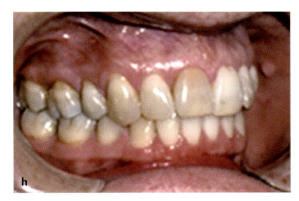
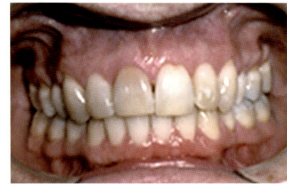
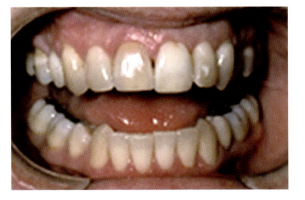

Fig. 3.5
- **d** Lateral cephalometric analysis before serial extraction (B.SEXT.), 8 years of age, 1962. Note the retrognathic mandible (SNB, 68°). Red: objective axial inclination of mandibular incisors.
- **e** Superimposition before serial extraction (B.SEXT.) and after treatment (A. T.). Note the dramatic mandibular response, SNB increasing from 68° to 76°. Note also the improvement in the soft-tissue profile and the uprighting of the mandibular incisors.
- **f** Lateral cephalometric analysis after treatment (A. T.), 13 years of age, 1967. SNB has increased by 8° from 68° to 76°. This has produced a significant improvement in the dentition and in the profile.
- **g** Lateral cephalometric analysis 9 years after treatment (9A. T.), 22 years of age, 1976. SNB is 79°, now within the normal range. The total improvement in the SNB is 11°. That is treatment complementing growth and development, one of the objectives of The Tweed Foundation.
- **h** Patient's dentition 28 years after treatment, 41 years of age, 1995. Although not perfect, this dentition is remarkably stable, indicating only minor discrepancies in the final occlusion after an extended period of time without retention appliances.

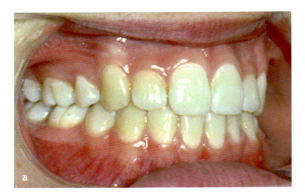
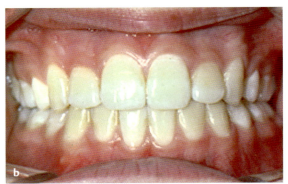

Fig. 3.6 **A Tale of Two Patients —Part 1.** In the final analysis, who would you rather be if you were just beginning the sensitive teenage period at 13 years of age: the young woman here, who benefited from interceptive guidance of occlusion including serial extraction, followed by the edgewise appliance, or the patient in Fig. 3.7, who did not?

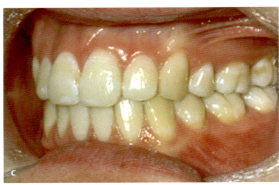

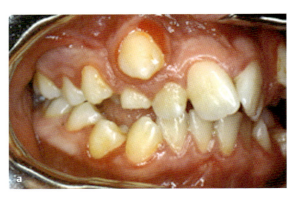
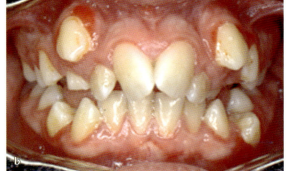

Fig. 3.7 **A Tale of Two Patients —Part 2.** This patient came into the office at 13 years of age to begin three years of edgewise treatment at the same time the patient in Fig. 3.6, who also originally had a crowded dentition, was leaving with a beautiful alignment, occlusion, and smile.

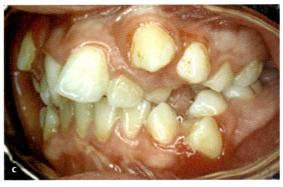

Conclusion

I have practiced my particular interpretation of "early treatment" for 48 years, and I have concluded that there are three major benefits of this treatment:

1. Beginning early and completing treatment just prior to the sensitive teenage period is appreciated by parents and patients alike. It is especially appreciated by the patients because it occurs at a very important stage in their lives. It is much more acceptable to leave the orthodontist's office with a beautiful smile at 13 years of age than to come in at that age for three years of "braces," as depicted in the Tale of Two Patients illustrated in Figures 3.6 and 3.7.
2. I have traced hundreds of cephalometric radiographs of my patients during the past 48 years, and I have observed, with very few exceptions, a favorable counterclockwise (upward and for-

ward) response of the mandible. I am convinced that the favorable mandibular response is even more pronounced with the early treatment patients because it has been encouraged to happen over a longer period of time by vertical control. Balance and harmony of the soft tissue and a well proportioned profile are the result. This is depicted in **Case Studies 3.2** and **3.3** and Figures 3.**1**, 3.**2**, and 3.**5**.
3. I have practiced in the same location for 48 years. This has provided an opportunity for me to observe my results many years after treatment has been completed.

An estimated 40% of my practice, at the present time, consists of patients whose parents I treated many years ago. I therefore have the chance to take long-range records of the parents to study the stability of their results.

I never dismiss my patients; I encourage them to continue coming to our office as long as they wish to come. One of the primary sources of gratification at this stage in my career is to observe the remarkable stability when I examine these patients who have been in the practice for so many years.

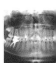

References

Bunon R. Essay sur les maladies des dents; ou l'on propose les moyens de leur procurer une bonne confirmation des la plus tendre enfance, et d'en assurer la conservation pendant tout le cours de la vie. Paris; 1743.

Burlington Orthodontic Research Project, University of Toronto, Faculty of Dentistry, report no. 3, 1957.

Dale JG, Dale HC. Interceptive guidance of occlusion with emphasis on diagnosis. In: Graber TM, Vanarsdall RL Jr. Orthodontics, current principles and techniques. 3rd ed. St Louis: Mosby; 2000: 375–469.

Dewel BF. Serial extractions in orthodontics; indications, objections, and treatment procedures. Int J Orthod. 1954; 40: 906.

Dewel BF. A critical analysis of serial extraction in orthodontic treatment. Am J Orthod. 1959; 45: 424.

Dewel BF. Serial extraction, its limitations and contraindications in orthodontic treatment. Am J Orthod. 1967; 53(12): 904–921.

Dewel BF. Extraction in orthodontic: premises and prerequisites. Angle Orthod. 1973; 43(1): 65–87.

Fanning EA. Longitudinal study of tooth formation and root resorption. NZ Dent J. 1961; 57: 202.

Fanning EA: Effect of extraction on deciduous molars on the formation and eruption of their successors. Angle Orthod. 1962; 32: 44.

Fanning EA, Hunt EB. Linear increments of growth in the roots of permanent mandibular teeth. J Dent Res. 1964; 43(suppl): 981.

Gebek TR, Merrifield LL. Orthodontic diagnosis and treatment analysis—concepts and values: Part I. Am J Orthod Dentofac Orthop. 1995; 107: 434–443.

Graber TM. Serial extraction: a continuous diagnostic and decisional process. Am J Orthod. 1971; 60(6): 541–575.

Graber TM, Vanarsdall RJ, Vig K, eds. Orthodontics, current principles and techniques. 4th ed. St. Louis: Mosby; 2005.

Gramling JF. A cephalometric appraisal of the results of orthodontic treatment on 50 unsuccessfully corrected difficult class II malocclusion. J Charles H. Tweed Found. 1987; 15: 102.

Gramling JF. A cephalometric appraisal of the results of orthodontic treatment on 50 unsuccessfully corrected difficult class II malocclusion. J Charles H. Tweed Found. 1987; 15: 112.

Grön AM. Prediction of tooth emergence. J Dent Res. 1962; 41: 573.

Heath J. The interception of malocclusion by planned serial extraction. NZ Dent J. 1953; 49: 77.

Heath J. Dangers and pitfalls of serial extraction. Eur Orthod Soc Trans. 1961; 37: 60.

Horn AJ. Facial height index. Am J Orthod Dentofac Orthop. 1992; 102: 180–186.

Hotz R. Active supervision of the eruption of teeth by extraction. Eur Orthod Soc Trans. 1947–1948: 34.

Hotz R. Guidance of eruption versus serial extraction. Am J Orthod. 1970; 58: 1.

Kjellgren B. Serial extraction as a corrective procedure in dental orthopedic therapy. Eur Orthod Soc Trans. 1947–1948: 134.

Lloyd ZB. Serial extraction as a treatment procedure. Am J Orthod. 1956; 42: 728.

Mayne WR. Serial extraction. In: Graber TM, ed. Orthodontics, current orthodontic concepts and techniques. Philadelphia: WB Saunders; 1969: Chapter 4.

Merrifield LL. The profile line as an aid in critically evaluation facial esthetics. Am J Orthod. 1966; 52: 804.

Merrifield LL. Differential diagnosis with total space analysis. J Charles H. Tweed Found. 1978; 6: 10.

Merrifield LL. The systems of directional force. J Charles H. Tweed Found. 1982; 10: 15.

Merrifield LL. Dimensions of the denture: back to basics. Am J Orthod Dentofac Orthop. 1994; 106: 535–542.

Merrifield LL, Gebek TR. Orthodontic diagnosis and treatment analysis-concepts and values: Part II. Am J Orthod Dentofac Orthop. 1995; 107: 541–547.

Merrifield LL, Klontz HK, Vaden JL. Differential diagnostic analysis system. Am J Orthod Dentofac Orthop. 1994; 106: 641–648.

Moorrees CFA. Growth changes of the dental arches—a longitudinal study. J Can Dent Assoc. 1958; 24: 449.

Moorrees CFA. The dentition of the growing child; a longitudinal study of dental development between 3 and 18 years of age. Cambridge, MA: Harvard University Press; 1959.

Moorrees CFA. Dental development—a growth study based on tooth eruptions as a measure of physiologic age. Eur Orthod Soc Trans. 1964; 40: 92.

Moorrees CFA. Changes in dental arch dimensions expressed on the basis of tooth eruption as a measure of biologic age. 1965; J Dent Res. 44: 129.

Moorrees CFA. Normal variation in dental development determined with reference to tooth eruption statistics. J Dent Res. 1965; 44: 161.

Moorrees CFA. Variability of dental and facial development. Ann NY Acad Sci. 1966; 134: 846.

Moorrees CFA, Chadha JM. Crown diameters of corresponding tooth groups in deciduous and permanent dentition. J Dent Res. 1962; 41: 466.

Moorrees CFA, Chadha JM. Available space for the incisors during dental development; a growth study based on physiological age. Angle Orthod. 1965; 35: 12.

Moorrees CFA, Reed RB. Biometrics of crowding and spacing of the teeth in the mandible. Am J Phys Anthropol. 1954; 12: 77.

Moorrees CFA, Reed RB. Correlations among crown diameters of human teeth. Arch Oral Biol. 1964; 9: 685.

Moorrees CFA, Thompson S, et al. Mesiodistal crown diameters of the deciduous and permanent teeth in individuals. J Dent Res. 1957; 36: 39.

Moorrees CFA, Fanning EA, Grön AM, Lebret J. Timing of orthodontic treatment in relation to tooth formation. Eur Orthod Soc Trans. 1962; 38: 87.

Moorrees CFA, Fanning EA, Grön AM. Consideration of dental development in serial extraction. Angle Orthod. 1963; 33: 44.

Moorrees CFA, Fanning EA, Hunt EB Jr. Age variation of formation stages for ten permanent teeth. J Dent Res. 1963; 42: 1490.

Moorrees CFA, Fanning EA, Hunt EB Jr. Formation and resorption of three deciduous teeth in children. Am J Phys Anthropol. 1963; 21: 99.

Moorrees CFA, Reed RB, Chadha JM. Growth changes of the dentition defined in terms of chronologic and biologic age, Am J Orthod. 1964; 50: 789.

Tweed CH. The Frankfort-mandibular plane angle in orthodontic diagnosis classification, treatment planning, and prognosis. Am J Orthod Oral Surg. 1946; 32: 175.

Tweed CH. The Frankfort-mandibular incisor angle in orthodontic diagnosis treatment planning and prognosis. Angle Orthod. 1954; 24: 121.

Tweed CH. Pre-orthodontic guidance procedure, classification of facial growth trends, treatment timing. In: Kraus BS, Riedel RA, eds. Vistas in orthodontics. Philadelphia: Lea & Febiger; 1962: Chapter 8.

Tweed CH. Treatment planning and therapy in the mixed-dentition. Am J Orthod. 1963; 49: 900.

Tweed CH. Clinical orthodontics. St. Louis: Mosby; 1966.

Tweed CH. The diagnostic facial triangle in the control of treatment objectives. Am J Orthod. 1969; 55: 651.

Vaden JL, Dale JG, Klontz HK. The Tweed-Merrifield edgewise appliance: philosophy, diagnosis and treatment. In: Graber TM, Vanarsdall RL Jr. 3rd ed. Orthodontics, current principles and techniques. St. Louis: Mosby; 2000: 647–707.

4 Functional Orthodontic and Functional Orthopedic Treatment

Thomas Rakosi

The functional appliances were considered by most authorities to be primarily orthopedic tools to influence the facial skeleton of the growing child in the condylar and sutural area so as to achieve a skeletal improvement. However, these appliances can also exert orthodontic effects in the dentoalveolar region. The uniqueness of the functional appliances lies in their mode of efficacy. They do not act on the teeth in a similar manner to conventional mechanical appliances, but rather transmit muscular forces while guiding the growth process and the eruption of the teeth by utilization, activation, and inhibition of natural forces–which signify the growth potential, the eruption potential, and the muscular forces.

The Principles of Functional Appliances

The influences of natural forces and functional stimulation on form were first reported by Roux in 1883 as result of studies performed on the tail fins of dolphins. Roux described the characteristics of functional stimuli as they build, mold, remold, and preserve the tissues (see Roux 1895). His working hypothesis became the biomechanical background of both general orthopedics and functional jaw orthopedics. Wolf (1892), Benninghof (1934), and Pauwels (1960) also described the biomechanics and the interaction between mechanical function and morphological design.

The clinical aspects of the Roux hypothesis had already been applied by Robin (1902), treating children with his "monobloc" as indicated in cases with glossoptosis. Andersen used a similar appliance termed a "working retainer" for children going away on long holidays in Norway. Häupl (1938) saw the potential of Roux's hypothesis and applied his concepts to the correction of jaw and dental arch deformities using functional stimuli.

According to Häupl, functional jaw orthopedics can only be performed with appliances that are "passive" and that transmit only the muscular stimulus. Because of their abilities to transfer muscular forces from one area to another, the functional orthopedic appliances were considered transformators.

Despite this biological approach, the principle of Häupl and its application to activator therapy produced some detrimental consequences for the development of orthodontics in Europe. Many orthodontists were convinced that only treatment with "passive" appliances is tissue preserving. Reitan (1951) showed that no special histological outcome resulted from the use of functional appliances. Now we know that there exists no "passive" force. The force can be mechanical or muscular in origin (artificially activated muscle force), with the same result—strain of the tissues. The results of the foregoing research necessitate alteration of the original treatment concept. The clinician can combine various therapeutic methods either consecutively or simultaneously. None of these methods produces a unique quality of reaction.

Forces

The forces employed in orthodontic and orthopedic procedures include both tensile and shearing forces. Tensile forces cause stress and strain in functional therapy. They also alter the stomatognathic muscle balance. Both external (primary) and internal (secondary) forces can be observed in each force application. External forces include forces acting on the dentition include both occlusal and muscular forces. Internal forces are the reaction of tissues to the primary forces. They strain the contiguous tissues, leading to the formation of an osteogenic guiding structure. This reaction is important for secondary tissue adaptation.

Treatment Principles

Applied forces may be compressive or tensile. Depending on the type of force applied, two treatment principles can be differentiated: force application and force elimination.
1. In *force application*, compressive stress and strain act on the structures involved, resulting in a primary alteration in form with a secondary adaptation in function.
2. In *force elimination*, disturbing and restrictive environmental influences are eliminated, allowing optimal development. Function is rehabilitated and this is followed by a secondary adaptation of tissues. During the elimination of pressure, a tensile strain can arise as a result of the viscoelastic displacement of periosteum and the bone-forming response in affected areas.

To achieve tooth movements, one of these force components can be eliminated (Fig. 4.1 left) or additional force can be used (right).

What is functional therapy?
- *Functional jaw orthopedics:*
  working with force application
- *Functional orthodontics:*
  working with force application or elimination
- *Function regulation:*
  working with force elimination
- *Interceptive therapy:*
  working with force elimination or application
- *Inhibitory treatment:*
  working with force elimination
- *Screening therapy:*
  working with force elimination

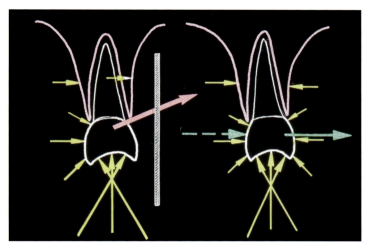

Fig. 4.1 **Various possibilities for tooth movement.** Natural forces are effective on the teeth from all directions. To achieve tooth movements, one of those components can be eliminated (left) or an additional force can be used (right).

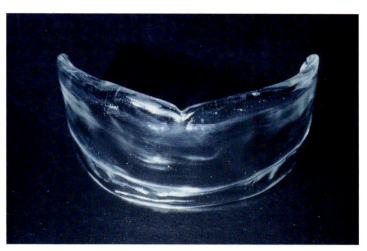

Fig. 4.2 **Vestibular screen.**

Functional Therapy by Force Elimination: Screening Therapy

A number of appliances influence primarily the lip, cheek, and tongue muscles. They can guide the stomatognathic function (as does the Fränkel regulator) or can work solely by eliminating unwanted muscular influences to enable undisturbed development of the orofacial system (as in the vestibular screen and its modifications). The application of protective barriers in the path of abnormal muscle forces has also been termed inhibitory treatment because its purpose is to inhibit the deformative influences of the soft tissues. In any case, the possibilities and limitations of orthodontic treatment determine the reaction and adaptation of the soft tissues and function. This means that stability depends on the limits of soft-tissue adaptation, and we can differentiate between "adapters" showing stability and "nonadapters" showing relapse. Screening therapy is indicated only in cases with normal hereditary pattern, which means an environmental malocclusions. To give a normal hereditary pattern the best chance to express itself, or to correct the effects of environmental insult, interceptive therapy must be started early so that it has the greatest opportunity for adaptation and the greatest amount of growth with which to work. The therapeutic measures interrupt the abnormal reflex pattern and reestablish normal exteroceptive and proprioceptive engrams, to promote an inherently normal developmental pattern. For example, in cases of habitual mouth breathing, both the anterior and posterior oral seals are not closed, and the tongue is low and flat. By treating this nonphysiological reflex pattern of habitual mouth breathing with a vestibular screen, the clinician provides a substitute for the anterior lip seal and aids the subsequent establishment of the lip seal with the therapy.

The goals of treatment with vestibular screen are:
1. Elimination of the noxious influences of the soft tissues.
2. Change of the equilibrium between the intraoral and perioral muscle groups.
3. Elimination of the pressure of some muscles, thereby strengthening the force of the antagonists.

The scope of functional orthodontics is movements of the teeth during or after their eruption:
- Actively, with guiding planes of the activator.
- Passively, by elimination of the harmful forces hindering tooth eruption with the screening appliance.

The preconditions for screening therapy are:
- Normal endogenous developmental tendency.
- To treat while there is still a good growth potential in the orofacial system, which means causal and early treatment during the period of high potential for growth.

Appliance Construction

The Vestibular Screen

The basic appliance for screening therapy is the vestibular screen (Fig. 4.2). Common modifications include the lower lip shield, the tongue crib, a combination of vestibular screen and tongue crib, and the vestibular screen with breathing holes. The inner arch of the headgear, the lip bumper, and the buccinator loop of the bionator have a screening side-effect.

The effectiveness of the vestibular screen depends on its correct construction. The construction bite is an edge-to-edge bite, taken without consideration of the facial pattern. In activator therapy the mandible is guided into a predetermined position by the construction bite, and exact planning is required to achieve this relationship. In contrast, the construction bite for the screening treatment does not predetermine a precise mandibular forward posture but should enable (or at least not hinder) a forward repositioning of the mandible. After elimination of abnormal perioral function, the mandible should return to its normal centric-relation balanced posture; the shield does not interfere with this process.

The vestibular shield extends into the vestibular sulcus to the labial fold. Care must be taken not to impinge on muscle attachments, the frenum, or other structures. The desired extension of the screen should be outlined with a pencil on the models (Fig. 4.3). The appliance extends vertically from the upper and lower fold and distally to the distal margin of the last erupted mo-

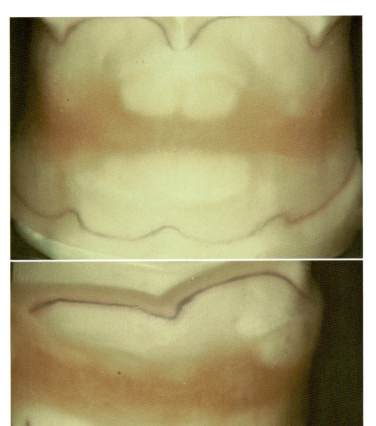

Fig. 4.3 **Casts in construction bite prepared for fabrication of vestibular screen and covered with a wax layer.** The extent of the appliance is marked.
a Lateral view – bottom.
b Frontal view – top.

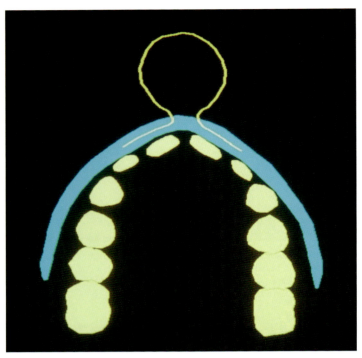

Fig. 4.4 **Incorrect construction of an old type of vestibular screen loading the upper incisors.**

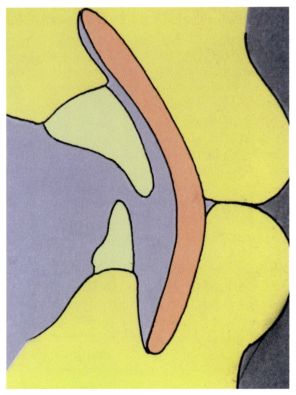

Fig. 4.5 **The anchorage of the vestibular screen is in the labial fold, but there should not be a contact with the alveolar process.**

lar. A comfortable lip seal must be maintained. During the treatment, the mandible, the alveolar process, and the teeth should be relieved (Fig. 4.4). To avoid contact with these structures, the articulated models are covered with a 2–3 mm wax layer over the labial surface of the teeth and alveolar process to ensure, that during fabrication of the shield, unwanted pressure is not generated (Fig. 4.5). The completed vestibular screen should be in contact only with the upper and lower labial fold, during the anterior positioning of the mandible. The shield is fabricated without a holding ring, which might interfere with the desired lip seal.

The appliance should be worn at night and at least 2–3 hours per day. Lip exercises can make the appliance a potent tool because they teach the patient the importance of an adequate lip seal.

The appliance is effective in eliminating sucking habits and lip and tongue dysfunctions. The shield interrupts the contact between the tip of the tongue and the lower lip, a vestige of the infantile swallowing pattern. This leads to a maturation of the deglutitional cycle and creates a somatic swallowing pattern. Some patients, however, persist in thrusting the tongue even with the screen in place. In such instances, a lingual restricting tongue screen in also needed and can be added to the vestibular screen (Fig. 4.6).

Many variations of the basic screen are available; the shield can be modified to specific needs and morphology, eliminating pressure in particular areas. However, all such constructions should follow the principles elucidated.

Functional Therapy by Force Elimination: Screening Therapy 71

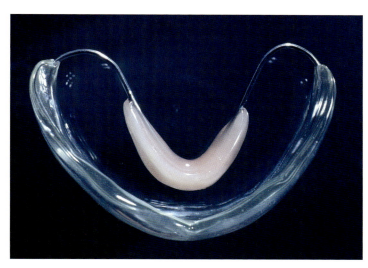

Fig. 4.6 Vestibular screen with tongue shield.

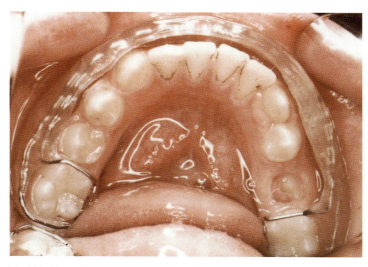

Fig. 4.7 Lower lip shield.

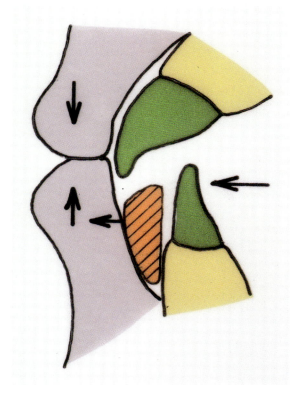

Fig. 4.8 Efficacy of the lower lip screen in the presence of labial movement. Reestablishment of the lip seal and contact between and the tip of the tongue and the lower lip is interrupted, without interference from anterior positioning of the tongue.

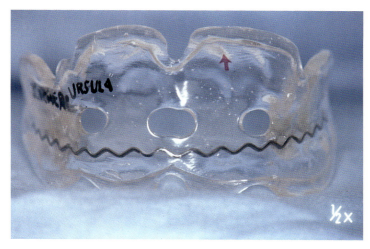

Fig. 4.9 Vestibular screen with holes.

Lower Lip Shield

The lower lip shield is actually the lower half of a full vestibular shield (Fig. 4.7). It is extended into the vestibular sulcus to the labial fold and the distal margin of the last molar. It is fabricated on the lower cast in which the wax layer has been placed. The shield makes contact only in the depth of the lower vestibular sulcus. The occlusal relationship should be considered. It extends superiorly to the incisal third of the lower teeth. However, if this relationship disturbs the occlusion, the margin must be reduced.

No contact should occur between the shield and the upper or lower incisors. Anchorage of the appliance can be improved after eruption of the permanent first molars by adding reverse Adams clasps.

The lower lip shield eliminates the persistence of hyperactivity of the mentalis muscle, which forces the lower lip into the overjet space.

The only indication for this type of appliance is elimination of abnormal lower lip function in Class II Division 1 malocclusions. The shield alters the functional equilibrium of the orofacial musculature, moving the lower lip anteriorly. However, if the incisors are tipped labially before treatment, the tongue activity can create undesirable procumbency. Thus, lower vestibular shields are contraindicated in patients in whom there is already excessive labial tipping of the lower incisors (Fig. 4.8).

Vestibular Screen with Breathing Holes

The use of three small holes at the interincisal level of the vestibular shield enhances wearability for patients who have difficulties breathing through the nose (Fig. 4.9). Habitual mouth breathers adjust better with this modification. The holes can be gradually reduced, which stimulates nose respiration. Many children con-

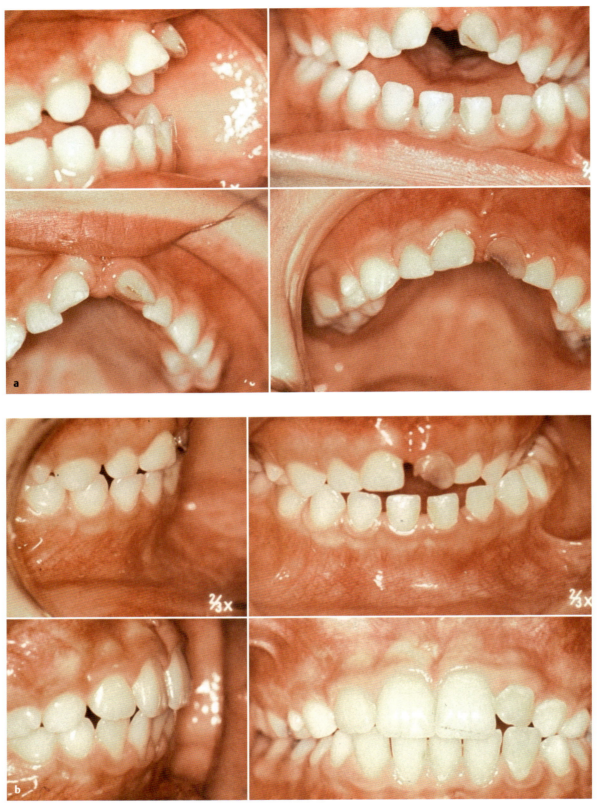

Fig. 4.10
a A 3-year-old boy with sucking habit, severe open bite, and crossbite (top). The upper dental arch before treatment and after treatment with the vestibular screen (bottom).
b The same patient after 5 month of treatment.

tinue mouth breathing after removal of adenoids; in such cases the adenoids can proliferate again. Thus the vestibular screen can be used at a critical time to break the habit and assist in conversion of a mouth breather to a nose breather, preventing the need for later surgery.

Indications for Screening Therapy

Screening appliances are to be used only in the deciduous and mixed dentition.

Indication in the Deciduous Dentition

Screening appliances intercept and eliminate all abnormal perioral and intraoral muscle functions in acquired malocclusions resulting from abnormal habits, and also mouth breathing. Open bites created by finger sucking and retained visceral deglutitional pattern tongue function can be helped with vestibular screens to improve the function.

For hyperkinetic children or for those with potential behavior problems who exhibit persistent finger sucking and concomitant tongue thrust, the use of vestibular screens first is more likely to be successful. One example of such benefits occurred in a 3-year-old boy with severe open-bite malocclusion and bilateral compressed upper arch (Fig. **4.10a**). Because the patient had an intense finger sucking habit and a crossbite in addition to the severe open bite, and because of the unfavorable family history (the sister had an open-bite malocclusion with a vertical growth pattern), treatment was begun at this early age. In spite of the crossbite, because of the severity of open bite and neuromuscular dysfunction, treatment was begun with a vestibular screen. The patient stopped the finger sucking habit, and the open bite and even the upper dental arch form improved within 5 months. The residual crossbite was corrected with an expansion plate (Fig. **4.10b**).

The vestibular screen can also be used in the deciduous dentition as a pretreatment device if an activator or active plate is going to be placed later.

Indication in the Mixed Dentition

The mixed dentition imposes more limitations on the ways in which a screen can be used. Usually a combination screen with an additional method of therapy is necessary.

Screening appliances in the mixed dentition can be used to eliminate the influence of abnormal perioral muscle function, before other treatment is started. Rapid improvement usually occurs in the initial stages of treatment. However, if treatment progress and improvement are minimal despite the elimination of abnormal perioral function, the etiological basis of the malocclusion may be caused by other nonenvironmental factors, requiring different treatment approaches.

Some appliances such as the activator have shortcomings because of their bulk and limited time of wearing during the day. In the presence of an abnormal habit pattern (particularly lip and tongue problems), nocturnal wear may not be sufficient to eliminate the abnormal functional influences and pressure. Patients with lip dysfunctions can wear a lower lip screen; those with tongue thrust problems can use an oral shield (tongue crib) during the day and activators may be worn at night.

The inner arch of the of the headgear and the bumper have a screening side-effect: an expansion of the dental arches. The 10-year-old girl illustrated in Fig. **4.11a,b**) was treated only with a headgear and a bumper. Besides the distalization in the upper and lower arches (Fig. **4.11c,d**) there is also an expansion of the upper and lower dental arches explained by the screening side-effect of both appliances.

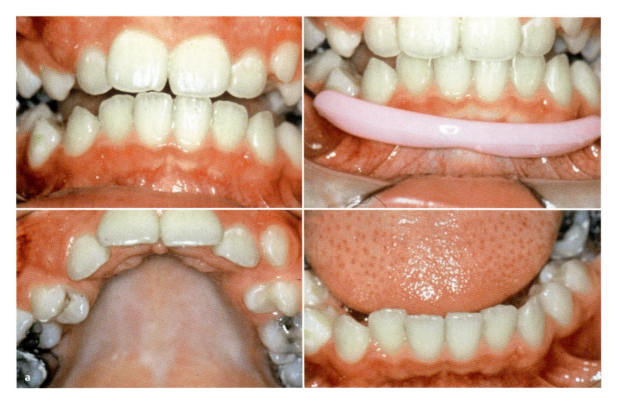

Fig. **4.11a** A 10-year-old girl with crowding in the upper and lower arch and slight open bite.

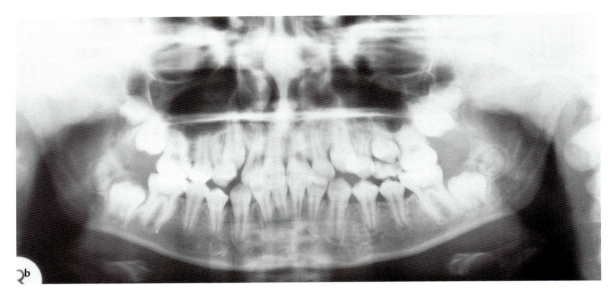

Fig. 4.**11 b** Radiograph of the patient before treatment.

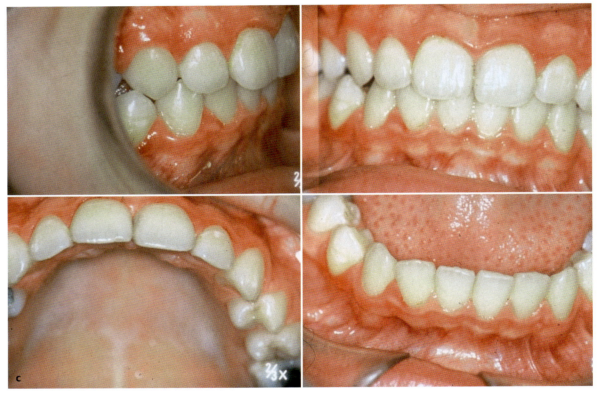

Fig. 4.**11 c** The same patient after treatment with bumper and headgear.

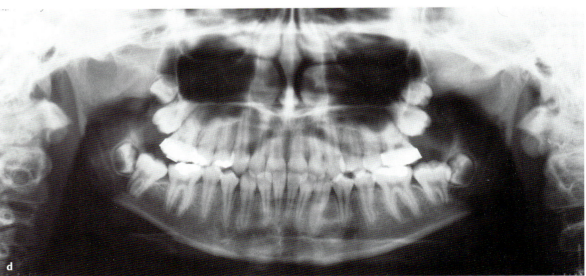

Fig. 4.**11 d** Radiograph of the patient after treatment.

The Activator

What does an activator activate?

An activator artificially activates the muscles of the stomatognathic system by changing the position of the mandible, moving the mandible from the rest position in anterior, posterior, vertical, or lateral directions.

The basic appliance is the activator of Andresen and Häupl, a bulky one-piece appliance—a monobloc—but each appliance that artificially activates mainly the muscles of mastication is an "activator." There are various modifications: one-piece appliances, but reduced in volume (such as the open activator of Klammt [1995] or the bionator of Balthers [1973]); the two-piece appliances connected with wires (such as the appliances of Stockfisch and Bimler [1949]), or the double plates (such as the plates of M. Schwarz, or Sanders, the twin block of Clark [1988]); even the Herbst appliance and the Jasper Jumper artificially activate the musculature.

In the regulation of craniofacial and occlusal development, the environment influences are also important. External influences act as modifiers of the genetic program. Most humans possess a genetic makeup that allows development of normal occlusion, given the correct environmental circumstances. External components of development can be influenced by therapeutic actions: bone and surrounding structures react to external influences.

The activator (and its modifications) are efficacious at the second and third levels of the craniofacial articulation (Moffett 1972) (Fig. 4.12). The third level is that of the sutural and condylar articulation, the area that can be influenced therapeutically by functional jaw orthopedics, exploiting the orthopedic efficacy of the activator.

Considering the **growth process**: growth at the sphenooccipital synchondrosis carries the anterior cranial base and maxilla upward and forward from the foramen magnum; the condylar growth translates the mandible downward and forward from the foramen magnum. These two divergent growths translate the jaw bases (Fig. 4.13). The orthopedic efficacy of the activator is to control the vector lines of growth and to control the translation of the basal bones. **Functional jaw orthopedics** is a treatment of skeletal dysplasia by repositioning of the mandible. The mechanism of treatment is the activated muscle force. The mode of action is dependent on the construction bite.

The goal of **functional orthodontics** is to control eruption (and some movement) of the teeth and apposition of alveolar bone filling between the two divergent growth vectors. The appliances for functional orthodontics are the activator and the screening appliance, and their modifications. The mechanism depends on the trimming of the activator and screening of the dysfunctions. Efficacy arises from the action through the guiding planes and the screening of noxious influences of the soft tissues.

Forces in Activator Therapy

While the functional appliance activates the muscles, various types of forces are created: static, dynamic, and rhythmic.

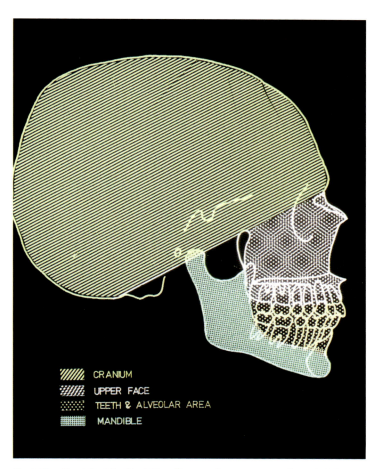

Fig. 4.12 **Craniofacial articulation.** Therapeutic measures can be undertaken with functional orthodontics at the occlusal and periodontal levels and with functional orthopedics at the sutural and condylar levels.

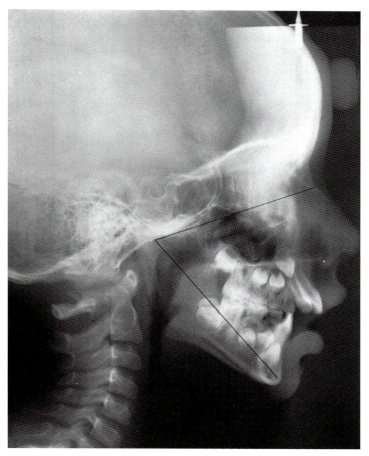

Fig. 4.13 **The two divergent growth vectors carrying the jaw bases anteriorly.**

1. *Static* forces are permanent and can vary in magnitude and direction. They do not appear simultaneously with movement of the mandible. The forces of gravity, posture, and elasticity of soft tissues and muscles are in this category.
2. *Dynamic forces* are interrupted and inconstant. They appear simultaneously with movements of the head, body, and mandible; they have greater magnitude than static forces. The frequency and magnitude of these forces depend on the design and construction of the appliance and on the patient's reaction. Swallowing, for example, produces dynamic forces.
3. *Rhythmic forces* are associated with respiration and circulation. They are synchronous with breathing, and their amplitude varies with the pulse. These trophic stimuli are important in stimulating cellular activity. The mandible transmits rhythmic vibrations to the maxilla.

The applied forces are intermittent and interrupted. Force application to the teeth and mandible is intermittent. Removal the activator from the mouth interrupts these forces.

The **types of forces** arising in activator therapy may be categorized as follows:
1. Growth guidance, including the eruption and migration of teeth, produces natural forces. These can be guided, promoted, and inhibited by the treatment.
2. Muscle contractions and stretching of the soft tissues initiate forces when the mandible is relocated from its postural rest position by the appliance. The activator stimulates and transforms these contractions. Whereas the forces may be functional (muscular) in origin, their activation is artificial. These artificially functioning forces can be effective in all three planes:
   - In the sagittal plane the mandible is propelled downward and forward, so that the muscle force is delivered to the condyles and a strain is produced in the condylar region. A slight reciprocal force can be transmitted to the maxilla.
   - In the vertical plane the teeth and alveolar processes are either loaded with or relieved of normal forces. If the construction bite is high, a greater strain is produced in the contiguous tissues. If transmitted to the maxilla, these forces can inhibit growth increment and direction and influence the inclination of the maxillary base (see later, mode of action II and "V" activator).
   - In the transverse plane, forces can also be created with midline correction, but only mandibular shift (skeletal) and never dental midline shift should be treated with the activator.
3. Various active elements (e.g., springs, screws) can be built into the activator to produce an active biomechanical type of force application. This mode of treatment is contradictory to the concept of Häupl, but from the research of Reitan we know that it is allowable to use mechanical elements in combination with the activator treatment.

Mode of action of the activator

Generally speaking, with the activator we can increase isometric muscle contractions, or increase the effect of myostatic reflex activity, and utilize the viscoelastic properties of the soft tissues and muscles. These viscoelastic properties are:

- Emptying of vessels
- Expression of interstitial fluid
- Stretching of fibers
- Elastic deformation of bone
- Bioplastic adaptation

The mode of action varies according to the construction of the appliance, especially depending on the mode of the construction bite. Depending on the construction of the appliance, we can differentiate between two modes of action:

Mode I. The forces generated in activator therapy are caused by muscle contractions and myostatic reflex activity. A loose appliance stimulates the muscles, and the moving appliance moves the teeth. The appliance applies intermittent forces utilizing the kinetic energy.

The preconditions for this mode of treatment are an anterior dislocated mandible with a low construction bite and a loose appliance (trimming of the appliance).

For this mode of treatment we construct the "horizontal" activator which is indicated in cases with horizontal growth pattern (see later).

Mode II. The appliance is squeezed between the jaws in a splinting action. The appliance exerts forces that moves the teeth in this rigid position. The stretch reflex is activated, inherent tissue elasticity is operative, and strain occurs without intermittent movements. The appliance works using potential energy. For this mode of action an overcompensation of the construction bite in the vertical plane is necessary (high construction bite). An efficient stretch action is achieved by overcompensation and exploitation of the viscoelastic properties of soft tissues.

For this mode of treatment we construct the "vertical" activator with a high and only slightly forward-postured construction bite. It is Indicated in cases with vertical growth pattern.

The **peculiarities** of the activator therapy
- Disocclusion of the dentition
- Maintenance of an anterior and inferior condylar position, depending on the construction bite
- Differential effect on the eruption of teeth, depending on trimming
- Use of forces that are no greater than those produced by the patient's own musculature. *Disocclusion:* The intercuspidation has the function of a "comparator" for the intermaxillary relationships. The disocclusion represents a deregulation, which promotes mandibular growth. The effect of disocclusion of the functional appliances is to promote mandibular growth, contrary to the fixed appliances without this effect.

Construction Bite

Before the construction bite is taken, an exact plane is necessary. In preparation, the clinician needs to make detailed study with plastic casts and cephalometric and panoral head films, and to analyze the patient's functional pattern. Patient compliance is essential. The patient's motivation should be also determined.

Study Model Analysis

The nature of midline discrepancy, if any, is to be identified: if the midlines are not coincident, a functional analysis should be made to determine the path of closure from postural rest to occlusion; if the midline changes, a functional problem amenable to correction in the appliance is likely. Dentoalveolar noncoincident midlines cannot be corrected by functional appliances.

Additionally, the symmetry of dental arches, the curve of Spee, and crowding should be examined.

Functional Analysis

1. Registration of the postural rest position in natural head posture. For the construction bite we activate the muscles from this position.
2. Path of closure from postural rest to habitual occlusion (any sagittal or transverse deviations are to be recorded). It is important to differentiate whether, for example, a Class II malocclusion is "true" (the postural rest position is posterior) or functional (the postural rest position is anterior). In the Class II malocclusion, an anterior rest position is favorable for functional treatment; a posterior rest position requires comprehensive treatment with a prolonged time of retention (Fig. 4.14).
3. Prematurities, point of initial contact, occlusal interferences, and resultant mandibular displacement: some of these can be eliminated with the activator treatment, but some require other therapeutic measures.
4. Examination of the TMJ. Some functional abnormalities of the TMJ necessitate modifications of the appliance design.
5. Interocclusal clearance or freeway space has two stages: a free stage (closing until the first occlusal contact) and an occlusal stage (from the first contact until full occlusion). This relationship should be checked.
6. Respiration. With disturbed nasal respiration or enlarged tonsils (Fig. 4.15) the patient cannot wear a bulky appliance; the respiratory abnormalities should be eliminated first (see vestibular screen with holes in habitual mouth breathing, Fig. 4.9).

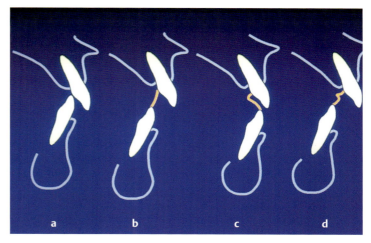

Fig. 4.14 During closing from the rest position, several relationships can occur. **a** Occlusal relationship; **b** normal hinge movement; **c** anterior postural rest position; **d** posterior postural rest position.

Cephalometric Analysis

The diagnostic tool of cephalometric analysis enables the clinician to identify the craniofacial morphogenetic pattern to be treated. The most important information required for planning the construction bite is the following:

1. The direction of the growth of the mandible can be average, vertical, or horizontal. The maxilla can be ante- or retro-inclined. The combination of the inclinations of the jaw bases is decisive for the treatment planning and possibilities. The growth pattern of the mandible can be vertical or there can be an anteinclination of the maxilla (Fig. 4.16). In these cases the treatment can be provided with a vertical activator. If there is a divergent growth pattern (a vertical growth pattern with anteinclination of the maxilla) a functional treatment with the activator is contraindicated.
2. Differentiation between position and size of the jaw bases. In a Class II malocclusion, for example, the mandible can be retrognathic because of a posterior position of a long mandible or because the mandible is short.
3. Morphological peculiarities, particularly of the mandible, may assist in determining the course of the development.

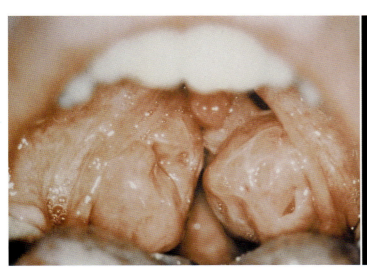
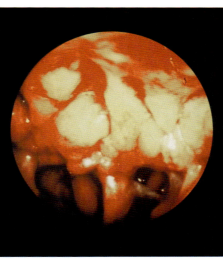

Fig. 4.15 Nasal respiration can be disturbed by enlarged tonsils or adenoids.

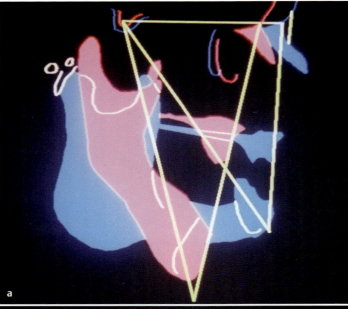

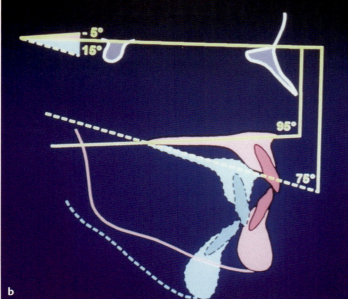

Fig. 4.16 **a** Vertical growth pattern of the mandible. **b** Anteinclination of the base of the maxilla.

4. Axial inclination and position of the upper and lower incisors provide important clues for determining the anterior positioning of the mandible required and particularly details of the appliance design for the incisor area.

Types of Construction Bites

1. Low construction bite with forward positioning of the mandible.
   Corresponds to the "H" activator with mode I of action.
2. High construction bite with slight forward posturing.
   Corresponds to the "V" activator with mode II of action
3. Bite without forward posturing
   - Moderate high
     indication: open bite, deep bite
   - Low
     indication: crowding, appliance with screws
4. Construction bite with retrusion of the mandible.
   For treatment of Class III malocclusion

Note:
1. The wax registration must be individualized depending on the configuration of the facial skeleton and the inclination of the incisors.
2. The trimming of the appliance must be according to an exact plane.

Rules for the two Variations of the Construction Bites

- Construction bite for the "H" activator: forward positioning 7–8 mm ahead of the postural rest position and opening only 2–4 mm. Mode of action I.
- Construction bite for the "V" activator: forward positioning 3–5 mm; opening of 4–6 mm below the postural rest position. Mode of action II.

Execution of the Construction Bite

A horseshoe-shaped wax rim is prepared for insertion between the maxillary and mandibular teeth. It should have proper arch form and size and adequate width and be 2–3 mm thicker than the planned construction bite. If the rim is placed on the lower arch, the mandible can be guided into the desired anterior position required for the treatment of the Class II malocclusion. If the wax rim is placed on the upper arch, the mandible can be moved into a retruded position required for the construction of a Class III activator. During the closing movement, the operator controls the edge-to-edge incisor relationship and the midline registration. The wax is carefully removed from the mouth and checked on the upper and lower models. The construction bite should always be taken on the patient and not on the models.

Low Construction Bite with Markedly Forward Positioning of the Mandible

The mandible is positioned anteriorly to achieve an edge-to-edge relationship parallel to the functional occlusal plane. In Class II retrusion cases that show posterior displacement from the postural rest position to habitual occlusion, the mandible can be positioned to a greater degree anteriorly than can be done in true Class II malocclusions with a normal (hinge axis) path of closure (with posterior postural rest position). The general rule is that the construction bite should be at most 3 mm posterior to the maximal protrusive position of the mandible.

The activator constructed with low vertical opening registration and a forward bite is appropriately designed the horizontal "H" activator (Fig 4.17 a, b). With this type of appliance (and the corresponding growth pattern), the mandible can be postured forward and the axial inclination of the incisors can be positioned upright. No additional dentoalveolar compensation is necessary as in cases with vertical growth pattern.

The 10-year-old girl illustrated in Fig. 4.18 had a biprotrusion with horizontal growth pattern (Fig. 4.18 a top – bottom); typical of cases with tongue thrust. The patient was treated with an "H" activator having upper and lower labial bows. Thanks to the horizontal growth pattern it was possible, during anterior positioning also to upright the lower incisors (from 105° to 96°) (Fig. 4.18 c, d).

High Construction Bite with Slightly Anterior Positioning of the Mandible

In the high construction bite the mandible is positioned less anterior (only 3–5 mm ahead of the habitual occlusal position). Depending on the magnitude of the interocclusal space (free-way space), the vertical dimension is opened a maximum of 4 mm beyond the postural rest–vertical dimension registration. Possibly stretching of the muscles and soft tissues elicits an additional force, causing a response in viscoelastic properties of the soft tissues involved. The activation of the stretch reflex with the increased vertical dimension may well influence the inclination of the maxillary base. The appliance is indicated in Class II cases with vertical growth pattern or anteinclination of the maxilla. It can be properly designated as the vertical "V" activator (Fig. 4.19 a, b).

The Class II malocclusion with vertical growth pattern cannot be significantly improved sagittally by anterior positioning of the mandible. The mandible can be moved only forward and downward. To achieve a good occlusal relationship, some additional compensatory mechanism are necessary: a dentoalveolar compensation and an adaptation of the maxilla to the lower dental arch—a retroinclination of the maxillary base.

The 9 years old girl depicted in Fig. 4.20 a was treated with a vertical activator. The results seem to be satisfactory (Fig. 4.20 b). The cephalometric analysis (Fig. 4.20 c, d) shows that although the mandible was postured forward (ANB angle from 8° to 3. 6°) and downward, because of the vertical growth pattern an additional dentoalveolar compensation was necessary by lingual tipping of the upper incisors and labial tipping of the lower incisors.

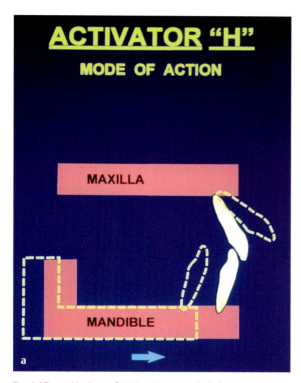

Fig. 4.17 **a Horizontal "H" activator** with slight opening, forward posturing of the mandible, and uprighting of the incisors.

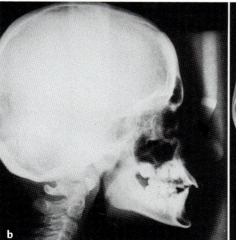 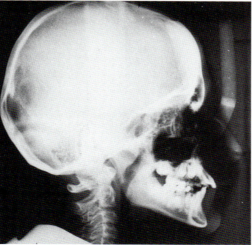 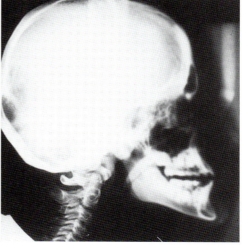

b The construction bite: *left*, occlusal position; *center*, postural rest position; *right*, construction bite position.

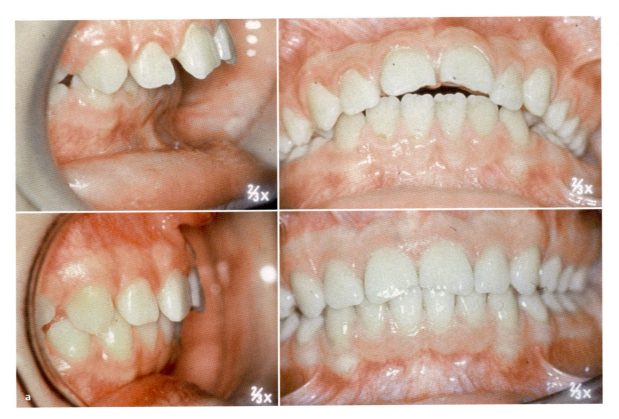

Fig. 4.18
a A 10-year-old girl with biprotrusion and horizontal growth pattern (Top). The same patient after 3 years of treatment with the "H" activator (Bottom).

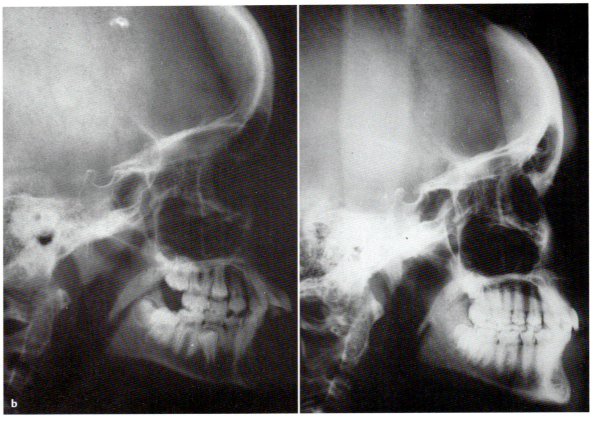

b Cephalograms of the patient before and after treatment.

The Activator

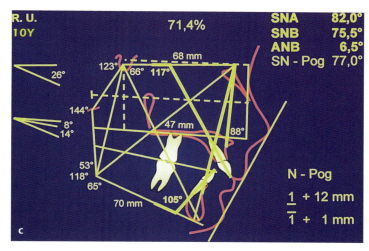

c The tracings of the patient before treatment.

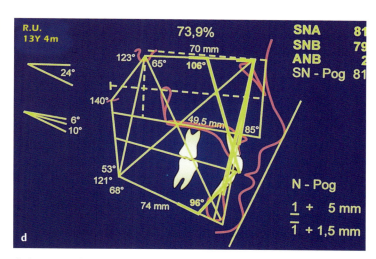

d The tracing after treatment. The lower incisors were uprighted during anterior posturing of the mandible.

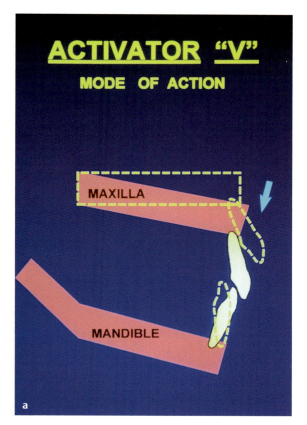

Fig. 4.19 a The vertical "V" activator with slight anterior-inferior posturing of the mandible, retroinclination of the maxillary base, and dentoalveolar compensation of the Class II relationship.

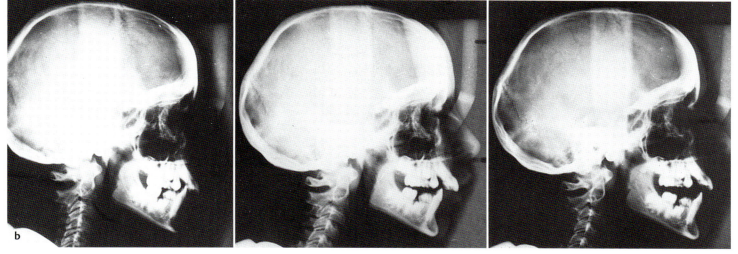

b The construction bite: *left*, occlusal position; *middle*, postural rest position; *right*, construction bite position.

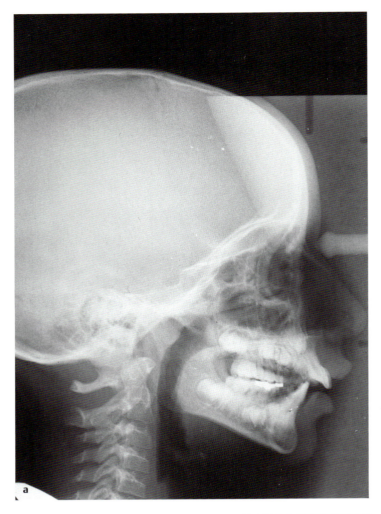
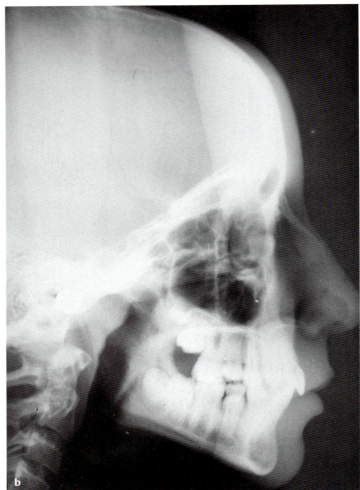
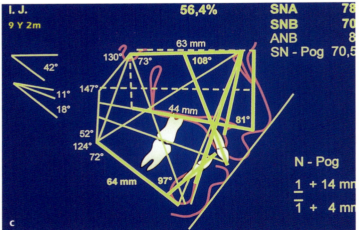
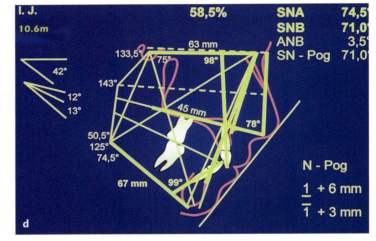

Fig. 4.20 **a** A 9-year-old girl treated with a vertical activator. **b** The results seem to be satisfactory. **c** Tracing of the same patient before treatment: a vertical growth pattern with labial tipping of the lower incisors. **c** Treatment with the activator was only possible, because of the retroinclination of the maxilla (partial compensation of the vertical growth pattern). **d** Tracing after the treatment: although the ANB angle improved, because of the vertical growth pattern the lower incisors could not be uprighted.

Construction Bite without Forward Positioning of the Mandible

Forward positioning of the mandible is not indicated in the activator construction if a correction in the sagittal plane is not necessary. Such appliances are used primarily in vertical dimension problems (deep overbite and open bite) and in selected cases of crowding.

Vertical Problems

Deep Overbite Malocclusion

Deep overbite malocclusion can be either dentoalveolar in origin or skeletal in nature. In dentoalveolar overbite, the deep overbite can be caused by infraocclusion of the buccal segments or supraocclusion of the anterior segments. Fig. 4.21 a shows a deep overbite caused by infraocclusion of the molars, Fig. 4.21 b caused by supraocclusion of the incisors. Functional treatment is indicated in cases with infraocclusion of the molars. The free-way space is large. The cause is mostly an interposition of the tongue. The activator can be trimmed to permit the extrusion of the molars, or with a bilateral screening appliance (Fig. 4.22) the tongue dysfunction can be eliminated.

In cases with supraocclusion of the incisors, the free-way space is small and an intrusion of the incisors should be the first step of the treatment, which can be provided only with multibracket appliances.

Open-Bite Malocclusion

Anterior positioning of the mandible is not necessary if the skeletal relationship is orthognathic. The dentoalveolar open bite can be treated with screening appliances or with proper trimming of the activator (Fig. 4.23). The bite is opened 4–5 mm below the postural rest position to develop sufficient elastic depressive force and load the molars that are in premature contact.

The skeletal open bite can be treated with the vertical "V" activator under the precondition that the growth pattern is not divergent (vertical growth pattern with anteinclination of the maxilla). Cases with divergent growth pattern require a difficult and long treatment, sometimes combined with orthognathic surgery.

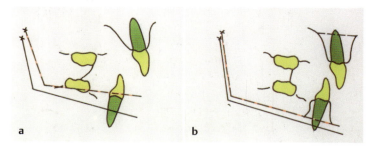

Fig. 4.21 **Dentoalveolar deep overbite** caused by (**a**) infraocclusion of the buccal segments with long interocclusal clearance, (**b**) supraocclusion of the incisors with short interocclusal clearance.

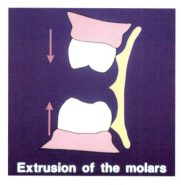 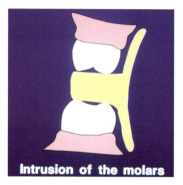

Fig. 4.22 Trimming of the activator for extrusion of the molars.

Fig. 4.23 Trimming of the activator for intrusion of the molars.

Arch Length Deficiency Problems

Malocclusions with crowding can sometimes be treated with the activator. In the mixed dentition period, problems with anchorage can occur with regular expansion plates. The activator can accomplish the desired expansion because of its intermaxillary anchorage.

The appliance works in a manner similar that of two active plates with jackscrews in the upper and lower parts (Fig. 4.24). The construction bite is low because jaw positioning and growth guidance are not desired. The treatment objective is expansion using an appliance stabilized by intermaxillary relationships. It is no longer a functional but an active-mechanical treatment. The

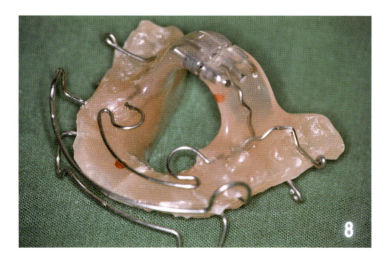

Fig. 4.24 Appliance with two jackscrews to expand the upper and lower dental arch.

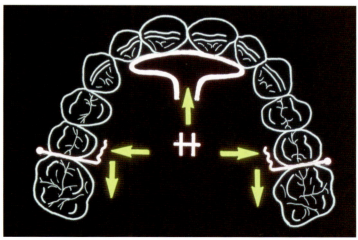

Fig. 4.25 Reciprocal force can be developed in the transversal and sagittal planes simultaneously.

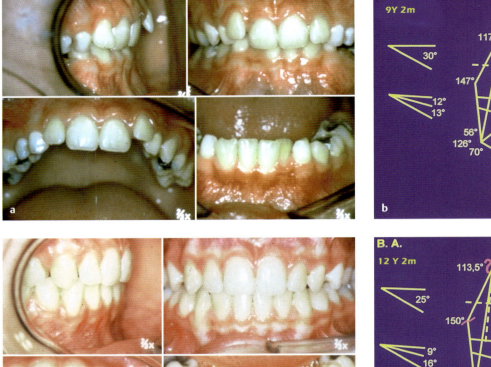
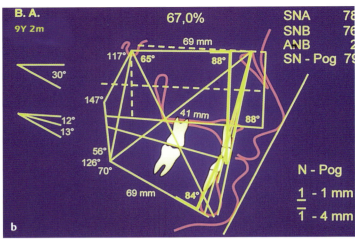
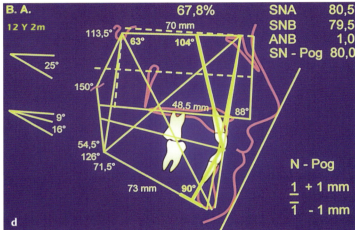

Fig. 4.26 **a** A 9-year-old girl with crowding and lingual tipping of the incisors. **b** Tracing of the patient shows a horizontal growth pattern, no sagittal problem, and lingual tipping of the incisors. **c** The patient 4 years later. **d** Tracing of the patient shows that the incisors are upright and the upper molars have moved distally, thanks to the reciprocal effect of the appliance.

force application of this type of appliance is reciprocal, an advantage in situations in which the demands are usually bilateral (Fig. 4.25). With the same appliance a reciprocal force also can be developed in the sagittal plane If the incisors are lingually declined and the molars must be moved distally to increase the arch length, a protrusive force loading the incisors can be directed onto the stabilizing wires, producing a molar distalization response.

In the 9-year-old girl with horizontal growth pattern shown in Fig. 4.26 a, b, there was crowding in the upper and lower dental arches, lingual tipping of the incisors, and mesial migration of the upper molars. The problem was solved with one appliance with reciprocal effect in the transversal and sagittal planes (Fig. 4.26 c, d).

Construction Bite with Opening and Posterior Positioning of the Mandible

The sagittal change of the construction bite depends on the malocclusion category and the treatment objectives. In Class III malocclusion the goal is a posterior positioning of the mandible, labial relationship with overjet of the upper incisors, and maxillary protraction. The construction bite is taken by retrusion of the mandible. An edge-to-edge bite relationship can be achieved only by opening the bite and the possibility of this opening is limited. If the retrusion of the mandible requires an extreme opening, treatment with the activator is not indicated. In a functional Class III malocclusion with a posterior rest position and anterior sliding in habitual occlusal position (Fig. 4.27), the prognosis is good especially in the deciduous and mixed dentition periods (Fig. 4.28). At this stage the skeletal manifestations are not usually severe, but the malocclusion develops progressively (Fig. 4.29). If it is possible to hold the mandible in a posterior position and guide the maxillary incisors into correct labial relationship with overjet, good incisal guiding can be established. If this is done in the early mixed dentition, the maxilla adapts to the prognathic mandible, creating a balanced relationship.

In Class III malocclusions in the early mixed dentition (Fig. 4.30 a), if there is crowding in the upper dental arch, systematic extractions in both arches are necessary. In this patient a good relationship of the incisors with the activator treatment was achieved (Fig. 4.30 b), because of the pretreatment lingual inclination of the upper incisors. The incisors were uprighted from 83° to 92° (Fig. 4.30 c, d) and the overbite can control the position of the mandible.

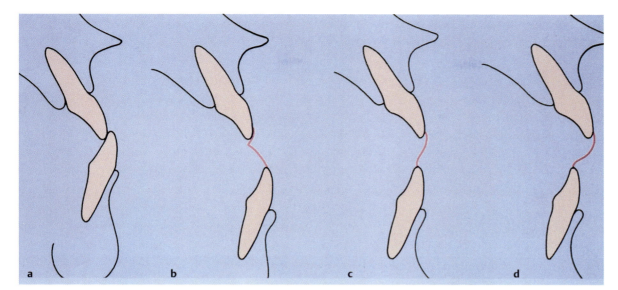

Fig. 4.27 Variations during closing from the postural rest position in the Class III malocclusions. **a** Occlusal relationship; **b** anterior rest position; **c** hinge movement; **d** posterior rest position.

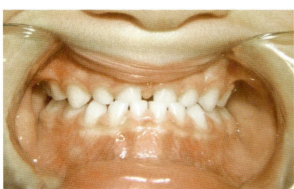
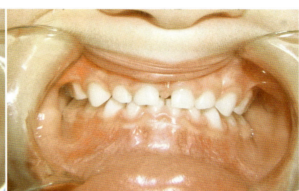

Fig. 4.28 **Class III malocclusion treated in the deciduous dentition.**

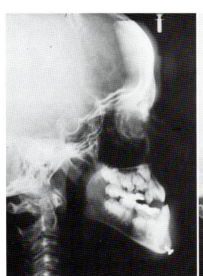
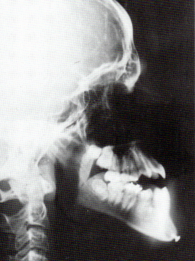
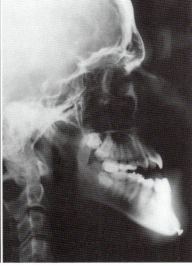

Fig. 4.29 **Progressive development of the Class III malocclusion in an untreated patient between 9 and 16 years of age.**

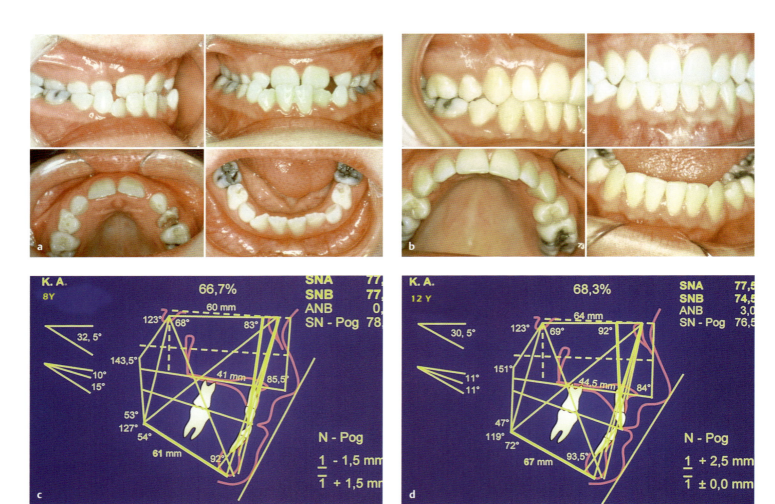

Fig. 4.30 a An 8-year-old patient with Class III malocclusion and crowding in the upper dental arch. b The patient 4 years later after systematic extractions in the upper and lower arch and treatment with a Class III activator. c Tracing before treatment; favorable axial inclination of the upper incisors for the Class III treatment. d Tracing after treatment; the mandible is postured posteriorly. ANB is increased from 0.5° to 3.0°.

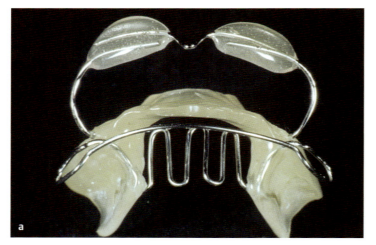
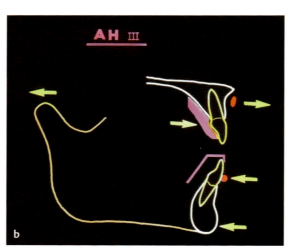

Fig. 4.31 a Activator for the early treatment of Class III malocclusions. b Efficacy of the Class III activator.

The appliance for the early treatment of the Class III malocclusion consists of an upper part contacting the upper incisors and a lower part that in the anterior region is open so as not to contact the incisors. To avoid tongue pressure, a lower lingual crib is incorporated. The pads in the upper fold have a growth-promoting effect in the upper anterior region. The lower labial bow controls the axial inclination of the incisors (Fig. 4.31 a, b). Treatment with functional appliances is not always possible or desirable in true skeletal Class III malocclusion with anterior rest position. The axial inclination of the incisors must be considered for possible dentoalveolar compensation. In general only a combined therapy, such as fixed and removable appliances and maxillary orthopedic protraction, is likely to be successful in severe skeletal Class III malocclusions.

The **most frequent failures in activator therapy** are:
- False indication
- False construction of the appliance
- Oral respiration
- Oral irritation
- Sleeping habits
- Poor motivation

The **preconditions for a successful activator therapy** are:
- The appropriate indication
- Optimal age of the patient
- Appropriate construction of the appliance

The appliance can either be well tolerated or because of some irritation or respiratory problem, the patient can lose it.

Dentoalveolar Effect of the Activator

Therapeutic Trimming for Tooth Guidance

The goal of trimming is to have an appliance without splinting effect, to guide the eruption, and to a limited extent to move the teeth. The guiding planes of the activator can provide movements of the incisors (protrusion, retrusion, intrusion and extrusion) and movements of the molars (intrusion, retrusion, distal, mesial, and transversal movements).

With a loose appliance, guidance of the movements and eruption of selected teeth can best be achieved by grinding away areas of the acrylic that contact the teeth to move the teeth in the desired direction. Any undercut acrylic surface that might interfere with the planed tooth guidance must be removed. The magnitude of force delivered can be estimated by determining the amount of acrylic contact with the tooth surfaces. Force delivered to a small portion of the tooth surface is greater than if broad contact occurs between the acrylic and a larger tooth surface. Acrylic surfaces that transmit the desired intermittent force and contact the teeth are called *guide planes*.

Trimming the Activator for Vertical Control

Two movements occur in the vertical plane: intrusion and extrusion. Some teeth are selectively prevented from erupting, whereas others are free to erupt and are stimulated to do so by acrylic guide planes.

Intrusion of Teeth

Intrusion of incisors can be achieved by loading the incisal edges of these teeth (Fig. 4.**32**). If they are ground properly, they become loaded only on contacting surfaces, with no other contact between the incisors and acrylic, even in the alveolar area. The contact between the labial bow wire and the incisors is below the greatest convexity or on the incisal third. This location does not interfere with intrusive movement of the incisors. Such intrusive loading is indicated in deep overbite cases.

Intrusion of the molars is achieved by loading only the cusps of these teeth (see Fig. 4.**23**). The acrylic detail is ground away from the fossae and fissures to eliminate any possible inclined stimulus to molar movement if only a vertical depressing action is re-

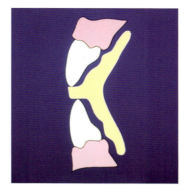
Fig. 4.**32** Intrusion of the incisors.

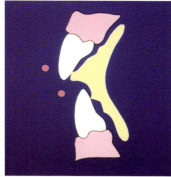
Fig. 4.**33** Extrusion of the incisors.

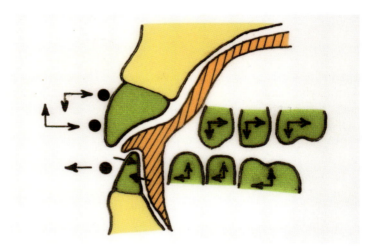
Fig. 4.**34** Various positions of the active and passive labial bow.

quired. Molar depression loading is indicated in open-bite problems if minimal interocclusal clearance is apparent.

Extrusion of Teeth

Extrusion of incisors requires loading their lingual surfaces above the area of greatest concavity in the maxilla and below this area in the mandible (Fig. 4.**33**). The labial bow should be placed above the greatest convexity. Such extrusion modifications are indicated for open-bite problems.

Extrusion of the molars can be facilitated by loading the lingual surfaces of these teeth above the area of greatest convexity in the maxilla and below this area in the mandible (see Fig. 4.**22**). Molar extrusion is indicated in deep overbite problems. The treatment is successful in cases with long free-way space.

Trimming of the Activator for Sagittal Control

Protrusion and retrusion of the incisors can be accomplished only through grinding of the acrylic and guide planes and adjustment of the labial bow wires. If the labial bow touches the teeth, it can either tip them lingually or retain them in position. In these cases it is called an active labial bow. If it is positioned away from the teeth and prevents soft-tissue contact, it is termed a passive labial bow (Fig. 4.**34**). The labial bow does not work as a spring force, however; it is fabricated from relatively thick (0.9 mm) wire and is activated only when the mandible closes in the construction bite position. By relieving pressure and muscle strains placed on

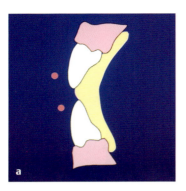
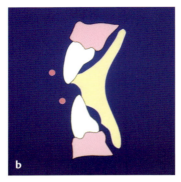

Fig. 4.36 Retrusion of the incisors.

Fig. 4.35 a Protrusion of the incisors. b Labial tipping of the incisors.

the dentition by the lips and cheeks, the passive bow permits labial and buccal movements of teeth.

Protrusion of the Incisors

The incisors can be protruded by loading their lingual surfaces with acrylic contact and screening away the lip strain with passive labial bow or lip pads. The loading can be achieved by either of two methods:
1. The entire lingual surface is loaded (Fig. 4.35a). Only the interdental acrylic projections are trimmed to avoid opening spaces between the teeth. This method allows the incisors to be moved labially with a low magnitude of force because the applied force is spread over a large surface.
2. The incisal third of the lingual surface is loaded (Fig. 4.35b). This variation results in labial tipping of the incisors with a greater degree of force, because the contact surface is small.

Retrusion of the Incisors

The acrylic is trimmed away from the back of the incisors to be retruded. The active labial bow, which contacts the teeth during functional movements, provides the force for moving these teeth.

The acrylic can be completely ground away from behind the incisors and alveolar process (Fig. 4.36). If the labial bow touches the teeth in the incisal margin region, the center of rotation approaches the apex. If the labial bow contacts the gingival third of the incisors, they move coronally toward the junction of the apical and middle third. The gingival position can elongate the incisors depending on the degree of labial convexity. This type of effect is desirable only in open-bite cases, in which both retrusion and elongation are desired. In labially inclined incisor problems with deep bites, every attempt should be made to minimize extrusion of the incisors while they are being axially uprighted.

If an axis of rotation in the middle third of the incisors is desired, the acrylic is trimmed away only in the coronal region, leaving a cervical contact point or fulcrum. The labial bow contacts the incisal third of the labial surfaces, preventing extrusion of the incisor during retraction.

Design of the Activator for the Lower Incisor Area

The conventionally made appliance loads the lingual surfaces of the lower incisors and tips these teeth labially, because of the reciprocal intermaxillary reaction built into the construction bite. This movement is desirable if lingual inclination of the lower incisors has occurred because of the hyperactive mentalis function and lip trap habits.

If the lower incisors are tipped labially before treatment is started in Class II malocclusion, conventional activator therapy is contraindicated. Further protrusion of the incisors not only worsens the axial inclination and lip line profile but also prevents a successful correction of the Class II sagittal malrelationship. Such result is unstable because:
- If the lower incisors are excessively procumbent, they may contact the lingual surface of the maxillary incisors, eliminating the overjet before the buccal segment sagittal malrelationship is corrected.
- If the mandible cannot be adequately postured anteriorly, dental compensation of original skeletal discrepancy occurs. This is acceptable only in cases of vertical growth patterns. With average or horizontal growth vectors, it is a poor treatment regimen for the mixed dentition period.
- If in a horizontal growth pattern, the mandible continues to grow after the treatment is finished (overgrowing the maxilla), a crowding of the lower incisors (the so called secondary crowding) can arise.

Treatment Possibilities

Depending on the axial inclination and position of the incisors, three treatment options are available:
1. Labial tipping of the lower incisors
2. Holding of the incisors in their initial positions
3. Uprighting of the lower incisors while positioning the mandible anteriorly

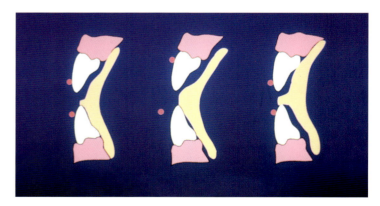

Fig. 4.37 Various design of the acrylics and various position of the labial bow for the incisors.

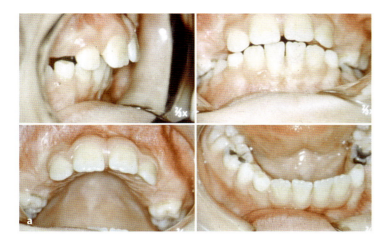
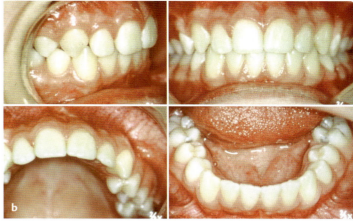

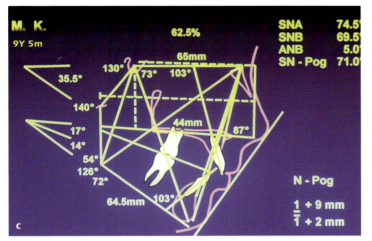
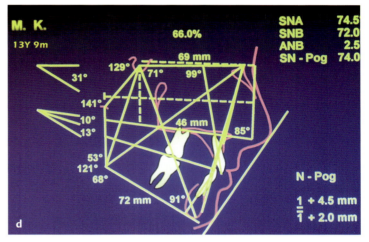

Fig. 4.**38** **a** A girl of 9 years 5 months with small retrognathic mandible and labial tipping of the lower incisors. **b** The same patient 4 years later. **c** Tracing before treatment. **d** Tracing after treatment shows anterior posturing of the mandible with simultaneous uprighting of the lower incisors.

Proclining of the incisors it can be done by loading the entire lingual surface or only the incisal third.

If retrusion or upright of the incisors is required during anterior positioning of the mandible, the design of the lower incisor area should be managed in a more sophisticated manner (Fig. 4.**37**). No contact should occur between the teeth and the acrylic on the lingual surface of the incisors, not even during functional movements of the mandible. An acrylic labial cap holds the incisors. In deep overbite cases, the incisal edges are loaded only from the labial side, creating a lingual movement component through the inclined plane of action while preventing the extrusion. With the labial bow, the incisors can be held or uprighted.

In a 9-year-old girl with retrognathic mandible, the overjet was partially compensated by extreme labial tipping of the lower incisors (Fig. 4.**38a, c**). With the horizontal activator, the mandible was postured anteriorly and simultaneously the incisors were uprighted from 103° to 91° (Fig. 4.**38b, d**).

Design of the Activator for the Upper Incisor Area

In deep overbite cases, the incisal edges are loaded with the acrylic rim. In open-bite cases, the acrylic is ground away to enable the teeth to extrude.

A special design for the upper incisor area is required for retrusive movements in the construction of the vertical activator. In the vertical activator the design for the upper incisor area is similar to that required for retrusion and deep overbite cases, but there are some differences:
1. The labial acrylic cap is extended to the area of greatest convexity at the junction of the incisal and middle thirds of the labial surface (Fig. 4.**39**).
2. The acrylic is completely ground away on the lingual of the incisors and away from the palatogingival tissue contiguous with the incisor alveolar support area.
3. The labial bow contacts the teeth on the gingival third.

This design has a twofold objective: it should influence the axial inclination of the teeth and effect a retroinclination of the anteinclination of the maxillary base.

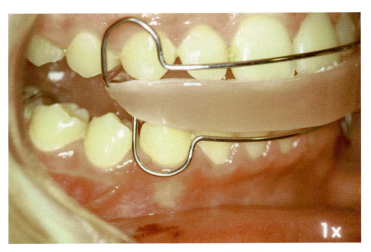

Fig. 4.39 Capping of the incisors in treatment of deep bite overbite.

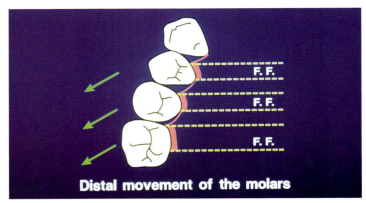

Fig. 4.40 Trimming of the activator for distal movement of the buccal teeth.

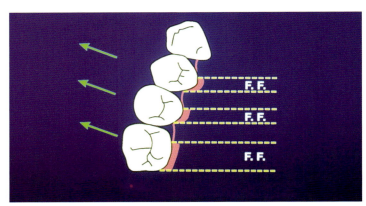

Fig. 4.41 Trimming of the activator for mesial movement of the buccal teeth.

Movements of the Posterior Teeth in the Sagittal Plane

The buccal segments can be moved mesially or distally by the activator. Although large mesiodistal bodily movements are not possible with the activator, modest movements of teeth can be achieved.

For distalizing movements, the guide planes load the molars on the mesiolingual surfaces (Fig. 4.40). The guide plane extends only to the areas of greatest convexity in the mesiodistal plane. A distalizing movement is indicated for the maxillary arch in Class II nonextraction problems. For mesial movements, the guide plane loads the molars on the distolingual surfaces. Mesial movement is indicated for the maxillary arch in Class III malocclusions (Fig. 4.41).

The restoration of normal function is a major contribution to improvement of the morphofunctional interrelationship. If treatment objectives require more orthodontic guidance, functional therapy can continue or a fixed or a removable appliance may be used in the permanent dentition.

The limitations of functional orthodontic therapy should be recognized. First, it should not be considered a stand-alone regimen, a method for full correction of all malocclusions. The elimination of abnormal perioral muscle function and guidance of growth and eruption of the teeth are important treatment objectives, but other facets of malocclusion respond better to other biomechanics and can be addressed separately or with activators and their modifications. The degree of success in treating skeletal problems depends on growth timing and magnitude. Dentoalveolar changes are best accomplished during the eruption of teeth.

The functional appliance is quite effective in treating mandibular retrognathism in patients with horizontal growth pattern. It is less effective in influencing maxillary prognathism or a vertical growth pattern: it is contraindicated in some instances and requires special modifications in others.

A popular and effective modification of the activator is the bionator, introduced by Balthers. This will be discussed because of its special design and anchorage considerations and unique trimming technique. There are some confusions and misapprehensions about the construction of and indications for the bionator. Differences between the activator and bionator are often not stressed sufficiently or sufficiently clearly; accordingly, the principles of construction of and indications for the bionator will be described in some detail.

The Bionator

Principles of Bionator Therapy

The bulkiness of the activator and its limitation to nighttime wear have deterred clinicians interested in attaining the greatest potential of functional growth guidance. In response to the bulkiness of the activator, appliances have been made less bulky and more elastic modifications have been introduced that improve the efficiency of the activator and facilitate daytime use.

The bionator is the prototype of a less bulky appliance. Its lower portion is narrow, and its upper part has only lateral extensions, with a crosspalatal stabilizing bar. The palate is free for proprioceptive contact with the tongue: the buccinator loop of the labial bow holds away potentially deforming muscular action (Fig. 4.42). The appliance may be worn continuously, except during meals. Balthers (1973) developed the original appliance during the early 1950. Although the theoretical principles of the bionator are based on the works of Robin (1902), Andresen (1938) and Häupl (1938), it is different from the activator.

Balthers believed that only the role of the tongue is decisive. According to Balthers, the equilibrium between the tongue and

The Bionator

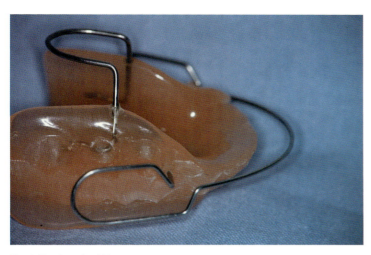

Fig. 4.**42** Standard bionator.

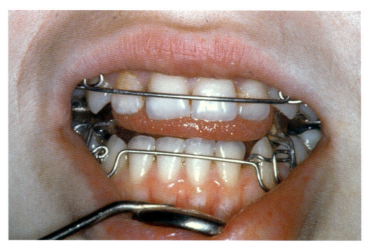

Fig. 4.**44** If an activator with high construction bite is anteriorly open, the patient can acquire a tongue-thrust habit.

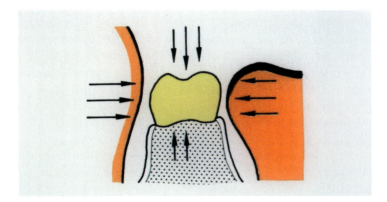

Fig. 4.**43** Equilibrium between the tongue and circumoral muscles.

the circumoral muscles is responsible for the shape of the dental arches and intercuspidation (Fig. 4.**43**). The functional space for the tongue is essential to the normal development of the orofacial system. This hypothesis supports the early function and form concept of van der Klaauw (1946) and the later functional matrix theory of Moos (1960). For Balthers, the tongue (as the center of reflex activity in the oral cavity) was the most important factor in the etiology and therapy of malocclusions. A discoordination of its function could lead to actual deformations. The purpose of the bionator is to establish good functional coordination and eliminate deforming, growth-restricting aberrations.

Balthers thought that the position of the tongue should be considered carefully in planning the therapy, because it is responsible for certain types of malocclusions: posterior displacement of the tongue could lead to Class II relationship; low anterior displacement of the tongue could cause Class III relationship; narrowing of the arches with resultant crowding—particularly of the upper dental arch—is a result of diminished outward pressure of the tongue during postural rest position and function, as opposed to the perioral forces of the buccinator mechanism; open bite is the consequence of hyperactivity and forward posturing of the tongue.

Convinced of the tongue's dominant role, Balthers designed his appliance to take advantage of the tongue posture. He constructed it to position the mandible anteriorly, with incisors in edge-to-edge relationship, which he considered important for natural bodily orientation and to control the tongue's position, because the forward posturing of the mandible enlarged the oral space, bringing the dorsum of the tongue into contact with the soft palate and helping to accomplish lip closure.

The principle of treatment with the bionator is not primarily to activate the muscles but rather to modulate muscle activity, thereby enhancing normal development of the inherent growth pattern and eliminating abnormal and potentially deforming environmental factors. In this light, the bionator falls between a screening appliance and an activator.

Unlike the construction bite of the activator, that of the bionator cannot make allowances for facial pattern and growth direction by variation in vertical opening as the mandible is postured forward. The bite cannot be opened and must be positioned in an edge-to-edge relationship. If the overjet is too large, the forward posturing can be done step-by-step, but it will still not open the bite. Balthers reasoned that a high construction bite could impair the tongue function and the patient could actually acquire a tongue-thrust habit (Fig. 4.**44**).

Because no allowance is made for the vertical component except in guiding the eruption of the posterior teeth, the indication is limited for this appliance. The labial bow and the palatal bar directly influence the behavior of the lips and tongue. Nevertheless, the main consideration is to influence the function of the tongue, in contrast, for example, with the Fränkel appliance, whose main aim is to influence the outer neuromuscular envelope.

Recent functional analysis of the orofacial system shows that abnormal tongue function can be secondary, adaptive, or compensatory because of skeletal maldevelopment. A primary tongue dysfunction is usually a consequence of habits or prolonged bottle feeding. Balthers did not consider this in the original version of his appliance.

The main advantage of the bionator lies in its reduced size, which allows it to be worn day and night. The appliance exerts a constant in magnitude and continuous in time influence on the tongue and perioral muscles. Because unfavorable muscular forces are prevented from exerting undesired and restrictive effects on the dentition for a longer wearing time, the bionator's action is faster than that of the classic activator.

The main disadvantage of the bionator lies in the difficulty of correctly managing it, which stems from the simultaneous requirements of stabilization of the appliance and selective grinding for guidance of eruption. Unlike the activator, the volume-reduced bionator is dentally anchored (the activator is dentoalveolar), hence the necessity of selective trimming. Normalization of function can occur only if the inherent growth pattern is normal. With skeletal disturbances, the effectiveness of the bionator is limited. Activators can be modified for different growth directions, but this possibility is lacking in bionator therapy. A further potential disadvantage is vulnerability to distortion, which occurs because far les acrylic support exists in the alveolar and incisal region. Of course, the bionator can be modified to satisfy some of these criticisms.

Bionator Types

Three basic bionator constructions are common: the standard or Class II appliance, the open-bite appliance, and the reversed or Class III appliance.

Standard Appliance

The standard appliance (Fig. 4.45) consists of a lower horseshoe-shaped acrylic lingual plate extending from the distal surface of the last erupted molars. For the upper arch, the appliance has only a posterior lingual extension that covers the molar and premolar regions. The anterior portion is open from canine to canine. The upper and lower parts, which are joined interocclusally in the correct construction bite relationship, extend respectively 2 mm above the gingival margin and 2 mm below the lower gingival margin. The upper anterior portion is kept free to prevent interference with tongue function. However, tongue function is controlled by the edge-to-edge incisal contact relationship, leaving no space for thrusting activity. If some space exists between the upper and lower incisors in the construction bite, the acrylics can be extended to cap the lower incisors. This does not hinder the potential procumbency of these teeth, because the labial bow does not contact them and the capping is only partially successful in preventing labial tipping—a limitation of the bionator, particularly if lower incisors are already labially inclined.

The posture and function of the lips, cheeks, and tongue are guided by the palatal bar and labial bow with extensions. The palatal bar is formed of 2.1 mm hard steel wire extending from the top of the edges of the lingual acrylic flanges in the middle area of the deciduous first molars. It lies approximately 1 mm away from the palatal mucosa and runs distally as far as a transpalatal line between the distal portions of the maxillary permanent first molars to form an oval, posteriorly directed, loop that reinserts on the opposite side.

The transpalatal bar stabilizes the appliance and simultaneously orients the tongue and mandible to achieve a normal relationship. The forward orientation of the tongue, according to Balthers, is accomplished by stimulating its dorsal surface with the palatal bar. This is the reason for the posterior curve of the palatal bar.

The labial bow (according to Balthers, the "lip bar"), made of 0.9 mm hard stainless-steel wire, begins between the contact points between the canines and deciduous upper molars (or premolars). It then runs vertically, making a rounded 90° bend to the distal along the middle of the crowns of the posterior teeth, and extends as far as the embrasure between the deciduous second molars and permanent first molars. Making a downward and forward curve, it runs anteriorly at about the same position with respect to the buccal surfaces of the lower posterior teeth as far as the lower canines. From there, it extends at a sharp angle obliquely upward toward the canines, and bends to the level line at approximately the incisal third of the upper incisors.

The incisal portion of the bow should be separated from the incisors by approximately the thickness of a sheet of paper. This position of the wire produces a negative pressure, with the wire supporting lip closure. The posterior portions of the labial bow are designed as buccinators loops, screening muscle forces in the vestibule (Fig. 4.46). The buccinators loops screen the buccinator muscles, and the lingual acrylic parts prevent both the cheeks and the tongue from interposing in the interocclusal space.

Open-Bite Appliance

The open-bite appliance is used to inhibit false posture and function of the tongue (Fig. 4.47). The construction bite is as low as possible, but a slight opening allows the interposition of posterior acrylic bite blocks for the posterior teeth to prevent their extrusion. To inhibit tongue movements, the acrylic portion of the low-

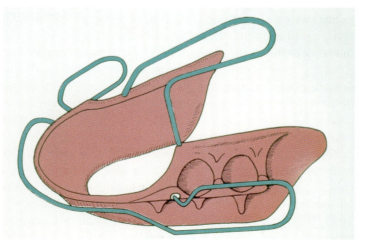

Fig. 4.45 Standard or Class II bionator.

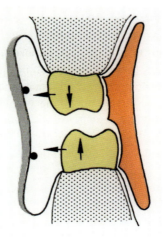

Fig. 4.46 The buccinators loop.

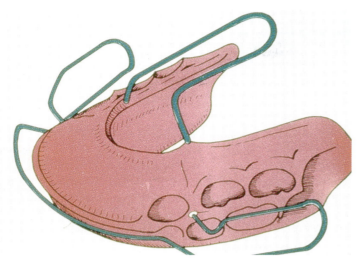

Fig. 4.**47** The bionator for treatment of open bite malocclusions.

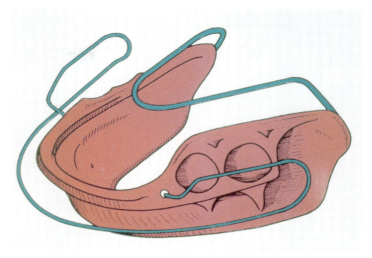

Fig. 4.**48** The Class III bionator.

er lingual part extends into the upper incisor region as a lingual shield, closing the anterior space without touching the upper teeth. The palatal bar has the same configuration as the standard (or Class II) bionator, with the goal of moving the tongue into a more posterior or caudal position.

The labial bow is similar in form to that of the standard appliance, differing only in that the wire runs approximately between the incisal edges of the upper and lower incisors. The labial part of the bow is placed at the height of the correct lip closure, thus stimulating the lips, to achieve a competent seal and relationship. The vertical strain on the lips tends to encourage the extrusive movement of the incisors after elimination of the adverse tongue pressure.

Class III or Reversed Bionator

The Class III or reversed bionator (Fig. 4.**48**) is used to encourage the development of the maxilla. The construction bite is taken in the most retruded position possible, to allow labial movement of the maxillary incisors and simultaneously exert a slight restrictive effect on the mandible. The lower acrylic portion is extended incisally from canine to canine. This extension is positioned behind the upper incisors, which are stimulated to glide anteriorly along the resultant inclined plane. The acrylic is trimmed away behind the lower incisors, to prevent tipping the lower incisors labially. This effect of the bionator is primarily dentoalveolar, compensating the Class III relationship.

The palatal bar configuration runs forward instead of posteriorly, with the loop extending as far as the deciduous first molars or premolars. The tongue is supposedly stimulated to remain in a retracted position in its proper functional space. The tongue should contact the anterior portion of the palate, encouraging the forward growth of this area.

The labial bow runs in the front of the lower incisors. The labial part runs along the lower incisors, without bending in the canine region. The wire touches the labial surfaces slightly.

Anchorage of the Appliance

Because the bulk, volume, and extension of the appliance are reduced, there are special requirements for anchorage. At the start of treatment with the bionator, trimming of all guiding planes simultaneously for all areas is not possible. Acrylic surfaces are used to stabilize the appliance; others can be ground as needed to effect the desired stimulus for tooth movement. During the treatment the loading areas and areas for tooth guidance require an alteration. The loading of the appliance is obtained from the following areas:

1. Incisal margins of the lower incisors, by extending the acrylic over the incisal margin and cap.
2. Loading areas: the cusps of the teeth fit into the respective grooves in the acrylic.
3. Deciduous molars, which can always be used as anchor teeth.
4. Edentulous areas, after premature loss of deciduous molars.
5. Acrylic noses in the upper and lower interdental spaces, particularly mesial to the first permanent molars.
6. The labial bow, which, when correctly placed, prevents posterior displacement of the appliance.

Trimming of the Bionator

As with the activator, trimming of the occlusal surfaces on the bionator is essential to allow certain teeth to erupt further while fully erupted teeth are prevented from further eruption through contact with the acrylics. Balther's terminology refers to stimulation of eruption as unloading or promotion of growth and prevention of eruption as loading or inhibition of growth. Trimming of the acrylic "tooth beds" and elimination of the influences of tongue and cheeks allow the teeth to erupt until they reach the articular plane. Once there, they should prevented from erupting further so that the loading can be accomplished by addition of self-curing acrylics. The appliance can be trimmed periodically until the teeth reach the desired relationship with the articular plane. Thus, periodic loading and unloading of the same area are necessary. The alternating loading and unloading of certain areas is the difficulty in managing the classic bionator (Fig. 4.**49**).

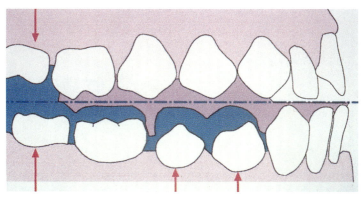

Fig. 4.49 Alternative loading and unloading the teeth in the course of the treatment.

Indications for Bionator Therapy

Opinions vary widely on the clinical usefulness of the bionator as Balthers envisioned and used. Some clinicians believe the appliance to be less effective than the activator; others hold that it can be used in every type of malocclusion.

The treatment of the Class II, Division 1 malocclusion with a bionator is indicated under the following preconditions:
1. The dental arches are originally well aligned.
2. The mandible is in a posterior position; i.e., functional retrusion.
3. The skeletal discrepancy is not severe.
4. A labial tipping of the upper incisors is evident.

The bionator is not indicated in the following situations:
1. The Class II relationship is caused by maxillary prognathism.
2. A vertical growth pattern is present.
3. Labial tipping of the lower incisors is evident. Anterior posturing of the mandible with simultaneous uprighting of the incisors cannot be performed with the bionator.

Our palatographic examinations (Rakosi et al. 1983) have shown that the palatal bar usually only flattens the dorsum of the tongue and does not move it anteriorly (Fig. 4.50) whether the loop is open anteriorly or posteriorly is of no consequence. The reverse appliance seems to tip the maxillary incisors labially, but does not stimulate the forward movement of the maxillary basal bone.

In conclusion, it can be stated that the bionator is effective in treating functional and mild skeletal Class II malocclusions in the deciduous and mixed dentitions, provided that the appliance is chosen after careful diagnostic study, that it is made properly and managed properly by loading and unloading different areas, and that the patient complies in both daytime and nighttime wear.

Functional Jaw Orthopedics and Class II Malocclusions

Functional jaw orthopedic management is mostly provided in treatment of the Class II malocclusion. In the treatment protocol of this most frequent of all malocclusions, there are still many myths and misapprehensions. Such a misapprehension is the belief that each Class II in the mixed dentition period can be treated with an activator. There are still clinicians treating every Class II malocclusion with activators and waiting on the results. In cases of good results, the patient is good; if the treatment fails, the patient is bad. But not the patient is necessarily "bad" or not cooperative, if the clinician is using "universal" appliances without exact diagnosis and indication.

A new paradigm for the present millennium is to differentiate and individualize. For this challenge, the historic Angle term "Class II malocclusion" is no longer appropriate. The Class II category is a dental, skeletal, or functional relationship of the 6-year molars; it is one symptom that is present in a great variety of malocclusions. A more appropriate term would be "Class II relation-

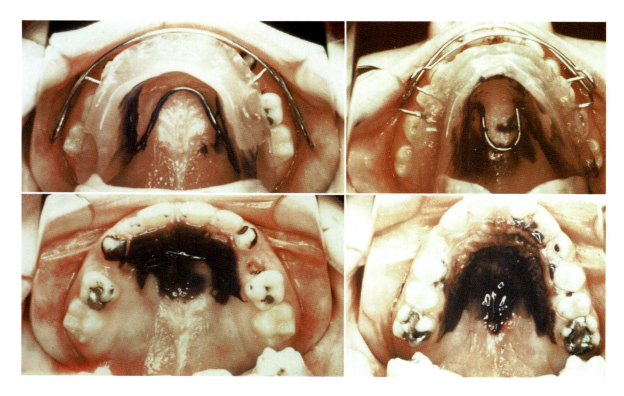

Fig. 4.50 Reaction of the tongue under influence of the palatal bar. Palatographic examination. Position of the tongue with appliance (top) and without appliance (bottom).

ship" or at least "Class II malocclusions." There is a great variety of Class II malocclusions: the mandible can be retrognathic and small or even long. The maxilla can be prognathic or there may be a combination of retrognathic mandible and prognathic maxilla. The treatment requirements are different: it may require growth promotion with the activator, or only an expansion of the upper arch. Sometimes jumping of the bite is indicated, or treatment with a headgear possibly in combination with an activator. The activator is the best choice for conventional functional therapy, but in many other cases the facial morphology is not suited to conventional therapy or the goal of the treatment is not identical with those of the functional therapeutic concept.

The most frequent errors in the treatment protocol of the Class II malocclusions are:
- False interpretation of the Class II. It is only one symptom.
- The belief that the only goal of the treatment is the production of a long mandible.
- While treatment with an activator and waiting on a growth spurt, it is possible, that no spurt is coming or it is not helping for anterior posturing of the mandible, even in many cases it is not necessary at all.

Many evidence-based publications put various Class II malocclusions in one pot; they measure and statistically evaluate gained mms in size of the mandible without differentiation. Also in evidence-based publications the samples do not include all types of Class II malocclusions or children, and the conclusions cannot be extended to patients with different problems; for example, those with combined anterior-posterior and vertical problems.

Retrognathic and Small Mandible

A growth promotion with therapeutic growth spurt is desirable in cases with small, retrognathic mandible (so called "anatomical mandibular retrusion"), with well aligned dental arches. Critical to therapy, though, is the question "Which type of growth pattern has the malocclusion?" In horizontal growth pattern, the reaction is favorable with functional treatment. In malocclusions with vertical growth pattern, the growth direction is unfavorable and the growth increments are low; there must be a compromise in the goal of the treatment.

Petrovic (1981) reported Class II malocclusions treated for 2 years with the Fränkel appliance; in the horizontal growth pattern, the growth increments was 8.58 mm, but was only 2 mm increments in the vertical pattern. In the control groups, the growth increment in the horizontal pattern was 3.05 mm, in the vertical pattern only 1.3 mm. If we were to compare a treated vertical group with an untreated horizontal group the result would be more growth without treatment. Exact diagnosis, differentiation, and individualization are thus preconditions for successful treatment.

Most publications examining the efficacy of functional treatment do not differentiate between the innate growth pattern variations. It is in any case difficult to differentiate between displacement and therapeutically induced growth increment. Coza et al. (2004) found a 3 mm anterior displacement of the mandible during activator treatment, but the length increase of the mandible did not differ from that of the control group. In addition, a more

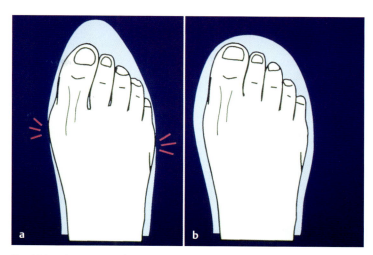

Fig. 4.51 The "narrow slipper" analogy of Körbitz.

posteriorly directed condylar growth (for example, as in treatment with the Herbst appliance) can increase the overall length of the mandible, which cannot be interpreted solely as a growth increase.

Retrognathic Mandible with Normal Length

The posterior position of the mandible is a forced bite with an anterior postural rest position and posterior sliding in full intercuspidation. This is a functional retrusion of the mandible. There are two variation of this relationship:

1. The maxilla is narrow—there is a posterior transverse interarch discrepancy (PTID)—with posterior displacement of an average size mandible. This variation was described by Körbitz in 1909. He compared this situation with a narrow slipper, in which the foot (the mandible) cannot move forward (Fig. 4.51). The same situation was described more recently by Tollaro, McNamara (2000) and Gianelly (2000) again using an example of shoes. After maxillary expansion, the mandible moves forward. If the maxilla is extremely narrow the condition can be designated as maxillary deficiency syndrome with: crossbite, dental crowding, and lingually flared upper and buccally flared lower molars.

In the 9-year-old boy depicted in Fig. 4.52, there was a functional retrusion of the mandible with extremely narrow maxilla. The growth pattern was horizontal; the upper incisors were inclined labially and the lower lingually. After expansion of the upper dental arch, a convenient case for a treatment with a "H" activator the mandible moved (Fig. 4.52 a, b) forward.

About 30% of Class II malocclusions belong in this category.

2. Posterior displacement of the mandible of normal size because of functional disturbances (Fig. 4.53). Various dysfunctions, such as interposition of the lip, the infantile type of swallowing with hyperactivity of the perioral muscles, tongue thrust syndrome, or even some occlusal disturbance (such as preliminary contact with posterior sliding), can increase the overjet and force the mandible in a posterior direction.

After elimination of the disturbing factors or neuromuscular aberration, the dentoalveolar and skeletal changes are partially or fully reversible. Angle (1920) had already stressed that "the habits of the tongue and lips are harmful and powerful in produc-

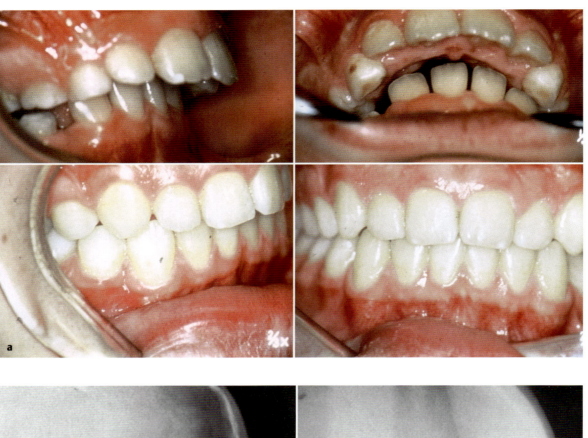
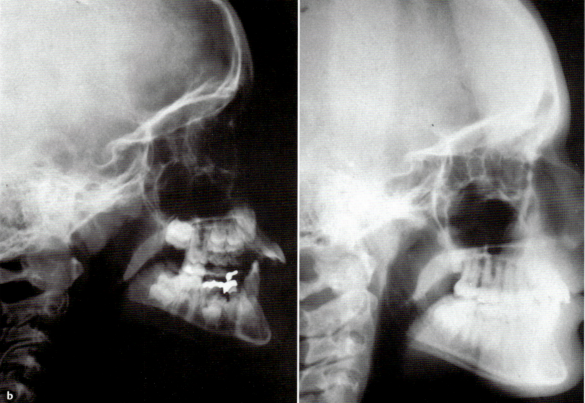

Fig. 4.52
a A 9-year-old boy with functional retrusion of the mandible because of narrow upper arch (top) and the same patient after expansion of the upper arch (bottom).
b Cephalograms of the same patient before and after treatment.

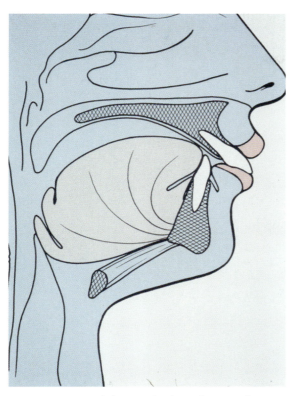

Fig. 4.53 Functional Class II malocclusion because of interposition of the lower lip.

tion of anomalies. As long as these habits are not eliminated, there is little prospect for success in a treatment." In many cases of Class II malocclusion (about 10–15%), early elimination of the noxious influences enables a normal development of the dentition.

In the 10-year-old girl described in Fig. 4.**54a, b**), an early elimination of the neuromuscular aberration induced a "jumping of the bite" during activator treatment. With the use of a second activator the occlusion was seated (Fig. 4.**54c, d**).

Prognathic Maxilla with Orthognathic Mandible

In this case a distal force against the maxillary teeth and orthopedic growth inhibition of the maxilla are indicated. The position of the mandible must not be altered. About 15–20% of cases of Class II malocclusion have a prognathic maxilla. Differential diagnosis is imperative. In combined cases, a combined treatment can be used, probably an activator with headgear.

Thus about 60% of the Class II malocclusions do not need therapeutic growth promotion of the mandible. In the remaining 40% of cases, should the clinician wait until the pubertal growth spurt to introduce the treatment?

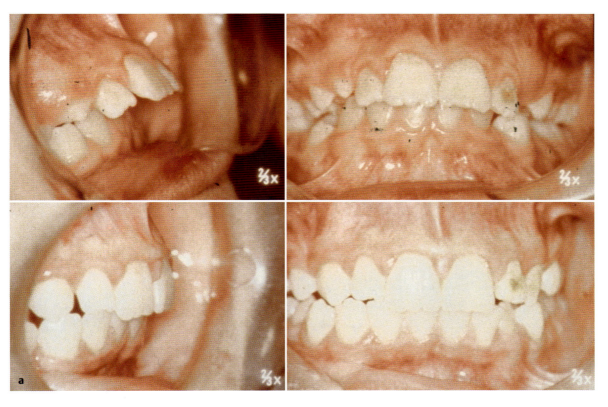

Fig. 4.**54**
a Functional Class II malocclusion with anterior postural rest position before treatment (top) and after jumping the bite (bottom).
b–d see next pages

Functional Orthodontic and Functional Orthopedic Treatment

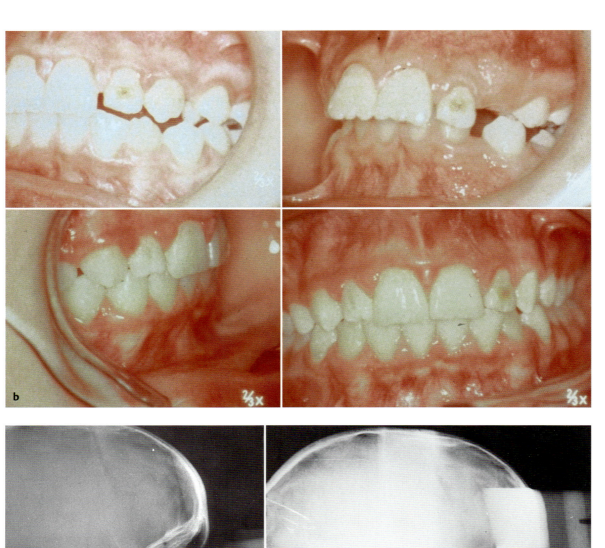

Fig. 4.54
b The patient before jumping (top right), after jumping the bite (top left), and after seating of the occlusion (bottom).

c Cephalograms of the patient before and after jumping.

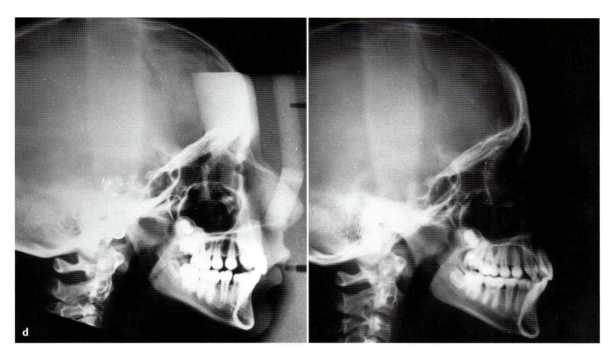

Fig. 4.54
d Cephalograms of the patient after jumping and after seating of the occlusion.

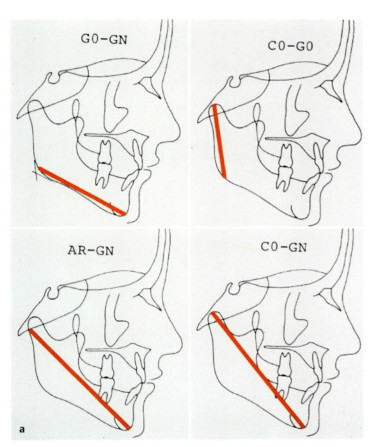
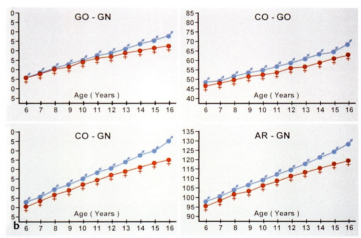

Fig. 4.55 a Various measurements of the length of the mandible after Riolo.
b All these measurements showed a continuous growth without growth spurts.

The Pubertal Growth Spurts

Riolo et al. (1974) and Bishara et al. (1981) have reported that there are no significant growth spurts of the mandible, but only a gradual increase in dimensions. Riolo found that pubertal growth spurts in the mandible are uncommon and that, when they occur, they are unpredictable. Some correlations can be significant, but none are clinically significant or predictive in any way (Fig. 4.55 a, b).

The literature does not agree on (1) the existence of facial growth spurts, (2) the timing and magnitude of such spurts, or (3) the predictability of changes in the facial dimensions relative to general somatic or skeletal events. Waiting on the pubertal growth peak means that:

- The permanent teeth are mostly erupted.
- The deviations in the start, course, and extent of the peak are great.
- The concept is of limited use in practice.

Lischer (1912) had already stressed that "irreparable damage is done by waiting until the permanent teeth erupted before beginning correction of the malocclusions."

According to Fränkel (1967), the pubertal growth peak is without significance for the development of the alveolar process. The growth-promoting factor is the genetically conditioned eruption potential of the teeth. We need to consider other mechanisms by which functional appliances correct Class II malocclusions: unlike in laboratory experiments with the difference between experimental and control groups limited to the single factor to be investigated, an orthodontic appliance is only one of the variables affecting the outcome. It is difficult to interpret whether differences are due to differences in the treatment or differences in the patients. The biological concept of normal occlusion includes a range of variation that is compatible with acceptable oral health and unhindered function. Perhaps integration of the mechanobiology with the gene–environment interaction can in future improve the treatment possibilities. Hereditary and mechanical modulation of growth and development share a common pathway via genes, so the length of the mandible can be increased under influences of both genes and environmental cues.

The goal of functional treatment cannot be the creation of long mandible, but is rather to achieve a harmonious jaw relationship —a harmony of the skeletal relationship with well-aligned dental arches. This harmony need not always be an orthognathic relationship: it also can be retrognathic or prognathic in a straight face.

References

Andresen V. Funktions-Kieferorthopädie. Leipzig: H. Meusser; 1938.
Angle EH. Orthodontia. Dent Cosmos. 1920: 11.
Araujo AM, Buschang PH, Melo AC. Adaptive condylar growth and mandibular remodeling changes. Eur J Orthod. 2004; 26: 515–522.
Balthers W. Eine Einführung in die Bionator Methode. Heidelberg: Herman Verlag; 1973.
Benninghoff A. Architektur der Kiefer und ihre Weichteilbedeckung. Paradentium. 1934; 6: 48.
Bimler HP. Die Elastischen Gebissformer. Zahnärtzl Welt. 1949; 19: 499.
Bishara SE, Jamison JE, Peterson LC, DeKock WH. Longitudinal changes in standing height and mandibular parameters between the ages of 8 and 17 years. Am J Orthod. 1981; 80: 115–135.
Clark WJ. The twin block technique. A functional orthopedic appliance system. Am J Orthod Dentofacial Orthop. 1988; 93: 1–18.
Cozza P, Polimeni A, Ballanti F. A modified monobloc for treatment of obstructive sleep apnoea. Eur J Orthod. 2004; 26: 523–530.
Fränkel R. Funktionskieferorthopädie und der Mundvorhof als apparative Basis. Berlin: VEB Verlag; 1967.
Gianelly AA. Evidence based treatment strategies: an ambition for the future. Am J Orthod Dentofacial Orthop. 2000; 117: 543-4544.
Graber TM. Orthodontics: principles and practice. Philadelphia: Saunders; 1972.
Graber TM, Rakosi T, Petrovic A. Dentofacial orthopedics with functional appliances. St. Louis: Mosby; 1997.
Häupl K. Gewebsumbau und Zahnveränderung in der Funktionskieferorthopädie. Leipzig: J.A. Barth; 1938.
Klammt G. Der offene Aktivator. Stomatol DDR. 1955; 5: 332.
Körbitz A. Kursus der Orthodontia. Berlin: 1909.
McNamara JA. Maxillary transverse deficiency. Am J Orthod Dentofacial Orthop. 2000; 117: 567–570.
Moffet BC. A research perspective on craniofacial morphogenesis. Acta Morphol Neerl Scand. 1972; 10: 91.
Moos ML. Functional analysis of human mandibular growth. J Prosthet Dent. 1960; 10: 1149.
Pauwels F. Theorie über den Einfluss mechanischer Reize auf Differenzierung des Stützgewebes. Z Anat Entwicklungsgesch. 1960; 121: 478.
Petrovic A, Stutzmann J, Gasson N. The final length of the mandible: is it genetically predetermined? In: Carlson DS, ed. Craniofacial Biology. Monograph No. 10, Craniofacial Growth Series. Ann Arbor, MI: Center for Human Growth and Development, The University of Michigan; 1981: 105–126.
Rakosi T. An atlas and manual of cephalometric radiography. Philadelphia: Lea & Febiger; 1982.
Rakosi T, Jonas I, Graber TM. Orthodontic diagnosis. Color atlas of dental medicine. Stuttgart–New York: Thieme; 1993.
Reitan K. Tissue behaviour during orthodontic tooth movement. Acta Odontol Scand. 1951; 9 (Suppl. 6).
Riolo ML, McNamara JA, Moyers RA, Hunter WS. An atlas of craniofacial growth. Ann Arbor: Center for Human Growth and Development, University of Michigan; 1974.
Roux W. Gesammelte Abhandlungen der Entwicklungsmechanik der Organismen. Leipzig: 1895.
Van der Klauw CI. Cerebral skull and facial skull. Arch Neerl Zool. 1946; 7: 16.
Wolf J. Das Gesetz der Transformation des Knochens. Berlin: 1892. Functional Orthodontic and Functional Orthopedic Treatment.

5 The Twin Block Technique

William Clark

The occlusal inclined plane is the functional mechanism of the natural dentition, but this fundamental force mechanism has not previously been exploited fully in the correction of malocclusion. Twin blocks modify the occlusal inclined plane using occlusal bite blocks to guide the mandible forward into the correct occlusion (Fig. 5.1).

Twin blocks utilize and modify the forces of occlusion to correct the malocclusion. This means that the patient eats with the appliances in the mouth, and the forces of mastication are harnessed to maximize the functional response to treatment.

Proprioceptive Stimulus to Growth

In normal development, the inclined plane plays an important part in the development of the dentition by determining the cuspal relationship of the teeth as they erupt into occlusion. A functional equilibrium is established under neurological control in response to repetitive tactile stimuli. Occlusal forces, transmitted through the dentition, provide constant proprioceptive stimuli to influence the rate of growth and the trabecular structure of the supporting bone.

The proprioceptive sensory feedback mechanism controls muscular activity and provides a functional stimulus or deterrent to the full expression of mandibular bone growth. The unfavorable cuspal contacts of distal occlusion represent an obstruction to normal forward mandibular translation in function and, as such, do not encourage the mandible to achieve its optimum genetic growth potential.

The occlusal inclined plane acts as a guiding mechanism, causing the mandible to be displaced downward and forward. Twin blocks use the occlusal inclined planes to promote protrusive function to correct the maxillo-mandibular relationship.

The primary goal in developing the twin block approach to treatment was to maximize the growth response to functional mandibular protrusion by using a full-time functional appliance system that is simple, comfortable, and esthetically acceptable to the patient for full-time wear.

Twin blocks are constructed to a protrusive bite that effectively modifies the occlusal inclined plane by means of acrylic inclined planes on occlusal bite blocks. The purpose is to promote protrusive mandibular function for correction of the skeletal Class II malocclusion.

Twin Blocks

Twin blocks (Fig. 5.2) are interlocking occlusal bite blocks designed for full-time wear so that they can take advantage of all functional forces acting on the dentition, including the forces of mastication. The bite blocks occlude on inclined planes at a 70° angle, covering the upper and lower teeth in the buccal segments and causing the mandible to occlude in a forward position, thus altering the distribution of occlusal forces and providing a positive stimulus to mandibular growth in order to correct the malocclusion.

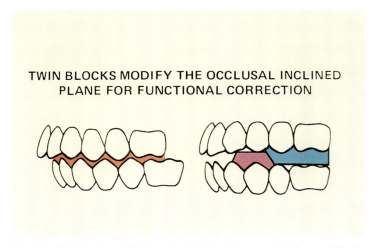

Fig. 5.1 Twin blocks modify the occlusal inclined plane to guide the mandible forward into correct occlusion.

Case Selection

Functional Treatment Objective (FTO)

What You See Is What You Get

Case selection, with particular reference to the growth response and the anticipated facial change, is an important aspect of treatment planning. Clinical examination provides the fundamental guidelines in case selection for functional therapy. The profile is first examined with the teeth in occlusion to confirm that the mandible is retrusive, relative to the maxilla. The patient is then instructed to advance the mandible and close the lips together. If the profile improves with the mandible advanced, this represents a preview of the end result. The advantage of clinical examination is that the anticipated facial change can be viewed in profile, full-face and ¾ views. This is a reliable guide to the changes observed during treatment (Fig 5.3).

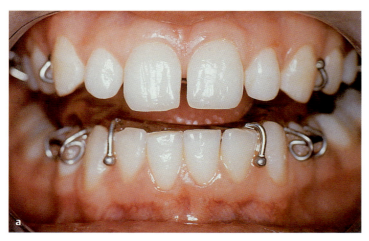
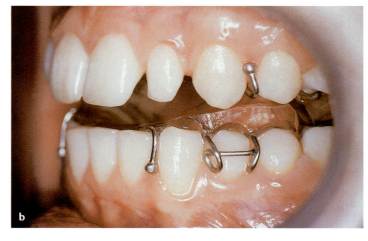

Fig. 5.2 Twin block appliances: **a** front view; **b** side view.

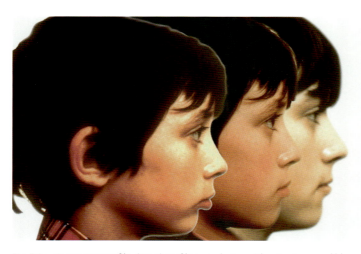

Fig. 5.3 Composite profile. (*Front*) Profile in occlusion with retrusive mandible. (*Middle*) Profile improves with mandible advanced. (*Rear*) Profile after 11 months' treatment.

Conversely, the same clinical guideline can be used to identify patients who will not respond well to functional correction, when the profile does not improve as the mandible is advanced. When the growth pattern is unfavorable for functional correction, the limitations are evident upon clinical examination with the mandible protruded. This helps to identify contraindications for functional mandibular advancement. Examples of good and poor responses are shown in the case reports at the end of this chapter.

Activation

Bite Registration for Deep Overbite

A typical construction bite in Class II Division 1 malocclusion with an overjet of up to 10 mm is registered edge to edge on the incisors with a 2 mm interincisal clearance, provided the patient can posture forward comfortably to maintain full occlusion on the appliances in that position. This enables full correction of the overjet and distal occlusion to be achieved with a single activation.

Control of the vertical dimension is important for correction of deep overbite. In the vertical dimension, a 2 mm interincisal clearance is equivalent to approximately 5 or 6 mm clearance in the first premolar region. This usually leaves 2 mm clearance distally in the molar region and ensures that space is available for vertical development of posterior teeth to reduce the overbite. The blocks are normally 5–6 mm thick between the first premolars or deciduous molars. It is a common mistake to make the blocks too thin.

The vertical activation must open the bite beyond the freeway space (interocclusal clearance) to ensure that the patient cannot drop the mandible into rest position and thus lose the functional response of the inclined planes. Opening the bite beyond the freeway space is an important factor in ensuring that the appliance is active when the patient is asleep.

Overjets exceeding 10 mm invariably require partial correction, followed by reactivation after the initial correction is complete (Fig. 5.4).

It is necessary to register a larger interincisal clearance of 4 or 5 mm in treatment of reduced overbite, in order to accommodate blocks of adequate thickness (5 or 6 mm) between upper and lower premolars or deciduous teeth. The increased vertical activation helps to control the vertical dimension by encouraging intrusion of the posterior teeth.

Progressive Activation of Twin Blocks

Recent research (Rabie et al 2003) confirms the findings of Petrovic and Stutzman in animal experiments that, in some cases, progressive activation may be more effective in maximizing the mandibular growth response. In animal experiments, Rabie (2001, 2003) relates the growth response to the cell count of mesenchymal cells with the capacity to be transported to growth sites to synthesize additional cartilage or bone. This is a genetic factor, which would help to explain the variation in individual response to functional mandibular protrusion. The clinical implication is that patients with a low mesenchymal cell count have a limited growth response to the functional stimulus. This study suggests that the potential growth response appears to improve when the protocol of progressive activation is adopted, and that patients with a low mesenchymal cell count may benefit from this protocol.

Screw Advancement System   **103**

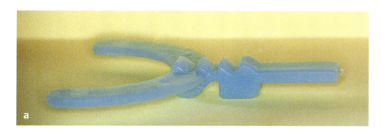

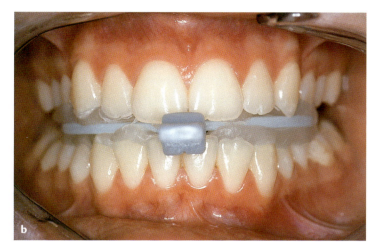

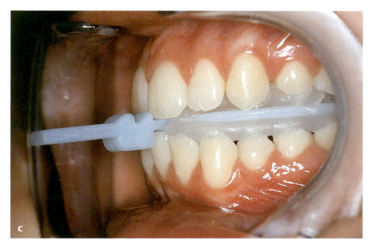

Fig. 5.**4**   **a–c** Bite registration for deep overbite.

Screw Advancement System

Carmichael, Banks, and Chadwick (1999) described a modification that enables controlled progressive advancement of the twin block. The activating mechanism uses a conical screw installed in a housing incorporated in the upper block. A laboratory kit includes components for installation and alignment and is supported by a chairside kit with cylindrical copolymer spacers of different sizes for progressive advancement.

Geserick et al. (2006) described an occlusal screw with an inclined plane attached as an alternative method for progressive advancement of the Twin Block (Fig 5.**5**). The following are indications for use of these mechanisms:
- Stepwise advancement is indicated to facilitate reactivation in the treatment of large overjets in excess of 10 mm.
- Patients with vertical growth patterns are not able to tolerate large mandibular advancements. In such cases, stepwise mandibular advancement may be more effective.

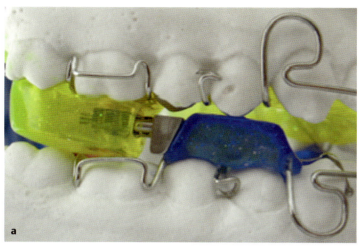

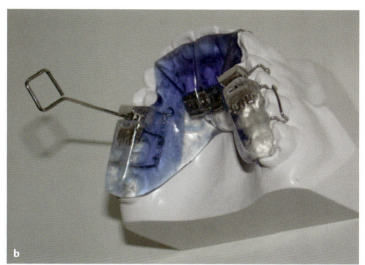

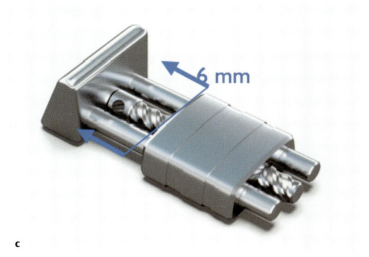

Fig. 5.**5**   **a–c** Screw advancement system for progressive advancement of twin blocks.

- Smaller adjustments are possible to improve patient tolerance and compliance.
- Stepwise activation may produce an improved mandibular response in patients with limited growth potential.
- The system may be adapted for progressive activation of reverse twin blocks in correction of Class III malocclusion.

Appliance Design

Comfort and esthetics are significant factors in appliance design when it comes to patient acceptance. "Patient friendly" appliances remove obstacles to compliance and motivate the patient to cooperate in treatment. Twin blocks meet a wide range of requirements for correction of different types of malocclusion for patients throughout the age range from childhood to adulthood. A functional appliance with separate components in the upper and lower arches can be adapted to resolve problems in both arches independently.

Twin block appliances are tooth- and tissue-borne. In order to limit individual tooth movements, the appliances are designed to link the teeth together as anchor units. In the lower arch, peripheral clasping, combined with occlusal cover, exerts three-dimensional control on anchor teeth and limits tipping and displacement of individual teeth. In the lower arch, anchorage is increased by extending clasps around the labial and buccal segments. Where indicated, additional clasps may be placed on lower incisors but, in practice, it is found that ball-ended clasps mesial to the lower canines are usually effective in controlling the lower labial segment. Some operators prefer to use incisal capping to control lower incisor angulation, or, alternatively, an acrylic labial pad may be added, supported by a bow with U-loops for adjustment.

The component parts of twin blocks appliances are common to conventional removable appliances, with the addition of occlusal inclined planes. Appliance design is modified by the addition of screws and springs or bows to move individual teeth. Arch development and alignment of individual teeth can proceed simultaneously with correction of arch relationships in the horizontal and vertical dimensions. Midline screws are used routinely for transverse expansion in the upper arch and additional screws or springs may be added for sagittal arch development (Fig. 5.6).

The modified design for correction of anterior open bite and treatment of vertical growth patterns is described on p. 107 and is illustrated in Figs. 5.10 – 5.12.

Twin Block Construction

Good impressions and an accurate construction bite are the basic necessities for accurate appliance construction. The appliance prescription should include details required for correction of the individual malocclusion. Variations in design should be specified. The construction bite is recorded in a suitable modeling wax that retains its dimensional stability after it is removed from the mouth. Any excess wax extending over the buccal surfaces of the teeth should be removed to allow the models to seat correctly into the construction bite. In the laboratory, the models are mounted on an articulator that registers the construction bite prior to constructing the occlusal bite blocks.

Occlusal Bite Blocks

The base plate and occlusal bite blocks may be constructed from heat-cured or cold-cure acrylic. Heat-cured acrylic is stronger and better able to resist breakage when the upper block is trimmed distal to the inclined plane. Making the appliances in wax first allows the blocks to be formed with greater precision.

Cold-cure acrylic has the advantage of speed and convenience, but sacrifices something in strength and accuracy. It is essential to use a top-quality cold-cure acrylic to avoid problems with breakage, especially as the blocks are progressively trimmed during treatment. The inclined planes can lose their definition as a result of wear if a soft acrylic is used. The disadvantages of cold-cure acrylic can be overcome by using preformed blocks made from good-quality heat-cured acrylic.

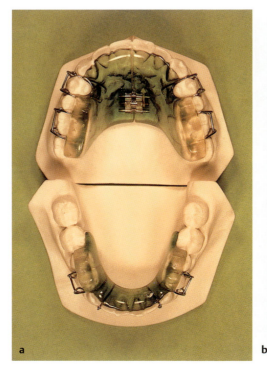 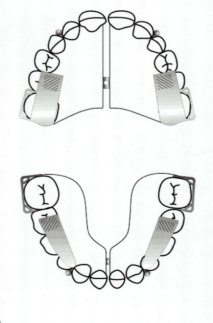 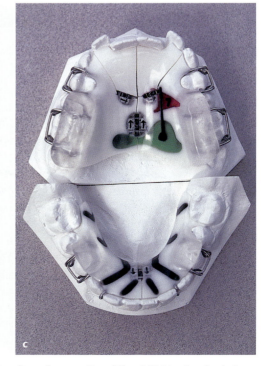

Fig. 5.6 **a** Appliance design for treatment of typical Class II Division I malocclusion with no crowding. **b** Twin block Schwarz appliances for independent expansion in both arches and correction of arch relationships in mixed dentition. **c** A twin block sagittal appliance for correction of Class II Division 2 malocclusion, designed for combined transverse and sagittal arch development.

The Delta Clasp

The delta clasp retains the basic elements of the Adams clasp, namely, interdental tags, retentive loops, and a buccal bridge. The crucial difference is that the retentive loops are triangular, circular, or oval in shape, as opposed to an open U-shaped arrowhead as in the Adams clasp. The advantage of the closed loop is that the clasp does not open with repeated insertion and removal and, therefore, maintains its shape better, requires less adjustment, and is less subject to breakage. A further advantage is that the clasp gives excellent retention on lower premolars, and is suitable for use on most posterior teeth (Fig. 5.**7**).

Stages of Treatment

Stage 1—Active Phase—Twin Blocks

During the active phase of treatment, twin blocks are worn full-time. The objectives are to correct arch relationships simultaneously in the anteroposterior, vertical, and transverse dimensions. Normally, the overjet and overbite are corrected within six months, and the lower molars have erupted into occlusion within nine months. The average time in twin blocks is nine months.

Stage 2—Support Phase—Anterior Inclined Plane

The aim of the second stage of treatment is to retain the corrected incisor relationship until the buccal segment occlusion is fully established. To achieve this objective, an upper removable appliance is fitted with an anterior inclined plane to engage the lower incisors and canines. This is worn full-time initially to allow the buccal segment occlusion to settle and then is used as a retainer.

The lower twin block appliance is left out at this stage and the removal of posterior bite blocks allows the posterior teeth to erupt. Full-time appliance wear is necessary to allow time for internal bony remodeling to support the corrected occlusion as the buccal segments settle into occlusion.

The occlusion is normally established within four to six months. Full-time appliance wear continues during the support phase for a further three to six months to allow functional reorientation of the trabecular system (Harvold, 1968), before reducing appliance wear during the retention period (Fig. 5.**8**).

Stability is excellent after twin block treatment, and this can be partly attributed to the support phase, when a functional retainer is used to stabilize the corrected incisor relationship, while the buccal teeth settle fully into occlusion. The support phase may be as important as the active phase in achieving stability after functional mandibular advancement.

Clinical Management

Temporary Fixation of Twin Blocks

Patient compliance is crucial in functional therapy, and any means of improving compliance contributes to the success of treatment. The two-piece design enables twin blocks to be fixed in the mouth temporarily for up to two weeks to ensure that the patient wears the appliance 24 hours per day. There are several possible methods of fixation during the initial stages of appliance wear. Composite may be added to bond the clasps to the teeth to ensure rigid retention. Alternatively, band cement may be used under the bite blocks for secure fixation, or glass ionomer cement may be added to the outer edges of the bite blocks to establish a peripheral seal. This allows the orthodontist the same degree of control as with a fixed appliance during the period when the patient is adapting to the twin blocks. After two weeks of full-time wear, the patient is normally more comfortable with the appliance in the mouth than without it, and the appliance can be detached from the teeth and removed for cleaning. By this time, the patient has adapted to wearing the appliance full-time, even during meals. Problems of poor cooperation are consistently resolved by adopting the protocol of temporary fixation of twin blocks.

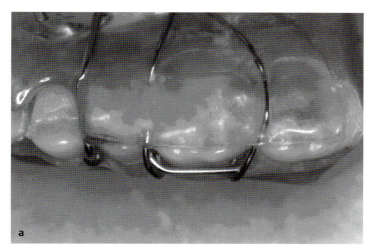 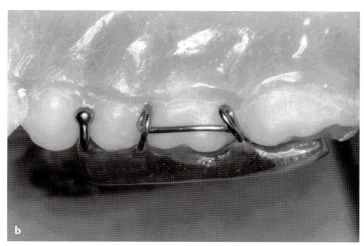

Fig. 5.**7** **a, b** The delta clasp.

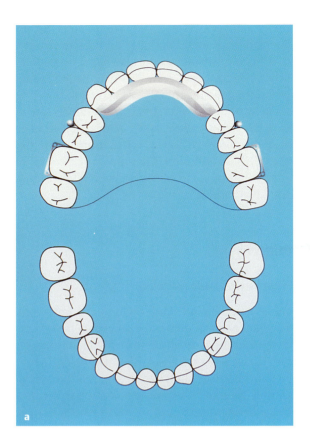

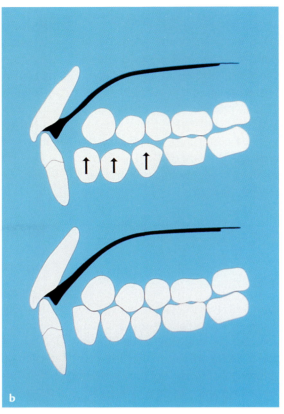

Fig. 5.**8**
a Support appliance with anterior inclined plane.
b Anterior inclined plane supports corrected occlusion; lower premolars are free to erupt.

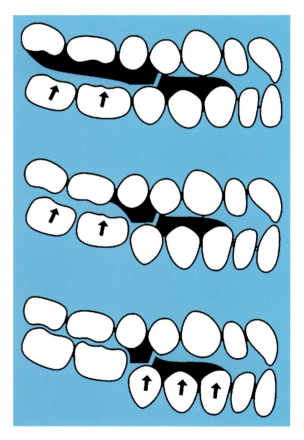

Fig. 5.**9** Sequence of trimming of blocks to reduce deep overbite.

Management of Deep Overbite

In treatment of deep overbite, vertical development of the lower molars is encouraged from the beginning of the active phase of treatment by progressively trimming the upper bite block occlusodistally to allow the lower molars to erupt. The inclined plane is moved forward to the mid point of the lower second premolar. The previous illustration shows a small inclined plane after trimming to allow eruption of the molar. This was vulnerable to breakage and I moved the inclined plane forward to retain a stronger lower block after trimming for molar eruption. At the end of the active phase, the incisors and the molars should be in correct occlusion.

At this stage, an open bite is still present in the premolar region because of the presence of the bite blocks. As a final adjustment at the end of the twin block stage, the upper surface of the lower block is trimmed to allow reduction of the open bite in the premolar region before progressing to the support phase. It is important to maintain adequate interlocking wedges to maintain the anteroposterior correction of arch relationships (Fig. 5.**9**).

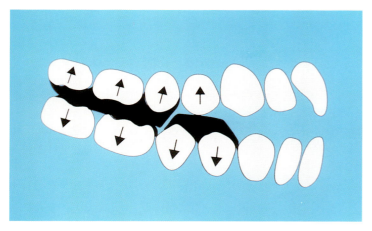

Fig. 5.**10** Occlusal cover is maintained over the posterior teeth to prevent eruption in treatment of anterior open bite.

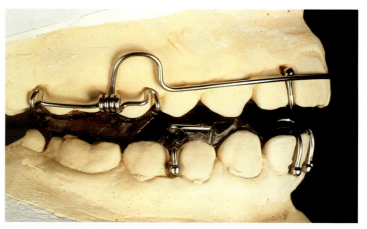

Fig. 5.**11** Twin block modified to accommodate a facebow for high-pull extraoral traction to intrude upper posterior teeth.

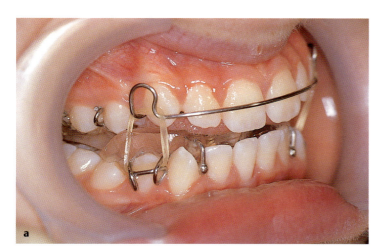

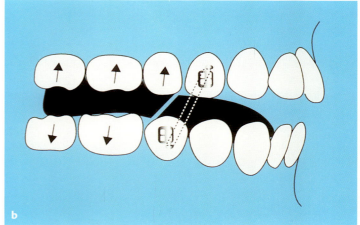

Fig. 5.**12** **a, b** Vertical elastics are effective in intruding upper molars in treatment of anterior open bite and vertical growth patterns.

Management of Anterior Open Bite

Management of reduced overbite or anterior open bite requires a different approach. Vertical growth patterns and anterior open bite require careful management to prevent eruption of the posterior teeth. It is important to maintain occlusal contact of all erupted teeth on the opposing bite-blocks in order to encourage intrusion, especially of the upper molars (Fig. 5.**10**).

If second molars erupt during the active phase, occlusal cover or occlusal rests should be extended to prevent overeruption of these teeth. These patients often have a weak musculature with restricted forward mandibular posture and may require stepwise advancement of the mandible. The screw advancement system is therefore appropriate in treatment of anterior open bite and vertical growth patterns.

Clasps are placed on lower molars to prevent their eruption, while the appliances are left clear of the anterior teeth to encourage eruption of the incisors. In addition, a vertical-pull headgear may be used to apply an intrusive force to the upper molars to reduce the vertical component of growth. The appliance design is modified to incorporate a tube to accommodate a facebow in the molar region to apply high-pull traction (Fig. 5.**11**).

Christine Mills, in orthodontic practice in Vancouver, Canada developed an approach using vertical intraoral elastics to reduce anterior open bite. The elastics are applied bilaterally and pass from the upper arch to the lower arch in the premolar region. They may be attached to the twin block appliances, or to buttons or brackets on opposing teeth. The vertical elastics intrude the upper molars by encouraging the patient to bite into the appliances consistently. This is an effective method of treatment for patients with vertical growth patterns who have weak musculature and do not close consistently on the appliance (Fig. 5.**12**) (Clark 2002).

Clinical Case Studies

Individual variation in the response to functional therapy has long been recognized and is a significant factor in case selection for functional mandibular protrusion. Patients with brachyfacial and mesofacial growth patterns have good potential for horizontal mandibular growth and respond well to mandibular advancement. In contrast, the dolichofacial pattern indicates a vertical growth tendency and, typically, the profile does not improve as the mandible is advanced. The direction of growth along the facial axis is therefore an important indicator of the likely response treatment. The facial axis angle, measured relative to the pterygoid vertical, represents the gradient of growth of the chin. The following case reports illustrate both favorable and unfavorable responses to functional correction, showing the importance of the clinical guideline in case section for functional therapy.

Response to Treatment

Case Study 5.1   Patient E. F., Age 12 years 3 months

The girl presents a typical Class II Division 1 malocclusion with a large overjet of 13 mm and deep overbite. The growth pattern is brachyfacial with good horizontal growth potential. The upper archform is narrow and there is mild crowding in the lower premolar region. An initial activation of 8 mm achieved partial correction of the overjet and distal occlusion, followed by reactivation of the occlusal inclined planes to complete mandibular advancement in two stages. Selective trimming of the upper block to encourage eruption of the lower molars during the twin block stage assisted in correction of the deep overbite.

The lower appliance included bilateral sagittal screws to open space for the lower premolars, and the upper arch was expanded by a midline screw. Twin block treatment extended over 15 months, followed by nine months retention.

A good growth response resulted in a satisfactory correction of the malocclusion with a favorable improvement in facial balance.

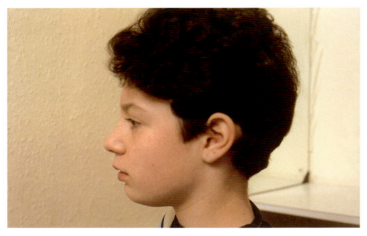

Fig. 5.1.1   **Profile before treatment.**

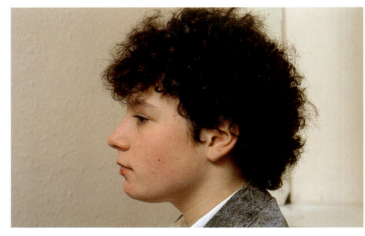

Fig. 5.1.2   **Profile after treatment.**

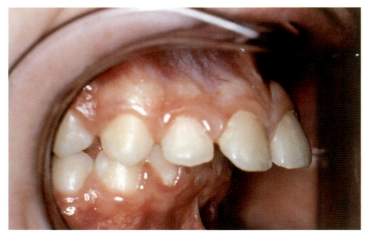

Fig. 5.1.3   **Archform before treatment (1).**

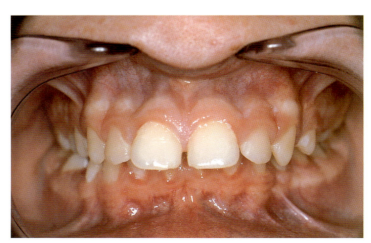

Fig. 5.1.4   **Archform before treatment (2).**

Clinical Case Studies

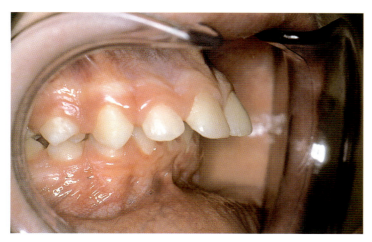

Fig. 5.1.**5** Occlusion before treatment (1).

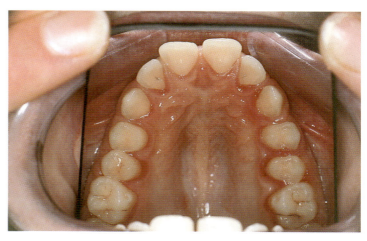

Fig. 5.1.**6** Upper archform before treatment (2).

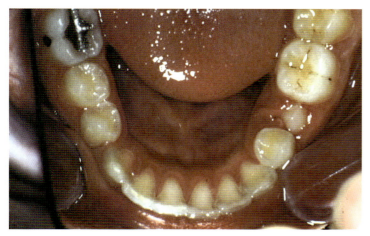

Fig. 5.1.**7** Lower archform before treatment (3).

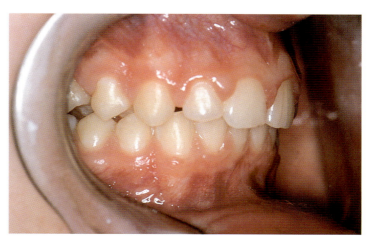

Fig. 5.1.**8** Occlusion after treatment (1).

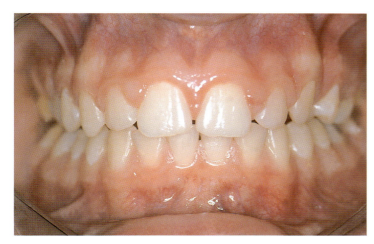

Fig. 5.1.**9** Occlusion after treatment (2).

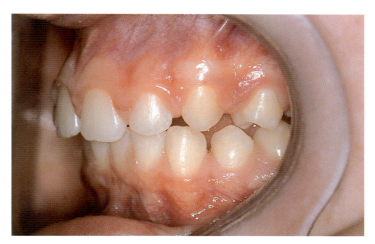

Fig. 5.1.**10** Occlusion after treatment (3).

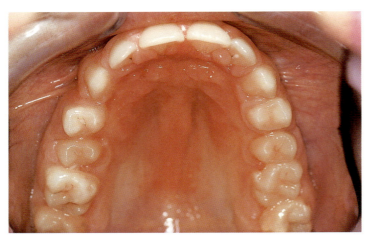

Fig. 5.1.**11** Archform after treatment (1).

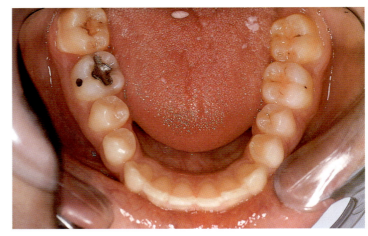

Fig. 5.1.**12** Archform after treatment (2).

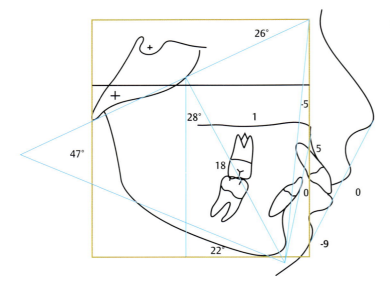

Fig. 5.1.**13** Cephalometric tracing before treatment.

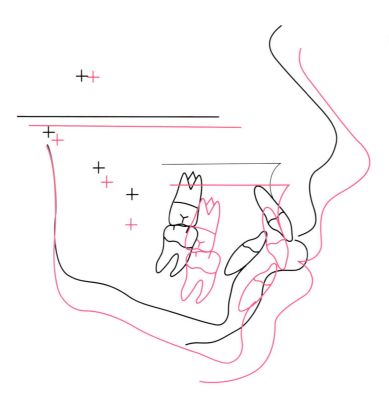

Fig. 5.1.**14** Before and after treatment.

Case Study 5.2 Patient A. P., Age 12 years 4 months

A subdivision of Class II Division 1 malocclusion presents a single retroclined upper incisor, and shows some features of Class II Division 2 malocclusion. The lower lip rests between the upper central incisors, causing one to be proclined and the other retroclined. Occlusal interference from the retroclined incisor is responsible for trapping the mandible in a distal occlusion. The facial type is severe brachyfacial with a convexity of 2 mm, indicating a Class I skeletal base relationship. The approach to treatment is simply to advance the retroclined incisor and release the mandible forward to correct the distal occlusion.

Twin blocks were activated edge to edge on the proclined incisor with 2 mm interincisal clearance, and a lingual spring is added to advance the retroclined incisor. In view of the strong horizontal growth pattern, a rapid improvement in facial appearance is observed after two months' treatment, by which time the lips are closing comfortably over the upper incisors as the mandible is released from distal occlusion. Twin block treatment was completed in seven months and followed by use of a retention appliance with an anterior inclined plane.

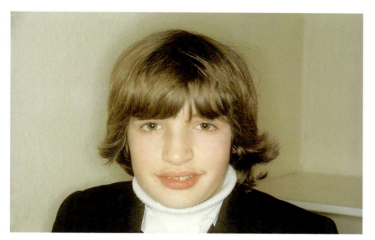

Fig. 5.2.**1** **Facial appearance before treatment.**

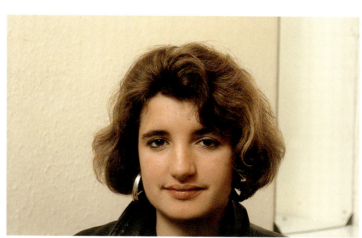

Fig. 5.2.**2** **Facial appearance at age 19 years.**

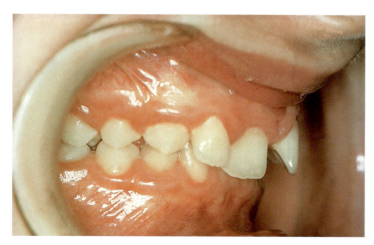

Fig. 5.2.**3** **Occlusion before treatment (1).**

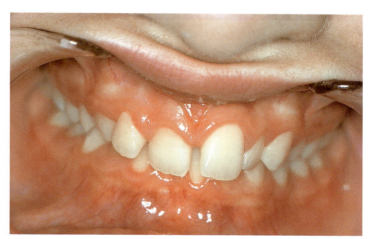

Fig. 5.2.**4** **Occlusion before treatment (2).**

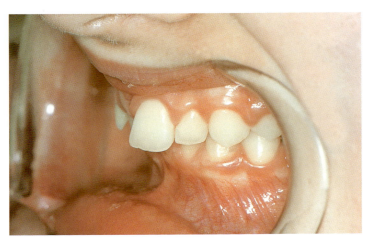

Fig. 5.2.**5** Occlusion before treatment (3).

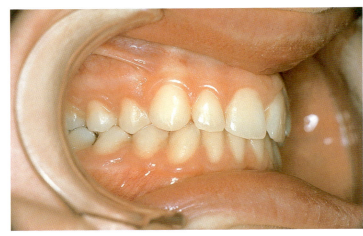

Fig. 5.2.**6** Occlusion 2 years out of retention (1).

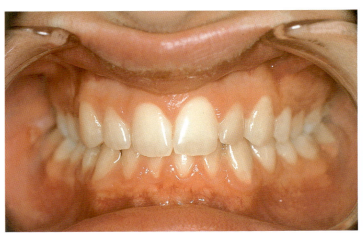

Fig. 5.2.**7** Occlusion 2 years out of retention (2).

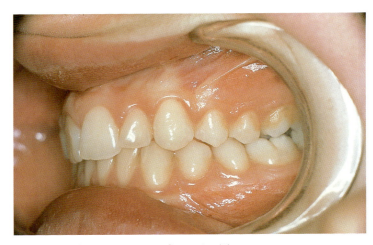

Fig. 5.2.**8** Occlusion 2 years out of retention (3).

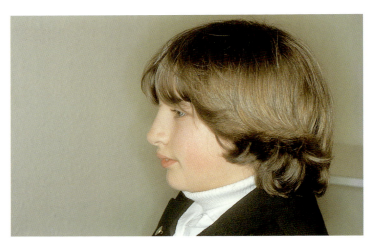

Fig. 5.2.**9** Profile (1).

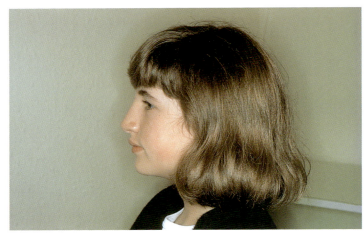

Fig. 5.2.**10** Profile (2).

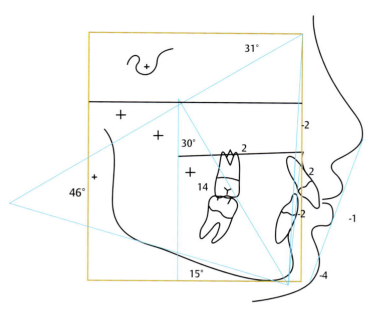

Fig. 5.2.**11** Cephalometric tracing before treatment.

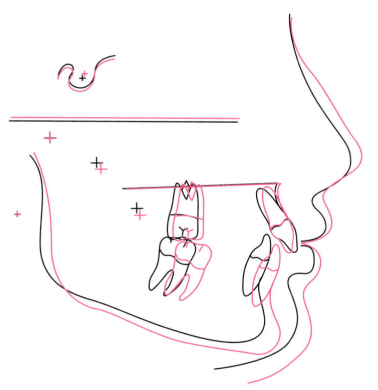

Fig. 5.2.**12** Before and after treatment.

Case Study 5.3 Patient P.McL., Age 12 years

An example of a Class II Division 1 malocclusion treated with twin blocks in early permanent dentition. This young girl presents a slight dental and facial asymmetry with displacement of the mandible to the left side, resulting in displacement of the lower center line to the left. The occlusion reflects the asymmetry as the distal occlusion is more pronounced on the left side. The facial type is retrognathic, with a convexity of 5 mm indicating a moderate Class II skeletal relationship. Severe protrusion of the upper incisors is partly responsible for an increased overjet of 8 mm and is associated with a deep overbite.

The soft-tissue pattern is not favorable in this case, as the lower lip is everted and slightly protrusive, while the upper lip is flaccid and slightly rounded, resulting in an obtuse nasolabial angle. When the profile is examined with the mandible advanced to correct the mandibular retrusion, the lower lip advances beyond the esthetic plane. Ideally the nasolabial angle should not exceed 90° for the best esthetics, and the lower lip should lie slightly behind the esthetic plane, defined by a line tangent to the nose and chin.

In this case, the lower lip appeared to be too protrusive in this position. The construction bite was therefore modified to limit the amount of mandibular advancement. A small mandibular advancement may not produce sufficient muscle activity to correct the malocclusion. In order to compensate for the reduced anterior activation, the vertical activation is increased by registering a 4 mm interincisal clearance. Clasps are placed on lower first molars to prevent eruption in this case, so as not to elongate the lower face. The dental asymmetry is eliminated by correcting the center lines in the construction bite. This increases the activation of the appliance on the left side, helping correct the distal occlusion, and restores symmetry.

A midline screw and a lower labial bow were included in the lower appliance to upright the lower incisors slightly during treatment. Brackets are added to the upper anterior teeth to correct alignment during the twin block phase. Correction of the distal occlusion, reduction of the overjet and overbite, and correction of the midline lines was achieved in six months. This was followed by upper and lower fixed appliances. Treatment was completed in 22 months, followed by retention. Final records show the position two years out of retention.

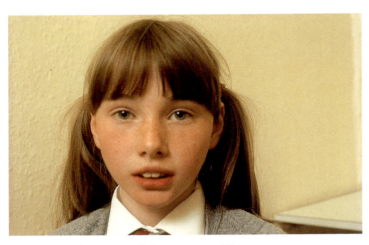

Fig. 5.3.1 **Facial appearance before treatment (1).**

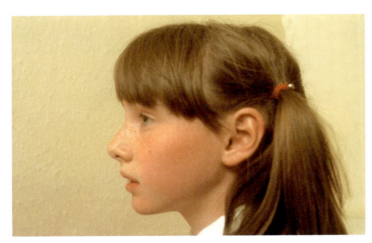

Fig. 5.3.2 **Facial appearance before treatment (2).**

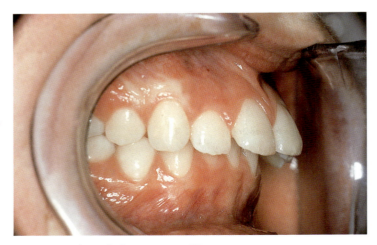

Fig. 5.3.3 **Occlusion before treatment (1).**

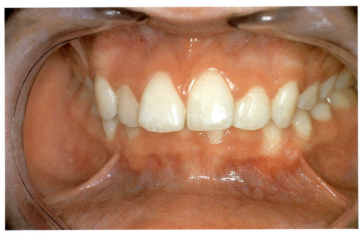

Fig. 5.3.4 **Occlusion before treatment (2).**

Clinical Case Studies

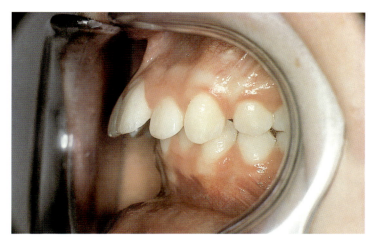

Fig. 5.3.**5**   Occlusion before treatment (3).

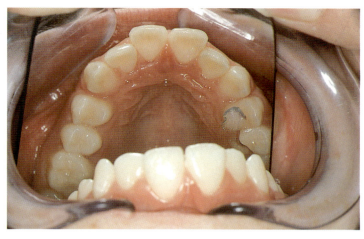

Fig. 5.3.**6**   Upper archform before treatment (1).

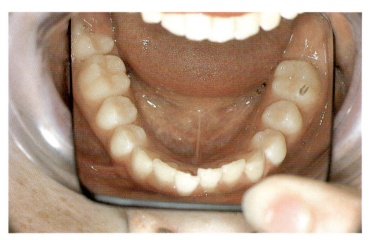

Fig. 5.3.**7**   Lower archform before treatment (2).

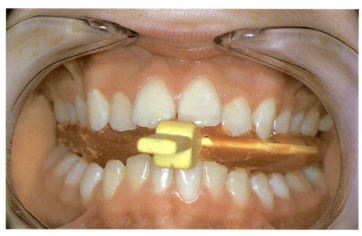

Fig. 5.3.**8**   Bite registration (1).

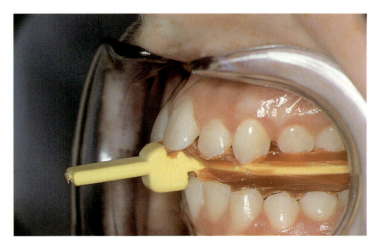

Fig. 5.3.**9**   Bite registration (2).

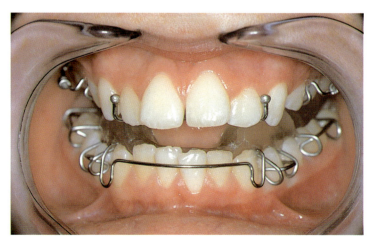

Fig. 5.3.**10**   Twin block appliances (1).

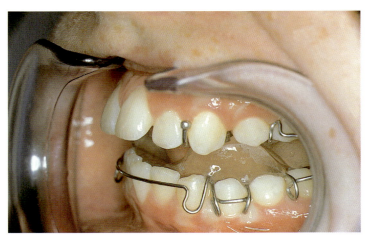

Fig. 5.3.11 Twin block appliances (1).

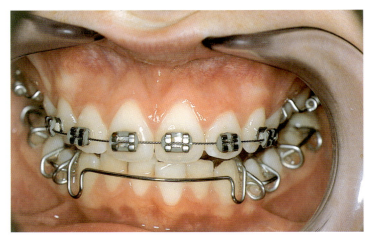

Fig. 5.3.12 Brackets are added to align the upper anterior teeth during the twin block phase.

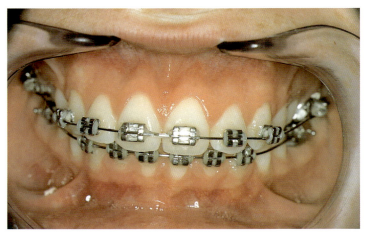

Fig. 5.3.13 Upper and lower fixed appliances.

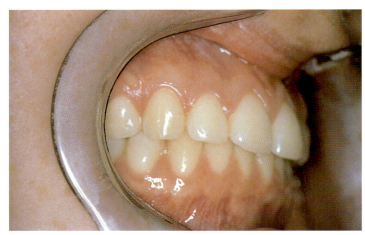

Fig. 5.3.14 Occlusion 2 years out of retention (1).

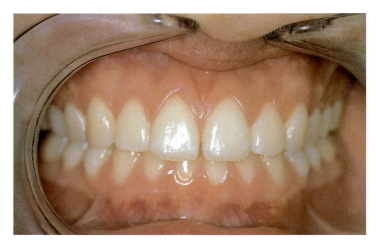

Fig. 5.3.15 Occlusion 2 years out of retention (2).

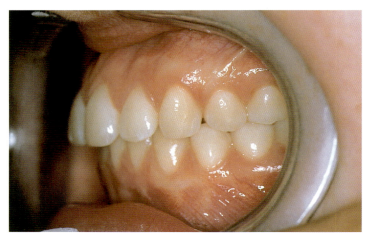

Fig. 5.3.16 Occlusion 2 years out of retention (3).

Clinical Case Studies

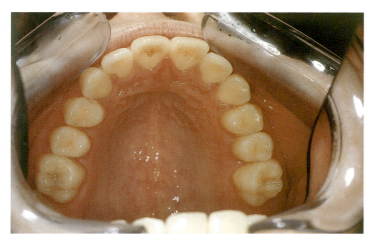

Fig. 5.3.**17** Archform after treatment (1).

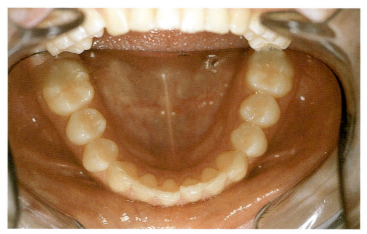

Fig. 5.3.**18** Archform after treatment (2).

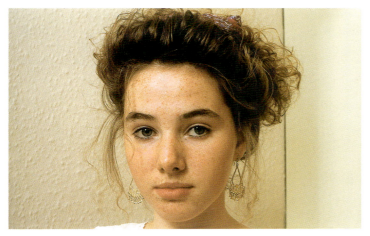

Fig. 5.3.**19** Facial appearance 2 years after treatment (1).

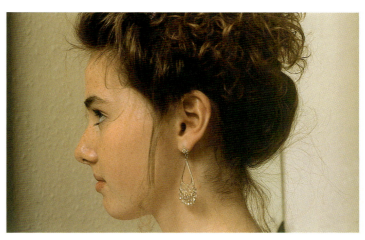

Fig. 5.3.**20** Facial appearance 2 years after treatment (2).

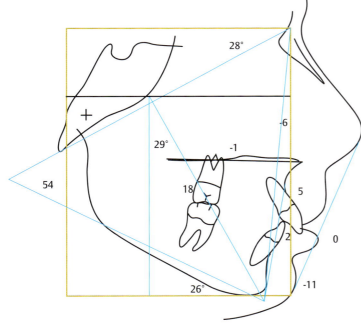

Fig. 5.3.**21** Cephalometric tracing before treatment.

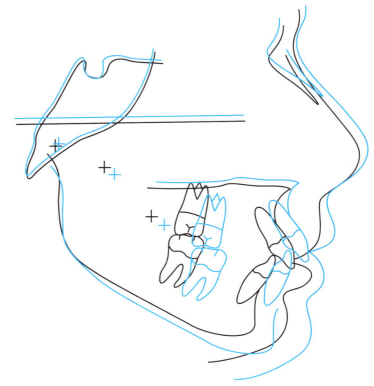

Fig. 5.3.**22** Before and after treatment.

Case Study 5.4 Patient A. C., Age 11 years 2 months

This girl presents a severe Class II Division 1 malocclusion with an overjet of 9 mm and a full unit distal occlusion. The growth pattern is dolichofacial with a retrognathic profile, as both maxilla and mandible are retrusive.

The occlusion was corrected following 10 months' treatment with twin blocks, followed by retention. Although the profile remains retrognathic after treatment, the improvement in facial appearance resulting from a simple course of treatment is satisfactory.

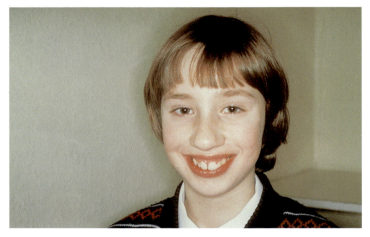

Fig. 5.4.**1** Facial appearance before treatment (1).

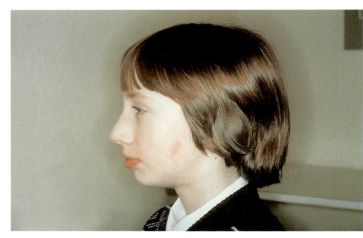

Fig. 5.4.**2** Facial appearance before treatment (2).

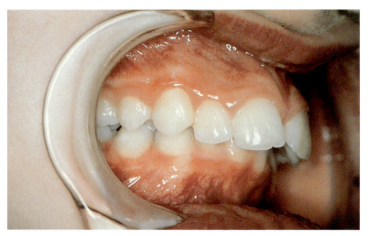

Fig. 5.4.**3** Occlusion before treatment (1).

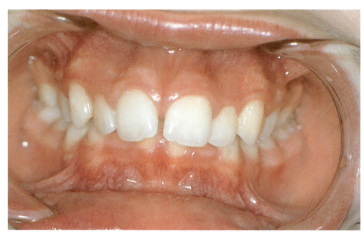

Fig. 5.4.**4** Occlusion before treatment (2).

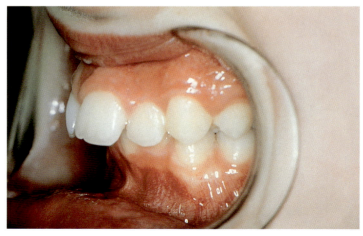

Fig. 5.4.**5** Occlusion before treatment (3).

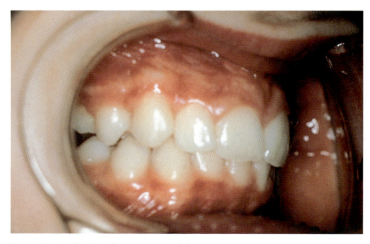

Fig. 5.4.**6** Occlusion after treatment (1).

Clinical Case Studies

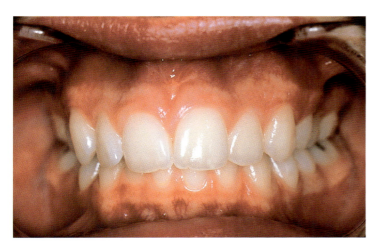

Fig. 5.4.7 Occlusion after treatment (2).

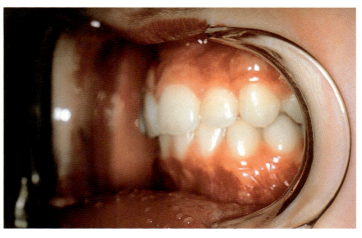

Fig. 5.4.8 Occlusion after treatment (3).

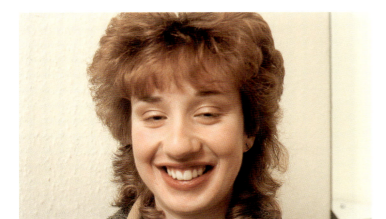

Fig. 5.4.9 Facial appearance after treatment (1).

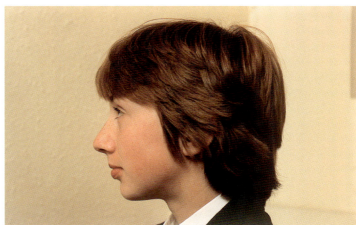

Fig. 5.4.10 Facial appearance after treatment (2).

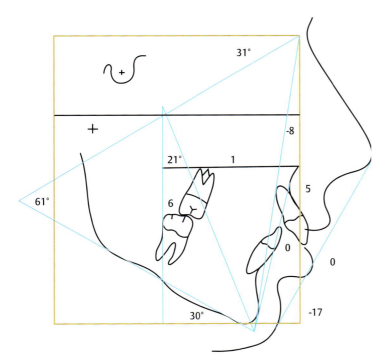

Fig. 5.4.11 Cephalometric tracing before treatment.

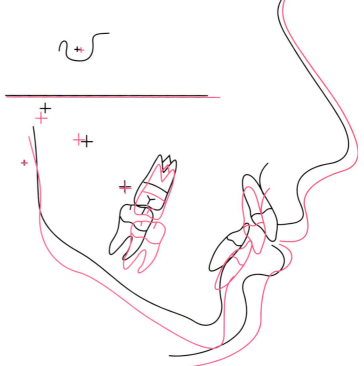

Fig. 5.4.12 Before and after treatment.

Limited Response to Functional Mandibular Advancement

Not all facial types respond well to functional treatment by mandibular advancement. The following two cases are examples of the limited response to be achieved when the growth pattern is not favorable.

Case Study 5.5   Patient S. L., Age 9 years 7 months

This is an example of treatment of a retrognathic profile where mandibular growth during treatment does not compensate for the amount of Class II skeletal discrepancy.

Cephalometric analysis confirms that both the maxilla and mandible are retrognathic, and mandibular retrusion is severe. A facial axis angle of 25° indicates a moderate vertical growth pattern, and the chin is not well developed. The lips are protrusive beyond the aesthetic plane, and this pattern does not significantly improve during treatment, despite achievement of a satisfactory dental correction. On review of the position four years after treatment, the retro-slanting profile is still evident, although the dental occlusion is stable.

The absence of a chin eminence may be anticipated in such cases by examining the profile before treatment with the mandible advanced. A genioplasty may produce a satisfactory esthetic improvement in the profile.

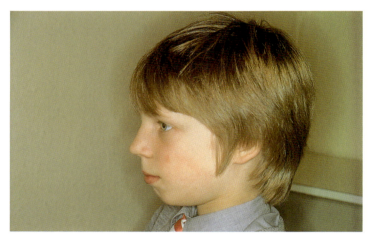

Fig. 5.5.1   Profile before treatment; age 9 years 7 months.

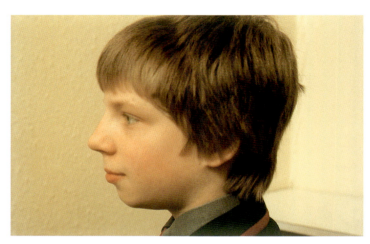

Fig. 5.5.2   Profile after treatment; age 11 years 5 months.

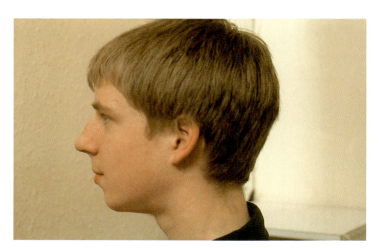

Fig. 5.5.3   Profile 4 years out of retention; age 15 years 3 months.

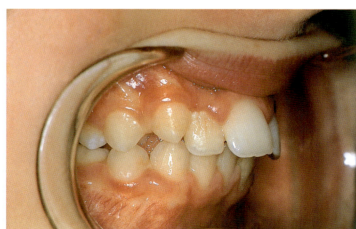

Fig. 5.5.4   Occlusion before treatment (1).

Clinical Case Studies

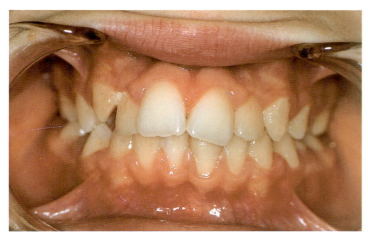

Fig. 5.5.5 Occlusion before treatment (2).

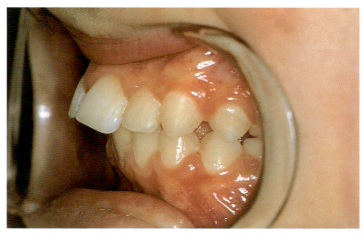

Fig. 5.5.6 Occlusion before treatment (3).

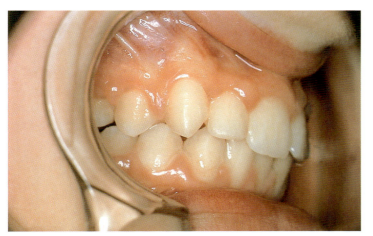

Fig. 5.5.7 Occlusion after treatment (1).

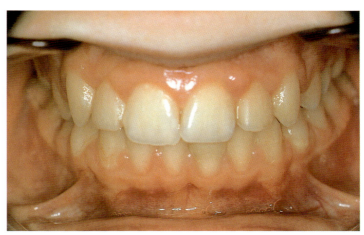

Fig. 5.5.8 Occlusion after treatment (2).

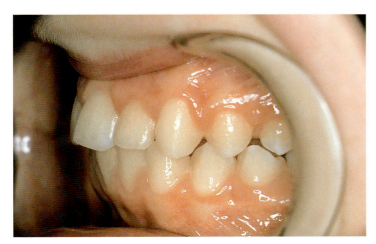

Fig. 5.5.9 Occlusion after treatment (3).

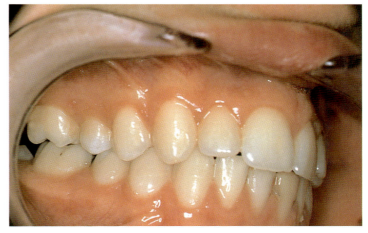

Fig. 5.5.10 Occlusion 4 years out of retention (1).

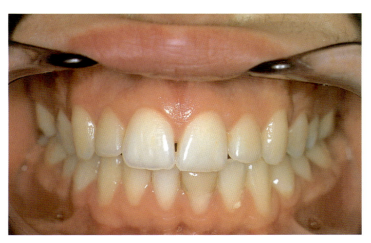

Fig. 5.5.**11** Occlusion 4 years out of retention (2).

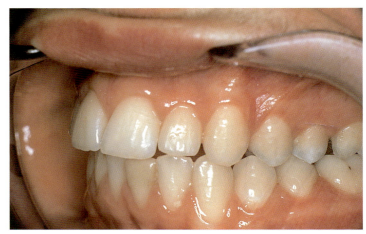

Fig. 5.5.**12** Occlusion 4 years out of retention (3).

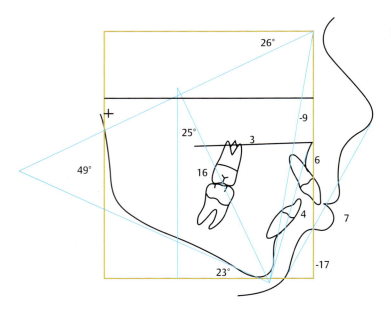

Fig. 5.5.**13** Cephalometric tracing before treatment.

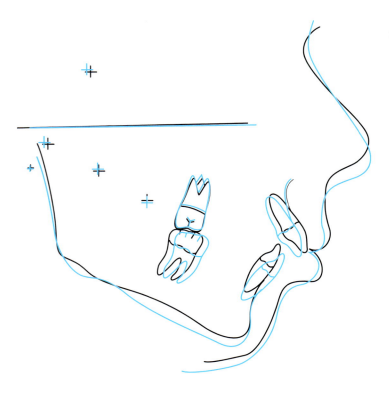

Fig. 5.5.**14** Before and after treatment.

Case Study 5.6   Patient M. B., Age 13 years 5 months

This boy is small for his age and did not grow well during treatment. Unfavorable or slow growth during treatment limits the possibility for improvement in the facial profile.

Cephalometric analysis confirms that a severe skeletal discrepancy of 10 mm convexity is due to significant maxillary protrusion combined with mandibular retrusion. Late dental development is associated with severe crowding and proclination of upper and lower incisors. The lower first premolars were extracted before treatment to accommodate buccally displaced lower canines. Two upper premolars were extracted during treatment to allow retraction of proclined upper incisors. Although dental correction is achieved, the facial improvement is a compromise, and the appearance of mandibular retrusion remains after treatment.

In this early example of twin block treatment, extraoral traction was added to restrict forward maxillary growth and reduce the maxillary protrusion. The headgear effect in the maxilla is often associated with an autorotation in the mandible and can negate the effects of mandibular advancement. Taking this into account, the author has not used extraoral traction for the past 20 years.

This patient was a late developer, which accounts for the slow growth during treatment. Posttreatment growth partly compensated for the limited response during treatment. The posttreatment records show the position five years after completion of treatment.

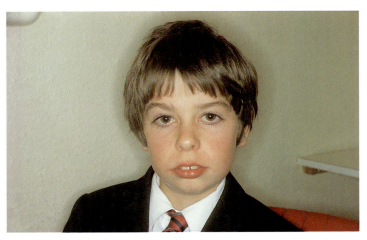

Fig. 5.6.1   Facial appearance before treatment; age 13 years 5 months.

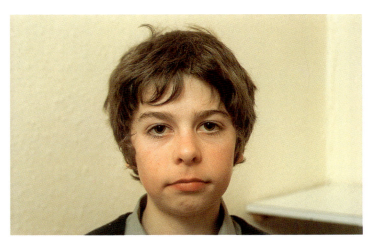

Fig. 5.6.2   Facial appearance after treatment; age 15 years.

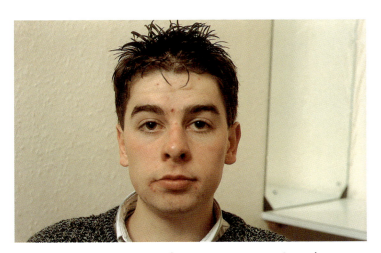

Fig. 5.6.3   Facial appearance out of retention; age 19 years 8 months.

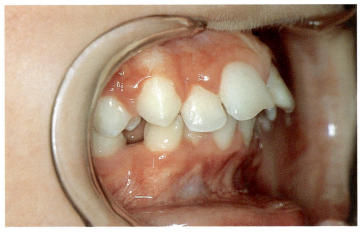

Fig. 5.6.4   Occlusion before treatment (1).

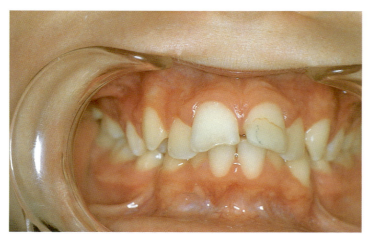

Fig. 5.6.5   Occlusion before treatment (2).

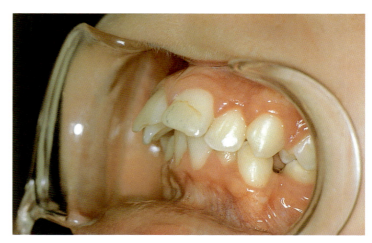

Fig. 5.6.6   Occlusion before treatment (3).

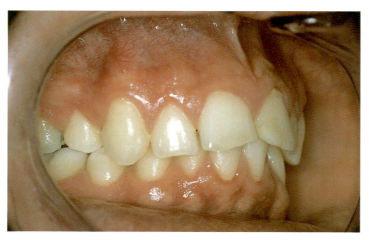

Fig. 5.6.7   Occlusion 5 years out of retention (1).

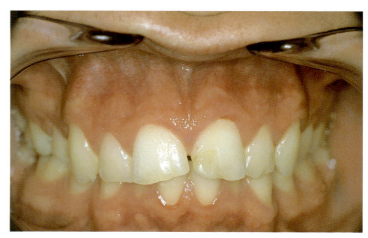

Fig. 5.6.8   Occlusion 5 years out of retention (2).

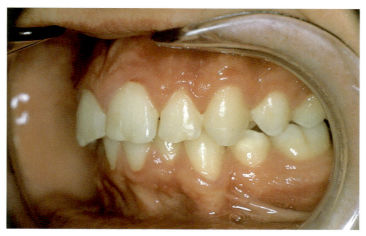

Fig. 5.6.9   Occlusion 5 years out of retention (3).

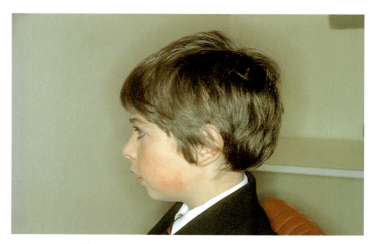

Fig. 5.6.10   Profile at 13 years 5 months.

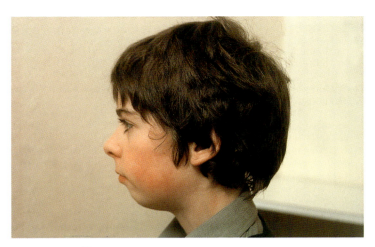

Fig. 5.6.**11** Profile at 15 years.

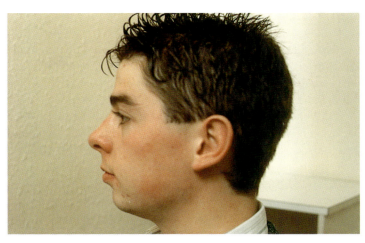

Fig. 5.6.**12** Profile at 19 years 8 months.

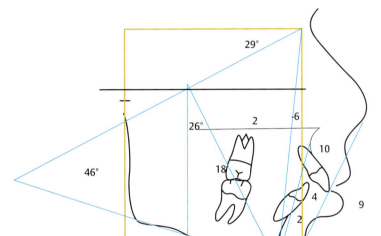

Fig. 5.6.**13** Cephalometric tracing before treatment.

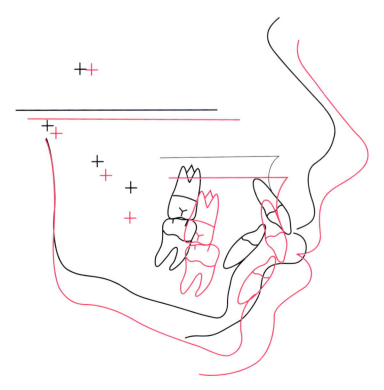

Fig. 5.6.**14** Before and after treatment.

Conclusion

The twin block technique is an extremely efficient full time functional mechanism. The main advantage is that twin blocks can be worn comfortably full time, including for eating, and it thus produces rapid results that prove to be stable out of retention.

While the majority of Class II malocclusions with mandibular retrusion respond well to treatment with twin blocks, especially when associated with a mesofacial or brachyfacial growth pattern, there are exceptions as with all functional techniques. A more limited response should be anticipated in vertical growth patterns. In some cases, there is insufficient chin eminence to significantly improve the profile after mandibular advancement. The latter may sometimes be related to bimaxillary dental protrusion.

Correct case selection is achieved by examining the facial change when the mandible is advanced with the lips closed together. The perceived change in the profile provides a reliable clinical guideline representing a preview of the anticipated change in facial appearance that will result from functional mandibular advancement.

References

Carmichael GJ, Banks PA, Chadwick SM. A modification to enable progressive controlled advancement of the twin block appliance. Br J Orthod. 1999; 26 (1): 9–13.

Clark WJ. Twin block functional therapy: Applications in dentofacial orthopaedics. 2nd ed. London: Mosby; 2002.

Clark WJ. The twin block technique. In: Graber TM, Rakosi T, Petrovic AG, eds. Dentofacial orthopedics with functional appliances. St. Louis: Mosby Year Book; 1997.

Clark WJ. The twin block traction technique. Eur J Orthod 1982; 4: 129–138.

Clark WJ. The twin block technique. Am J Orthod Dentofac Orthop. 1998; 93: 1–18.

Harvold EP, The role of function in the aetiology of malocclusion. Am J. Orthod. 1968; 54: 883.

Harvold EP, Altering craniofacial growth: force application and neuromuscular-bone interaction. In Clinical Alteration of the Growing Face, Monograph 14, Craniofacial Growth Series. University of Michigan

Geserick M, Olsburgh SR, Petermann D: The bite-jumping screw for modified twin-block treatment. J Clin Orthod 2006; 40: 423–425.

McNamara JA, Brudon WL. The twin block appliance. In: Orthodontics and dentofacial orthopedics. 2nd ed. Ann Arbor: Needham Press; 2001.

Mills CM, McCulloch KJ. Treatment effects of the twin block appliance: a cephalometric study. Am J Orthod Dentofacial Orthop. 1998; 114: 15–24.

Mills CM, McCulloch KJ. Post treatment changes following successful correction of Class II malocclusions with the twin block appliance. Am J Orthod Dentofacial Orthop. 2000; 118: 24–33.

Rabie ABM, Zhao Z, Shen G, Hagg GU, Robinson W, Osteogenesis in the glenoid fossa in response to mandibular advancement. Am. J. Ortho Dentofacial Orthop. 2001; 119: 390–400.

Rabie ABM, She TT, Hagg GU, Functional appliance therapy accelerates and enhances condylar growth. Am. J. Ortho Dentofacial Orthop. 2003; 123 (1): 40–48.

Rabie ABM, Wong L, Tsai M, Replicating mesenchymal cells in the condyle and the glenoid fossa during mandibular forward positioning. Am. J. Ortho Dentofacial Orthop. 2003; 123 (1): 49–57.

Rabie ABM, Wong L, Hagg GU, Correlation of replicating cells and osteogenesis in the glenoid fossa during stepwise advancement.. Am. J. Ortho Dentofacial Orthop. 2003; 123 (5): 521–533.

Singh GD, Clark WJ. Localisation of mandibular changes in patients with Class II Division 1 malocclusions treated with the twin-block appliance: Finite element scaling analysis. Am J Orthod Dentofacial Orthop. 2001; 119(4): 419–425.

6 The Functional Magnetic System

Alexander Vardimon

Tom Graber—A Man of Extraordinary Vision. I am happy that this book is a "Tom Graber Memorial Edition". I was honored to work with him at the American Dental Association Research Institute for 6 years in which we investigated the use of magnetic forces in orthodontics. A great scientist needs knowledge, analytic ability and vision. Numerous textbooks and scientific papers are evidence of Tom's depth of knowledge and immense analytic ability. Less known is his great vision. Shortly after Tom's nomination as Editor-in-Chief of the "American Journal of Orthodontics", he changed the name to the "American Journal of Orthodontics Dentofacial Orthopedics". When asked why he changed the name, he answered that today (1985) rapid maxillary expansion justifies the addition of Dentofacial Orthopedics to the name of our journal, but tomorrow other orthopedic procedures will emerge, expanding the framework of our profession. The recent introduction of distraction osteogenesis, miniscrew implants, accelerated osteogenic orthodontics, and the following chapter, are just a few examples, which demonstrate that Tom was "a man of extraordinary vision".

The Functional Magnetic System

The term "functional appliance" was first used to describe Robin's "monoblock," Kingsley's "jumping the bite appliance," and their derivatives such as the Activator introduced by Andresen and Häupl (Andresen et al. 1936). The use of this popularized label describe a family of orthodontic appliances employed in the treatment of Class II malocclusions ignored the fact that their orthopedic mechanism of action was spatial displacement of the lower jaw.

Myth and Reality

This nomenclature originated in the early decades of the last century when European orthodontics was subdivided according to the use of one type or another of removable appliance. The first group employed active removable appliances that were affixed to one dental arch by means of clasps and included active elements such as springs and screws. Appliances in the second group were known as functional appliances. These lacked clasps and allowed free jaw movement when oral functions are performed (i.e., deglutition and speech) (Weise 1988).

The rationale of requiring free jaw movement adjunctive to mandibular spatial displacement was based on Roux's concept that myofunctional activity (e.g., jaw movements) can stimulate osteogenesis (i.e., by shaking of the bones) (Roux 1985). When these appliances were supplemented with clasps to the upper molars or screws (Miethke et al. 1996) or modified into nonrigid tissue-borne appliances (e.g., the Fränkel functional regulator) (Fränkel 1973), they were sharply criticized as violating the biological principles of functional appliances. However, it was demonstrated that a "functional response" could be accomplished even when these principles did not adhere to Roux's concept.

It has been shown that the response to wearing of functional appliances is diurnal in nature (Ahlgren 1978). However, it was also demonstrated that response to nocturnal wearing of functional appliances results in a more favorable functional correction, although jaw movements are profoundly reduced during sleep when compared to waking hours (Petrovic and Stutzmann 1997; Rakosi 1997; Graber 2000). Moreover, when the Herbst appliance was introduced as a hybrid of fixed and functional appliances (Herbst 1934), it was initially referred to as a pseudo functional appliance (Schwarz 1934). Reports ascribing good functional response to this appliance balanced these initial reservations, however (Pancherz 1997).

During the 1970's, evidence began to amass that called into question Roux's earlier concept based on "function." These studies theorized that prolonged "jaw displacement" was the mechanism driving response to these appliances (Sergl 1983; Bass 1987; Clark 1997; Eckhart 1998; Jasper et al. 2000). The term "functional appliance" has nevertheless persevered, although the time has come to debate its validity.

In addition to the effect on jaw position credited to these appliances, Harvold and Woodside promoted a concept by which guidance of tooth eruption was performed while increasing bite clearance beyond the freeway-space. They proposed that this stabilized the functional appliance (bite registration is taken 4 mm beyond the rest position) (Woodside 1974; Harvold 1975). However, as bite clearance increases, maximal advancement is reduced (Vardimon et al. 1997). It was also demonstrated that, when these vertical stipulations were ignored, a functional correction still took place even with minute bite clearance, as long as an anteroposterior jaw displacement was maintained (Sander and Schmuth 1979).

Another misleading idea was the necessity of accomplishing functional treatment during "peak growth." It was theorized that, in order to maximize the efficacy of the functional response (maximal exploitation of mandibular growth potential), functional therapy should be undertaken during a period of acceleration in total body development. However, it has been demonstrated that the only requirement is no cessation of growth potential. Success in functional correction has been documented in early childhood, childhood, early juvenile, and adolescent periods (Hansen et al. 1991; Hamilton 1997; Baccetti et al. 2000); that is, both pre and post "peak growth" periods are potentially appropriate for functional correction.

The wearing time and duration during which functional appliances achieve their greatest response have not been appropriately investigated. A wearing period of 10–12 hours per day has been recommended (Vargervik and Harvold 1985). Simply wearing the appliance, however, is not yet a guarantee of effective functional correction. In nonproductive appliance wearing, the patient opens the mouth and the mandible is not only not placed in an advanced position but rotated backward, aggravating the Class II malocclusion. Based on a daily average 1200–3000 swallows, each lasting 638 milliseconds (Kydd and Neff 1964; Gibbs et al. 1981), maximal intercuspation is 8–20 minutes per day (Lear et al. 1965, Sheppard and Markus 1962). It is during these short periods that maximal effective functional correction occurs. Moreover, during sleep, maximal intercuspation contact decreases to 1–2 per minute (Lear et al. 1965; Powell 1965). Most patients studied were found to sleep with their mouths open due to muscle relaxation, causing inferior location of the rest position from 1–3 mm during the day to 5–12 mm during the night (Manns et al. 1981; Rugh and Drago 1981; Peterson et al. 1983; Van Sickels et al. 1985). This means that conventional functional appliances are not operating in full mandibular advancement, especially during nocturnal wear.

Thus, three requirements are imperative for maximizing functional correction:
1. Patient displays some degree of somatic growth potential
2. Anterior propulsion of the mandible (with concomitant bite clearance)
3. Extended "efficacious wearing time"

The functional magnetic system (FMS) fulfills each of these requirements.

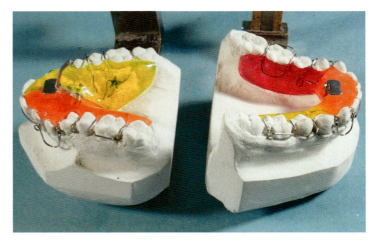

Fig. 6.**1** **The functional magnetic system (FMS) is composed of upper and lower removable appliances.** A magnetic unit is incorporated into each appliance in such a way that the poles of the upper magnetic unit face the opposite poles of the lower magnetic unit, so that the two units are oriented in a magnetically attractive pole configuration (courtesy B. Leibovitch and S. Rellu).

FMS Design

The functional magnetic system (FMS) comprises upper and lower removable appliances, each containing a magnetic unit arranged in an attractive pole orientation (Fig. 6.**1**). The upper FMS unit includes a magnetic housing, an expansion screw, and a prong (Figs. 6.**2**). Two cylindrical rare-earth magnets (samarium–cobalt; Sm_2Co_{17}) magnetized along their long axis are sealed by laser welding in a stainless-steel housing. This protects them from salivary fluids, a necessary precaution due to the high corrosive susceptibility of rare earth magnets. The stainless steel layer of the magnetic housing is only 0.2 mm thick so as not to interfere with the maximal magnetic attractive force when the upper and lower FMS units approximate each other (at less than or equal to a 0.4 mm gap).

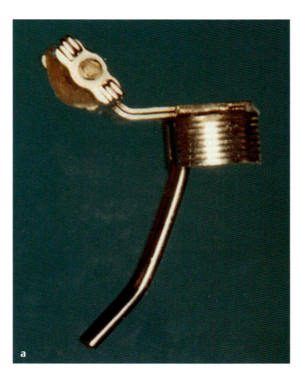

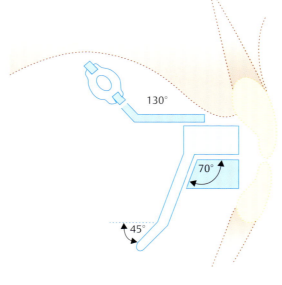

Fig. 6.**2** **Upper FMS unit.**
a The upper FMS unit is composed of three elements: the prong, which guides the lower jaw into anterior displacement; the magnet, which guides and constrains the lower jaw in this position; and the expansion screw, which expands the constricted upper arch.
b An extension arm with a 130° bend connects the magnetic housing to the expansion screw. The prong is inclined 70° to the magnetic interface, which is parallel to the occlusal plane.

FMS Design   129

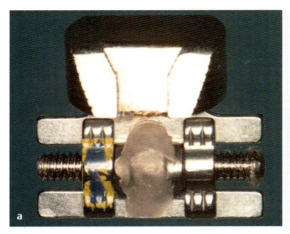
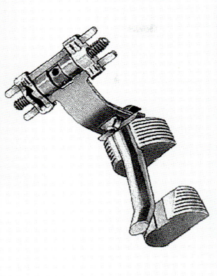
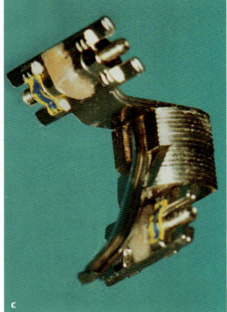

Fig. 6.**3** **Lower FMS unit.**
a The lower FMS unit.
b The posterior wall of the lower magnetic housing is oriented in an oblique plane.
c Upon mouth closure into edge-to-edge incisal contact, the prong slides along a funneled groove in the oblique plane of the lower magnetic housing.

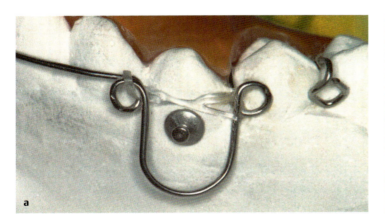
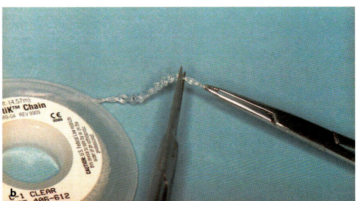
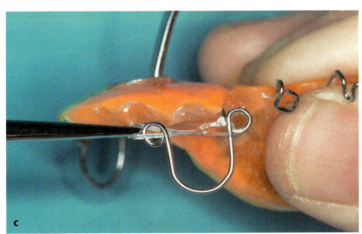
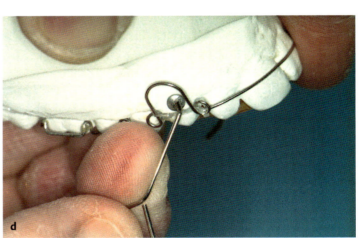
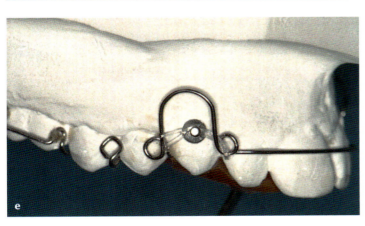

Fig. 6.**4** **The elastic clasp.**
a Two helices are bent at the occlusal ends of the vertical legs of the U-loops, which places them 2 mm occlusal to the button.
b A unit of two elastomeric rings is cut from a roll of elastomeric chain.
c The chain unit (medium-size power chain) is stretched between the two helices, so that each elastomeric ring is wrapped around one helix and the connecting elastic span is stretched between.
d The patient places the elastic span in the gingival undercut of the button using a screw-key.
e The elastic span increases the retention of the FMS units, counteracting the magnetic force that tends to dislodge the FMS appliance toward the occlusal plane. Disruption of the elastomeric chain occurs infrequently. However, the patient can obtain a longer elastomeric ring unit for self use and be instructed to replace the out-of-order piece by first installing two elastomeric rings on the helices of the elastic clasp and then cutting the excess chain (courtesy B. Leibovitch and S. Rellu).

The upper and lower magnets are oriented in an attractive configuration with a maximal magnetic force of 3 newtons (N) (Vardimon et al 1977). The expansion screw is connected to the magnetic housing by an extension arm (Fig. 6.2 b). The mid-sagittal position of the magnetic housing does not change upon activation of the expansion screw.

The lower FMS unit contains a magnetic housing and an expansion screw (Fig. 6.3 a). The posterior wall of the lower magnetic housing formed the oblique plane to receive the prong of the upper magnetic housing (Fig. 6.3 b, c). Two cylindrical rare-earth magnets are positioned in the magnetic housing in opposite pole orientation to the upper magnets. As in the upper FMS unit, the midsagittal position of the lower magnetic housing does not change upon activation of the lower expansion screw.

Both upper and lower FMS appliances are anchored to the dental arches by means of Adams and triangular clasps and a specially designed labial bow with two elastic-bearing clasps (Figs. 6.1, 6.4). The elastic clasps counterbalance the tendency of both FMS appliances to be dislodged by the magnetic attractive force pulling toward the occlusal plane (Fig. 6.4 e). Usually, the elastic clasp is placed in the canine region. Prior to taking the working model impression, button attachments are bonded to the canine labial crown surface at midcrown width close to the gingival margin.

FMS Fabrication

It is recommended to take the upper and lower alginate impressions after attachment placement (Figs. 6.5, 6.6). The bite registration is taken at edge-to-edge (max 7 mm mandibular advancement). If occlusal clearance at the molar region is less than 2 mm, then registration is taken with no incisor contact. The upper and lower midlines should usually coincide. Midline deviation is corrected during bite registration in the case of functional or mandibular skeletal shift. Midline is not coincident if the deviation was caused by a dental shift.

If overjet is greater than 7 mm, a one step mandibular advancement may produce muscle pain. Two-stage mandibular advancement is then recommended (Remmelink and Tan, 1991). This is of major interest because patient compliance can be gained if no initial pain is present (light initial discomfort is always present). After 1–3 months, a second advancement is done. The upper and lower impressions are taken with appliances in the mouth (elastic chains are removed prior to impression and a hole is made in the upper tray for the prong). A new bite registration (working bite) is taken in the new advanced position. The lower magnetic unit is detached from the lower FMS appliance prior to this.

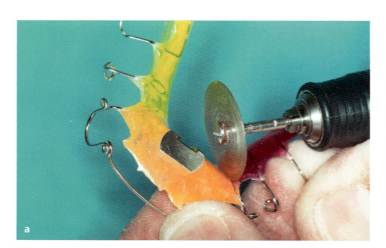
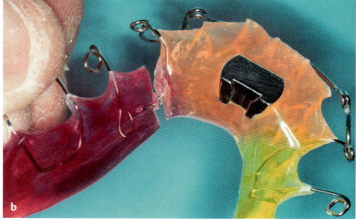
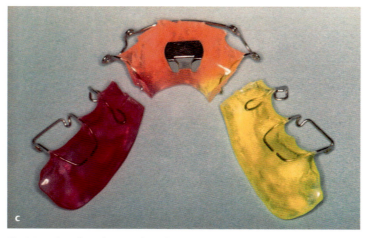
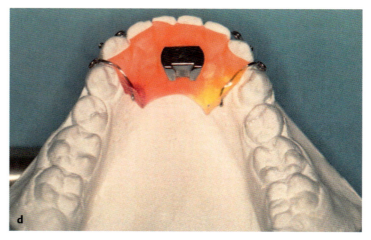

Fig. 6.5 a–d **After Class I molar relationship is established, the lower FMS appliance is cut distal to the canines and the two posterior segments of the appliance are removed from the mouth.** The absence of the posterior segments (only the anterior segment of the lower appliance remains in the mouth) results in a posterior bite clearance that allows guided eruption of the lower posterior segments (courtesy B. Leibovitch and S. Rellu).

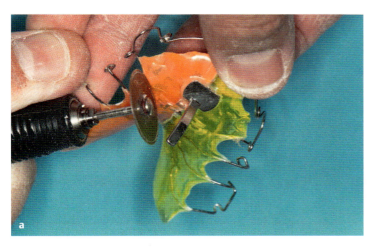
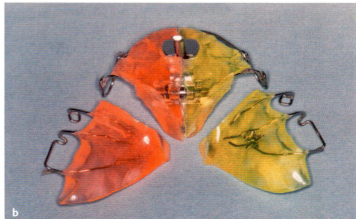
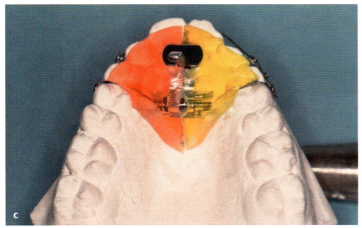
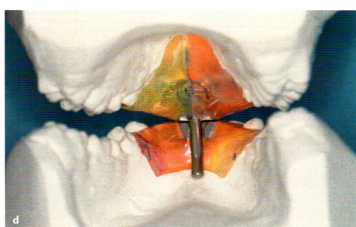

Fig. 6.**6a–d** It is of major importance to start the removal of the posterior segments in the lower FMS appliance and to wait 2–4 months before repeating the procedure in the upper appliance. Guidance of eruption is mainly required in the lower dental arch to correct deep bite (lower molar eruption) and level the curve of Spee (lower premolar eruption). For this reason, the contribution of the upper posterior dental arch to the vertical correction is secondary and should follow after the full potential of lower guidance of eruption is completed (courtesy B. Leibovitch and S. Rellu).

FMS Modus Operandi

The major advantage of using attractive magnetic forces to drive mandibular propulsion over conventional purely muscle-driven or elastic forces is the unique force versus distance ratio exhibited by the former (Fig. 6.7). As the points of force origin approximate each other, as in mouth closure, the magnetic force increases inversely to the square of the distance, while Class II elastic force decreases. This increase in magnetic force at short distances counterbalances the weaker vertical support of the oral musculature and allows an increase in the "efficacious wearing time."

The initial guidance of the mandible into the protrusive closure position is produced by the slide of the lower inclined plane along the upper prong (from mouth opening of 8.5 mm to 3 mm) (Fig. 6.**8a, c**). Final guidance is controlled mainly by the magnets (from mouth opening of 3 mm to 0 mm, i.e., from 0 to 3 N) (Fig. 6.**8b, d**).

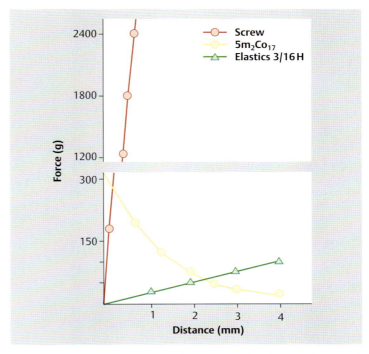

Fig. 6.7 **The magnetic force is inversely proportional to the second power of the distance ($F \sim 1/d^2$).** In contrast, forces exhibited by Class II elastics or screws are directly proportional to the distance ($F \sim d$).

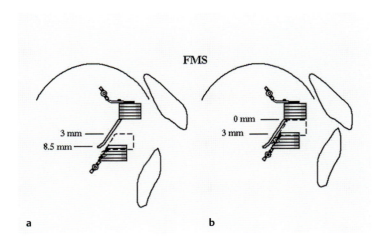

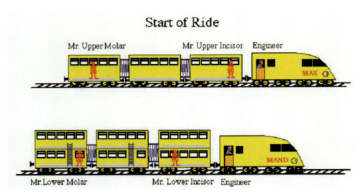

Fig. 6.9 **Rules of the functional correction ride.**
1. Maxillary train and passengers are ahead of the mandibular train and passengers.
2. Both trains move in a forward direction, and the mandibular train also downward.
3. The passengers are free to walk during the ride forward and upward in the mandible (to the upper deck) and backward in the maxillary train.
4. At the end of the trip all passengers remain in their new positions.
(Fig. 6.**9**–**20** courtesy Mrs. Ana Behar)

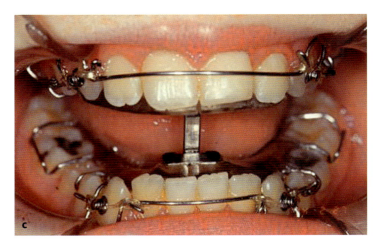

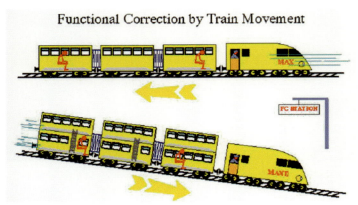

Fig. 6.**10** The result of the functional correction ride accomplished by the movement of the trains with the passengers staying stationary.

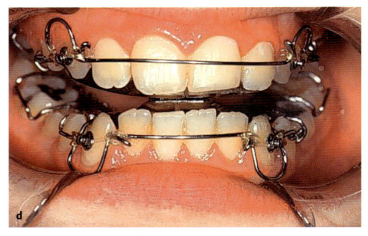

Fig. 6.8 **Guidance into the final position.**
a Initial guidance of the mandible into the protrusive closure position is provided by the lower incline and upper prong (from mouth opening of 8.5 mm to 3 mm).
b The final guidance is provided by the attractive magnets (from mouth opening of 3 mm to 0 mm, i.e., from 0 to 3 N).
c Intraoral initial prong guidance.
d Intraoral final magnetic guidance.

Mechanism of Functional Correction

The biological principles of functional correction were well described (Meikle, 2007). However, the reciprocated interaction between the dental and skeletal units needs a thorough elucidation. To understand the mechanism of functional correction, let us use an analogy involving two trains. One train is the mandible and the other the maxilla. Each train has two passengers, Mr. Molar and Mr. Incisor. The third person in each train is the train's engineer. The two trains start the journey from a Class II position and end up when the passengers are in Class I relationship. There are, however, certain rules to consider before starting the journey (Fig. 6.**9**).

Both trains and passengers have a common objective—reaching the station with the molar passengers in Class I relationship. This objective can be reached by the movement of the trains with the passengers staying in an entirely stationary position (Fig. 6.**10**), by the movement of the passengers with no movement of the trains (Fig. 6.**11**), or by a combination of the two.

Appropriate questions to ask about this hypothetical excursion are:
1. What is the percentage of train motion in the functional correction ride and what is the contribution of the passengers' movement?
2. Does the maxillary engineer accelerate or decelerate his train in accordance with the backward movement of his passengers? Conversely, is the backward movement of the maxillary passengers regulated by the speed of the maxillary train?
3. Does the mandibular engineer slow down or speed up his train in response to a forward movement of his passengers? How do the mandibular passengers react to an advancement of the mandibular train?

Mechanism of Functional Correction 133

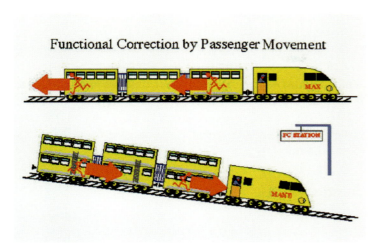

Fig. 6.**11** The result of the functional correction ride accomplished by movement of the passengers with no movement of the trains.

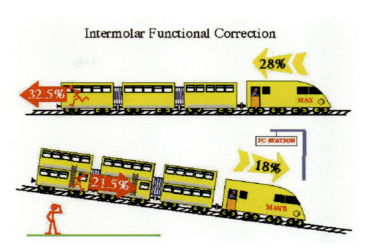

Fig. 6.**13** Functional correction of intermolar relationship as seen by an observer not riding on any of the trains.

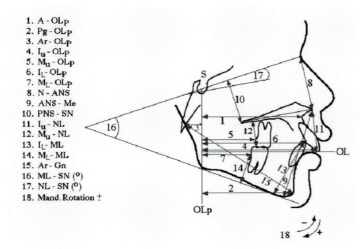

Fig. 6.**12** The pretreatment and 1-year interval lateral cephalometric radiographs superimposed according to Pancherz's method.

1. A–OL$_P$ – A point to the perpendicular to the occlusal line passing through sella point (OL$_P$)
2. Pg–OL$_P$ – Pogonion to OL$_P$
3. Ar–OL$_P$ – Articulare to OL$_P$
4. IU–OL$_P$ – Upper incisor to OL$_P$
5. MU–OL$_P$ – Upper molar to OL$_P$
6. I$_L$–OL$_P$ – Lower incisor to OL$_P$
7. M$_L$–OL$_P$ – Lower molar to OL$_P$
8. N–ANS – Nasion to anterior nasal spine
9. ANS–Me – Anterior nasal spine to menton
10. PNS–SN – Posterior nasal spine to sella nasion line
11. I$_U$–NL – Upper incisor to nasal line
12. M$_U$–NL – Upper molar to nasal line
13. I$_L$–ML – Lower incisor to mandibular line
14. M$_L$–ML – Lower molar to mandibular line
15. Ar–Gn – Articulare to gnathion
16. ML–SN – Mandibular line to sella nasion line (angle)
17. NL–SN – Nasal line to sella nasion line (angle)
18. Mandibular rotation – (+) clockwise rotation (–) counter clockwise rotation

4. Does the engineer of the first train react to the movement of the second train?
5. Do analogous passengers synchronize their movement? That is, does the travel of Mr. Lower Molar depend on the movement of Mr. Upper Molar, or do the two move independently?
6. How do passengers compensate for the slope in the lower railway?

To answer these questions, we took 60 subjects with a mean age of 10.8 ± 0.8 years and divided them into three groups of 20 subjects each (Vardimon et al. 2001). Group 1 (GCl I) and group 2 (GCl II) were untreated and served as controls. The third group (GFMS) had Class II malocclusions and received FMS treatment. Serial cephalometric radiographs of each subject were evaluated for skeletal and dental changes (Fig. 6.**12**).

The results of this study shed light on all of the above six questions relating to the rail travel analogy.

Question 1

It was found that an observer standing at the molar-end of the tracks (Fig. 6.**13**) would report that passengers Mr. Upper Molar and Mr. Lower Molar have now been transported into a Class I occlusion. Of this change, 28% was found to be due to a slow-down of the maxillary train speed (maxillary growth restraint), and 32.5% to the backward movement of Mr. Upper Molar (upper molar distalization). The mandibular train contributed 18% of the molar correction through an increase in train speed (mandibular growth augmentation) and 21.5% through the forward movement of Mr. Lower Molar (lower molar mesialization). That is, the maxillary train with its posterior passenger contributed 60.5% of the correction, while the mandibular train with its posterior passenger contributed only 39.5% of the correction. The skeletal to dental ratio was 46% to 54% respectively.

Another observer placed by the front side of the railway (Fig. 6.**14**) during the same trip would report that the journey of the upper and lower incisors had transported them into an improved interincisal relationship. Of this improvement, 21% can be attributed to a slow-down (maxillary growth restraint) of the maxillary train speed and 43.5% to the backward movement (retroclination) of Mr. Upper Incisor. In addition, the mandibular train's forward movement (mandibular growth acceleration) contributed 13.5% to the correction, and the forward movement (proclination) of Mr. Lower Incisor contributed 22%. Thus, similarly to the intermolar correction, 64.5% of the interincisor relationship was accomplished by the maxillary train with its anterior passenger, and 34.5% by the mandibular train with its anterior passen-

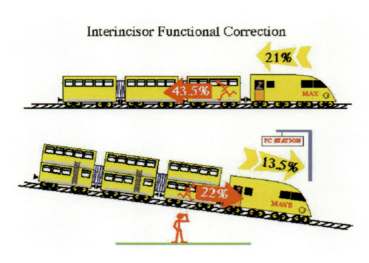

Fig. 6.14 Functional correction of interincisor relationship as seen by an observer not riding on any of the trains.

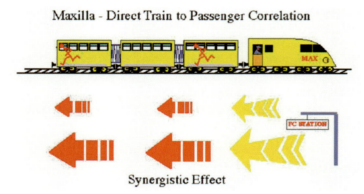

Fig. 6.15 In the maxilla, a direct correlation developed between the dental and skeletal reaction to functional correction (synergistic reaction). The less the forward movement of the maxillary train (i.e., greater backward maxillary restraint), the greater the backward movement of Mr. Upper Molar or Mr. Upper Incisor.

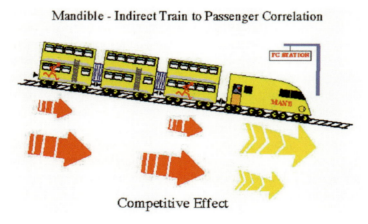

Fig. 6.16 In the mandible, an indirect correlation developed between the dental and skeletal reaction to functional correction (competitive reaction). The greater the forward movement of the mandibular train, the less Mr. Lower Molar and Mr. Lower Incisor will move forward, and vice versa. That is, the greater the forward movement of Mr. Lower Molar, the less the advancement of the mandibular train.

ger. In this instance the skeletal to dental ratio is 34.5% to 65.5% respectively (Fig. 6.14).

The major difference between the two observers concerns the ratio of train movement to passenger movement, i.e., skeletal to dental correction. The molar observer reported a ratio close to 1:1, while the incisor observer reported a ratio closer to 1:2. That is, up to twice as much passenger (dental correction) as train (skeletal correction) movement was observed from the incisal vantage point.

Questions 2–5

To answer these questions, a Pearson's test of correlation was carried out between pairs of skeletal parameters (i.e., maxillary train vs. mandibular train), skeletal vs. dental parameters (i.e., mandibular train vs. Mr. Lower Molar), and dental vs. dental parameters (i.e., Mr. Upper Molar vs. Mr. Lower Molar). If the correlation between two parameters was found to be significant, treatment changes occurring in one parameter were dependent on treatment changes occurring in the other parameter, and vice versa. Likewise, if a comparison of two parameters was not found to be significant, this indicated that they occurred independently of one another. Further, if an increase in one parameter caused an increase in the second, the two are described as being related in a positive (direct) correlation. If an increase in one parameter was found to cause a decrease in the second, the two are said to be related in a negative (inverse) correlation.

The findings showed that dependent correlations were almost always related to at least one skeletal parameter. Most of the independent correlations occurred between dental parameters. These findings suggest that the skeletal parameters are the regulating factors controlling the functional correction process in spite of their modest contribution. In other words, the train moves a small distance and the passengers move a greater distance, but the ones who regulate the system are the train engineers. Thus, the principal criterion of functional correction is the *presence* of a skeletal response and not its magnitude. These findings support the notion that functional correction occurs so long as there is a skeletal contribution, no matter how small.

Question 2

In the maxilla (Fig. 6.15), the dental reaction was found to be significant and directly correlated with the skeletal reaction. This implies that the greater the maxillary growth restraint (less forward movement of the maxillary train, i.e., decrease in A–OL$_P$), the greater the distalization of the upper dental arch (greater backward movement of Mr. Upper Molar or Mr. Upper Incisor; i.e., decrease in M_U or I_U). Thus, the skeletal to dental reaction was synergistic in the maxilla (Fig. 6.15).

Question 3

In the mandible (Fig. 6.16), the dental reaction was significantly but inversely (negatively) correlated with the skeletal reaction. This indicates that the greater the mandibular growth (more forward movement of the mandibular train; i.e., increase in Pg–OL$_P$), the less the mesialization of the lower dental arch (less forward

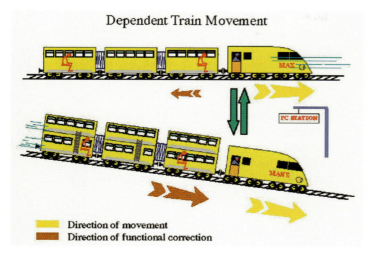

Fig. 6.**17** **The interaction between the trains is directly correlated.** A favorable mandibular skeletal advancement is coupled with an increase in maxillary growth, that is, a decrease in maxillary growth restraint.

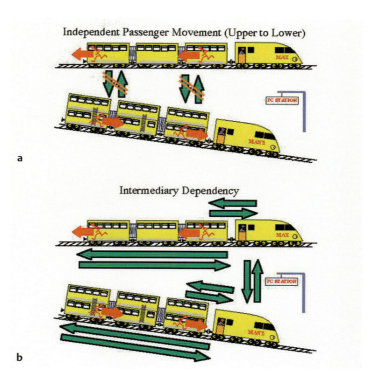

Fig. 6.**18** **Independent movement (a) and intermediary dependency (b).**
a Dental parameters were independent of each other; i.e., the movements of Mr. Lower Molar and Mr. Upper Molar are not related.
b However, the dental reaction between their respective arches has a degree of dependence on skeletal changes (intermediary dependency: trains react as intra-arch and inter-arch mediators). That is, each train dictates the movement of its passengers, and the two trains exchange information by a direct correlation.

movement of Mr. Lower Molar or Mr. Lower Incisor; i.e., decrease in M_L or I_L). Thus, the skeletal to dental reaction was competitive in the mandible (Fig. 6.**16**).

Question 4

The interaction between the trains (i.e., the interjaw skeletal reaction: A–OL_P and Pg-OL_P) was found to be a significant direct correlation (Fig. 6.**17**). This suggests that the two train engineers react to each other and change their speeds in the same direction (but inversely to their functional correction effect). Favorable mandibular skeletal advancement is coupled with an increase in maxillary growth, which is to say that a smaller restraint of maxillary growth or favorable maxillary growth restraint is linked to weak mandibular skeletal advancement. This again emphasizes that the whole system is operated by the train engineers. The degree of functional skeletal reaction varies between individuals, however.

Question 5

As noted, dental parameters were found to be independent of one another. Thus, the movements of Mr. Lower Molar and Mr. Upper Molar were not synchronized (Fig. 6.**18a**). This is an incomplete answer, however, as these were found to be related to their skeletal parameters (directly in the maxilla [see Question 2] and indirectly in the mandible [see Question 3]), and the two trains themselves were related (see Question 4). This implies that the movement of two upper and lower passengers is regulated via the supervision of the two train engineers (Fig. 6.**18b**).

Question 6

The slope of the railway is about 2°. Therefore, to compensate for the separation between the passengers of the upper and lower trains, Mr. Upper Molar should move inferiorly and Mr. Lower Molar superiorly. However, it was found that only Mr. Lower Molar moved superiorly (2 mm) (Fig. 6.**19**). This guidance of eruption is performed by removing the posterior clasps and their acrylic support distal to the canines in the lower FMS appliance only. Guidance of eruption is undertaken once a stable anteroposterior relationship is established. It is extremely important to achieve a well-interdigitated posterior occlusion. This requirement is necessary to prevent dental and skeletal relapse once treatment is terminated.

To summarize the modus operandi of the FMS functional correction:

1. There is an orthopedic response with every functional correction.
2. The skeletal response regulates the functional correction reaction. Although the skeletal response is less than the dental response, the system will not operate without at least a minute skeletal response.
3. The dental response in the upper arch reacts synergistically with the maxillary orthopedic response. That is, the greater the upper molar distalization, the more restraint of maxillary sagittal growth was observed.

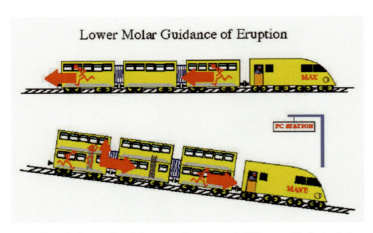

Fig. 6.**19** **The forward and downward movement of the mandibular train is compensated by the mesiosuperior movement of Mr. Lower Molar (guidance of eruption).**

4. The dental response in the lower arch reacts competitively to the mandibular orthopedic reaction. That is, with greater lower molar mesialization there was less mandibular sagittal growth.
5. There is an inverse interaction between the maxillary and mandibular functional skeletal responses. That is, an increase in one skeletal response (e.g., strong mandibular advancement) was found to cause a decrease in the other (e.g., weak maxillary growth restraint).
6. The vertical clearance that developed between the dental arches as a consequence of the posteroanterior functional correction is compensated by a guidance-of-eruption mechanism of the lower posterior dentition.

Clinical Case Studies

Analysis of Treatment Results

In general, the philosophy of orthodontic treatment seeks to accomplish facial harmony, dental symmetry, balanced occlusion, and Andrews' six keys of occlusion (Andrews 1972). FMS treatment addresses the treatment goals of facial and musculoskeletal harmony, and the first and last of Andrew's six keys (molar classification and curve of Spee). The use of fixed orthodontic appliances following FMS treatment allows one to satisfy the remaining treatment goals (i.e., leveling and alignment, angulation, inclination, torque, etc.). Cases Studies 6.1 to 6.4 demonstrate this treatment approach. Treatment results are assessed according to seven cephalometric parameters (Fig. 6.20).

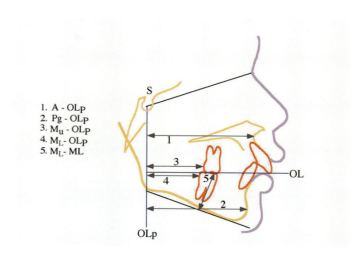

Fig. 6.**20** The seven parameters used to assess the FMS treatment results:
1. Maxillary base sagittal = $A–OL_P$
2. Mandibular base sagittal = $Pg–OL_P$
3. Upper molar skeleto-dental sagittal = $M_U–OL_P$
4. Lower molar skeleto-dental sagittal = $M_L–OL_P$
5. Lower molar skeleto-dental vertical = $M_L–ML$
6. Upper molar dental sagittal = (3) – (1) = $(M_U–OL_P) – (A–OL_P)$
7. Lower molar dental sagittal = (4) – (2) = $(ML–OL_P) – (Pg–OL_P)$.

Case Study 6.1 Patient I. G.

This is a 13-year-old boy presenting with a severely retrognathic mandible (SNB = 70°, Pg to N⊥ = – 14 mm or Pg to N⊥ = – 14 mm), and a slightly retrognathic maxilla (SNA = 77°), 10 mm overjet, and incomplete bite (Figs. 6.1.**1–4**). After nine months of FMS treatment, a Class I molar relationship was achieved *[5–8]*, and the cephalometric changes listed in Table 6.**1** were noted. However, since the open bite was aggravated due to the incompetent lip seal caused by protruded incisors (Figs. 6.1.**5–8**), it was decided to extract four first premolars prior to a second stage of treatment using edgewise appliances (Figs. 6.1.**9–12**).

The intermolar correction of patient I. G. at the end of the FMS treatment is presented in (Fig. 6.1.**13**). The dark blue arrows represent the treatment outcome, including the effects of growth. The light blue arrows illustrate the net treatment change after subtracting the average growth that occurred during this period. This is not the individual growth change but a mean growth change (1 year) of untreated Class II patients. That is, the resultant net treatment change is only an approximation since a patient cannot serve as the control for himself or herself for the same given period. With this limitation, the net treatment changes exhibited by patient I. G. demonstrate that in patient I. G. only the mandibular dental and skeletal components contributed to the functional correction, while the maxillary components aggravated the malocclusion. The mandibular contribution was greater than the maxillary impairment, however.

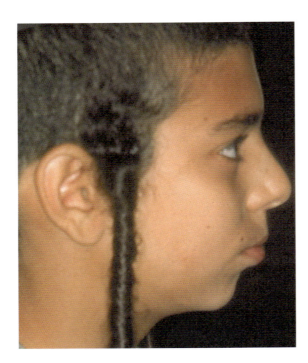

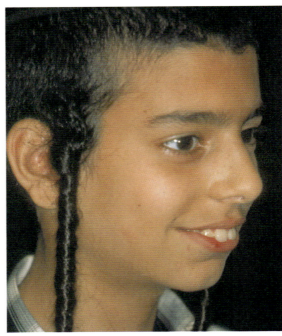

Fig. 6.1.**1** **Pre-treatment.** Profile with a severely retrognathic mandible. (Courtesy Dr. Diego Grinblat.)

Fig. 6.1.**2** **Pre-treatment.** Smile, with everted lower lip. (Courtesy Dr. Diego Grinblat.)

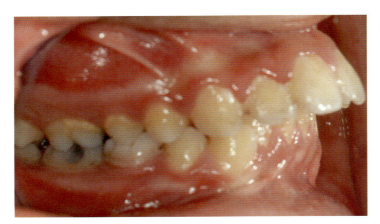

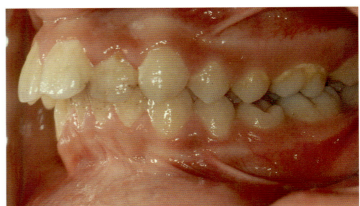

Fig. 6.1.**3** **Pre-treatment.** Occlusion with Class II molar.

Fig. 6.1.**4** **Pre-treatment.** Canine relationship, 10 mm overjet, and incomplete bite. (Courtesy Dr. Diego Grinblat.)

Table 6.1.**1** Patient I. G. Cephalometric changes

Parameter	Before Treatment (mm)	After FMS Treatment (mm)	Treatment Change (After – Before) (mm)	Growth Change (mm)	Net Change (Treatment – Growth) (mm)
$A-OL_P$	77	80	3	1.93	1.07
$Pg-OL_P$	72	80	8	2.59	5.41
M_U-OL_P	40	46	6		
M_L-OL_P	37	47	10		
M_L-ML	30	33	3	1.04	1.96
M_U			−3*	0.77	2.23
M_L			2	0.19	1.81

* A negative value represents distal movement; a positive value represents mesial movement.
$A-OL_P$, distance from point A to occlusal line perpendicular.
$Pg-OL_P$, distance from pogonion to occlusal line perpendicular.
M_U-OL_P, distance from upper molar to occlusal line perpendicular.
M_L-OL_P, distance from lower molar to occlusal line perpendicular.
M_L-ML, vertical distance mandibular line to mesial cusp tip of lower molar
M_U, M_L, The difference (after minus before) of ($M_{U,L}-OL_P$ minus $A-OL_P$)
Growth Change, change that occurred in untreated Class II patient during 1 year
Net Change, difference between treatment change and growth change

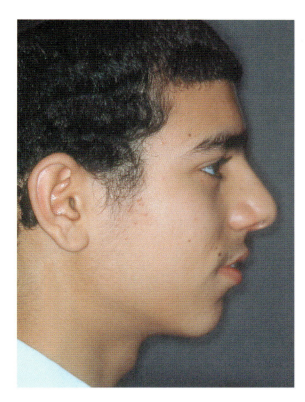
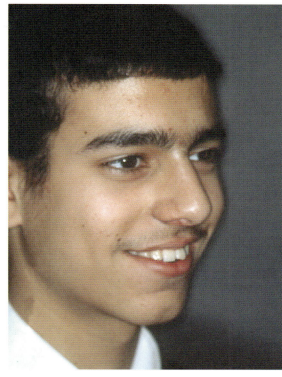

Fig. 6.1.**5** **FMS treatment stage.** Profile; note the reduction in soft ANB angle as compared to the pretreatment profile in 6.1.**1**. (Courtesy Dr. Diego Grinblat.)

Fig. 6.1.**6** **FMS treatment stage.** Smile; lower lip eversion was reduced as compared to the pretreatment smile in Fig. 6.1.**2**. (Courtesy Dr. Diego Grinblat.)

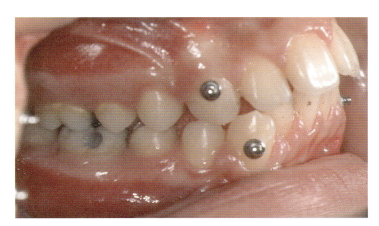
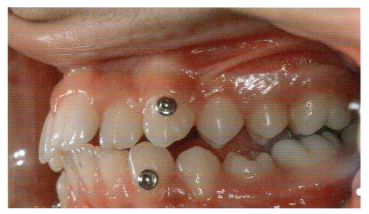

Fig. 6.1.**7** **FMS treatment stage.** Occlusion, a Class I molar and canine relationship was accomplished on both sides. However, an incomplete bite developed. (Courtesy Dr. Diego Grinblat.)

Fig. 6.1.**8** **FMS treatment stage.** Occlusion, a Class I molar and canine relationship was accomplished on both sides. However, an incomplete bite developed. (Courtesy Dr. Diego Grinblat.)

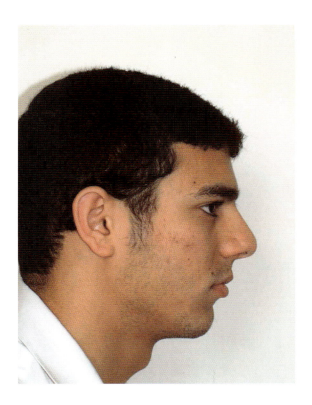
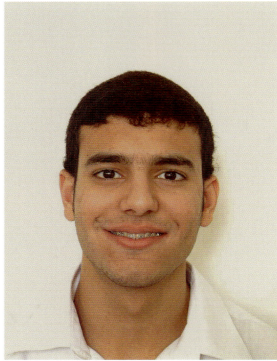

Fig. 6.1.**9** **Edgewise treatment stage with four premolar extractions.** Profile; a complete lip seal was established as compared to pretreatment Fig. 6.1.**1** and post-FMS treatment stage Fig. 6.1.**5**. (Courtesy Dr. Iliana Stavrinidou.)

Fig. 6.1.**10** **Edgewise treatment stage with four premolar extractions.** Smile; lower lip eversion was deleted as compared to pretreatment smile Fig. 6.1.**2** and post-FMS treatment stage Fig. 6.1.**6**. (Courtesy Dr. Iliana Stavrinidou.)

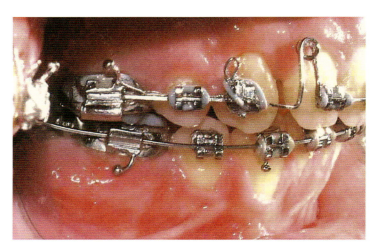
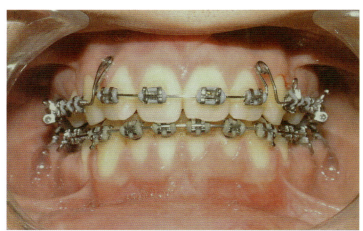

Fig. 6.1.**11** **Edgewise treatment stage with four premolar extractions.** Occlusion; the incomplete bite was eliminated with a substantial improvement in anterior overbite. (Courtesy Dr. Iliana Stavrinidou.)

Fig. 6.1.**12** **Edgewise treatment stage with four premolar extractions.** Occlusion; the incomplete bite was eliminated with a substantial improvement in anterior overbite. (Courtesy Dr. Iliana Stavrinidou.)

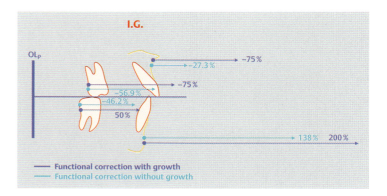

Fig. 6.1.**13** **For patient I.G., only the mandibular dental and skeletal components contributed to the functional correction, while the maxillary components aggravated the malocclusion (a minus value refers to a change in opposite direction to the functional correction).** However, the mandibular contribution was greater than the maxillary detraction.

Case Study 6.2 Patient F. N.

F. N. was a boy of 11.3 years at the time of initiation of FMS treatment. His Class II malocclusion was mostly due to a prognathic maxilla and a mildly retrognathic mandible (A–N⊥ = 4 mm, Pg–N⊥ = − 8 mm, SNA = 80°, SNB = 72°) (Figs. 6.2.**1–6**). First-stage treatment with FMS lasted nine months (Figs. 6.2.**7–12**) and was followed by a stage of edgewise appliance therapy (Figs. 6.2.**13–20**). Table 6.**2**.1 shows the cephalometric functional correction changes.

Fig. 6.2.**21** illustrates the percentage correction of each component. Without adjusting for the influence of normal growth, it was found in this patient that 75% of the change observed in the molar occlusion was due to upper molar distalization. After subtracting the influence of growth, however, the mandibular skeletal contribution decreased to 10.5% and the maxillary dental contribution (molar distalization) increased to 96.2%.

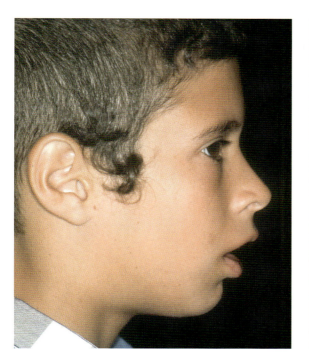

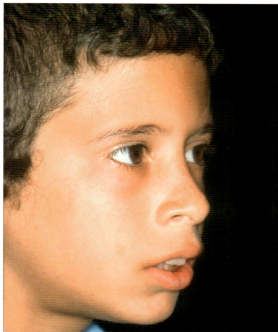

Fig. 6.2.**1** Pretreatment record. Profile, with mildly retrognathic mandible, prognathic maxilla, and incompetent lips.

Fig. 6.2.**2** Pretreatment record. Smile. (Courtesy Dr. Abraham Kyriakides.)

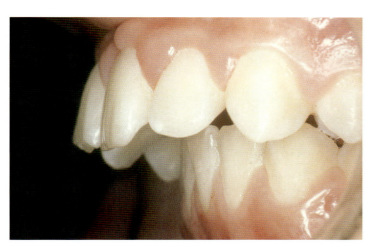

Fig. 6.2.**3** Pretreatment record. Overjet; the severe sagittal discrepancy produced a scissor-bite of the first upper premolar. (Courtesy Dr. Abraham Kyriakides.)

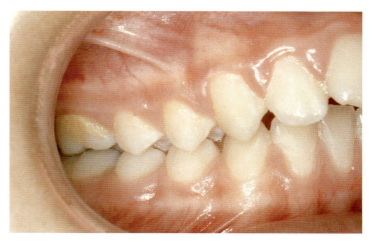

Fig. 6.2.**4** Pretreatment record. Right occlusion with Class II molar and canine relationship. (Courtesy Dr. Abraham Kyriakides.)

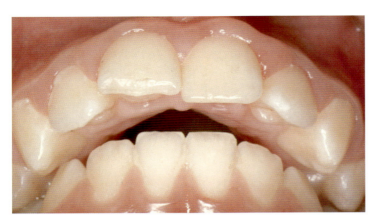

Fig. 6.2.**5** **Pretreatment record. Frontal view with incomplete bite.** (Courtesy Dr. Abraham Kyriakides.)

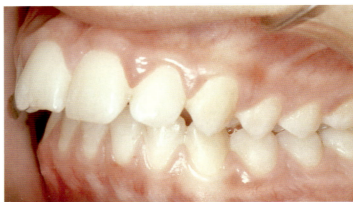

Fig. 6.2.**6** **Pretreatment record. Left occlusion;** the severe sagittal discrepancy produced, similarly to the right occlusion, a scissors-bite of the first upper premolar. (Courtesy Dr. Abraham Kyriakides.)

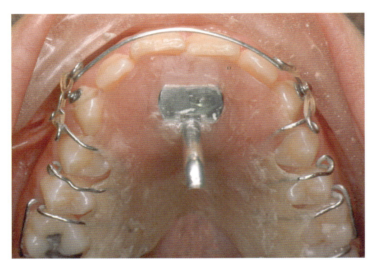

Fig. 6.2.**7** **FMS treatment stage.** Upper FMS appliance. (Courtesy Dr. Abraham Kyriakides.)

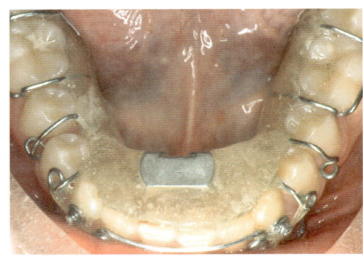

Fig. 6.2.**8** **FMS treatment stage.** Lower FMS appliance; in both FMS appliances the acrylic support on the palatal/lingual side of the canines prevents extrusion of these abutment teeth by the elastic clasp. (Courtesy Dr. Abraham Kyriakides.)

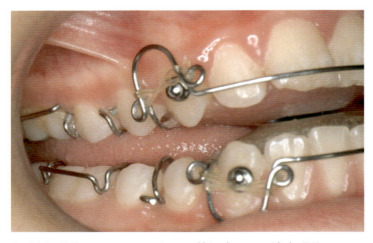

Fig. 6.2.**9** **FMS treatment stage.** Increased bite clearance with the FMS. (Courtesy Dr. Abraham Kyriakides.)

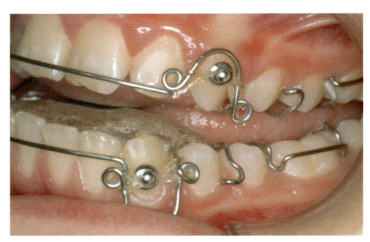

Fig. 6.2.**10** **FMS treatment stage.** Increased bite clearance with the FMS. (Courtesy Dr. Abraham Kyriakides.)

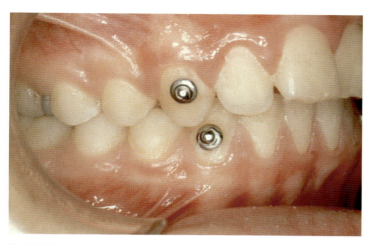

Fig. 6.2.**11 FMS treatment stages.** End of FMS treatment; a Class I molar and canine relationship was established with residual spaces and mild overjet. (Courtesy Dr. Abraham Kyriakides.)

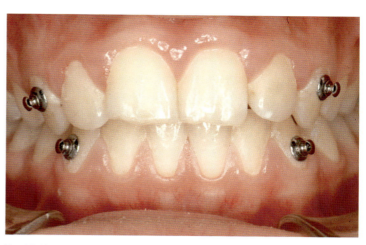

Fig. 6.2.**12 FMS treatment stages.** End of FMS treatment; a Class I molar and canine relationship was established with residual spaces and mild overjet. (Courtesy Dr. Abraham Kyriakides.)

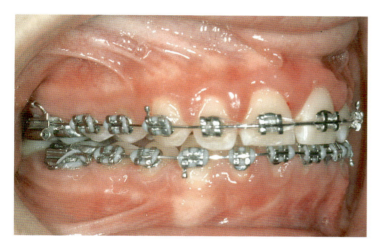

Fig. 6.2.**13 Edgewise treatment stage.** During treatment, closing residual spaces. (Courtesy Dr. Eleni Dre.)

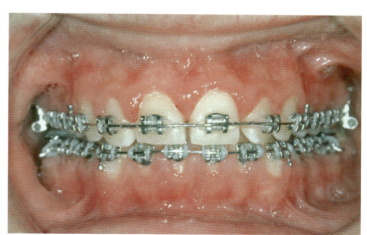

Fig. 6.2.**14 Edgewise treatment stage.** During treatment, closing residual spaces. (Courtesy Dr. Eleni Dre.)

Table 6.2.1 Patient F. N. Cephalometric changes

Parameter	Before Treatment (mm)	After FMS Treatment (mm)	Treatment Change (After – Before) (mm)	Growth Change (mm)	Net Change (Treatment – Growth) (mm)
A–OL$_P$	77	80	3	1.93	1.07
Pg–OL$_P$	72	75	3	2.59	0.41
M$_U$–OL$_P$	50	50	0		
M$_L$–OL$_P$	47	51	4		
M$_L$–ML	30	34	4	1.04	2.96
M$_U$			–3*	0.77	–3.77*
M$_L$			1	0.19	0.81

* A negative value represents distal movement; a positive value represents mesial movement.
A–OL$_P$, distance from point A to occlusal line perpendicular.
Pg–OL$_P$, distance from pogonion to occlusal line perpendicular.
M$_U$–OL$_P$, distance from upper molar to occlusal line perpendicular.
M$_L$–OL$_P$, distance from lower molar to occlusal line perpendicular.
M$_L$–ML, vertical distance mandibular line to mesial cusp tip of lower molar
M$_U$, M$_L$, The difference (after minus before) of (M$_{U,L}$–OL$_P$ minus A–OL$_P$)
Growth Change, change that occurred in untreated Class II patient during 1 year
Net Change, difference between treatment change and growth change

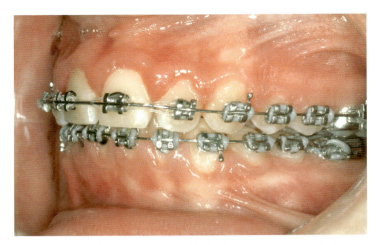

Fig. 6.2.**15** **Edgewise treatment stage.** During treatment, closing residual spaces. (Courtesy Dr. Eleni Dre.)

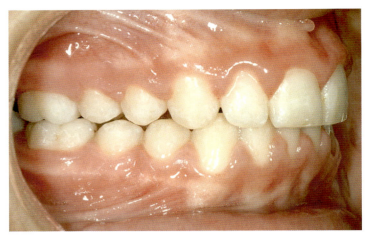

Fig. 6.2.**16** **Edgewise treatment stage.** Post treatment, a solid Class I molar and canine relationship was established with no overjet. (Courtesy Dr. Eleni Dre.)

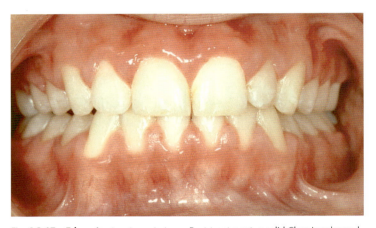

Fig. 6.2.**17** **Edgewise treatment stage.** Post treatment, a solid Class I molar and canine relationship was established with no overjet. (Courtesy Dr. Eleni Dre.)

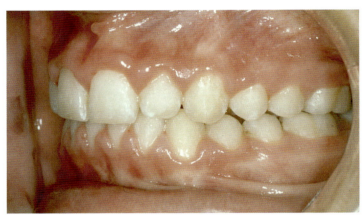

Fig. 6.2.**18** **Edgewise treatment stage.** Post treatment, a solid Class I molar and canine relationship was established with no overjet. (Courtesy Dr. Eleni Dre.)

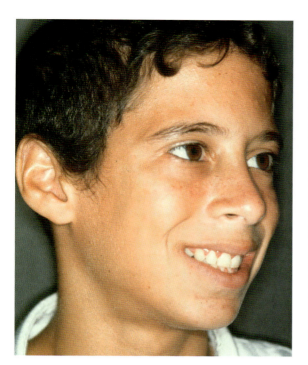
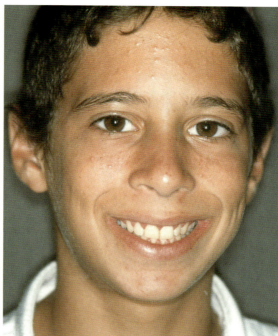

Fig. 6.2.**19** **Edgewise treatment stage.** Post-treatment profile and smile. (Courtesy Dr. Eleni Dre.)

Fig. 6.2.**20** **Edgewise treatment stage.** Post-treatment profile and smile. (Courtesy Dr. Eleni Dre.)

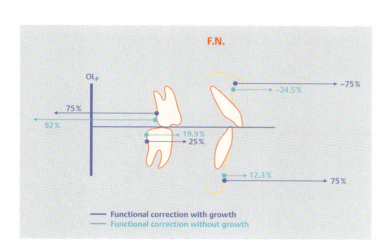

Fig. 6.2.**21** After accounting for the effects of growth, the mandibular skeletal contribution dropped to 12.3% and the maxillary dental contribution (molar distalization) increased to 92%. The sum of the positive contribution (104.3%) is greater than 100% since additionally negative contribution took place (−4.3%).

Case Study 6.3   Patient J. M.

J. M. is a 12.6-year-old boy presenting with a Class II malocclusion comprising a retrognathic mandible (SNB = 71°, Pg–N⊥ = − 17 mm), a 9 mm overjet associated with a deep overbite, and hypoplasia of the maxillary lateral incisors (Figs. 6.3.**1–4**). He was treated for an extended 24-month period with the FMS due to initial poor compliance, a treatment program that included bonding the appliance for three weeks (Figs. 6.3.**5–10**). The upper central incisors served as abutments for the FMS appliance due to delayed eruption of the upper canines (Figs. 6.3.**7, 8**). The bite clearance was increased to facilitate guidance of eruption of the posterior segment (Figs. 6.3.**9, 10**). After the FMS stage of therapy (Table 6.**3**), the upper arch was banded and bonded in order to open spaces around the lateral incisors (Figs. 6.3.**11–15**) for restorative recontouring with composite (Figs. 6.3.**12–14**). The gingival hypertrophy was expected resolve after bracket debonding.

The majority of intermolar occlusal correction was accomplished by lower molar mesialization (63.6%) and mandibular advancement (45.5%) (Fig. 6.3.**15**). As in the case of F. N., mandibular skeletal contribution was reduced by half (from 45.5% to 22.1%) when growth was detracted from the treatment outcome (Fig. 6.3.**19**). For J. M., however, this was associated with an increase (from 27.3% to 34.5%) in upper molar distalization (Fig. 6.3.**14**).

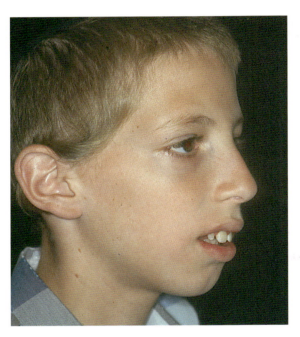
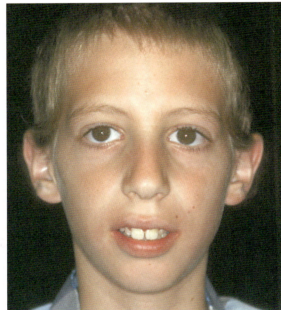

Fig. 6.3.**1** **Pretreatment records.** Profile; a retrognathic mandible. (Courtesy Dr. Costas Ergatoudes.)

Fig. 6.3.**2** **Pretreatment records.** Smile; with incompetent lips. (Courtesy Dr. Costas Ergatoudes.)

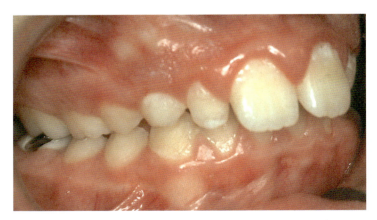

Fig. 6.3.**3** **Pretreatment records.** Right occlusion. with a 9 mm overjet. (Courtesy Dr. Costas Ergatoudes.)

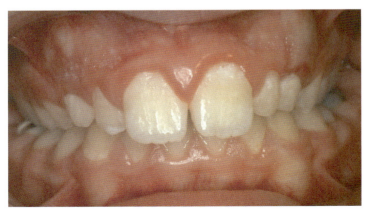

Fig. 6.3.**4** **Pretreatment records.** Frontal view; a deep overbite associated with hypoplasia of the maxillary lateral incisors. (Courtesy Dr. Costas Ergatoudes.)

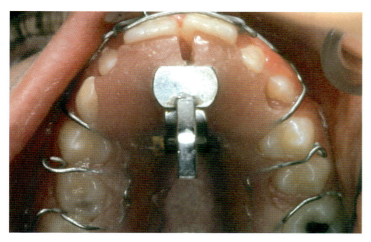

Fig. 6.3.**5** **FMS treatment stage.** Upper FMS appliance. (Courtesy Dr. Costas Ergatoudes.)

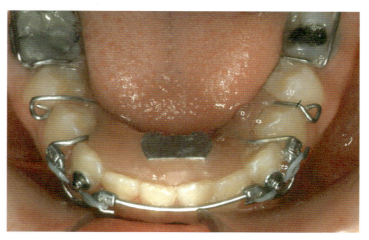

Fig. 6.3.**6** **FMS treatment stage.** Lower FMS appliance; due to initial poor compliance the upper and lower FMS appliances were bonded for three weeks by adding bonding material around the buccal extension of the Adam's clasps. (Courtesy Dr. Costas Ergatoudes.)

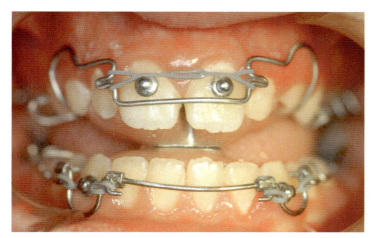

Fig. 6.3.**7** **FMS treatment stage.** Upper attachments were bonded to the central incisors, since the canines were not fully erupted. (Courtesy Dr. Costas Ergatoudes.)

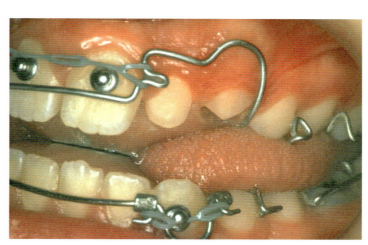

Fig. 6.3.**8** **FMS treatment stage.** Upper attachments were bonded to the central incisors, since the canines were not fully erupted. (Courtesy Dr. Costas Ergatoudes.)

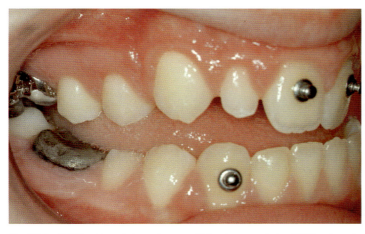

Fig. 6.3.**9** **FMS treatment stage.** Increased bite clearance during FMS treatment. A temporary overcorrection was achieved at the end of the bonding period, which was augmented due to the hypoplasia of the maxillary lateral incisors. (Courtesy Dr. Costas Ergatoudes.)

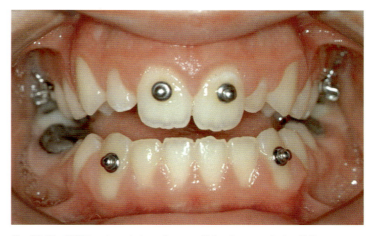

Fig. 6.3.**10** **FMS treatment stage.** Increased bite clearance during FMS treatment. A temporary overcorrection was achieved at the end of the bonding period, which was augmented due to the hypoplasia of the maxillary lateral incisors. (Courtesy Dr. Costas Ergatoudes.)

Table 6.3 Patient J.M. Cephalometric changes

Parameter	Before Treatment (mm)	After FMS Treatment (mm)	Treatment Change (After – Before) (mm)	Growth Change (mm)	Net Change (Treatment – Growth) (mm)
A–OL$_P$	80	84	4	1.93	2.07
Pg–OL$_P$	74	79	5	2.59	2.59
M$_U$–OL$_P$	46	47	1		
M$_L$–OL$_P$	44	56	12		
M$_L$–ML	33	38	5	1.04	3.96
M$_U$			– 1.5*	0.77	– 3.77*
M$_L$			– 2*	0.19	6.81

* A negative value represents distal movement; a positive value represents mesial movement.
A–OL$_P$, distance from point A to occlusal line perpendicular.
Pg–OL$_P$, distance from pogonion to occlusal line perpendicular.
M$_U$–OL$_P$, distance from upper molar to occlusal line perpendicular.
M$_L$–OL$_P$, distance from lower molar to occlusal line perpendicular.
M$_L$–ML, vertical distance mandibular line to mesial cusp tip of lower molar.
M$_U$, M$_L$, The difference (after minus before) of (M$_{U, L}$–OL$_P$ minus A–OL$_P$).
Growth Change, change that occurred in untreated Class II patient during 1 year.
Net Change, difference between treatment change and growth change.

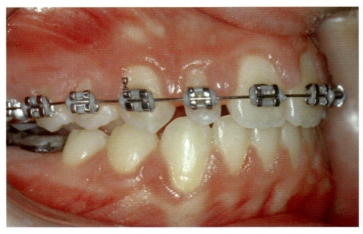

Fig. 6.3.**11** **Edgewise treatment stage.** A preparatory for upper lateral incisor restoration. (Courtesy Dr. Vasilis Kalamatas.)

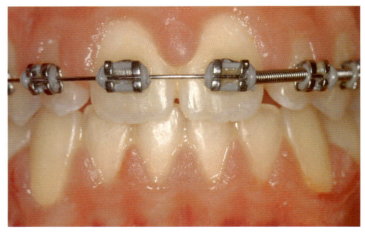

Fig. 6.3.**12** **Edgewise treatment stage.** A preparatory for upper lateral incisor restoration. (Courtesy Dr. Vasilis Kalamatas.)

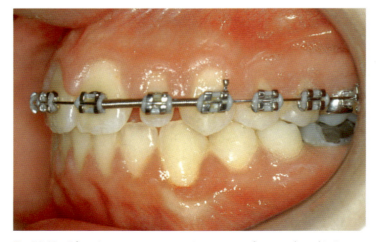

Fig. 6.3.**13** **Edgewise treatment stage.** A preparatory for upper lateral incisor restoration. (Courtesy Dr. Vasilis Kalamatas.)

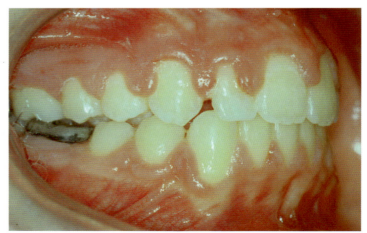

Fig. 6.3.**14** **Edgewise treatment stage.** Posttreatment occlusion with restored lateral incisors. (Courtesy Dr. Vasilis Kalamatas.)

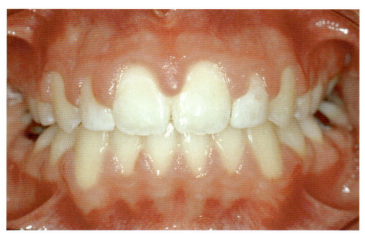

Fig. 6.3.**15** **Edgewise treatment stage.** Posttreatment occlusion with restored lateral incisors. (Courtesy Dr. Vasilis Kalamatas.)

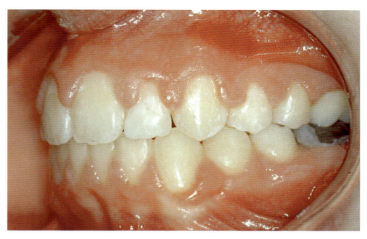

Fig. 6.3.**16** **Edgewise treatment stage.** Posttreatment occlusion with restored lateral incisors. (Courtesy Dr. Vasilis Kalamatas.)

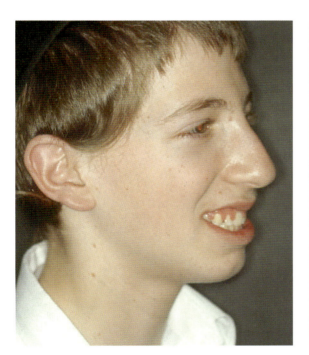

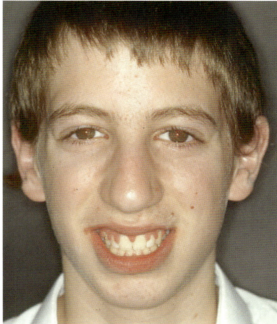

Fig. 6.3.**17** **Edgewise treatment stage.** Posttreatment profile and smile. (Courtesy Dr. Vasilis Kalamatas.)

Fig. 6.3.**18** **Edgewise treatment stage.** Posttreatment profile and smile. (Courtesy Dr. Vasilis Kalamatas.)

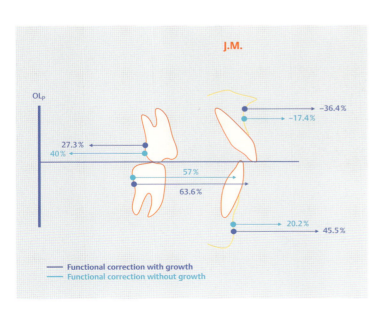

Fig. 6.3.**19** After accounting for the effects of growth, mandibular skeletal contribution was reduced by half (from 45.5% to 22.1%), followed by increase in distalization contribution of the upper molar (from 27.3% to 34.5%).

Case Study 6.4 Patient N. F.

N. F. was a boy of 14.3 years presenting with a severe Class II malocclusion comprising a slightly retruded maxilla (SNA = 76°) and severely retruded mandible (SNB = 67°) (Figs. 6.4.**1, 2**). Other relevant clinical findings included a 10 mm overjet, deep overbite, a narrow upper arch with crossbites of the right molar and second premolar associated with a functional midline deviation towards the crossbite side (Figs. 6.4.**3, 4**).

His treatment was divided into three stages, the first being use of a quad helix [5, 6] to establish an improved maxillary transverse dimension and to eliminate cross bites which would become aggravated with functional correction. The quad helix was augmented by the bonding of palatal buttons to the upper premolars to hinder occlusal slippage of the appliance lateral arms (Fig. 6.1.**5**).

Second, the FMS was used to correct sagittal and vertical discrepancies (Figs. 6.4.**7, 8**). This was carried out in two steps due to the strain on the musculature associated with the deep bite. The initial FMS application was prepared using a mandibular advancement to an edge-to-edge incisor relationship resulting in an edge-to-edge molar relationship (Figs. 6.4.**9, 10**). This initial stage of FMS therapy lasted four months and was followed by a second mandibular advancement to a 2 mm negative overjet. This second advancement brought the molars into Class I relationship but the canines were still in slight Class II (12 months).

Lastly, a fixed appliance was placed in order to accomplish all remaining dental objectives. This third stage corrected the canine position after four months using Class II elastics (Figs. 6.4.**11–13**). The mandibular advancement improved the profile allowing a balanced lip seal. The major contributor at the end of the FMS treatment was the mandibular bone (128.5%), which remained substantial even after deducting growth (92.6%) (Table 6.**4**; Fig. 6.4.**14–18**).

The four cases presented demonstrate the variation in response to functional correction. Even so, they also show that functional correction using the FMS is a feasible procedure. Further, the data indicate that a minor skeletal response is a mandatory prerequisite for this correction. It should also be noted that in order to complete all occlusal requirements, functional correction required an adjunctive fixed appliance treatment phase. This combined application provides a powerful synergistic tool that should be carried out in a logically ordered fashion, according to the individual treatment requirements of each patient.

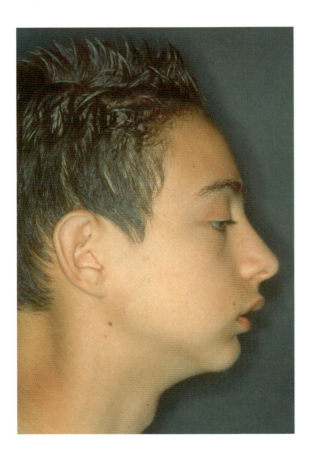

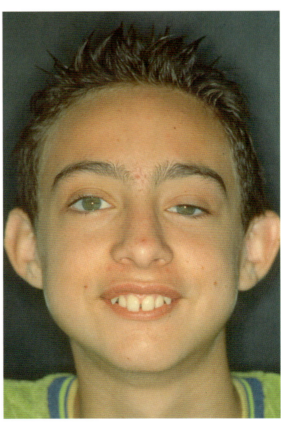

Fig. 6.4.**1 Pretreatment records.** Profile. (Courtesy Dr. Stefan Beckmann.)

Fig. 6.4.**2 Pretreatment records.** Smile; incompetent lip seal with everted lower lip. (Courtesy Dr. Stefan Beckmann.)

Clinical Case Studies   **151**

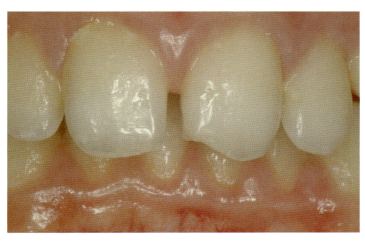

Fig. 6.4.**3 Pretreatment records.** Frontal view; excessive deep bite. (Courtesy Dr. Stefan Beckmann.)

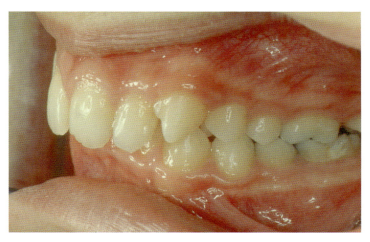

Fig. 6.4.**4 Pretreatment records.** Left occlusion, a full Class II molar and canine relationship. (Courtesy Dr. Stefan Beckmann.)

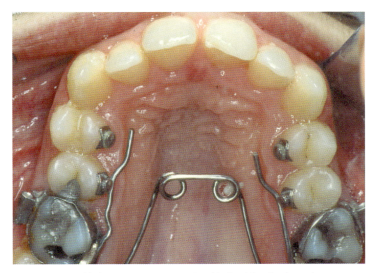

Fig. 6.4.**5 Quad helix treatment stage.** Quad helix with palatal attachments to prevent slippage of expansion arms. Initially, the molars and second premolars were expanded by the Quad helix and subsequently the first premolars. (Courtesy Dr. Stefan Beckmann.)

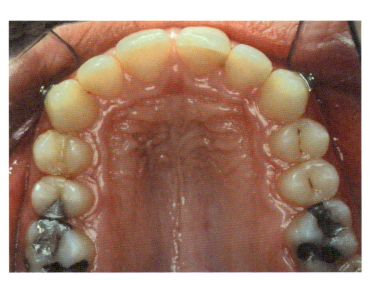

Fig. 6.4.**6 Quad helix treatment stage.** Occlusal view of the upper arch after expansion and removal of the Quad helix. Transverse discrepancy was corrected, and canine crowding was unraveled. (Courtesy Dr. Stefan Beckmann.)

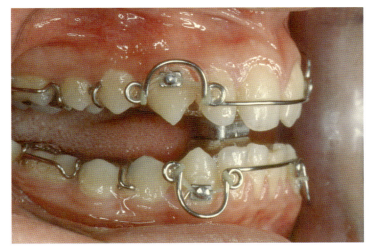

Fig. 6.4.**7 Increased bite clearance with the FMS appliance.** (Courtesy Dr. Stefan Beckmann.)

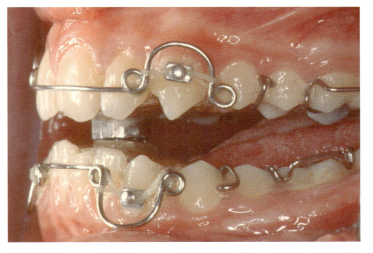

Fig. 6.4.**8 Increased bite clearance with the FMS appliance.** (Courtesy Dr. Stefan Beckmann.)

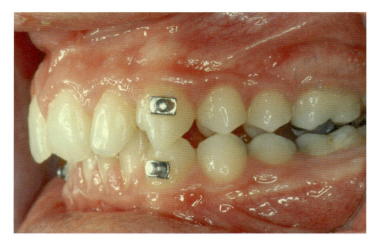

Fig. 6.4.9 Left occlusion and frontal view after first step of FMS advancement. An edge-to-edge canine and molar relationship was accomplished. (Courtesy Dr. Stefan Beckmann.)

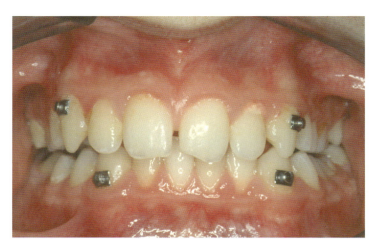

Fig. 6.4.10 Left occlusion and frontal view after first step of FMS advancement. An edge-to-edge canine and molar relationship was accomplished. (Courtesy Dr. Stefan Beckmann.)

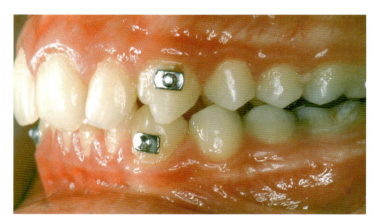

Fig. 6.4.11 Left occlusion and frontal view after second step of FMS advancement. A weak Class II canine relationship and an almost Class I molar relationship was accomplished. (Courtesy Dr. Stefan Beckmann.)

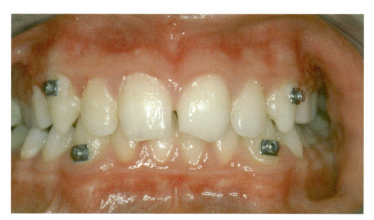

Fig. 6.4.12 Left occlusion and frontal view after second step of FMS advancement. A weak Class II canine relationship and an almost Class I molar relationship was accomplished. (Courtesy Dr. Stefan Beckmann.)

Table 6.4 Patient N. F. Cephalometric changes

Parameter	Before Treatment (mm)	After FMS Treatment (mm)	Treatment Change (After – Before) (mm)	Growth Change (mm)	Net Change (Treatment – Growth) (mm)
A–OL_P	83.5	85	1.5	1.93	−0.43
Pg–OL_P	87	96	9	2.59	6.41
M_U–OL_P	51	51	0		
M_L–OL_P	42	49	7		
M_L–ML	31	35	4	1.04	2.96
M_U			−1.5	0.77	−2.27*
M_L			−2	0.19	−2.19*

* A negative value represents distal movement; a positive value represents mesial movement.
A–OL_P, distance from point A to occlusal line perpendicular.
Pg–OL_P, distance from pogonion to occlusal line perpendicular.
M_U–OL_P, distance from upper molar to occlusal line perpendicular.
M_L–OL_P, distance from lower molar to occlusal line perpendicular.
M_L–ML, vertical distance mandibular line to mesial cusp tip of lower molar
M_U, M_L, The difference (after minus before) of ($M_{U,L}$–OL_P minus A–OL_P)
Growth Change, change that occurred in untreated Class II patient during 1 year
Net Change, difference between treatment change and growth change

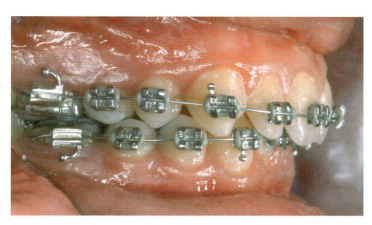

Fig. 6.4.**13** **Edgewise treatment stage.** Right occlusion. (Courtesy Dr. Stefan Beckmann.)

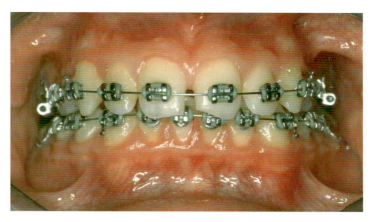

Fig. 6.4.**14** **Frontal view during treatment;** a full Class I canine and molar relationship was accomplished. (Courtesy Dr. Stefan Beckmann.)

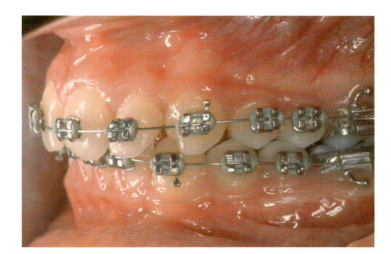

Fig. 6.4.**15** **Left occlusion;** a full Class I canine and molar relationship was accomplished. (Courtesy Dr. Stefan Beckmann.)

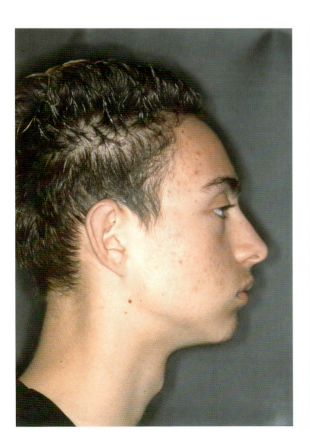

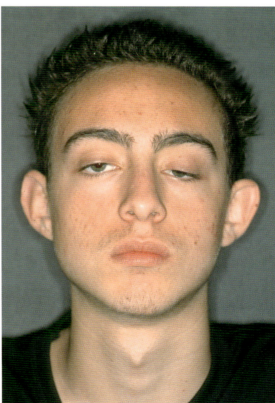

Fig. 6.4.**16** **Profile.** (Courtesy Dr. Stefan Beckmann.)

Fig. 6.4.**17** **Balanced lip seal after debonding.** (Courtesy Dr. Stefan Beckmann.)

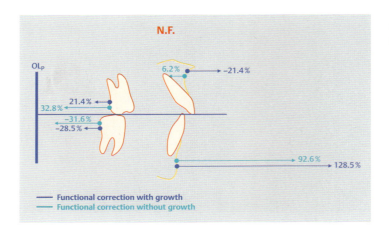

Fig. 6.4.**18** Mandibular repositioning was the major contributor, even after deducting growth (92.6%).

References

Ahlgren J. Early and late electromyographic response to treatment with activators. Am J Orthod. 1978; 74: 88–93.
Andresen V, Häupl K, Petrik L. Funktionskieferorthopädie – die Grundlagen des norwegischen Systems. 2nd ed. Leipzig: Meusser; 1936.
Andrews LF. The six keys to normal occlusion. Am J Orthod. 1972; 62: 296–309.
Baccetti T, Franchi L, Toth LR, McNamara JA Jr. Treatment timing for twin-block therapy. Am J Orthod Dentofacial Orthop. 2000; 118: 159–170.
Bass NM. Orthopedic appliance system. Part 2. Diagnosis and appliance prescription. J Clin Orthod. 1987; 21: 312–320.
Clark W. The twin block technique. In: Graber TM, Rakosi T, Petrovic AG, eds. Dentofacial orthopedics with functional appliances. St. Louis: Mosby; 1997: 268–298.
Eckhart JE. Introducing the MARA. Clinical impressions. 1998; 7: 2–5.
Fränkel R. Technick und Handhäbung der Funktionsregler. Berlin: VEB Verlag; 1973.
Gibbs CH, Mahan PE, Lundeen HC, et al. Occlusal forces during chewing-influences of biting strength and food consistency. J Prosthet Dent. 1981; 46: 561–567.
Graber TM. Functional appliances. In: Graber TM, Vanarsdall RL eds. Orthodontics, current principles and techniques. St. Louis: Mosby; 2000: 473–520.
Hamilton DC. Early treatment—the emancipation of dentofacial orthopedics. In: Graber TM, Rakosi T, Petrovic AG, eds. Dentofacial orthopedics with functional appliances. St. Louis: Mosby; 1997: 319–335.
Hansen K, Pancherz H, Hagg U. Long-term effects of the Herbst appliance in relation to the treatment growth period: a cephalometric study. Eur J Orthod. 1991; 13: 471–481.
Harvold E. The activator in interceptive orthodontics. St. Louis: Mosby; 1975.
Herbst E. Dreißigjährige Erfahrungen mit dem Retentionscharnier. Zahnärztl Rundschau. 1934; 43: 1515–1524, 1563–1568, 1611–1616.
Jasper JJ, McNamara JA Jr., Mollenhauer B. The modified Herbst appliance (Jasper Jumper). In: Graber TM, Vanarsdall RL, eds. Orthodontics, current principles and techniques. St. Louis: Mosby; 2000: 367–378.
Kydd WL, Neff CW. Frequency of deglutition of tongue thrusters compared to sample population of normal swallowers. J Dent Res. 1964; 43: 363–369.
Lear CSC, Flanagan JB, Moorrees CFA. The frequency of deglutition in man. Arch Oral Biol. 1965; 10: 83–99.
Manns A, Miralles R, Guerrero F. The changes in electrical activity of the postural muscles of the mandible upon varying the vertical posture. J Prosthet Dent. 1981; 45: 438–445.
Meikle MC, Remodeling the Dentofacial Skeleton: The Biological Basis of Orthodontics and Dentofacial Orthopedics. J Dent Res. 2007: 86: 12–24.
Miethke RR, Drescher D. Kleines Lehrbuch der Angle-Klasse II,1 unter besonderer Berücksichtigung der Behandlung. Berlin: Quintessenz; 1996.
Pancherz H. The modern Herbst appliance. In: Graber TM, Rakosi T, Petrovic AG, eds. Dentofacial orthopedics with functional appliances. St. Louis: Mosby; 1997: 336–366.
Peterson TM, Rugh JD, McIver JE. Mandibular rest position in subjects with high and low mandibular plane angles. Am J Orthod. 1983; 83: 318–320.
Petrovic AG, Stutzmann JJ. Research methodology and findings in applied craniofacial growth studies. In: Graber TM, Rakosi T, Petrovic AG, eds. Dentofacial orthopedics with functional appliances. St. Louis: Mosby; 1997: 13–63.
Powell RN. Tooth contact during sleep: association with other events. J Dent Res. 1965; 44: 959–967.
Rakosi T. Fabrication and management of the activator. In: Graber TM, Rakosi T, Petrovic AG, eds. Dentofacial orthopedics with functional appliances. St. Louis: Mosby; 1997: 189–193.
Remmelink HJ, Tan BG. Cephalometric changes during headgear-reactivator treatment. Eur J Orthod. 1991; 13: 466–470.
Roux W. Gesammelte Abhandlugen über Entwicklungsmechanik der Organismen. Vols. I, II. Leipzig: Engelmann; 1985.
Rugh JD, Drago CJ. Vertical dimension: a study of clinical rest position and jaw muscle activity. J Prosthet Dent. 1981; 45: 670–675.
Sander FG, Schmuth GPF. Der Einfluss verschiedener Bißsperren auf die Muskelaktivität bei Aktivatorträgern. Fortschr Kieferorthop. 1979; 40: 107–111.
Schwarz M. Erfahrungen mit dem Herbstschen Scharnier zur Behandlung des Distalbisses. Zahnärztl Rundschau. 1934; 43: 47–54, 91–100.
Sergl HG. Tierexperimentelle Untersuchungen zur Erschütterungstheorie. Fortschr Kieferorthop. 1983; 44: 28–38.
Sheppard IM, Markus N. Total time of tooth contacts during mastication. J Prosthet Dent. 1962; 12: 460–463.
Van Sickels JE, Rugh JD, Chu GW, Lemke RR. Electromyographic relaxed mandibular position in long-faced subjects. J Prosthet Dent. 1985; 54: 578–581.
Vardimon AD, Drescher D, Bourauel C, Schmuth GPF, Graber TM. The magnetic functional system. In: Graber TM, Rakosi T, Petrovic AG, eds. Dentofacial orthopedics with functional appliances. St. Louis: Mosby; 1997: 299–318.
Vardimon AD, Koklu S, Iseri H, Shpack N, Fricke J, Mete L. An assessment of skeletal and dental responses to the functional magnetic system (FMS). Am J Orthod Dentofacial Orthop. 2001; 120: 416–426.
Vargervik K, Harvold EP. Response to activator treatment in Class II malocclusion. Am J Orthod. 1985; 88: 242–251.
Weise W. Die kieferorthopädische Behandlung. In: Schmuth G, ed. Kieferorthopädie II. Band 12: Praxis der Zahnheilkunde. München: Urban & Schwarzenberg; 1988: 2–27.
Woodside DG. The activator. In: Salzmann JA, ed. Orthodontics in daily practice. Philadelphia: Lippincott; 1974: 556–591.

7 Early Maxillary Expansion

M. Ali Darendeliler

Transverse maxillary deficiency requiring maxillary expansion is the result of a multitude of factors: genetic, environmental, traumatic, and iatrogenic. Many constricted maxillae are caused by abnormal function such as mouth breathing and sucking behaviors (Harvold et al. 1972; Graber and Swain 1975) which have been shown to create a characteristic malocclusion with a narrow maxilla and posterior cross bite, anterior open bite, proclined maxillary incisors and retroclined mandibular incisors (Warren and Bishara 2002)

Narrow maxillary dental arches and increased facial heights in rhesus monkeys were created by converting them from nasal to obligatory oral respiration by blocking the nose thus changing their breathing pattern (Harvold et al. 1973). The same applies to humans with mouth breathing habits, with the open mouth posture altering the equilibrium between the cheeks and the tongue leading to narrowing of the maxillary arch and a vertical growth pattern (Linder-Aaronson and Backstrom 1960).

From the time of Angell's (1860) description of maxillary expansion in the treatment of transverse deficiencies to the present, investigators have used a variety of maxillary expanders with differing force levels and durations (Haas 1961; Krebs 1964; Reitan 1964; Stockfisch 1969; Hicks 1978; Howe 1982). Their conclusions were that, depending upon the age, sex, and growth potential of the patient, this application could have orthodontic and orthopedic influences, but individual variations were unpredictable (Krebs 1958; Haas 1961, 1965; Wertz 1970; Hicks 1978; Linder-Aronson and Lindgren 1979; Timms 1981; Mossaz-Joëlson and Mossaz 1989).

Research done on the stability of the maxillary expansion gave contradictory results. Skeletal maxillary expansion and the increase in width of the nasal cavity were found to be stable in growing patients (Haas 1970, 1980; Hartgerinck et al. 1987). Timms (1968) reported significant relapse after an out-of-retention period of at least one year; but these results were criticized due to the lack of the rigidity of the appliance. However, the age of the patient during maxillary expansion was found to be correlated with the relapse potential. While the accumulated evidence appears to support a treatment rationale of early correction using a slow expansion procedure, individual variables must be considered in determining an expansion protocol that will optimally affect the quantity and quality of the expansive changes.

Growth and Anatomy

It is well known that the maxilla articulates with the following 10 bones: frontal, nasal, lacrimal, ethmoid, sphenoid, zygoma, palatine, vomer, mandible (teeth), and the other maxilla (McMinn et al. 1981). Therefore, any orthopedic change in the maxillary structures will inevitably affect the surrounding hard and soft tissues.

The midpalatal suture has always been heavily emphasized in the literature on maxillary expansion. Growth at the midpalatal suture was previously thought to cease at the age of 3 years (Latham 1971) however, by means of implants, it was found that growth at the suture could occur as late as 17 years of age (Bjork 1966). In a study on 24 cadavers, it was found that only 5% of the suture was obliterated by age 25. The variation was such that one 15-year-old cadaver had an ossified suture while a 27-year old cadaver had an unossified suture (Persson and Thilander 1977).

Rapid maxillary expansion (RME) also referred to as rapid palatal expansion (RPE), in both adolescents and adults may involve fracturing of the bony interdigitations. It should be noted that the main bony resistance to maxillary expansion derives mainly from the lateral sutures and not from the midpalatal suture as previously thought. Evaluations of the relationship between RME and cyclic nucleotides in the suture led to the conclusion that older animals are less responsive to the applied forces than younger animals. This thus decreased the ability of the older group to adapt to the forces of RME (Brin et al. 1981). Most investigators agree that RME with midpalatal splitting can be achieved with both youths and adults, though the sutures become more tortuous and interdigitated with advancing maturity and thus limit the extent and stability of the expansion (Krebs 1959; Isaacson and Ingram 1964; Zimring and Isaacson 1965; Wertz 1970). Although Bishara and Staley (1987) defined the optimal age for expansion as before 13–15 years, it would still be advisable to expand the maxilla at early ages, depending on the severity as well as the origin of the constriction.

Clinical and Radiological Diagnosis

The diagnosis of transverse dental or skeletal maxillary deficiency is apparent in the presence of different types of posterior crossbites, which may be unilateral or bilateral. In rare situations, the crossbite can be related to a wide mandible. This topic will not be discussed in this chapter.

Posterior crossbites can be due to a dental transverse deficiency, a skeletal transverse maxillary deficiency, or a combination of

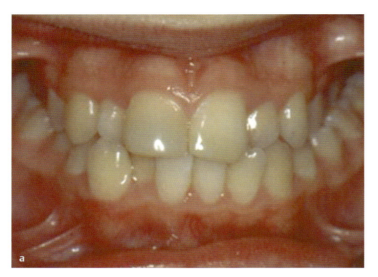
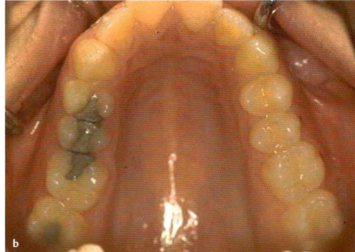
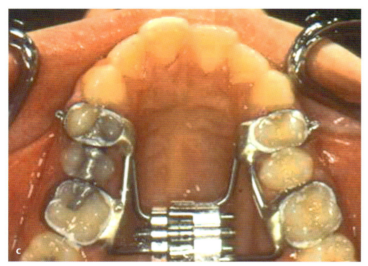

Fig. 7.1 Differential diagnosis of the dental versus skeletal maxillary deficiency in the clinic is based on the angulation of the posterior teeth, severity of the crossbite and the shape of the palatal vault (**a** and **b**). A skeletal maxillary deficient case treated using a banded Hyrax appliance (**b–d**).

the two. Since the type of appliance and expansion technique used will depend mainly upon the origin of the problem, determination of the dental and/or skeletal component of maxillary deficiency is the first step before treatment.

Clinical Diagnosis

Three points should be considered during the clinical differential diagnosis of dental versus skeletal transverse deficiency.

Angulation (Buccopalatal) of the Posterior Teeth

If the posterior teeth crowns are of normal angulation in the presence of a unilateral or bilateral posterior crossbite, a skeletal deficiency is evident. As a consequence, orthopedic correction using a rapid or slow maxillary expander should be considered. However, if the posterior teeth are palatally angulated, the discrepancy is dental in origin. The aim of treatment is to correct the compensation by dental uprighting, which will eliminate the crossbite.

Severity of the Crossbite

Severe crossbites are almost always an indicator of skeletal transverse maxillary deficiencies. A bilateral posterior crossbite that involves multiple teeth with an increased maxillomandibular arch width discrepancy usually reflects an underlying skeletal problem (Fig. 7.1). It is very rare for a bilateral crossbite to be solely the result of a dental deficiency.

Morphology of the Palatal Vault

A deep and "V" shaped palatal vault is often a viable indication of a skeletal deficiency (Fig. 7.1b). The morphology of the palatal vault is shallower and flatter in a crossbite of dental origin.

In maxillary transverse deficiency cases with mixed origin these clinical signs will be less pronounced depending on the ratio of dental versus skeletal discrepancy.

Radiological Diagnosis

Radiological diagnosis of transverse maxillary skeletal deficiency is only possible by assessment of a postero-anterior (PA) head film. Betts et al. (1995) described a comprehensive method for evaluation, from which the need for orthopedic, surgical, or surgically assisted maxillary expansion could be determined (Fig. 7.2). In their analysis, they used a two-step evaluation:

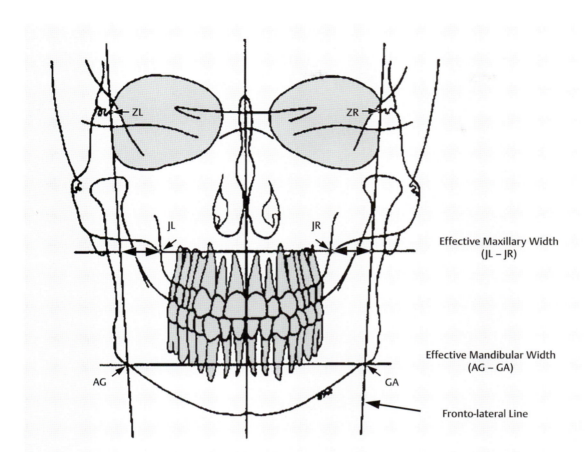

Fig. 7.2 Reference lines and maxillary and mandibular landmarks on the postero-anterior head film according to Betts et al. (1995).

Step 1: Assessment of maxillomandibular width differential.
The aim of this first step is to determine the total skeletal discrepancy between maxillary mandibular widths and demonstrate whether the deficiency is unilateral or bilateral. If the distance between right and left maxillary landmarks (JL and JR) and the vertical reference lines (ZL–AG and ZR–GA) is bigger than 10 ± 1.5 mm, a maxillomandibular transverse deficiency is present. Unilateral or bilateral skeletal deficiencies can also be defined by comparing right and left distances.

Step 2: Assessment of maxillomandibular transverse differential index. The aim of the second step is to determine the discrepancy between the actual and the expected maxillomandibular width difference. A discrepancy greater than 5 mm from the normal index, as described by Ricketts (1981), is an indication for skeletal expansion. Maxillo-mandibular width difference is the difference in millimeter between the distances AG–Ga and JL–JR. According to Ricketts in a normal case the maxillomandibular width difference should be 14 mm at age 9, 15.6 mm at age 11, 17.2 mm at age 13, 18.8 mm at age 15 and 19.6 mm in adults.

Timing of Maxillary Expansion

One of the greatest challenges faced by the clinician is to determine the timing of the maxillary expansion. Three factors must be taken into account in deciding when the expansion should be started:
- Functional shifts
- Cooperation of the patient
- Need for dental versus skeletal expansion and stability

Functional Shifts

Maxillary transverse deficiency is most frequently the sole factor causing a lateral functional shift, which necessitates early intervention. When a lateral functional shift is present, due to a maxillary transverse deficiency, the maxilla should be expanded as soon as it is diagnosed. Frequently a symmetrical mandible shifts laterally and sometimes anteriorly upon closing due to interference in the posterior region and occasionally in the canine area as the patient shifts his or her mandible to obtain the maximum interdigitation. Although some authors have reported self-correction in 45 % of cases (Kurol and Berglund 1992), others have noted that this was unlikely (Thilander et al. 1984). If the premature contact causing the interference is at the canines, some authors recommend selective grinding of the primary canines to eliminate the shift (Kurol and Berglund 1992). However, this correction has its limitations and can be a traumatic experience for the child. It involves careful consideration.

In a randomized clinical study that included patients in late deciduous or early mixed dentition with unilateral posterior cross bite and functional mandibular shift, it was shown that the control group exhibited no spontaneous self-healing tendencies. The treatment group who received a bonded expander followed by a U-bow activator showed significant reduction in condylar deviation and improvement in occlusion. It was recommended that early orthodontic treatment may also be described as "temporomandibular functional prophylaxis" (Lippold et al. 2009).

In a young patient, if the functional shift is not corrected, the continuous lateral position of the mandible can result in an asymmetric growth of the mandible and facial asymmetry. This was

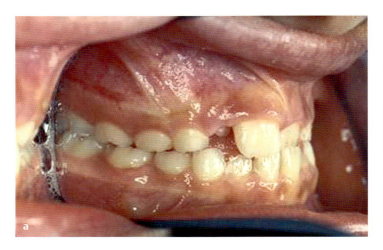
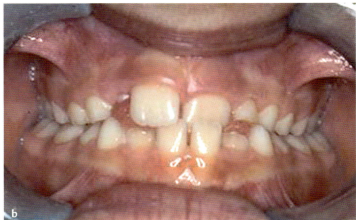
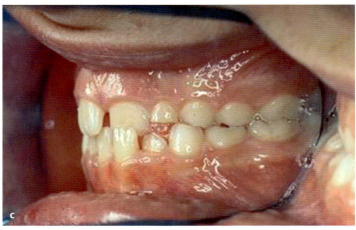
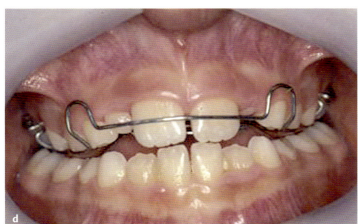
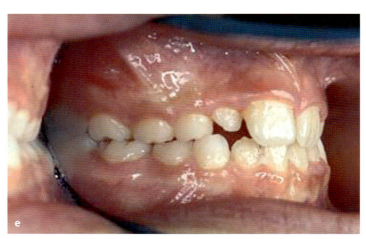
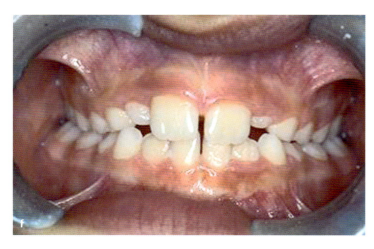
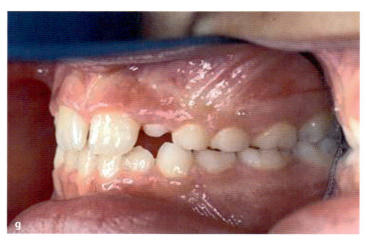

Fig. 7.**3** A unilateral frontal cross-bite with a lateral shift of the mandible treated with a removable expansion plate. Initial intra-oral views (**a–c**), expansion plate with posterior occlusal acrylic cover (**d**), intra-oral views after the expansion (**e–g**), note the correction of the mandibular shift.

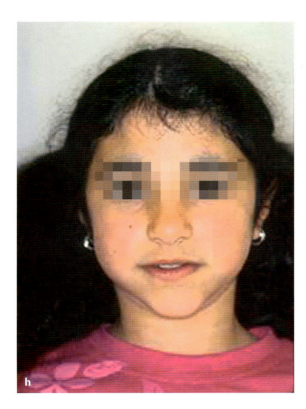
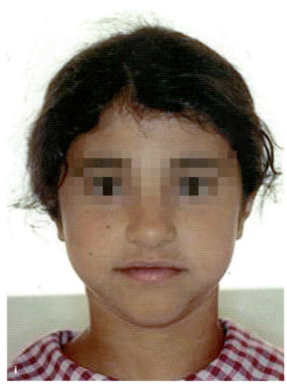

Fig. 7.3 Frontal extra-oral views before and after expansion (h, i).

demonstrated by creating lateral shifts in rabbit mandibles by unilateral grinding of the right molars, which produced dimensional and angular differences between the right and left sides of the mandible and maxilla in the experimental animals after a test period of 40 days (Poikela et al. 1995). Inclination of the articular surfaces of the right and the left glenoid fossae was also found to be shallower in the group with asymmetrical mandibular function.

Dental and skeletal asymmetry was investigated by examining adults with unilateral lingual posterior cross bite (Langberg et al. 2005). It was concluded that unilateral posterior cross bite in adults was primarily due to dentoalveolar asymmetry and positional deviation of the mandible and not simply to right–left skeletal asymmetry of the mandible. The data suggests that untreated unilateral posterior cross bites in children might lead to progressive asymmetric compensation of the condyle-fossa relationship and result in a positional deviation of the mandible, which, along with a distinct dentoalveolar asymmetry, maintains the crossbite occlusion in adults. The mechanism behind that compensatory growth modification is identical to that of functional orthopedic treatment. In an MRI study, which evaluated the effects of functional cross bite treatment, it was shown that with expansion the asymmetric morphology and position of the mandible and condyles were eliminated, and the stomatognathic system functions were normalized (Kecik et al. 2007). Expansion of the maxilla will eliminate the functional shift as the transverse dimensions of the maxillary and the mandibular arches will be coordinated. This allows the mandible to reach intercuspation in the midsagittal plane (Fig. 7.3). The maxillary-mandibular relationship will then be normalized in all three planes, and the dentition will develop normally. It was shown that in cases with unilateral posterior cross bites the condylar and ramal heights on the cross bite side were smaller than those on the non-crossbite side (Kilic et al. 2008). It is rare that the crossbite will redevelop in the permanent dentition. However, if there is no shift but a skeletal discrepancy is evident, the correction can be left for later intervention during the early mixed dentition.

Patient Co-operation

Even if early expansion is critical in the case of lateral functional shifts, the age and cooperation of the patient are important factors to be considered with regard to the timing of the expansion. Although the expansion may begin as early as 5–6 years of age, the clinical need to proceed must be weighed against the maturity and personality development of such young patients. The choice of the appliance type, removable or fixed, is not only an issue when considering dental and skeletal effects but must also be taken into consideration in the clinical management of very young patients. In case of absence of co-operation and maturity, one can wait another 6 to 12 months before correcting the maxillary deficiency. If the first molars are half erupted it is also advisable to wait until their full eruption for clinical practicality (design and retention of the appliance) and vertical control of the molars.

Dental versus Skeletal Discrepancy and Stability

The amount of dental versus skeletal expansion is a function of age and skeletal maturity and the type of appliance used. The timing of the expansion is also important when skeletal expansion is needed. As will be discussed later, the degree of skeletal expansion and its stability decreases with age. Therefore, if a severe skeletal discrepancy exists, earlier maxillary expansion is recommended.

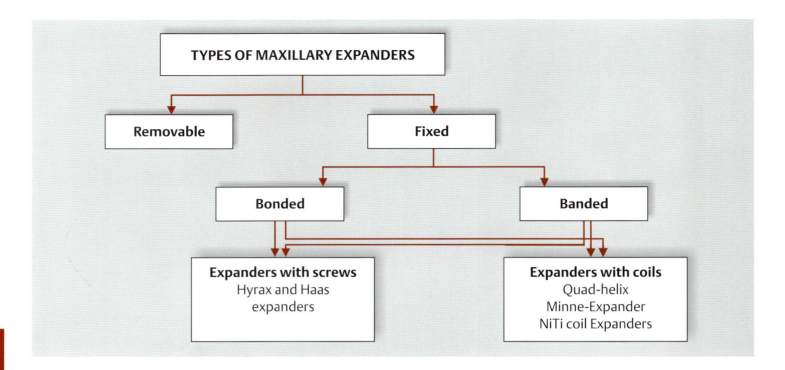

Types of Maxillary Expanders

Generally, expanders fall into one of two categories: removable and fixed.

Removable Maxillary Expanders

Removable maxillary expanders are designed to produce slow maxillary expansion. They are mainly used for unilateral or localized dental arch expansion. General applications include the correction of single tooth crossbite to unilateral or bilateral crossbite. The activation of the screw produces a heavy force that always decays rapidly. Rapid reactivation of the screw may cause dislodging of the appliance therefore maximum rate of expansion should not exceed one turn per every 5 days. The rate of expansion using removable appliances may also depend on the shape of the palate; in cases of a shallow palate, slower expansion, of a high palate, up to one turn per every 5 days should be adopted.

Fixed Maxillary Expanders

Fixed maxillary expanders are designed to produce rapid maxillary expansion. They are mainly used for unilateral or bilateral skeletal expansion. Fixed expanders can be retentive on bands (banded expander) (Fig. 7.**4a, c, d**) or on acrylic blocks (bonded expander) (Fig. 7.**4b**).

The design of the appliance should depend on the stage of dental development. A bonded type of expander may be used in any stage of the dentition except in the late mixed phase. A bonded expander can be used in the latter if the deciduous molars and canines have adequate root length to provide the necessary anchorage. Otherwise a banded expander taking anchorage from the first molars or from the first premolars and molars is recommended in the late mixed phase.

Bonded expanders require little chair-time and only two clinical procedures, impression taking and cementing of the appliance. Its use eliminates the need for placement and removal of separation elastics, band adaptation and transfer to the impression, precision wire bending, and soldering. Thus, the time and cost spent with a banded expander is not justified if there is no special requirement for it. The placement may be extremely difficult and painful for the patient when the anchorage teeth are not parallel to each other.

With the introduction of contemporary glass ionomer cements, the retention of bonded expanders has improved significantly and there is no longer a need to use composite or acrylic-based materials that require acid-etching procedures. However the design of the appliance is extremely critical. The acrylic component of the plate should cover the crowns of the teeth, leaving only 1 mm of clearance at the gingival margins along the buccal and palatal aspects. This ensures a maximum surface area for retention and sufficient clearance at the gingival margins to allow maintenance of good oral hygiene (Fig. 7.**5**). The acrylic extensions should have a chamfer finish to minimise food retention. Acrylic occlusal coverage does not need to be more than 1 to 2 mm in thickness and holes should be drilled into it to allow excessive cement to escape. In openbite cases the presence of the acrylic block will help in controlling the vertical dimension.

Fixed maxillary expanders have two types of force delivery mechanisms: screw expansion or coil spring expansion.

Expanders with Screws

The Hyrax expander (Fig. 7.**1c**, 7.**4a**) and Haas expander (Fig. 7.**6**) are the most commonly used maxillary expansion appliances. Both involve banding of first premolars and first molars. The Haas expander has additional acrylic pads on the palatal side to increase bony anchorage (Fig. 7.**6a**). A bonded modification can also be used.

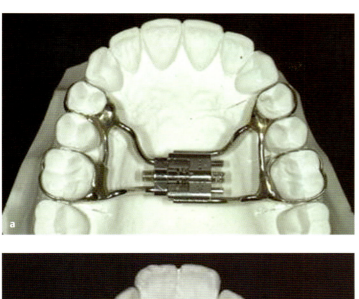
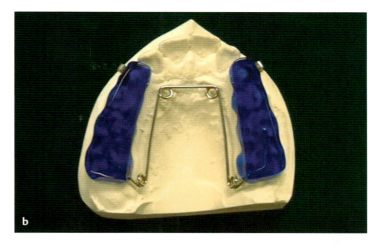
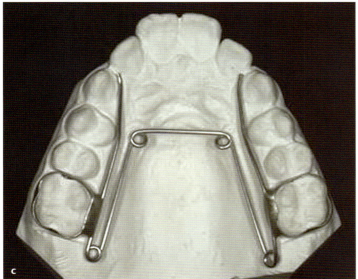
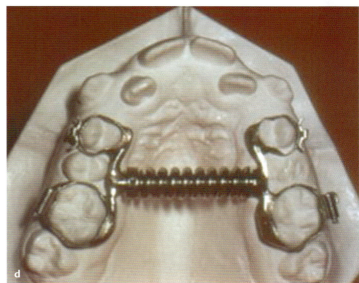

Fig. 7.4 Fixed Expanders; a banded Hyrax expander (**a**), a bonded Quad-helix (**b**) a banded Quad-helix with molar bands (**c**), a banded Minne-Expander on premolar and molar bands (**d**).

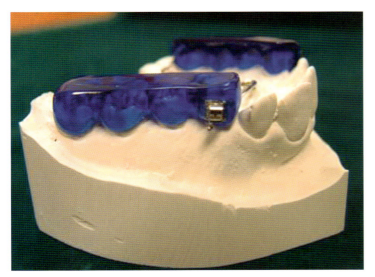

Fig. 7.5 Bonded Quad-Helix; Acrylic component of the plate covering the crowns of the teeth, leaving only 1 mm of clearance at the gingival margins along the buccal and palatal aspects to increase the retention of the appliance and still allow maintenance of good oral hygiene.

With the Haas expander, when the impression is taken, the palatal contour on the plaster model represents the contour of the mucosa, not the bone. This means that during the early stages of expansion, the lateral forces are not applied directly onto bone. It is thus questionable whether the Haas expander provides more skeletal expansion. It has been found that there was no significant difference on the skeletal effects of the Hyrax and the Haas expanders (Erverdi et al. 1993). Mucosal irritation and inflammation underneath the palatal acrylic and palatal gingival necrosis have been reported with the use of the Haas expander (Lanigan and Mintz 2002; Sardessai and Fernandesh 2003).

Another type of screw appliance is the bonded acrylic expander, which does not have any wire connections or bands (Fig. 7.7).

Early Maxillary Expansion

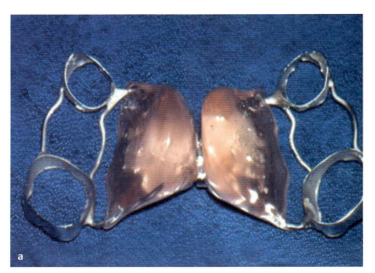
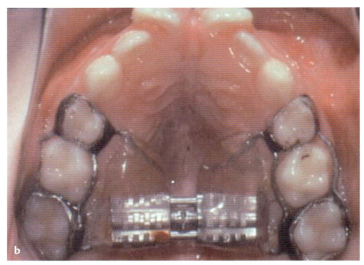

Fig. 7.6 Haas Expander has additional acrylic pads on the palatal side to increase bony anchorage. Before cementing (**a**) and after it was cemented on premolars and molars (**b**).

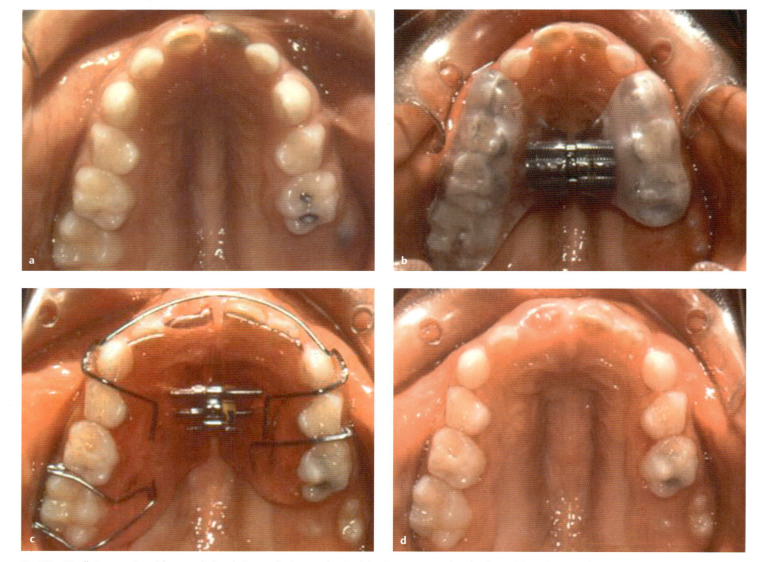

Fig. 7.7 Maxillary expansion with an acrylic bonded expander in an early mixed dentition case; initial occlusal view (**a**), acrylic expander after bonding (**b**), retention plate after expansion (**c**), occlusal view after expansion (**d**).

Expanders with Coils

The Quad-helix of Ricketts is a frequently used expander for dental and mild skeletal deficiencies. It can be used on molar bands or lateral acrylic blocks with occlusal coverage (Figs. 7.**4c**, 7.**8**). When used on molar bands, clinical management of the Quad-helix is simple; it is not very bulky, it rarely needs reactivation, and it does not rely on patient cooperation. In a randomized controlled trial to compare the effectiveness of quad-helix, expansion plate, and composite onlay (Petren and Bondemark 2008) on a mixed dentition unilateral cross-bite sample, it was found that one third of the treatments with expansion plates were unsuccessful, because of insufficient patient cooperation. The most successful results were obtained with a quad-helix.

The Minne Expander consists of a sliding pin and tube mechanism loaded with a heavy coil spring that applies 2 to 4 pounds of force (Fig. 7.**4d**). This mechanism, which is placed horizontally between the two hemi-maxillae, occupies more space than any other type of expander (Fig. 7.**9**). Re-compressing the coil by means of a nut reactivates the expander; thus force levels can be kept relatively constant by frequent activation (Figs. 7.**9b,c**).

The Minne Expander may be used on premolar and molar bands (banded Minne expander) or on lateral acrylic blocks with occlusal coverage (bonded Minne expander, Fig. 7.**9**). The dental and skeletal effects with banded and bonded expanders are very similar (Fig. 7.**10**) (Mossaz-Joëlson and Mossaz 1989).

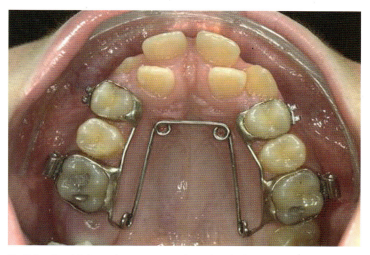

Fig. 7.**8**   Quad-Helix appliance on premolar and molar bands.

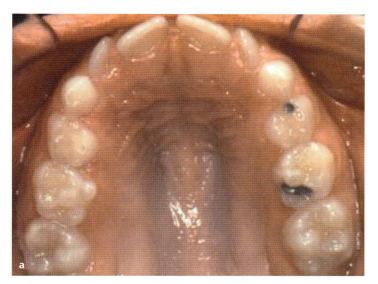
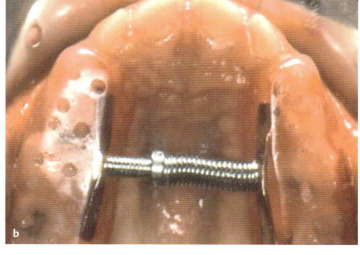
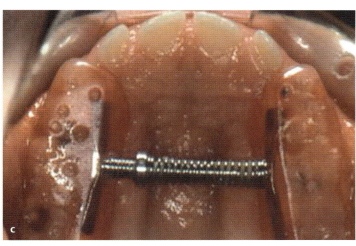
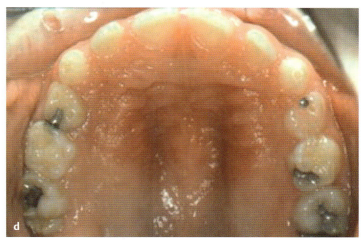

Fig. 7.**9**   A transverse maxillary deficiency case treated with a bonded Minne-Expander appliance; initial occlusal view (**a**), activation of the appliance by compressing the coil (**b**), six weeks later before the reactivation of the coil (**c**), occlusal view of the maxilla after expansion (**d**).

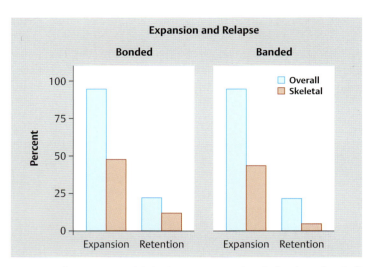

Fig. 7.**10** The percentage of skeletal expansion (G1E [Bonded] and G2E [banded]) and the percentage of overall and skeletal relapse(G1R [Bonded] and G2R [banded]) using bonded and banded Minne Expanders (adapted from Mossaz-Joëlson and Mossaz, 1989).

At present this type of appliance is not widely used because of its bulk in the palate. The coil spring has to be blocked at the end of the expansion phase by a ligature wire or composite, otherwise the coil continues to exert expansion forces. If the patient fails to attend the appointment at the end of the expansion period, continued and excessive expansion will result.

Using the same pin and tube concept, an auto blocking self-expander applying only 400 to 800 grams of force has been developed by Darendeliler and Lorenzon in 1996. The design consists of a blocking system on the central shaft to stop the expansion when the desirable correction is reached. The coil spring used is formed from Neo-Sentalloy wire (0.022 in. × 0.028 in.) (GAC, CA, USA), and it thus eliminates the need for reactivation (Fig. 7.**11**). Despite the low level of force, 25 to 75% of the result is skeletal expansion, the figure depending upon the age of the patient and the duration and amount of overall expansion. This design is not commercially available, however, it demonstrates the effects of light forces on skeletal structures in young patients.

Another fixed expansion appliance using NiTi wire delivered a uniform, slow continuous force for maxillary expansion and molar derotation using the shape memory and thermal phase transformation properties of NiTi wires (Corbett 1997).

The effects of the NiTi expansion appliance in a sample of primary and mixed dentition children showed an increase in maxillary arch width which was probably due to a combination of different effects: opening of the midpalatal suture, tipping of the alveolar process, and molar tipping. This resulted in completely corrected crossbites in all patients and symmetrical derotation of the anchorage teeth in a distal direction occurred in almost all children (Ferrario et al. 2003).

The comparison of the NiTi appliance to a conventional Quadhelix appliance, found that although both are effective in achieving the correction NiTi expanders tended to be less predictable and not as controlled. It was concluded that in most cases two activations were necessary and so the Quadhelix tended to be more cost effective. Thus NiTi expansion appliance is more effective in the correction of mild transverse deficiencies in young children (Donohue et al. 2004).

Force Produced with Maxillary Expanders

Clinical researchers have used various force levels to expand the maxilla and have focused on the amount of skeletal effects obtained. However, optimal force levels for different ages have yet to be established.

It is reported that, during rapid maxillary expansion, forces between 3 and 10 pounds are produced by a single activation of screw appliances. Multiple daily activations could result in cumulative loads of 20 pounds or more due to a corresponding linear increase in resistance from surrounding tissues (Isaacson and Ingram 1964; Zimring and Isaacson 1965). As a general pattern, higher resistance is produced in more mature patients compared to younger patients. Therefore, resistance to the expansion increases with increasing maturity and age. It has been shown that the major resistance to maxillary expansion does not come from the midpalatal suture but from the other sutures of the maxilla. Therefore, the retention of rapid maxillary expansion cases probably do not depend on the presence of bone in the opened midpalatal suture. It relies rather on the creation of a stable relationship of the other sutures of the maxilla; even deposition of new bone in the midpalatal suture does not necessarily ensure the stability of the expansion. As long as forces are present at adjacent maxillary sutures, it is possible that relapse forces can cause the resorption of this bone just as expansion forces caused its deposition. This important reaction is too often overlooked.

Considerable variations in force levels from patient to patient can occur increasing up to 120 N during maxillary expansion. After "rupture" of the midpalatal suture, the forces decrease. The remaining forces seemed to be the result from stress on soft tissue and bone (Sander et al. 2006).

More physiological expansion of the maxillary complex without the accumulation of a large residual load could be obtained by using slower rates of expansion (for example, light maxillary expansion [LME]). This was in agreement with Skieller (1964), who stated that the rate of midpalatal suture separation with slow expansion systems led to a more physiological response by the sutural elements than was seen with the relatively disruptive RME. In other studies, slow maxillary expansion showed the maintenance of sutural integrity, lower relapse potential and less dental tipping during reorganization of the maxillary complex compared to treatment using RME (Skieller 1964; Ohshiama 1972; Storey 1973; Hicks 1978; Timms 1981; Bell 1982). In a study comparing the effects of slow and rapid palatal expansion in the early (mean age 7.2 years) and late mixed dentition (mean age 9.9 years), it was revealed that there were no significant differences in relapse between the age groups and that the relapse was mainly due to the skeletal growth pattern of the mandible and to a lesser extent to the stability of the expanded maxilla (Bartzela and Jonas, 2007).

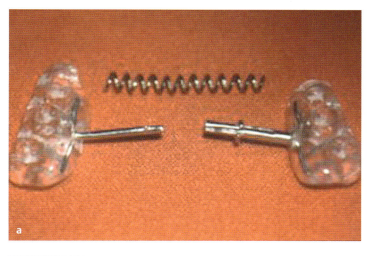
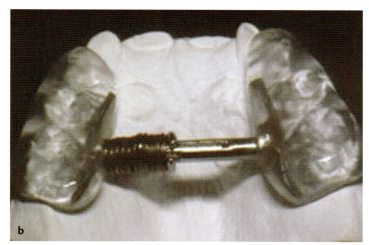
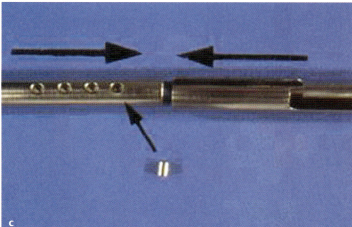
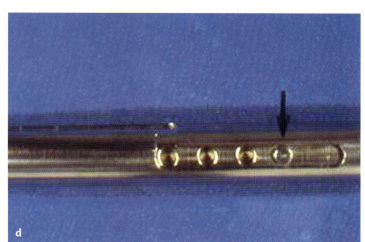
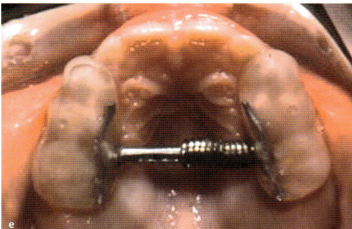
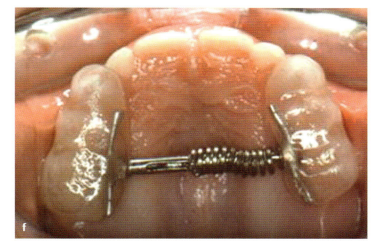

Fig. 7.11 The components and the use of the bonded auto-blocking self-expander; components (**a**), Self-expander on the plaster model (**b**), auto-blocking mechanism of the Self-expander (**c** and **d**), occlusal view on the day of cementation (coil active) (**e**), occlusal view 3 months after the necessary expansion was obtained (coil and the expansion stopped by the pin) (**f**) (from Darendeliler MA, Lorenzon C. 1996).

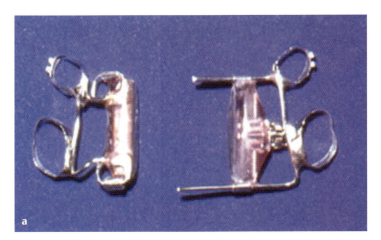
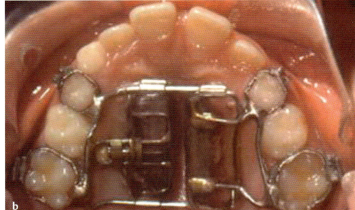
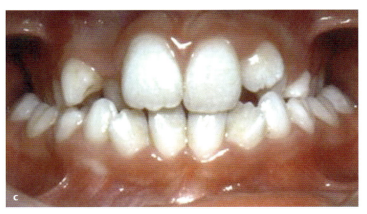
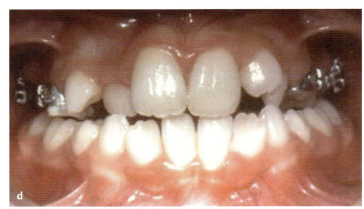
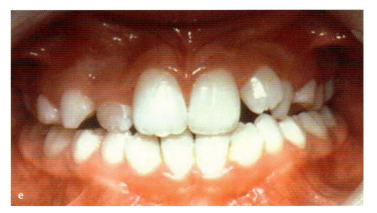

Fig. 7.**12** Banded Magnetic Expansion Device; right and left components carrying repulsive magnets (**a**), occlusal view on the day of cementation (**b**), frontal intra-oral view before (**c**), during (**d**) and after expansion (**e**).

Rate of Expansion and their Dental and Skeletal Effects

The rate of expansion varies depending upon the level of force applied and the rate of activation. There are four rates of maxillary expansion: slow (SME), light (LME) semi-rapid (SRME), and rapid maxillary expansion (RME).

Slow Maxillary Expansion (SME)

Slow maxillary expansion can be obtained by using functional appliances such as the Fränkel and the bionator as well as using removable plates.

When using Fränkel and Bionator type of functional appliances, an imbalance is created between the pressure produced by the buccal soft tissues and the tongue. Positive tongue pressure on dento-alveolar segments results in a more physiological expansion by bony deposition along the buccal borders of the dentoalveolar segments (Breiden et al. 1984). Although the expansion obtained is more stable, the use of functional appliances to expand the maxilla requires a relatively longer (75–80%) period of active treatment time (Fränkel and Fränkel 1989).

With the use of removable plates carrying expansion screws, the rate of expansion is usually 0.8 to 1.5 mm per month, obtained by activating the screw one turn every 5 to 7 days. More frequent activation of the screw may result in an undesirable effect. If it exceeds the threshold of elastic adaptation of the dentoalveolar bone, a removable plate will not allow the adaptation of the hard and soft tissues. The plate will therefore not fit, and expansion will not continue and may even relapse between two appointments. This requires the practitioner to re-set the screw, re-fit the plate, and re-start the expansion, especially in patients with a shallow palatal vault.

Light Maxillary Expansion

Lighter forces of 250 to 500 grams and 400 to 800 grams also produced skeletal expansion in patients less than 11 years old with a typical rate of expansion of 0.25 to 0.5 mm per week (Darendeliler et al. 1994; Darendeliler and Lorenzon 1996). The force was produced by either Neo-Sentalloy coils or repulsive magnets embedded in the Magnetic Expansion Device (MED) (Figs. 7.**11**, 7.**12**). Using maxillary implants in a limited number of patients with MED, researchers found an average skeletal expansion on the anterior and posterior regions of 40% and 38% of the overall expansion, respectively. Even though there are important variations between individuals, light forces might be effective in obtaining maxillary base expansion in growing patients. This work reflected the experimental results of Vardimon and Graber on primates (Vardimon et al. 1987). The expansion rate was slower than that found with the screw and coil spring activation.

Semi-rapid Maxillary Expansion (SRME)

Semi-rapid maxillary expansion can be obtained using coil-activated expanders such as the Quad-helix and the Minne expander or screws. Semi-rapid maxillary expanders are fixed by means of bands or acrylic blocks.

The mechanism of action of the Quad-helix and the Minne Expander is through the creation of continuous pressure on the hemi-maxilla, resulting in expansion. The rate of expansion is 2 to 2.5 mm per month, depending on the amount and frequency of activation, which is determined by the individual clinician.

Hicks (1978) evaluated the skeletal effects of the Minne expander using implants on five patients between the ages of 10 and 15 years, and found this to be 16–30% of the overall expansion. In a similar implant study involving 10 patients, Mossaz-Joëlson and Mossaz (1989) showed 50% skeletal expansion using the Minne expander with an expansion rate of 0.64 mm per week. However, their patient sample consisted of children from 8 to 12 years of age. Using a force of 2 pounds, they demonstrated that the two halves of the maxilla did not separate but tipped buccally by 5 to 6 degrees around a center of rotation located approximately at the frontomaxillary suture (Haas 1961, 1970; Wertz 1970).

A relatively new approach has been introduced with the hypothesis that it may stimulate the adaptation process in the naso-maxillary complex and thus would result in reduction of relapse in the postretention period on dentofacial structures in older adolescents and adults (Iseri et al., 2004). A rigid acrylic maxillary expander was used on patients of average 14.57 years old. The protocol for SRME was: RME of 5–7 days, followed by SME. The mean expansion time was 4 months, and the mean follow-up period was 2.68 years after retention. The findings of this study suggested that the dento-skeletal changes after the use of SRME were maintained satisfactorily in the long term in older adolescents and adults.

Rapid Maxillary Expansion (RME)

Rapid maxillary expansion can be obtained by using screw-activated expanders such as the Hyrax and the Haas expander. RME are fixed by means of bands or acrylic blocks. In 90% of the patients, the skeletal effect is found around 50% of the overall expansion, with a rate of 0.2 to 0.5 mm per day. However, 30% of the skeletal expansion relapsed after an average retention period of 18 months. Expansion of the nasal cavity is approximately 25% of the overall expansion (Krebs, 1964).

The mechanism of action of rapid maxillary expanders consists of creating intermittent accumulated force on the hemi-maxilla, resulting in expansion.

Generally, the Hyrax expander is used by including the first premolars and first molars in the appliance, creating a 4-point expander. Recently, the modification of the appliance to the 2-point expander by solely using the first molars was questioned. The results showed no differences in the amount of dental expansion however the 4-point RME showed 2.5 times greater suture separation and 6-fold larger arch perimeter increase. The use of the 2-point RME was recommended for mixed dentition cases with more posterior discrepancy (Lamparski et al. 2003, Davidovitch et al. 2005).

Skeletal effects, dental effects, and stability after RME, SRME and SME as well as after maxillary expansion with functional appliances and in combination with different surgical techniques, have been studied by several researchers. The average durations of expansion using RME, SRME, LME and SME are 1 to 1.5 months, 2 to 4 months, 4 to 8 months and 10 to 12 months respectively depending on the amount of expansion required. Nevertheless, the science behind maxillary expansion is not yet fully understood and the different findings with regard to the dental versus skeletal effects are contradictory (Chaconas et al. 1977; Schwarz et al. 1985; Warren et al. 1987).

Effects in Different Age Groups

It was believed for a long period of time that the main resistance to expansion came from the degree of fusion or interdigitation of the midpalatal suture. Currently it is considered that in older patients the resistance of the facial bones in general increases with age as the bone becomes less flexible and so offers greater resistance to expansion and thus greater relapse potential.

Wertz and Dreskin (1977) evaluated the effects of screw appliances on three different age groups: under 12 years, 12 to 18 years, and over 18 years old. The skeletal component of the overall expansion was 43.4% in the younger group (<12 years), 37% in the middle group (12 to 18 years), and 19% in the adult group (>18 years). During the retention period, the younger group continued with an average of 1 mm of transverse widening, the middle group did not show any change, and the adult group showed an average of 1 mm of skeletal relapse. The overall outcomes in the three different age groups were 50%, 45.6%, and 16%, respectively (Fig. 7.**13**).

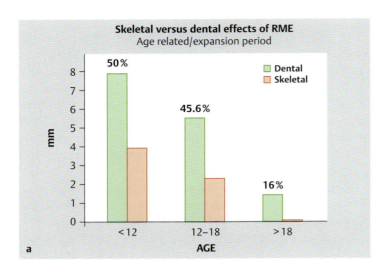
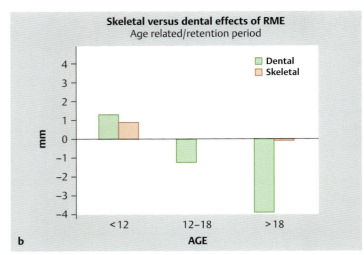
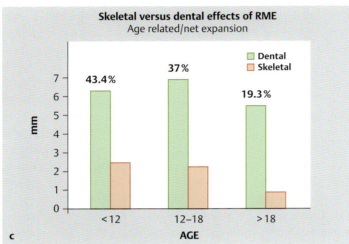

Fig. 7.13 Skeletal versus dental expansion in three different age groups (<12; 12–18; >18) using Hyrax Expander; During the expansion (**a**), retention (**b**) periods and net expansion (outcome) (**c**) (adapted from Wertz and Dreskin (1977).

In younger patients some clinicians face making the choice of expanding early in the mixed dentition to gain maximum skeletal benefits (Sari et al. 2003) and then going for a second phase of fixed appliance therapy while others may choose to wait for the eruption of the permanent teeth and to combine the expansion into a single phase of treatment. With the use of the Haas expander, the adults showed an 18% of the transmolar expansion by skeletal expansion at the height of the palate and the remainder with buccal displacement of the alveolus. On the other hand the children displayed 56% of the expansion by an increase at the height of the palate with the remainder due to displacement of the alveolus (Handelman et al. 2000).

Clinical Case Studies

Rapid Maxillary Expansion in Conjunction with the Treatment of Sagittal Maxillary Deficiency

The idea of influencing the mobile maxillae during and after expansion has been explored. Following RME, the orthopaedic response in many patients is increased by applying mesially and distally directed forces to the maxillae (Haas 1961).

Class II and Class III malocclusions are usually associated with transverse maxillary deficiency (Franchi and Baccetti 2005). The Class II is usually masked by bringing the mandible forward into a Class I relationship as the deficiency becomes apparent. Maxillary expansion is usually recommended before or alongside functional appliance therapy. On the other hand in Class III cases there is often an already visible transverse deficiency. Maxillary expansion is believed to serve more than one purpose in this case. In addition to correcting the transverse relationship it is believed that in some way it aids orthopedic sagital correction if a Reverse Headgear (Delaire mask) is used.

Comparing the effects of the Delaire mask with and without rapid maxillary expansion, the average sagital skeletal correction of the maxilla was 2.0 mm with maxillary expansion and only 0.9 mm without maxillary expansion (Baik 1995). The underlying reason behind this has been attributed to the mobilization of sutures and the maxillary complex thus responding better to the mesially directed extraoral forces. The expander used in combination with reverse headgear can be bonded or banded depending on the dentition phase (see Fixed Maxillary Expanders). In open bite or open bite tendency cases, the hooks on the expander should be placed as anteriorly and as high as possible without soft-tissue irritation. This is to reduce the bite opening effect of the reverse headgear. However, if there is a deep bite tendency, the hooks can be placed on the occlusal level (Case Study 7.**1**). Brackets can be incorporated in the acrylic to align the incisors and control the overjet and overbite (Case Study 7.**2**). In such cases bonded RME represents perfect anchorage against incisors.

A controlled randomized clinical trial to quantify the effects of maxillary protraction with or without palatal expansion was undertaken with children aged 5 to 10 years (Vaughn et al. 2005). Early facemask therapy, with or without palatal expansion, was effective to correct skeletal Class III malocclusions and that RME did not add a significant advantage. In another more recent study comparing the effects of maxillary protraction with or without maxillary expansion it was determined that both treatment options show significant differences compared to the control group but increases in CoA and SNA angle had no significant difference between the treatment groups (Tortop et al. 2007).

An alternative technique for growing Class III patients is to use a 2-hinged RME which disarticulates the maxilla by repetitive rapid expansions and constrictions (7 mm per week each for 4 and 5 times, respectively) and intraoral maxillary protraction springs for non-compliant protraction (Liou 2005). On average, the maxilla could be protracted for 5.8 mm in 3 months without using an extraoral appliance and the result remains stable at least 2 years later. The rationale for this technique is sutural expansion/protraction osteogenesis.

In a finite element study it was shown that biomechanically, maxillary protraction combined with maxillary expansion appeared to be a superior treatment modality for the treatment of maxillary retrognathia than maxillary protraction alone (Gautam et al. 2009).

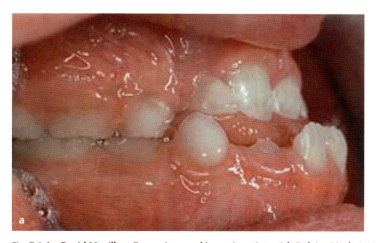
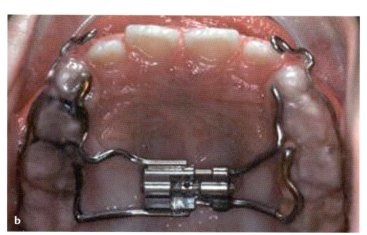

Fig. 7.1.**1** **Rapid Maxillary Expansion used in conjunction with Delaire Mask;** Initial lateral intra-oral view (**a**), occlusal intra-oral views at the end of expansion and maxillary protrusion phase (**b, c**).

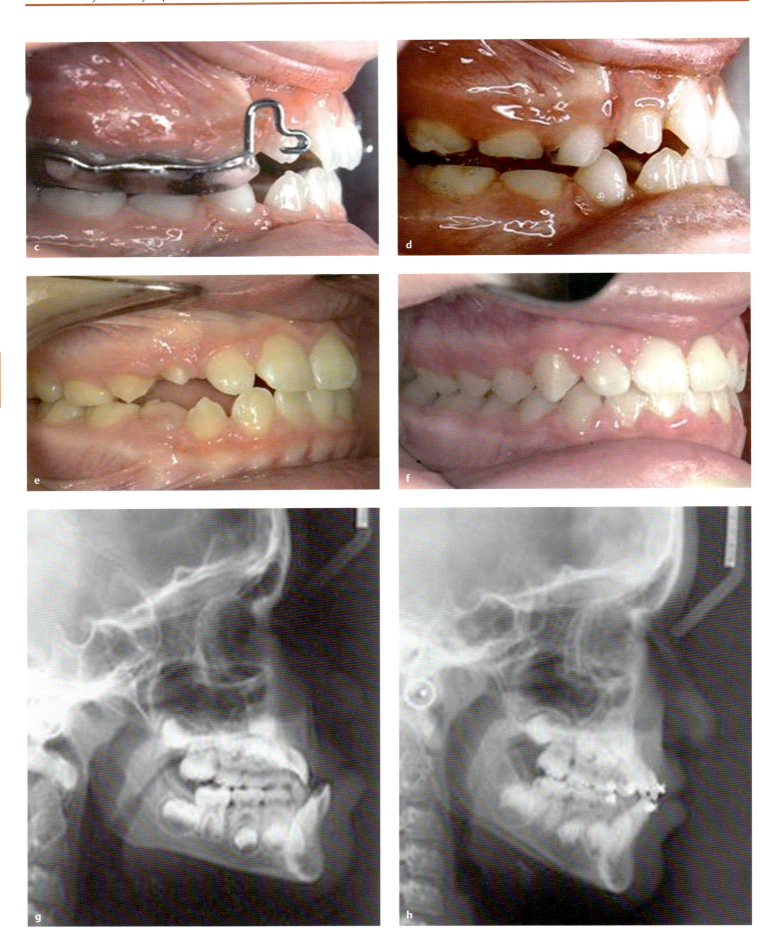

Fig. 7.1.1 **Rapid Maxillary Expansion used in conjunction with Delaire Mask;** After removal of the maxillary expander (**d**), intra-oral photo 2½ years post protraction following the removal of an upper 2 × 4 (**e**), intra-oral [photo at the end of full fixed appliances, 5 years post protraction (**f**) initial (**g**) and 2 years post-protraction (**h**) cephalometric x-rays.

Clinical Case Studies

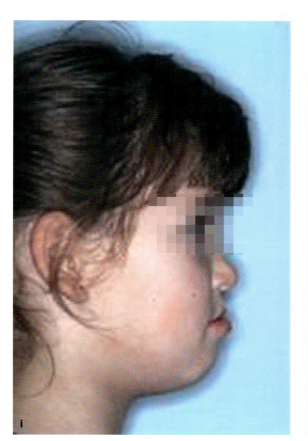
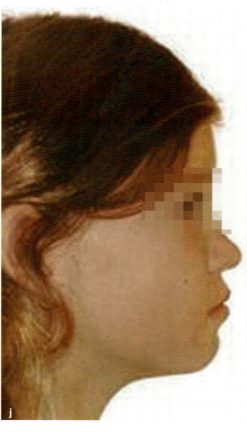
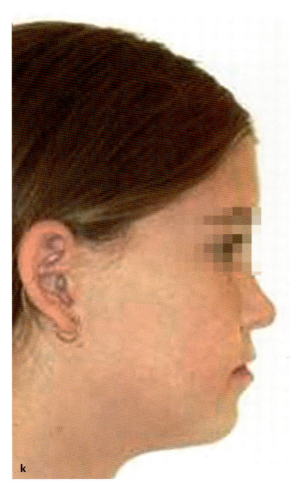
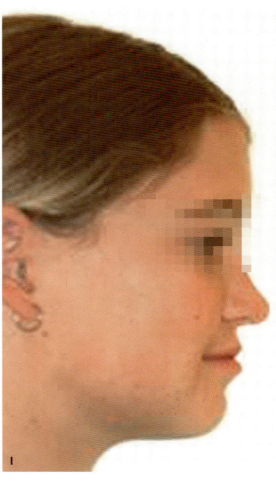

Fig. 7.1.**1** **Rapid Maxillary Expansion used in conjunction with Delaire Mask;** Initial (**i**), end of protraction (**j**) and 2½ years post protraction (**k**) and end of treatment (**l**) profile photos.

Early Maxillary Expansion

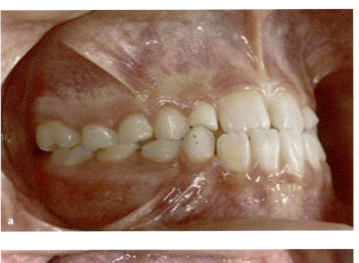
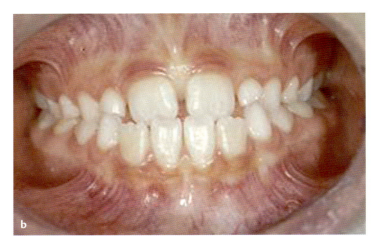
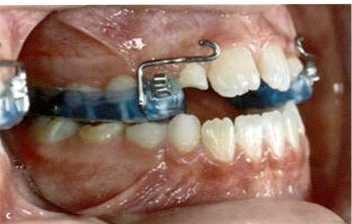
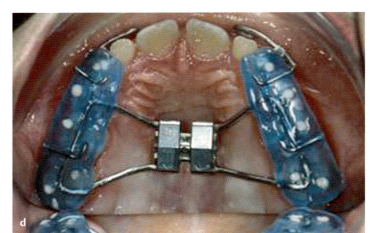
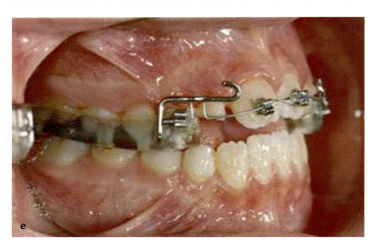
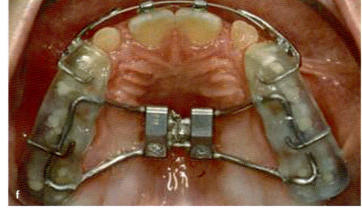

Fig. 7.2.**1** Brackets can be incorporated on both sides of the upper bonded plate to allow the alignment of the incisors and the serve to increase and secure the overbite. Intra-oral photos of a class III tendency case (**a** and **b**), lateral and occlusal views of the plate after cementation (**c** and **d**) alignment and extrusion of the incisors using plate anchorage (**e** and **f**). After the removal of the bonded plate and the brackets on the incisors (**g** and **h**),

Clinical Case Studies

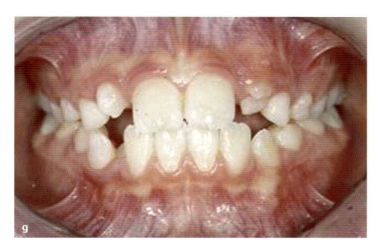
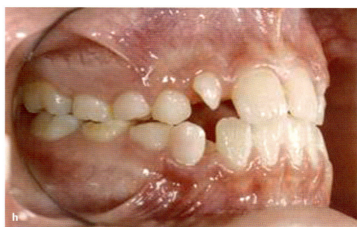
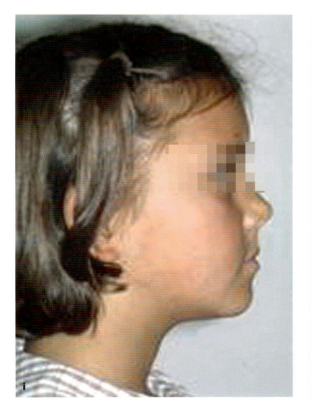
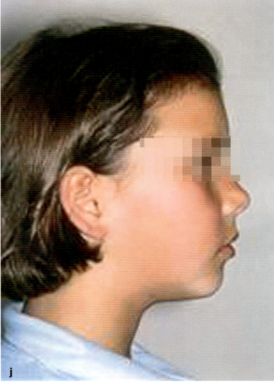

Fig. 7.2.1 **Brackets can be incorporated on both sides of the upper bonded plate to allow the alignment of the incisors and the serve to increase and secure the overbite.** Initial (**i**) and progress profile (**j**) photos.

Early or Late Treatment? Surgically Assisted Maxillary Expansion versus Orthopedic Expansion

It is evident that to obtain orthopedic expansion of the maxilla, the force applied must be sufficient to overcome the bioelastic resistance of the periodontium, alveolar bone, and sutural elements (Storey 1955).

Orthopedic effects on the maxillary complex are usually the result of mechanical repositioning, followed by an adaptive growth of the facial sutures depending on the age and growth potential of the patient. In the sagittal plane, forward or backward growth modifications of the maxilla were observed using forces between 400 and 2000 grams (Cleall et al. 1965; Storey 1973). These forces influenced the sutures of the nasomaxillary complex that are oriented in a similar, mostly sagittal, plane (Remmelink 1988). Because these sutures are oriented in this manner, one would assume there would be more resistance to forces applied during transverse orthopedic correction than during sagittal orthopedic correction. This may explain the preference for the use of heavy forces to expand the maxilla. It is also well known that the major resistance to expansion is not the midpalatal suture itself but other sutures of the maxilla (Bishara and Staley 1987; Gautam et al. 2008). Rapid or slow maxillary expansion using screw or coil spring-loaded appliances provide clinically acceptable results even in late-adolescent patients up to the age of 15 years. However, as shown by several authors, the skeletal effect decreases, and the relapse tendency increases with age. Resistance to maxillary expansion in adults could most effectively be reduced by carrying out a corticotomy procedure through the zygomatic buttress and the nasomaxillary and pterygomaxillary areas (Bell and Epker 1976; Kennedy et al. 1976).

The use of surgically assisted maxillary expansion in unilateral and bilateral crossbite cases demonstrated the unilateral corticotomy procedure in unilateral crossbite cases where the noncrossbite side was used as anchorage against the operated crossbite side (Mossaz et al. 1992).

Berger et al. (1998), in their study comparing maxillary and nasal expansion between orthopedically treated growing patients and adult patients treated using the surgically assisted maxillary expansion method, found no significant differences between the groups (Fig. 7.**14**). Thirteen per cent and 4% of relapse was observed in orthopedic and in surgical groups respectively and the net skeletal expansion obtained one year after removal of the expanders was in average 66% with orthopedic and 52% with surgically assisted maxillary expansion. This supports the view that both orthopedic and surgically assisted maxillary expansion methods are equally effective for the correction of transverse discrepancies when indicated. In a study that evaluated the stability in changes after two years follow-up, it was also shown that the dentoalveolar responses of RME and SARME were similar after orthodontic treatment and the amount of relapse was not significant after two years (Sokucu et al. 2009).

It was also shown in another study with a 6 year follow-up period evaluating the long term outcomes of surgically assisted maxillary expansion that the decreases in the transverse dimensions are most pronounced during the first 3 years post-treatment (Magnusson et al. 2009).

Rapid Maxillary Expansion and Obstructive Sleep Apnea (OSA)

Graber (1975) believed that the claims of improved nasal breathing apparently as a result of RME are most likely only temporary. He also noted that 12-year-old children have much more lymphoid tissue than adults do and the lymphoid tissues could act to block nasal breathing. Spontaneous regression of lymphoid tissues during growth may automatically improve nasal breathing, even if nothing is done to the palate. In some studies, the use of RME in widening nasal cavities was shown to be an efficient method to improve nasal breathing (Compadretti et al. 2006). An increase in nasal size was the eventual aftermath of maxillary expansion (Garib et al. 2005; Palaisa et al. 2007; Garrett et al. 2008). However in other studies, the individual variability was high and patients demonstrated reduction in nasal resistance following RME due to increase in nasal width. This increase was stable one year after the expansion (Hartgerink et al. 1987). It was also shown that with RME in children younger than 12 years of age,

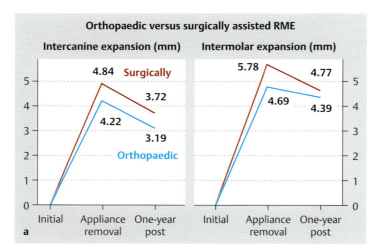
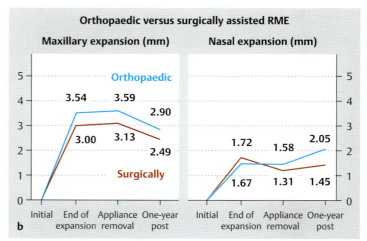

Fig. 7.**14** Dental and skeletal effects of the orthopedic and surgically assisted maxillary expansion; intercanine and intermolar changes (**a**), maxillary and nasal width changes (**b**), (adapted from Berger et al. (1998).

there is a significant improvement of nasal airflow, which remained stable after 1 year of expansion, along with the increase in posterior nasal space (Monini et al. 2009). However, in a study by Enoki et al. (2006) conducted on children between the ages 7–10 years, it was shown that RME did not change nasal geometry even though the nasal resistance lessened. So it was concluded that RME cannot be indicated for this purpose by itself.

The effects of RME on Obstructive Sleep Apnea (OSA) were evaluated recently. A clinically conclusive and key study assessed the change in apnea-hypopnea index (AHI) in children without adeno-tonsillar hypertrophy. The results showed that following RME, the AHI was less than 1 (which is considered normal in children) and stayed stable 6–12 months after treatment. The RME is therefore a valid treatment of OSA in children without adeno-tosillar hypertrophy (Pirelli et al. 2004, Villa et al. 2007). In another study on children (n = 32) with moderate OSA and requiring both adenoidectomy and orthodontic treatment, it was shown that both treatments were required to obtain complete resolution of OSA (Guilleminaut et al. 2008).

RME was also successful in 70 to 100% of the cases in treating nocturnal enuresis (NE) in children (Timms 1990; Kurol et al. 1998; Usumez et al. 2003). Treatment of NE may occur indirectly due to the treatment of OSA using RME. Children who had NE due to their sleeping disorder before RME could sleep well following the increase in their nasal airway after RME and have shorter periods of deep sleep so that children awaken more easily when the bladder is full.

Another suggested mechanism was that with the placement of an orthodontic appliance, whether or not it is activated, may change the awakening mechanism (Schütz-Fransson and Kurol 2008).

Retention and Stability

In general, following expansion, the RME or SME fixed appliance is used for at least three months for retention, followed by a removable plate for another six months. However, if the treatment continues with full fixed appliances, there is no need for the removable plate phase following the retention with the original expander. In some cases trans-palatal arches are incorporated or broader and expanded arch-wires are used.

Slow expansion seems less disruptive to the sutural systems allowing better soft tissue adaptation (Bell RA 1982). Tissue integrity needs 1–3 months of retention with slow expansion, which is significantly shorter than the 3–6 months recommended for RME.

The duration of retention with a fixed lower appliance in the posttreatment period did not appear to affect the long-term outcomes of the treatment protocol significantly. The amount of correction in both maxillary and mandibular intermolar widths equaled two-thirds of the initial discrepancy, whereas treatment eliminated the initial deficiency in maxillary and mandibular intercanine widths (McNamara et al. 2003).

After fixed retention was discontinued, substantial reduction in dental arch width could continue for up to five years Krebs (1959). The distance between implants in the infrazygomatic ridges decreased during the 3 months of fixed retention by an average of 10% to 15%. This relapse continues during retention with removable appliances. After an average period of 15 months, approximately 70% of the infrazygomatic maxillary width increase is maintained.

The amount of relapse is related to the method of retention after expansion.

With no retention, the relapse can amount to 45%, compared with 10 to 23% with fixed retention and 22 to 25% with removable retention in patients aged 8 to 12 years old (Hicks 1978). Stability of arch perimeter after RME followed by fixed appliances was evaluated and a net gain of 6 mm was achieved in the maxillary arch perimeter, whereas a net gain of 4.5 mm was found for the mandibular arch perimeter.

After orthodontic appliance removal, the dental tipping and alveolar bending components of transverse expansion tend to regress. Therefore, when orthopedic maxillary expansion is used to correct transverse maxillary deficiency, overcorrection is recommended. Even though some indicate as much as 50% (Betts et al. 1995) of overcorrection, 25–30% is a safe ratio. In a more recent study on younger group of patients (prepubertal and pubertal), at the end of the active phase of expansion, the buccal bone plate thickness of the supporting teeth showed a significant decrease of 0.4 and 0.2 mm (corresponding to mesial and distal roots, respectively) with no fenestration, dehiscence, or attachment loss. After a retention period of 6 months, recovery of both buccal and lingual plate thickness was observed. The results emphasized the importance of a retention period more than 3 months for the recovery of buccal and palatal bone thicknesses (Ballanti et al. 2009).

Side-Effects of Maxillary Expansion

Pathological effects such as root resorption, alveolar dehiscence and fenestration caused by appliances overpowering the biological boundaries have been reported by several authors (Rinderer 1966; Barber and Sims 1981; Vardimon et al. 1991). Histological examination of anchor teeth extracted from humans and animals has demonstrated root resorption following the application of heavy forces with RME (Dabbane 1958; Rinderer 1966; Starnbach et al. 1966; Moss 1968; Timms 1968; Timms and Moss 1971; Barber and Sims 1981; Langford and Sims 1982; Vardimon et al. 1991; Erverdi et al. 1994).

The mechanisms controlling external root resorption are related to the stress applied (force/surface area), environmental density, and the duration of force application. Root resorption mainly affects multirooted teeth, in particular, the mesiobuccal root, buccal surfaces, furcation areas, and apical root zones (Vardimon et al. 1991). Heavy orthodontic forces (225 grams) showed significantly ($p = 0.000$) more root resorption than light orthodontic forces (25 grams) after a duration of 28 days (Chan and Darendeliler 2005). However during RME the level of buccally directed forces may reach 9000 g on anchorage teeth. This implies that, if not used with precaution RME may cause tissue damage in some cases.

RME compresses the periodontal ligaments and affects the alveolar bone.

In a recent study, it is reported that the buccal bone plate thickness of supporting teeth is reduced by 0.6 to 0.9 mm and increased the lingual bone plate thickness by 0.8 to 1.3 mm. RME induced bone dehiscences on the anchorage teeth's buccal aspect

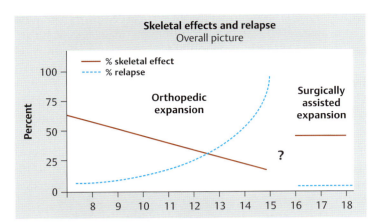

Fig. 7.15 An overview of the effect of maxillary expansion in relation to age.

(7.1 ± 4.6 mm at the first premolars and 3.8 ± 4.4 mm at the mesiobuccal area of the first molars), especially in subjects with thinner buccal bone plates (Garib et al. 2006). In a study that evaluated tongue posture after RME, it was suggested that normalization of tongue posture following ME in growing subjects without enlarged tonsils might enhance stability by balancing buccal pressure (Ozbek et al 2009). When expanding the maxilla, the status of the buccal hard and soft tissues also has to be taken into account. In adult patients, several authors suggested corticotomy with or without palatal osteotomy (Lines 1975; Bell and Epker 1976; Glassmann et al. 1984; Lehmann et al. 1984; Alpern and Yurosko 1987; Mossaz et al. 1992) in order to avoid root resorption, buccal alveolar bone fenestration, and dehiscence, to obtain skeletal effects and to ensure stability.

Although these undesirable effects have been reported with the use of RME, it is still unclear whether any pathological effect exists with slow maxillary expanders.

Discussion and Conclusion

Animal and clinical studies, although with different methodologies and sample selection, support increased orthopedic effect of maxillary expansion at early ages. The maturation of the bony structures and the sutural components around the maxillary complex seems to play an important role in the expression of skeletal versus dental effects during expansion. In a mature individual, the resistance to lateral forces in the maxillary complex is higher than to the sagittal forces. This is because of the orientation of most of the sutures articulating the maxilla to the other bony structures.

Selection of the type of appliance and the form of expansion, e.g., rapid or slow, should depend on the origin of the problem as well as the maturation of the patient. Early treatment, besides increased skeletal response in maxillary expansion, appears to allow the use of less complex and lower-force expansion systems to achieve increases in maxillary arch width. The early correction of transverse maxillary deficiency may bring about advantages of redirecting the erupting teeth into a normalized occlusion, correcting asymmetries of condylar position, and allowing normal vertical closure of the mandible without functional shifts to avoid occlusal interferences. Despite the length of treatment, the rate of midpalatal suture separation by slow expansion systems seem to allow a more physiologically tolerable response by the bony and the sutural elements than the disruptive nature of rapidly expanded maxillary segments. This more physiological transverse increase in maxillary dimension during slow expansion has been shown as the main reason for greater stability and less relapse potential during reorganization of the maxillary complex. Reduction of iatrogenic potential is of increasing importance in this litigious world.

The long-term benefits of allowing a more harmonious occlusion may at least theoretically, eliminate or minimize deleterious anatomic and functional growth factors due to pathological disturbances and parafunctional activities. The increased sutural and skeletal response has been related to growth periods of high cellular activity with increased reparability potential and treatment prior to the formation of bony interlocking at maxillary articulations. Older patients may require higher-force systems or surgical intervention to achieve palatal suture separation.

The detection of root resorption, dehiscence and fenestration, and gingival recession with the use of screw-type appliances, which apply heavy intermittent forces, has resulted in the emergence of a trend toward the use of more continuous and lighter forces. Forces used with semi-rapid and slow expansion devices were found to fall more within biological boundaries. Slow maxillary expanders such as the Quad-helix or Minne expander incorporate a force system that varies from several ounces to approximately 2 pounds.

In the management of the maxillary expansion, the following conclusions should be taken into account:
- When a functional lateral shift is present as a result of maxillary deficiency, expansion of the maxilla should be done as early as possible and is among the few conditions recommended for treatment in the primary dentition unless the permanent first molars are expected to erupt in less than 6 months.
- The percentage of skeletal effect decreases with age (Fig. 7.15).
- The percentage of relapse increases with age (Fig. 7.15).
- If an orthopedic expansion has not been done, surgically assisted maxillary expansion is indicated after 15 years of age. Then the amount of skeletal expansion achieved with orthopedic and surgically assisted maxillary expansion is similar to treatment at an earlier age (Fig. 7.15).
- The design of the fixed expansion appliance should depend on the stage of dental development:
  - In primary dentition: bonded expander
  - In early mixed dentition: bonded expander
  - In late mixed dentition: banded expander (on the molars or on the premolars and molars)
  - In permanent dentition: bonded expander
- 25 to 30% overexpansion of the maxilla is necessary to accommodate the relapse.
- High forces produced by screw loaded expanders can cause root resorption, dehiscence, fenestration, and gingival recession on anchorage teeth and careful initial evaluation of neighboring tissues is recommended.
- Clinically, with current appliance availability, the most practical and effective maxillary expander is the bonded Quad-helix appliance in growing children. This time-tested appliance allow for easy fabrication and insertion, reduced chair time, and minimal patient cooperation.

References

Alpern MC, Yurosko JJ. Rapid palatal expansion in adults with and without surgery. Angle Orthod. 1987; 57(3): 245–263.

Angell EC. Treatment of irregularities of the permanent or adult teeth. Dental Cosmos 1860; 1: 540–544, 599–601.

Baik HS. Clinical results of the maxillary protraction in Korean children. Am J Orthod Dentofacial Orthop. 1995; 108(6): 583–592.

Ballanti F, Lione R, Fanucci E, Franchi L, Baccetti T, Cozza P. Immediate and postretention effects of rapid maxillary expansion investigated by computed tomography in growing patients. Angle Orthod. 2009; 79(1): 24–29.

Barber AF, Sims MR. Rapid maxillary expansion and external root resorption in man: a scanning electron microscope study. Am J Orthod. 1981; 79(6): 630–652.

Bartzela T, Jonas I. Long-term stability of unilateral posterior crossbite correction. Angle Orthod. 2007; 77(2): 237–243.

Bell RA. A review of maxillary expansion in relation to the rate of expansion and patient's age. Am J Orthod. 1982; 81(1): 32–37.

Bell WH, Epker BN. Surgical-orthodontic expansion of the maxilla. Am J Orthod. 1976; 70(5): 517–528.

Berger JL, Pangrazio-Kulbersh V, Borgula T, Kaczynski R. Stability of orthopedic and surgically assisted rapid palatal expansion over time. Am J Orthod Dentofacial Orthop. 1998; 114(6): 638–645.

Betts NJ, Vanarsdall RL, Barber HD, Higgins-Barber K, Fonseca RJ. Diagnosis and treatment of transverse maxillary deficiency. Int J Adult Orthod Orthognath Surg. 1995; 10(2): 75–96.

Bishara SE, Staley RN. Maxillary expansion: clinical implications. Am J Orthod Dentofacial Orthop. 1987; 91(1): 3–14.

Bjork A. Sutural growth of the upper face studied by the implant method. Acta Odontol Scand. 1966; 24(2): 109–127.

Breiden CM, Pangrazio-Kulbersh V, Kulbersh R. Maxillary skeletal and dental change with Frankel appliance therapy-an implant study. Angle Orthod. 1984; 54(3): 226–232.

Brin I, Hirshfeld Z, Shanfeld JL, Davidovitch Z. Rapid palatal expansion in cats: effect of age on sutural cyclic nucleotides. Am J Orthod. 1981; 79 (2): 162–175.

Chaconas S, de Alba y Levy JA. Orthopedic and orthodontic applications of the quad-helix appliance. Am J Orthod. 1977; 72(4): 422–428.

Chan E, Darendeliler MA. Physical properties of root cementum: Part 5. Volumetric analysis of root resorption craters after application of light and heavy orthodontic forces. Am J Orthod Dentofacial Orthop. 2005; 127(2): 186–195.

Cleall JF, Bayne DI, Posen JM, Subtelny JD. Expansion of the midpalatal suture in the monkey. Angle Orthod. 1965; 35: 23–35.

Compadretti GC, Tasca I, Bonetti GA. Nasal airway measurements in children treated by rapid maxillary expansion. Am J Rhinol. 2006; 20(4): 385–393.

Corbett MC. Slow and continuous maxillary expansion, molar rotation, and molar distalization. J Clin Orthod. 1997; 31: 253–263.

Dabbane EF. A cephalometric and histologic study of the effect of orthodontic expansion of the midpalatal suture of the cat. Am J Orthod. 1958; 44: 187–219.

Darendeliler MA, Lorenzon C. Maxillary expander using light, continuous force and autoblocking. J Clin Orthod. 1996; 30(4): 212–216.

Darendeliler MA, Strahm C, Joho JP. Light maxillary expansion forces with the magnetic expansion device. A preliminary investigation. Eur J Orthod. 1994; 16(6): 479–490.

Davidovitch M, Efstathiou S, Sarne O, Vardimon AD. Skeletal and dental response to rapid maxillary expansion with 2- versus 4-band appliances. Am J Orthod Dentofac Orthop. 2005; 127(4): 483–492.

Donohue VE, Marshman LA, Winchester LJ. A clinical comparison of the quad-helix appliance and the nickel titanium (tandem loop) palatal expander: a preliminary, prospective investigation. Eur J Orthod. 2004; 26(4): 411–420.

Enoki C, Valera FC, Lessa FC, Elias AM, Matsumoto MA, Anselmo-Lima WT. Effect of rapid maxillary expansion on the dimension of the nasal cavity and on nasal air resistance. Int J Pediatr Otorhinolaryngol. 2006; 70(7): 1225–1230.

Erverdi N, Sabri A, Kucukkeles N. Cephalometric evaluation of Haas and Hyrax rapid maxillary expansion appliances in the treatment of the skeletal maxillary deficiency. J Marmara University Dental Faculty. 1993; 1(4): 361–366.

Erverdi N, Okar I, Kucukkeles N, Arbak S. A comparison of two different rapid palatal expansion techniques from the point of root resorption. Am J Orthod Dentofacial Orthop. 1994; 106(1): 47–51.

Ferrario VF, Garattini G, Colombo A, Filippi V, Pozzoli S, Sforza C. Quantitative effects of a nickel-titanium palatal expander on skeletal and dental structures in the primary and mixed dentition: a preliminary study. Eur J Orthod. 2003; 25(4): 401–410.

Franchi L, Baccetti T. Transverse maxillary deficiency in Class II and Class III malocclusions: a cephalometric and morphometric study on postero-anterior films. Orthod Craniofac Res. 2005; 8(1): 21–28.

Fränkel R, Fränkel C. Orofacial orthopedics with the function regulator. Basel: Karger, 1989.

Garib DG, Henriques JFC, Janson G, Freitas MR, Coelho RA. Rapid maxillary expansion—tooth tissue-borne versus tooth-borne expanders: a computed tomography evaluation of dentoskeletal effects. Angle Orthod 2005; 75: 548–557.

Garib DG, Henriques JF, Janson G, de Freitas MR, Fernandes AY. Periodontal effects of rapid maxillary expansion with tooth-tissue-borne and tooth-borne expanders: a computed tomography evaluation. Am J Orthod Dentofac Orthop. 2006; 129(6): 749–758.

Garrett BJ, Caruso JM, Rungcharassaeng K, Farrage JR, Kim JS, Taylor GD. Skeletal effects to the maxilla after rapid maxillary expansion assessed with cone-beam computed tomography. Am J Orthod Dentofacial Orthop. 2008; 134(1): 8–9.

Gautam P, Valiathan A, Adhikari R. Stress and displacement patterns in the craniofacial skeleton with rapid maxillary expansion: a finite element method study. Am J Orthod Dentofacial Orthop. 2007; 132(1): 5.e1–11.

Gautam P, Valiathan A, Adhikari R. Skeletal response to maxillary protraction with and without maxillary expansion: a finite element study. Am J Orthod Dentofacial Orthop. 2009; 135(6): 723–728.

Glassman AS, Nahigian SJ, Medway JM, Aronowitz HI. Conservative surgical orthodontic adult rapid palatal expansion: sixteen cases. Am J Orthod. 1984; 86(3): 207–213.

Graber TM, Swain BF. Current orthodontic concepts and techniques. 2nd ed. Philadelphia: WB Saunders; 1975.

Guilleminault C, Quo S, Huynh NT, Li K. Orthodontic expansion treatment and adenotonsillectomy in the treatment of obstructive sleep apnea in prepubertal children. Sleep. 2008; 31(7): 953–957.

Haas AJ. Rapid expansion of the maxillary dental arch and nasal cavity by opening the midpalatal suture. Angle Orthod. 1961; 31: 73–90.

Haas AJ. The treatment of maxillary deficiency by opening the midpalatal suture. Angle Orthod. 1965; 35: 200–217.

Haas AJ. Palatal expansion: just the beginning of dentofacial orthopedics. Am J Orthod. 1970; 57(3): 219–255.

Haas AJ. Long-term posttreatment evaluation of rapid palatal expansion. Angle Orthod. 1980; 50(3): 189–217.

Hartgerink DV, Vig PS, Abbott DW. The effect of rapid maxillary expansion on nasal airway resistance. Am J Orthod Dentofacial Orthop. 1987; 92(5): 381–389.

Harvold EP, Chierici G, Vargervik K. Experiments on the development of dental malocclusions. Am J Orthod. 1972; 61(1): 38–44.

Harvold EP, Vargervik K, Chierici G. Primate experiments on oral sensation and dental malocclusions. Am J Orthod. 1973; 63(5): 494–508.

Handelman CS, Wang L, BeGole EA, Haas AJ. Nonsurgical rapid maxillary expansion in adults: report on 47 cases using the Haas expander. Angle Orthod. 2000; 70(2): 129–144.

Hicks EP. Slow maxillary expansion a clinical study of the skeletal versus dental response to low magnitude force. Am J Orthod. 1978; 73(2): 121–141.

Howe RP. Palatal expansion using a bonded appliance. Report of a case. Am J Orthod. 1982; 82(6): 464–468.

Isaacson RL, Ingram AH. Forces produced by rapid maxillary expansion II. Forces present during treatment. Angle Orthod. 1964; 34: 261–270.

Jacobs JD, Bell WH, Williams CE, et al. Control of the transverse dimension with surgery and orthodontics. Am J Orthod. 1980; 50: 110–113.

Kecik D, Kocadereli I, Saatci I. Evaluation of the treatment changes of functional posterior crossbite in the mixed dentition. Am J Orthod Dentofacial Orthop. 2007; 131(2): 202–215.

Kennedy JW 3rd, Bell WH, Kimbrough OL, James WB. Osteotomy as an adjunct to rapid maxillary expansion. Am J Orthod. 1976; 70(2): 123–137.

Kilic N, Kiki A, Oktay H. Condylar asymmetry in unilateral posterior crossbite patients. Am J Orthod Dentofacial Orthop. 2008; 133(3): 382–387.

Krebs A. Expansion of the midpalatal suture studied by means of metallic implants. Eur Orthod Soc Rep. 1958; 163–171.

Krebs AA. Expansion of mid palatal suture studied by means of metallic implants. Acta Odontol Scand. 1959; 17: 491–501.

Krebs AA. Rapid expansion of midpalatal suture by fixed appliance. An implant study over a 7-year period. Trans Eur Orthod Soc. 1964; 141–142.

Kurol J, Berglund L. Longitudinal study and cost-benefit analysis of the effect of early treatment of posterior cross-bites in the primary dentition. Eur J Orthod. 1992; 14(3): 173–179.

Kurol J, Modin H, Bjerkhoel A. Orthodontic maxillary expansion and its effect on nocturnal enuresis. Angle Orthod. 1998; 68(3): 225–232.

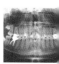

Lamparski DG Jr, Rinchuse DJ, Close JM, Sciote JJ. Comparison of skeletal and dental changes between 2-point and 4-point rapid palatal expanders. Am J Orthod Dentofac Orthop. 2003; 123(3): 321–328.

Langberg BJ. Arai K. Miner RM. Transverse skeletal and dental asymmetry in adults with unilateral lingual posterior crossbite. Am J Orthod Dentofac Orthop. 2005; 127(1): 6–15; discussion 15–16.

Langford SR, Sims MR. Root surface resorption, repair, and periodontal attachment following rapid maxillary expansion in man. Am J Orthod. 1982; 81: 108–115.

Lanigan DT, Mintz SM. Complications of surgically assisted rapid palatal expansion: review of the literature and report of a case. J Oral Maxillofac Surg. 2002; 60(1): 104–110.

Latham R A. The development, structure and growth pattern of the human mid-palatal suture. J Anat. 1971; 108: 31–41.

Lehmann JA Jr, Haas AJ, Haas DG. Surgical orthodontic correction of transverse maxillary deficiency: a simplified approach. J Plastic Reconstr Surg. 1984; 73: 62–68.

Linder-Aronson S, Backstrom A. A comparison between mouth breathers and nose breathers with respect to occlusion and facial dimensions. Odontol Revy. 1960; 11: 343–376.

Linder-Aronson S, Lindgren J. The skeletal and dental effects of rapid maxillary expansion. Br J Orthod. 1979; 6(1): 25–29.

Lines PA. Adult rapid maxillary expansion with corticotomy. Angle Orthod. 1975; 67(1): 44–56.

Liou EJ. Effective maxillary orthopedic protraction for growing Class III patients: a clinical application simulates distraction osteogenesis. Prog Orthod. 2005; 6(2): 154–171.

Lippold C, Hoppe G, Moiseenko T, Ehmer U, Danesh G. Analysis of condylar differences in functional unilateral posterior crossbite during early treatment– a randomized clinical study. Orofac Orthop. 2008; 69(4): 283–296.

McNamara JA Jr, Baccetti T, Franchi L, Herberger TA. Rapid maxillary expansion followed by fixed appliances: a long-term evaluation of changes in arch dimensions. Angle Orthod. 2003; 73(4): 344–353.

McMinn RMH, Hutchings RT, Logan BM. A colour atlas of head and neck anatomy. London: Wolfe Medical Publications; 1981.

Magnusson A, Bjerklin K, Nilsson P, Marcusson A. Surgically assisted rapid maxillary expansion: long-term stability. Eur J Orthod. 2009; 31(2): 142–149.

Mew JRC. Semi-rapid maxillary expansion. Br Dent J. 1977; 143(9): 301–306.

Monini S, Malagola C, Villa MP, Tripodi C, Tarentini S, Malagnino I, Marrone V, Lazzarino AI, Barbara M. Rapid maxillary expansion for the treatment of nasal obstruction in children younger than 12 years. Arch Otolaryngol Head Neck Surg. 2009; 135(1): 22–27.

Moss JP. Rapid expansion of maxillary arch. J Pract Orthod. 1968; 2: 168–171, 216–223.

Mossaz CF, Byloff FK, Richter M. Unilateral and bilateral corticotomies for correction of maxillary transverse discrepancies. Eur J Orthod. 1992; 14(2): 110–116.

Mossaz-Joelson K, Mossaz CF. Slow maxillary expansion: a comparison between banded and bonded appliances. Eur J Orthod. 1989; 11: 67–76.

Ohshiama O. Effect of lateral expansion force on the maxillary suture in cynomolgus monkey. J Osaka Dental University. 1972; 6: 11–50.

Ozbek MM, Memikoglu UT, Altug-Atac AT, Lowe AA. Stability of maxillary expansion and tongue posture. Angle Orthod. 2009; 79(2): 214–220.

Palaisa J, Ngan P, Martin C, Razmus T. Use of conventional tomography to evaluate changes in the nasal cavity with rapid palatal expansion. Am J Orthod Dentofacial Orthop. 2007; 132(4): 458–466.

Palmisano RG, Wilcox I, Sullivan CE, Cistulli PA. Treatment of snoring and obstructive sleep apnoea by rapid maxillary expansion. Aust NZ J Med. 1996; 26: 428–429.

Persson M, Thilander B. Palatal suture closure in man from 15 to 35 years of age. Am J Orthod. 1977; 72(1): 42–52.

Petrén S, Bondemark L. Correction of unilateral posterior crossbite in the mixed dentition: a randomized controlled trial. Am J Orthod Dentofacial Orthop. 2008; 133(6): 790.e7–13.

Pirelli P, Saponara M, Guilleminault C. Rapid maxillary expansion in children with obstructive sleep apnea syndrome.[see comment]. Sleep. 2004; 27(4): 761–766.

Poikela A, Kantomaa T, Tuominen M, Pirttiniemi P. Effect of unilateral masticatory function on craniofacial growth in the rabbit. Eur J Oral Sci. 1995; 103(2): 106–111.

Reitan K. Effects of force magnitude and direction of tooth movement on different alveolar bone types. Angle Orthod. 1964; 34: 244–255.

Remmelink HJ. Orientation of maxillary sutural surfaces. Eur J Orthod. 1988; 10(3): 223–226.

Ricketts RM. Perspectives in the clinical application of Cephalometrics. The first fifty years. Angle Orthod. 1981; 51(2): 115–150.

Rinderer L. The effects of expansion on the palatal suture. Trans Eur Orthod Soc. 1966; 365–377.

Sander C, Huffmeier S, Sander FM, Sander FG. Initial results regarding force exertion during rapid maxillary expansion in children. J Orofac Orthop. 2006; 67(1): 19–26.

Sardessai G, Fernandesh AS. Gingival necrosis in relation to palatal expansion appliance: an unwanted sequelae. J Clin Pediat Dent. 2003; 28(1): 43–45.

Sari Z, Uysal T, Usumez S, Basciftci FA. Rapid maxillary expansion. Is it better in the mixed or in the permanent dentition? Angle Orthod. 2003; 73(6): 654–661.

Schütz-Fransson U, Kurol J. Rapid maxillary expansion effects on nocturnal enuresis in children: a follow-up study. Angle Orthod. 2008; 78(2): 201–208.

Schwarz GM, Thrash WJ, Byrd LD, Jacobs JD. Tomographic assessment of nasal septum changes following surgical-orthodontic rapid maxillary expansion. Am J Orthod. 1985; 87(1): 39–45.

Skieller V. Expansion of the mid palatal suture by removable plates, analysed by the implant method. Trans Eur Orthod Soc. 1964; 143–157.

Sokucu O, Kosger HH, Bicakci AA, Babacan H. Stability in dental changes in RME and SARME: a 2-year follow-up. Angle Orthod. 2009; 79(2): 207–213.

Starnbach H, Bayne D, Cleall J, Subtelny JD. Faciosketelal and dental changes resulting from rapid maxillary expansion. Angle Orthod. 1966; 36(2): 152–164.

Stockfisch H. Rapid expansion of the maxilla—success and relapse. Rep Cong Eur Orthod Soc. 1969; 469–481.

Storey E. Bone changes associated with tooth movement: a histological study of the effect of force in the rabbit, guinea pig and rat. Aust Dent J. 1955; 59: 147–161.

Storey E. Tissue response to the movement of bones. Am J Orthod. 1973; 64(3): 229–247.

Thilander B, Wahlung S, Lennartsson B. The effect of early interseptive treatment in children with posterior cross-bite. Eur J Orthod. 1984; 6(1): 25–34.

Timms DJ, Moss JP. An histological investigation into the effects of rapid maxillary expansion on the teeth and their supporting tissues. Trans Eur Orthod Soc. 1971; 263–271.

Timms DJ. An occlusal analysis of lateral maxillary expansion with midpalatal suture opening. Dent Pract. 1968; 18(12): 435–440.

Timms DJ. Rapid maxillary expansion. Chicago: Quintessence Pub.Co., 1981.

Timms DJ. Rapid maxillary expansion in the treatment of nocturnal enuresis. Angle Orthod. 1990; 60(3): 229–233; discussion 234.

Tortop T, Keykubat A, Yuksel S. Facemask therapy with and without expansion. Am J Orthod Dentofacial Orthop. 2007; 132(4): 467–474.

Usumez S, Iseri H, Orhan M, Basciftci FA. Effect of rapid maxillary expansion on nocturnal enuresis. Angle Orthod. 2003; 73(5): 532–538.

Vardimon AD, Graber TM, Voss LR, Verrusio E. Magnetic versus mechanical expansion with different force thresholds and points of force application. Am J Orthod Dentofacial Orthop. 1987; 92(6): 455–466.

Vardimon AD, Graber TM, Voss L, Lenke J. Determinants controlling iatrogenic external root resorption and repair during and after palatal expansion. Angle Orthod. 1991; 61(2): 113–122. discussion 123–124.

Vaughn GA, Mason B, Moon HB, Turley PK. The effects of maxillary protraction therapy with or without rapid palatal expansion: a prospective, randomized clinical trial. [see comment]. Am J Orthod Dentofac Orthop. 2005; 128(3): 299–309.

Villa MP, Malagola C, Pagani J, Montesano M, Rizzoli A, Guilleminault C, Ronchetti R. Rapid maxillary expansion in children with obstructive sleep apnea syndrome: 12-month follow-up. Sleep Med. 2007; 8(2): 128–134.

Warren JJ. Bishara SE. Duration of nutritive and nonnutritive sucking behaviors and their effects on the dental arches in the primary dentition. Am J Orthod Dentofacial Orthop. 2002; 121(4): 347–356.

Warren DW, Hershev HG, Turvev TA, Hinton VA, Hairfield WM. The nasal airway following maxillary expansion. Am J Orthod Dentofacial Orthop. 1987; 91(2): 111–116.

Wertz RA. Skeletal and dental changes accompanying rapid midpalatal suture opening. Am J Orthod. 1970; 58: 41–66.

Wertz RA, Dreskin M. Midpalatal suture opening: a normative study. Am J Orthod. 1977; 71(4): 367–381.

Zimring JF, Isaacson RJ. Forces produced by rapid maxillary expansion III. Forces present during retention. Angle Orthod. 1965; 35(3): 178–186.

8 The Interarch Compression Spring in Orthodontics

John DeVincenzo

Since the interarch compression spring was first introduced as the Eureka Spring in 1996, its use has increased dramatically. In 1999 and 2000, two additional types, Twin Force (Ortho-Organizers) and Forsus (3 M Unitek), became available. Sales have increased rapidly, and widespread interest among orthodontists is evident because of the spring's versatility, the rapid tooth movements it can produce with minimal patient compliance, and their low rate of breakage.

It is the purpose of this chapter to compare the interarch compression spring (ICS) with more established approaches to the correction of anteroposterior discrepancies, to evaluate the force vectors and hence anchorage preparations required for successful treatment, to examine the various types available, and to present clinical applications.

The force mechanism in every ICS is a linear open coil spring. This spring can vary in material, wire diameter, number of windings per unit length, and overall outside dimension. Since these springs are loaded by linear compression, the forces generated are linear throughout the range of action. This linearity assures the same amount of deformation along the entire length of the spring. In contrast, the leaf spring and the closed coil curved spring, as used in the Jasper Jumper, experience variable amounts of deformation and are therefore subject to breakage in the area where the deformation is greatest.

This linearity of force can be seen in Figure 8.1, the data for which were obtained from actual measurements from a sample of Eureka springs. These springs were initially lightly loaded with 14 g of force so that the first millimeter of compression produced 32 g. Thereafter, every additional millimeter of compression produced approximately 18 g of force.

Force Vectors, Moments, and Analyses

Because the force of every ICS is derived from compression rather than expansion, a Class II correction with an ICS will appear to be in the direction of Class III elastics (Fig. 8.2). The ICS has an intrusive force component to both the mandibular anterior and maxillary posterior dentitions, while the Class II elastic delivers maxillary anterior and mandibular posterior extrusive forces (Fig. 8.2). As the dentition changes from Class II toward Class I, the intrusive component of the ICS lessens, while the extrusive component of the Class II elastic increases (Fig. 8.3, Table 8.1).

As shown in Table 8.1, the magnitude of the extrusive force of Class II elastics increases from 56 g to 75 g as the dentition changes from Class II to Class I. It has been reported (DeVincenzo and Winn 1987) that clinically significant maxillary incisor intrusion occurs with 56 g of continuous force. Therefore, it would not be unreasonable to assume that significant extrusion could also occur at this force level and that an additional 20 g of such force could be clinically significant as well. Contrast this with the 29–36 g of intrusive force produced by the ICS (Table 8.1), and a clinical difference in the vertical movement of teeth between these two force symptoms becomes compelling.

In mouth breathers, the difference becomes even more dramatic (Fig. 8.4, Table 8.2). If a patient maintains an open mouth position of 10 mm, the extrusive force on the maxillary anterior and mandibular posterior teeth is 134 g. If this is coupled with the 60 g of intrusive force generated by the ICS, a dramatic vertical force differential of 194 g exists. This should have significant clinical implications.

Herein lies the biggest fundamental difference between the Class II elastics and the ICS forces. The former have a clinically significant extrusive component in the force vector, while the latter deliver an intrusive component. In most facial types, and certainly in all dolichofacial patterns, the ICS should be the treatment of choice.

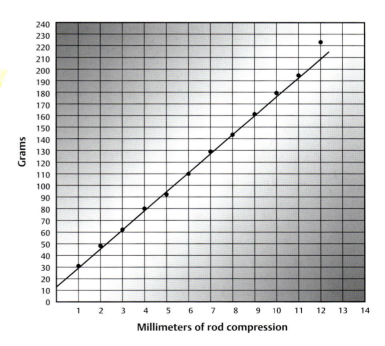

Fig. 8.1 **Force generated by compressing an interarch compression spring.** The linearity of the force permits the clinician to visually assess the amount presented at each appointment. (Eureka Spring model 23.)

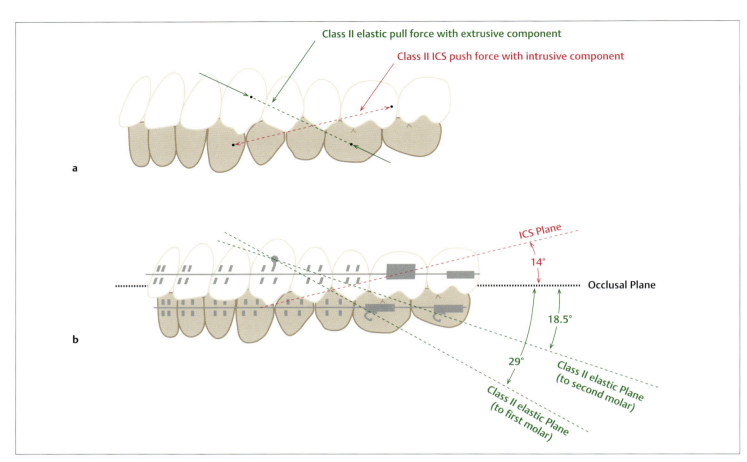

Fig. 8.2 **Force vectors comparing the Class II elastic with the Class II ICS (50% enlargement).**
a The vector of the Class II elastic compared to the Class II ICS. The ICS intrudes the dentition, while the Class II elastic has an extrusive component.
b The force vector can vary depending on the location of the attachment (50% enlargement).

Table 8.1 Changes in the force vectors of the Class II elastic and ICS when used in Class II and Class I malocclusions

Tooth Position	Vector	Force* (g)	Components	Force (g) + intrusive − extrusive
Class II	C: Class II elastic	150	C_x (horizontal)	142
			C_y (vertical)	− 56
Class II	D: Class II ICS	150	D_x (horizontal)	142
			D_y (vertical)	+ 36
Class I	E: Class II elastic	150	E_x (horizontal)	132
			E_y (vertical)	− 75
Class I	F: Class II ICS	150	F_x (horizontal)	143
			F_y (vertical)	+ 29

* Assuming clinical adjustments to maintain force at 150 g.

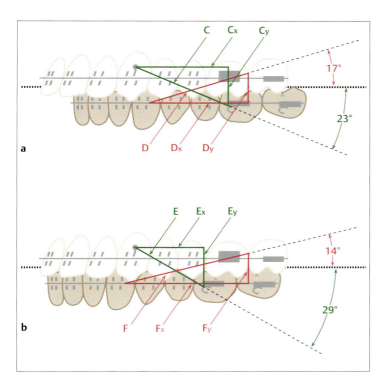

Fig. 8.**3** **Comparative vectors using the Class II elastic and the ICS in Class II and Class I malocclusion (actual size).**
a Complete Class II malocclusion. **C**, Class II elastic vector; C_x, C_y, horizontal and vertical components. **D**, Class II ICS vector; D_x, D_y, horizontal and vertical components.
b Class I malocclusion. **E**, Class II elastic vector; E_x, E_y, horizontal and vertical components. **F**, Class II ICS vector; F_x, F_y, horizontal and vertical components.

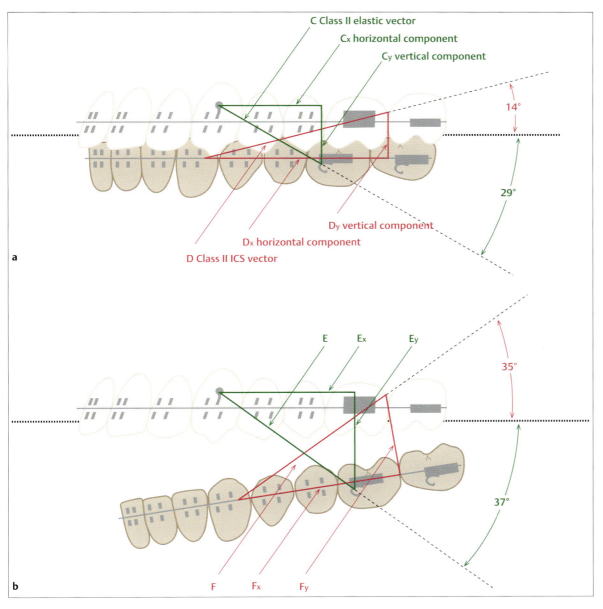

Fig. 8.**4** **Comparative vectors using Class II elastics and ICS in two mouth positions (50% enlargement).**
a Mouth closed. **C**, Class II elastic vector; C_x, C_y, horizontal and vertical components. **D**, Class II ICS vector. D_x, D_y, horizontal and vertical components.
b Mouth open 10 mm (assuming 2 mm of initial overbite). **E**, Class II elastic vector; E_x, E_y, horizontal and vertical components. **F**, Class II ICS vector; F_x, F_y, horizontal and vertical components.

Table 8.2 Changes in the force vectors between two mouth positions: closed and open 10 mm (see Fig. 9.4 for reference).

Mouth Position	Vector	Force* (g)	Components	Force (g) + intrusive − extrusive
Closed	C: Class II elastic	150	C_x (horizontal)	132
			C_y (vertical)	− 75
Closed	D: Class II ICS	150	D_x (horizontal)	143
			D_y (vertical)	+ 29
Open	E: Class II elastic	220	E_x (horizontal)	177
			E_y (vertical)	− 134
Open	F: Class II ICS	140	F_x (horizontal)	123
			F_y (vertical)	+ 60

* Assuming linearity of Class II elastic force.

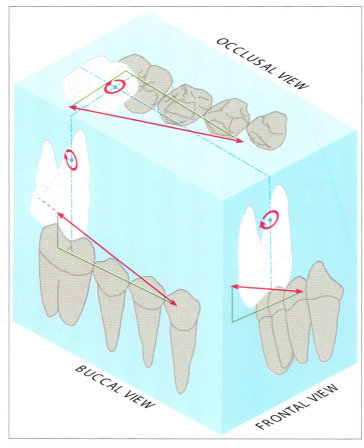

Fig. 8.5 **Three-dimensional diagrammatic representation of the vectors and resulting moments acting on the maxillary first molar from a Class II ICS.** The dark blue centerline represents the molars' original three-dimensional planes of rotation around the blue dot center of resistance. The light blue dashed line represents the moments resulting from the ICS class II vector (red line). The solid green lines represent the vertical and horizontal components.

Although the intrusive component of the ICS may well be the most important differentiating movement, other forces are also acting. The forces on the maxillary first molar are shown in Figure 8.5. There is obvious intrusion and distal tipping (buccal view), intrusion and buccal crown torque (frontal view), and expansion with mesiobuccal rotation (occlusal view). The combination of vectors and moments produces the three-dimensional force and hence movement of the maxillary first molar.

A more complete analysis of the transverse forces, as visualized in the occlusal view, is shown in Figure 8.6. Note the variation in force between the sagittal (y) and transverse (x) components depending on the type of malocclusion and ICS setup. A similar analysis could be performed from the frontal view.

It is observed clinically that, when all of the teeth are engaged in rectangular arch wires and a transpalatal bar is attached to the maxillary molars, when using the Class II ICS, or a lingual arch is used on the mandibular molars, with the Class III ICS, most of the moments and transverse forces are minimized. However, it is often beneficial to band second molars to diminish the intrusion component (see Fig. 8.3, vectors; Fig. 8.5, buccal and frontal views). Intrusion and buccal crown torque resulting from the ICS can be clinically significant (Figs. 8.7 and 8.8) and can be almost completely avoided by including the second molars, if the ICS force does not exceed 150 g. Vector forces in the 200–250 g range will demonstrate a clinically observable intrusive component, even if the second molars are incorporated.

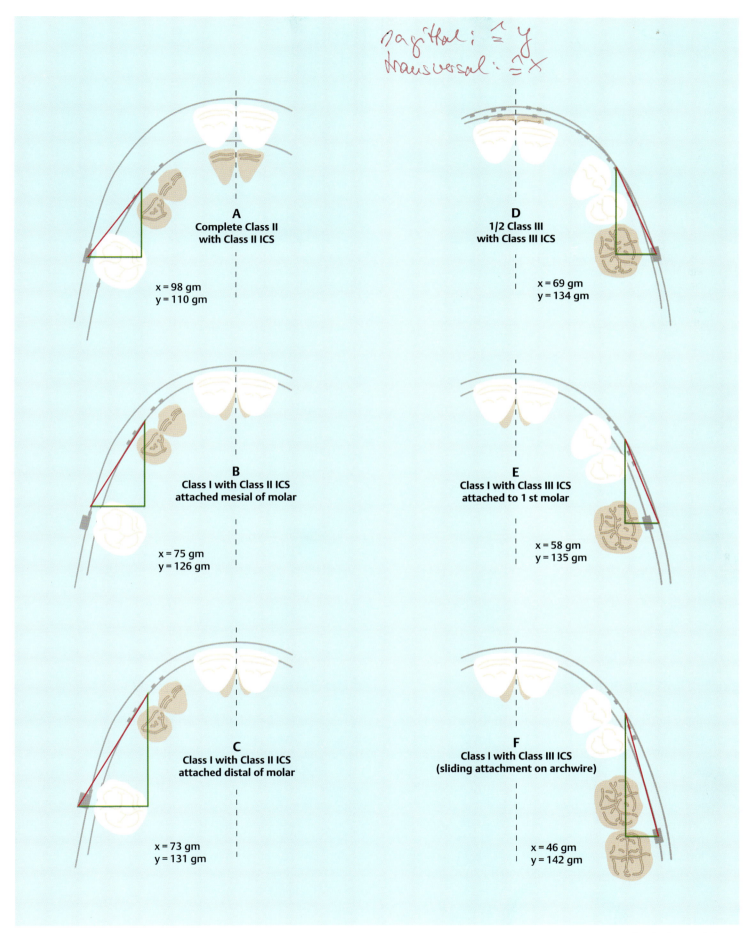

Fig. 8.6 **Transverse and sagittal forces generated by ICS in various malocclusions as viewed from the occlusal.** Red lines represent vectors at 150 g and green lines represent components. The y axis is the sagittal force while the x axis depicts transverse force. Class I, Class II, Class III represent types of malocclusions; light brown depicts mandibular teeth. Depending on the center of resistance of a single tooth or group of teeth, the moments can be visualized (50% enlargement).

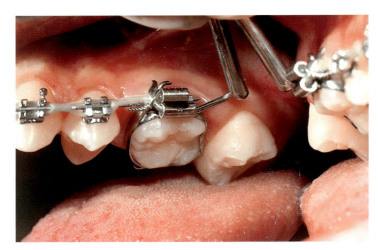

Fig. 8.**7** **Buccal occlusion after 6 months of Class II ICS without a transpalatal bar but with 15° of palatal crown torque to the maxillary molars.** Note the extent of intrusion, the effects of the moment-producing buccal crown rotation, and the importance of tying the arch together to prevent space from occurring mesial to the molar. (All intraoral photographs were taken by the author with the condyles seated in their most posterosuperior positions. This condylar position was also used for all cephalograms. The Eureka Spring was the ICS used in all the treatments described in this chapter.)

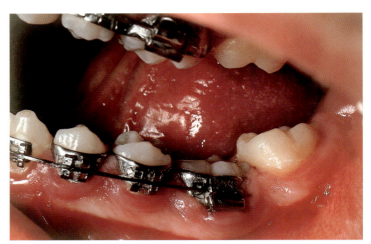

Fig. 8.**8** **Patient after one year of Class III ICS with a lingual arch.** Note the pronounced intrusion, the tipping of the occlusal plane, and the absence of buccal crown torque because of the lingual arch. Incorporating the second molars would have given additional valuable intrusive anchorage.

Table 8.**3** Comparison of ICS, Herbst and Jasper Jumper.

	ICS	Herbst	JJ
Special molar attachments	No	Yes	No
Use during finishing	Yes	No	Yes
Use in mixed dentition treatment	Yes	Yes	Yes
Cost (+ to +++)	+ to +++	+++	++
Claimed orthopedic response	No	Yes	Maybe
Requires condylar advancement for response	No	Yes	No
Adjustable vertical component of vector	Yes	No	No
Adjustable force	Yes	No	Yes

Comparison of ICS with Herbst and Jasper Jumper

The popular Herbst appliance, designed by Emil Herbst and reintroduced by Pancherz (1979), and the Jasper Jumper (Jasper and McNamara 1995) (American Orthodontics) also delivers an intrusive force, in contrast to conventional intermaxillary elastics. Since claims of lasting increases in mandibular length following functional appliance therapy have been challenged (DeVincenzo 1991; Wieslander 1993; Pancherz 1997), it seems increasingly clear that intrusive forces provided by these appliances may be more important than any temporary increase in mandibular length. A comparison of ICS, Herbst and Jasper Jumper appliances are presented in Table 8.**3**.

Description and Comparison of the Various ICS Appliances

There are three choices of ICS available to clinicians: the Eureka Spring, the Forsus, and the Twin Force. The Eureka Spring, the smallest and most compact of the three, was the first to be introduced (Fig. 8.**9**). It comes in two sizes and may be used on either the right or left side of the dental arches. Several force levels for spring module (A) are available, as well as a quick connect/disconnect model, permitting rapid insertion and removal of the spring module without removal of the arch wire. Should an additional tube not be available on the molars, which is frequently the case when Class III force is desired, an auxiliary sleeve can be used for insertion on the arch wire (Fig. 8.**10**).

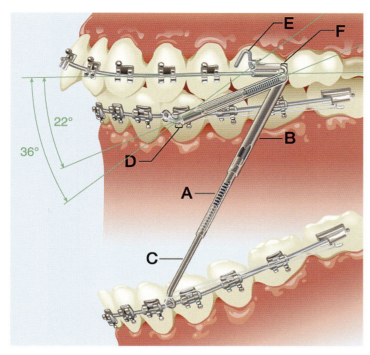

Fig. 8.9 **The Eureka Spring with the mouth closed in full Class II and open 50 mm.** The spring module (A) slides within a molar attachment tube (B). The compression spring is encased in the cylinder and drives the push rod (C) against the opposing anterior dentition. It is essential that the free distance (D) be at least 3 mm to reduce breakage of this ICS (50 % enlargement).

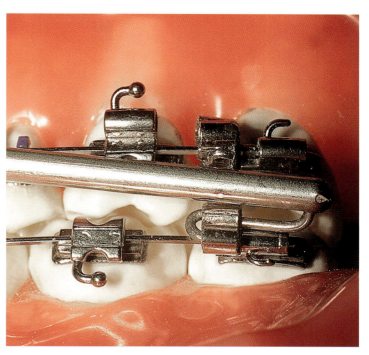

Fig. 8.10 **Auxiliary sleeve on arch wire for insertion of Class III Eureka Spring.** Note the similar but unused attachment on the maxillary arch.

Table 8.4 Physical characteristics of the individual ICSs.

	Eureka	Forsus	Twin Force
Largest outside diameter[a]	2.38 mm	3.33 mm	4.43 mm
Maximum extension[b]	66 mm	62 mm	72 mm
Maximum compression[b]	27 mm	35 mm	31 mm
Net extension[c]	33 mm	27 mm	41 mm
Force at full compression	225 g	250 g	225 g

[a] This would be diameter for Eureka Spring and Forsus and as an ellipse measured on its longest axis for Twin Force.
[b] Measured on the longest available model.
[c] Measured from maximum compression.

The Forsus (Fig. 8.11) can also be used on either the left or right side and requires four sizes to accommodate the range of mouth openings. It is only available in a 10-spring kit that offers a variety of lengths. Considerably larger then the Eureka Spring, its use is limited in some patients. Its most significant advantage lies in less breakage. A recent ingeneous molar attachment simplifies insertion.

The Twin Force (Fig. 8.12) is available in two sizes, is convertible into left or right, and has an inseparable ball-and-socket attachment to the arch wire in the anterior region. It can have either an attachment wire or a ball-and-socket attachment that can be placed mesial or distal of the first molar. The dual compression springs are encased to avoid irritation to the patient's tissue on breakage.

A visual comparison of physical characteristics of each ICS is presented in Figure 8.13, while Table 8.4 represents some quantitative assessments of each. Some comparative strengths and weaknesses of each ICS can be appreciated after examining Table 8.5. Some patients cannot tolerate much invasion of the buccal vestibule and, for these, the smaller the ICS the better. Occasionally, even the Eureka Spring causes sufficient vestibular irritation to necessitate removal. The Eureka Spring, which is initially the least expensive, can be even less costly since components can be purchased separately. When the Twin Force breaks, the entire appliance must be discarded.

Although the Eureka Spring, the Forsus, and the Twin Force are different in appearance, their mechanisms of action, force magnitudes, and vector analyses are similar. Because of this, the orthodontic and orthopedic responses to treatment also should be similar.

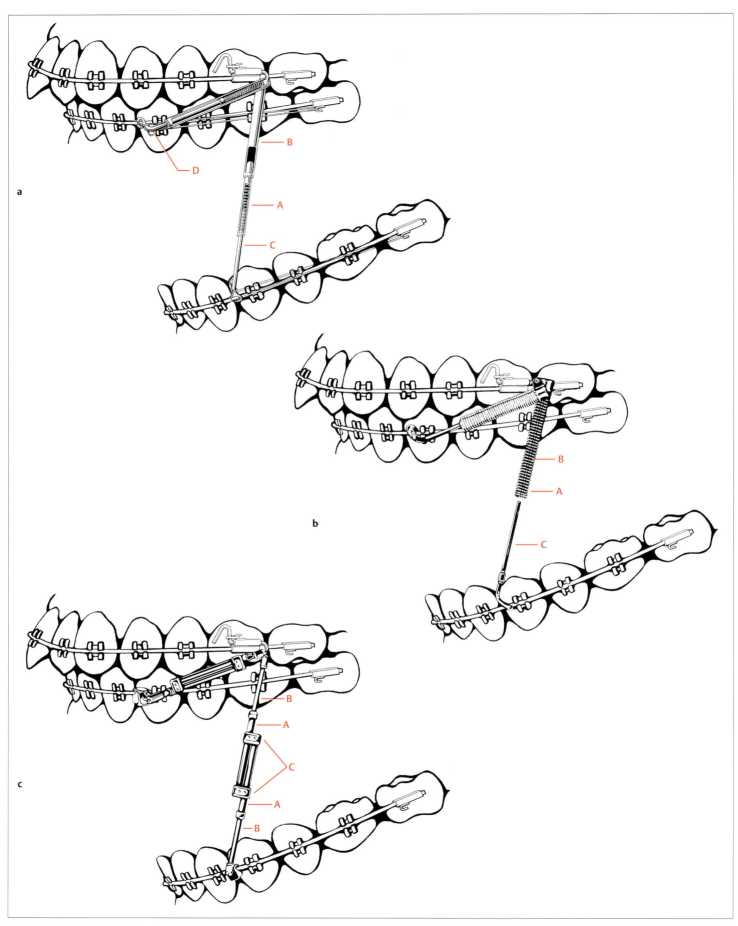

Fig. 8.**11** **The Forsus has the compression spring (A) wound around the outside of an expandable cylinder (B) with an internal sliding tube from which the push rod (C) extends.** Note the separation of the push rod from the tube at 50 mm of mouth opening. This is the result of its small net extension (see Table 8.**4**; 50% enlargement).

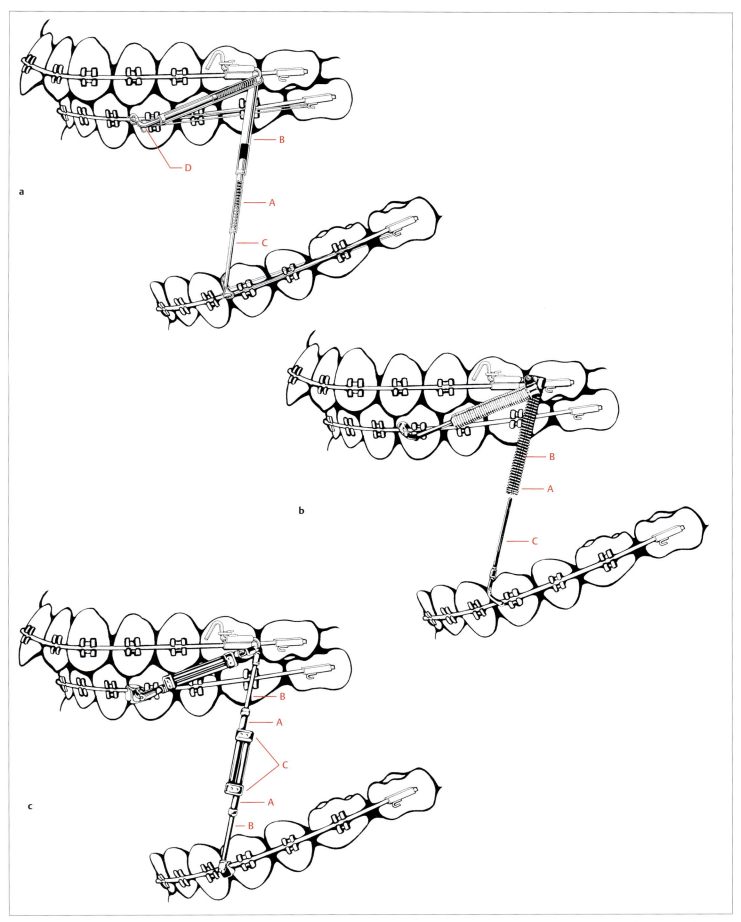

Fig. 8.**12** **The Twin Force has two cylinders (A), which contain compression springs, and two push rods (B) joined by a guiding bar (C), which is fixed to one cylinder while the other cylinder slides freely.** It has the greatest net extension of the three available ICS appliances, as seen in the open mouth position and as evident from Table 8.**4** (50% enlargement).

Table 8.5 Strengths and weaknesses of each ICS

ICS	Strengths	Weaknesses
Eureka Spring	• Small size, good patent acceptance • Variety of forces and attachments • Replacement components available • Can use with removable appliances • Least expensive	• Technically exacting to inset • Breaks more frequently than Forsus • Lacks an international sales force • Product availability variable at times
Forsus	• Least breakage • Technically easiest to insert • Backing of international orthodontic company • Unique molar attachment	• Smallest net extension • Not recommended for Class III correction • Tissue irritation in anterior vestibule • Most expensive
Twin Force	• Greatest net extension • Can use for Class III correction on some patients • Does not need a molar tube • Backing of international orthodontic company	• Breakage comparable to Eureka Spring • Breakage of one part requires disposal of entire unit • Occlusal interferes with some patients • Expensive

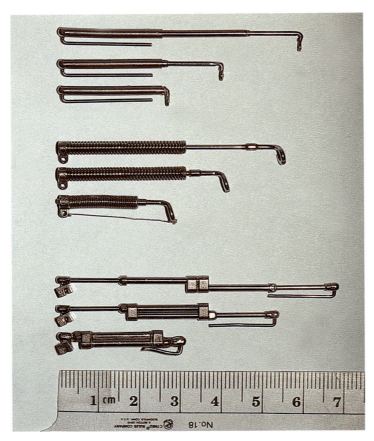

Fig. 8.13 **Visual comparison of the three ICSs.** (*Top*) Eureka Spring; (*middle*) Forsus; (*bottom*) Twin Force. Each ICS is shown at maximum extension (*upper*), passive extension (*middle*), and maximum compression (*lower*).

Table 8.6 Effects of Class II correction using the ICS[a]

- All changes were dentoalveolar
- No changes in the vertical dimensions regardless of facial type
- Rate of molar correction was 0.7 mm per month
- 3 mm of Class II correction resulted in:
  - 1.5 mm anterior movement of mandibular dentition
  - 1.5 mm posterior movement of maxillary dentition
  - 1.0 mm of maxillary molar intrusion
  - 2.0 mm of mandibular incisor intrusion
  - 3.5° of mandibular incisor tipping forward
  - 3.0° of maxillary incisor tipping backward

[a] Cephalometric evaluation of 37 consecutively treated, noncompliant patients using the Eureka Spring (Stromeyer et al. 2002)

Effects of ICSs on the Dentition

The first report on an ICS, which described the Eureka Spring and its application in Class II noncompliant patients, appeared in 1997 (DeVincenzo 1997). A cephalometric study evaluated the dental and skeletal changes that occurred during treatment with the Eureka Spring (Stromeyer et al. 2002). The conclusions of this study are presented in Table 8.6. One of the most interesting findings was the subgroup analysis of dolichofacial and brachyfacial patients. During ICS therapy, the mandibular plane angle and anterior face height did not change in either group. Although this would be expected, given the intrusive component in the Class II ICS vector, it was encouraging to actually detect no difference in vertical responses when comparing these two facially diverse subgroups.

Clinical Case Studies

Examples of the Use of the ICS in Various Clinical Settings

The speed and the response that occurs in clinical treatment utilizing the ICS is at first surprising and suspicious to the clinician. After use of the ICS for a while, it comes to be expected (Braga 2001). It should be emphasized that patient compliance, an absolute necessity with intermaxillary elastics, is no longer a significant factor. The constant light force produces more rapid tissue response with less iatrogenic potential. Additionally, since this Class II ICS force does not tend to rotate the mandible downward and backward, as occurs with Class II elastics, the rate of correction is further enhanced. This rapid movement can be seen in the following two patients.

The patient in Example 8.1 had bilateral Eureka Springs with Damon low-friction brackets while the patient in Example 8.2 had a unilateral ICS with conventional edgewise brackets. It is sometimes desirable to move certain teeth more than others. The use of differential anchorage and force can help the clinician achieve this.

Example 8.1: Eureka Springs with Damon low-friction brackets

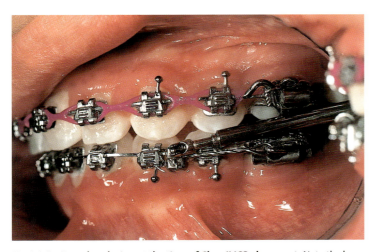

Fig. 8.1.1 **Buccal occlusion at the time of Class II ICS placement.** Note the low-friction Damon brackets, the extent of the overbite, and the free distance on the push rod.

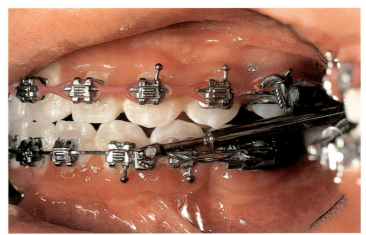

Fig. 8.1.2 **Buccal occlusion after two appointments and 10 weeks.** Note the reduction in overbite caused by the intrusive component of the Class II ICS vector and the increase in free distance on the push rod. Teeth may move faster with low-friction brackets. Differential movement could be obtained by low-friction brackets in one arch and standard edgewise brackets in the other.

Example 8.2: Unilateral ICS with conventional edgewise brackets

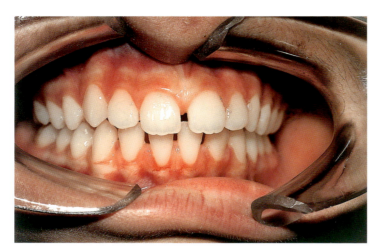

Fig. 8.2.**1** **Frontal view of initial unilateral malocclusion.**

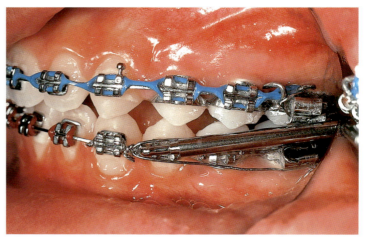

Fig. 8.2.**2** **Buccal view at insertion of Class II ICS and 16 × 22 rectangular arch wires.** At this time, bonds had been in place for three months.

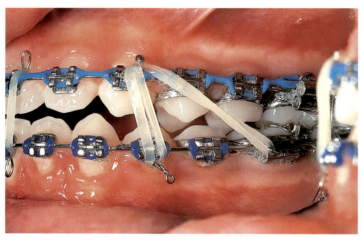

Fig. 8.2.**3** **Buccal view at the time of ICS removal three appointments and four months later.** Note the anterior open bite resulting from the intrusive component and a light Class II elastic to maintain the Class II correction while extruding the mandibular anterior teeth.

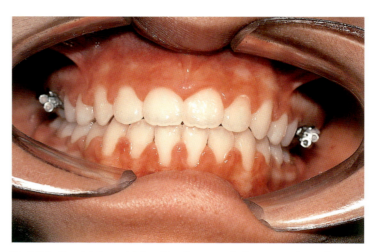

Fig. 8.2.**4** **Frontal view at debonding three months later.** Note the midline compared to Fig. 8.2.**1**.

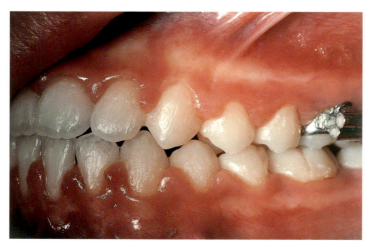

Fig. 8.2.**5** **Posterior intercuspation at bond/band removal.** Total active treatment time was 10 months. Note that the molar bands are still in place for extraoral anchorage to be utilized for the first four months of retention.

For example, low-friction brackets in one arch and high-friction brackets in the other will encourage differential movement. The use of varying amounts of anterior root torque, extraoral anchorage, the number of teeth incorporated into the appliance, and extraction of maxillary second molar (Waters and Harris 2001) all contribute to differential movement of maxillary or mandibular teeth. Likewise, varying the amount of force on each side, as in the unilateral case presented above, can produce differential movement.

The Noncompliant Patient

Probably no case provides the clinician with as much motivation to use the ICS as that of the noncompliant Class II patient who has already been under treatment for an extended time. The latest edition of *Orthodontics: Current Principles and Technique* (Graber and Vanarsdall 2000) contains a chapter on treatment options in noncompliant patients that gives many examples utilizing an ICS (Eureka Spring) (DeVincenzo 2000). The speed of correction and the predictable outcome in this most difficult group of patients is evident.

The patient depicted in Example 8.3 is representative of this all too large portion of every orthodontist's practice. The ICS works well in patients who miss appointments because the force diminishes as the malocclusion corrects. The use of differential forces as demonstrated here is sometimes helpful and can be obtained by either activating the ICS more or less on one side or by selecting a spring module (Fig. 8.9, see A) delivering a greater or lesser force.

Example 8.3: Noncompliant Class II patient already under treatment

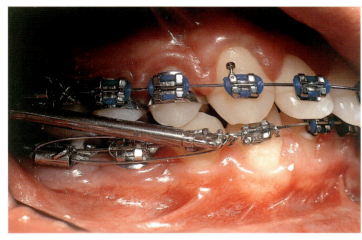

Fig. 8.3.**1** **Buccal occlusion after 11 months in treatment with a noncompliant patient.** During this interval, the patient missed eight appointments and kept only two.

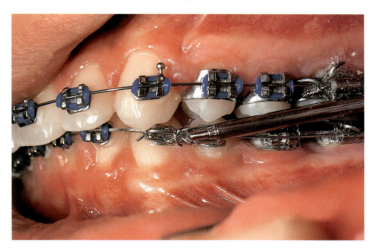

Fig. 8.3.**2** **Left buccal occlusion.** Note more severe Class II on this side. Because of this, a spring module that delivers 50% more force was used.

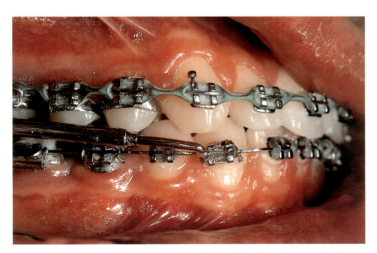

Fig. 8.3.**3** **Right buccal occlusion after eight months of ICS, during which time the patient missed six appointments and was seen only twice.**

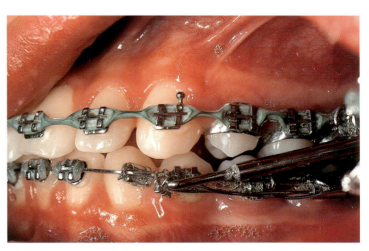

Fig. 8.3.**4** **Left buccal occlusion after the same interval.** Note the more rapid movement with the higher-force ICS, the increased free distance, and the decreased overbite.

Treatment Planning with the ICS

As the clinician gains confidence in the ICS, and as appreciation of the predictable nature of the results increases, treatment planning utilizing the ICS will naturally follow. The patients presented show a variety of treatment planning approaches centered around the diverse capabilities of the ICS.

Example 8.**4** presents a unilateral Class II in which only selected teeth were banded initially and the maxillary anterior bonds were in place for only the last eight months of treatment. Soldering the molar bands together increases the anchorage sufficiently to counteract most of the intrusion and moments that will be acting together on this body (Fig. 8.**5**). By doing this, the center of resistance is moved distally and nearer to the point of force application, thereby reducing the moments. The free distance of the push rod (Fig. 8.**9**, see C) permits the clinician to visually determine the magnitude of the initial force at 156 g. (If free distance is 3 mm and full compression produces 210 g, as shown in Figure 8.**1**, and, for every millimeter of push-rod extension, the force at the vector decreases 18 g, then the force vector will be 210 − 54 = 156). The lower anterior teeth were bonded to correct slight crowding and provide some anchorage to the anticipated canine–premolar transverse movement (Fig. 8.**6**). During the ensuing seven months and five appointments, the clinician changed the mandibular anterior wire and adjusted the free distance of the ICS so that the Class II force remained near 150 g.

Example 8.4: Unilateral Class II

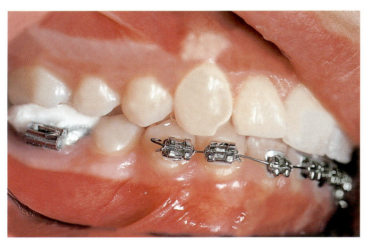

Fig. 8.4.**1** **Right buccal occlusion on the day of bonding.** Note the Ketac glass ionomer cement placed over the occlusal surface for bite opening.

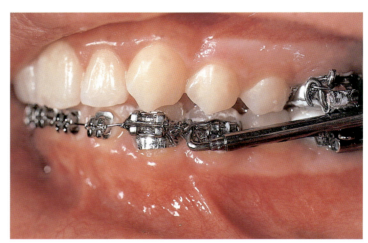

Fig. 8.4.**2** **Left Buccal occlusion on the day of bonding and placement of the ICS.** Bands had been selected the previous week for the left maxillary molars and mandibular canine and premolar. These bands were then soldered together in the laboratory. The ICS was placed at this bonding appointment, and the initial free distance of the push rod (see Fig. 8.**9**, C) can be seen.

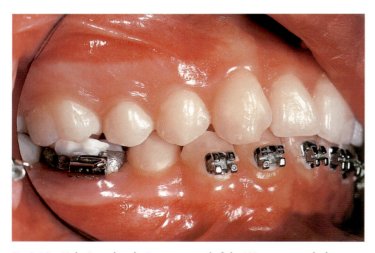

Fig. 8.4.**3** **Right Buccal occlusion at removal of the ICS seven months later.** Note the unchanged posterior relationships.

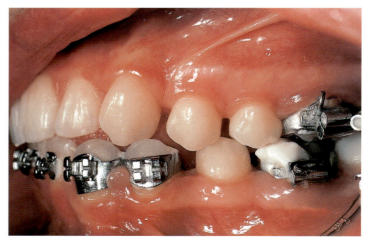

Fig. 8.4.**4** **Left buccal occlusion at removal of the ICS.** Note the slight intrusion of the mandibular anterior teeth and the lack of expected molar buccal crown torque. The molar bands are now removed, unsoldered, and cemented separately to improve hygiene in the interproximal area. The remaining bands/bonds were placed at this time.

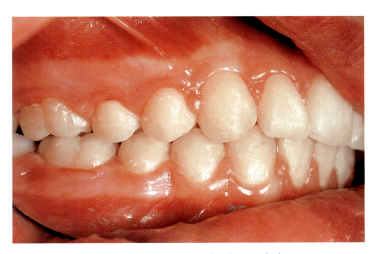

Fig. 8.4.**5** **Right buccal occlusion at removal eight months later.**

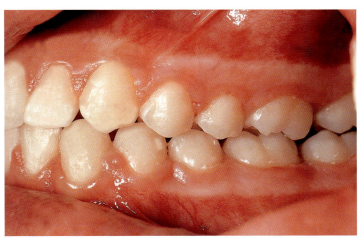

Fig. 8.4.**6** **Left buccal occlusion at appliance removal.** Total treatment time was 15 months.

Since the ICS provides dependable and easily quantifiable Class II and Class III force vectors, the clinician can use them in conjunction with intra-arch (Class I) forces. In Figure 8.**14**, the Class II ICS vector is used in conjunction with a Class I mandibular force within a complete Class II malocclusion. By varying the magnitude and duration of these two forces, a variety of dental responses can be obtained.

For example, if the Class I force exceeds the horizontal component of the Class II force vector, the mandibular incisors will be retruded during space closure. If the Class II force vector exceeds the Class I force, the lower incisors will be proclined during space closure. If the two forces are equal, the lower incisor position will remain stable in the sagittal dimension. Of course, this rests on the assumption that the anchorage units are equal. However, using progress cephalograms and visual assessments, the originally desired tooth positions can be realized by varying the applied forces.

If the patient has congenitally missing mandibular second premolars with a poor prognosis for retaining the mandibular deciduous second molars and a desirable position of the lower incisors, there are presently two treatment options. The first is bilateral three-unit bridges; the second is bilateral dental implants.

The patient depicted in Example 8.**5** chose a third option, namely mechanics set up as in Fig. 8.**14a**. Since the pretreatment position of the maxillary and mandibular incisors was acceptable, the force system was calculated such that the horizontal component of the Class II force equaled the Class I force protracting the mandibular molars. The beginning and end of ICS treatment cephalograms indicate that the pretreatment objectives were realized.

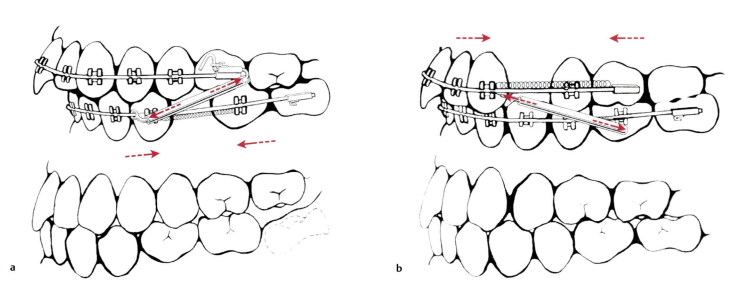

Fig. 8.14 **The hypothetical use of inter-arch and intra-arch forces of varying magnitude, represented as dotted portions of the arrows, to accomplish differential tooth movements.**

a With a complete Class II malocclusion, Class II ICS force is used in conjunction with Class I intraoral force to close the space resulting from a congenitally missing second bicuspid. At the same time, the maxillary dentition is retracted.

b With a partial Class II occlusion and some mandibular anterior crowding, Class III ICS force is used to intrude the maxillary incisors and distalize the mandibular molars while the Class I force protracts the maxillary molars into a Class II relationship. This is done in conjunction with extraction of the maxillary first premolars. (From Graber TM, Vanarsdall RL Jr., eds. *Orthodontics: Current Principles and Techniques*. St. Louis: Mosby; 2000.)

Example 8.5: ICS space closure of congenitally missing bicuspids

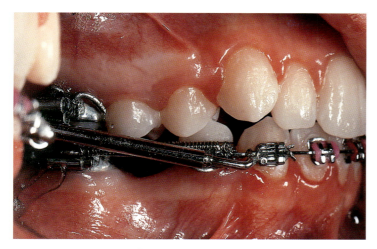

Fig. 8.5.**1** **Patient at time of ICS placement, as illustrated in Fig. 8.14a.** The four maxillary molars were soldered together with a transpalatal bar. The maxillary incisor roots showed blunting and foreshortening in the pretreatment radiographs and therefore were not bonded initially. The measured Class I force of the closed coil spring equaled the horizontal force component of the Class II ICS. An equalization of the two forces was chosen because no movement of the mandibular anterior teeth was desired.

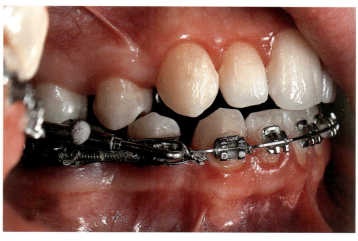

Fig. 8.5.**2** **Dental changes after six months.** Note the spaces in the maxillary arch, the protraction of mandibular molars, and little change in overjet.

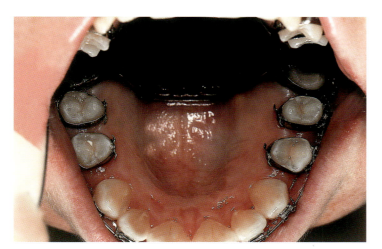

Fig. 8.5.**3** **The maxillary dentition after eight months of treatment and at the time the remaining bonds/bands were placed.** Although the initial transpalatal bar was made 2 mm away from the palatal mucosa, the intrusion force component of the ICS necessitated its removal at this time because of palatal impaction.

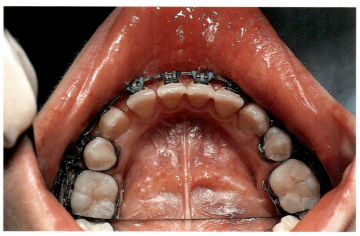

Fig. 8.5.**4** **The mandibular dentition after 11 months of combined Class II ICS and Class I forces.** Note the near-complete space closure.

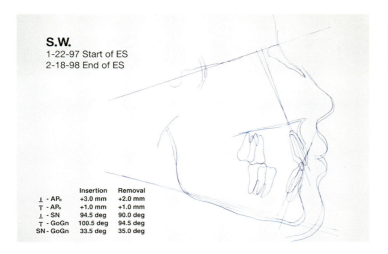

Fig. 8.5.**5** **Cephalometric measures after 13 months of treatment and at the termination of the ICS and the Class I force.** Note that the Class II and Class I forces were properly balanced with the combined anchorage in the two arches. The expected intrusion of the maxillary molars and mandibular incisors occurred.

S.W.
1-22-97 Start of ES
2-18-98 End of ES

	Insertion	Removal
$\underline{1}$ - APo	+3.0 mm	+2.0 mm
$\overline{1}$ - APo	+1.0 mm	+1.0 mm
$\underline{1}$ - SN	94.5 deg	90.0 deg
$\overline{1}$ - GoGn	100.5 deg	94.5 deg
SN - GoGn	33.5 deg	35.0 deg

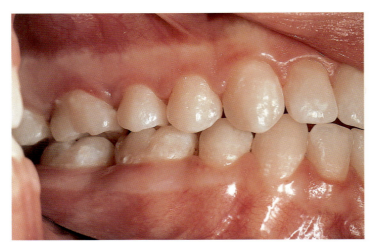

Fig. 8.5.**6** **Right buccal occlusion at completion.** Note the offset of the maxillary second premolar to enhance intercuspation when finishing with a Class III molar occlusion.

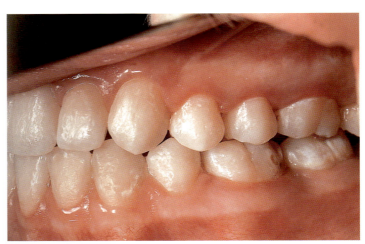

Fig. 8.5.**7** **Left buccal occlusion at completion.** The total active treatment time was 25 months.

A word of caution for those contemplating this treatment plan: be sure that well-positioned mandibular third molars are present. Additionally, maxillary second molars must be incorporated into the arch wires with sufficient palatal crown torque. Immediately after debanding, the second molars must be stabilized to prevent eruption until the mandibular third molars emerge. This can be done by banding or bonding the first and second molars together.

The young adolescent patient seen in Example 8.**6** presented with the right central incisor missing since age 7 years. The molar relationship was end-to-end, and the maxillary midline had shifted into the space of the missing central incisor. The treatment plan included moving the right lateral incisor into the position of the exfoliated central incisor, moving the left anterior teeth into the space created by extraction of the left first premolar, and obtaining bilateral Class II molar relationships.

Example 8.6: Missing right central incisor

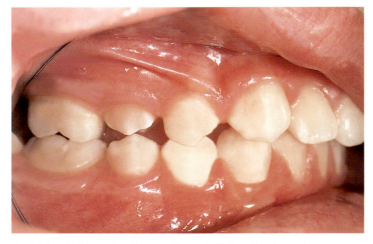

Fig. 8.6.**1** **Right buccal occlusion with one half Class II molar and more pronounced Class II canine relationships.**

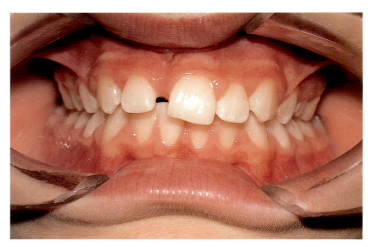

Fig. 8.6.**2** **Frontal view showing dental migration resulting from the exfoliation of the right central incisor at 7 years of age.**

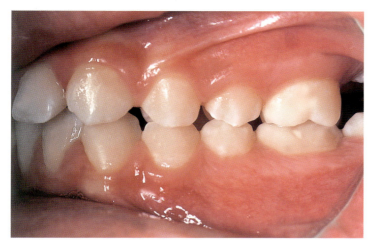

Fig. 8.6.**3** **Left buccal occlusion with end-to-end molar and canine relationships.**

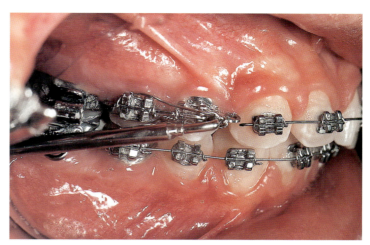

Fig. 8.6.**4** **At time of placement of the Class III ICS.** A lingual arch helped control mandibular molar tipping, the maxillary molar and both premolars were soldered together on the palatal surface, and a section of 16 × 22 wire was bent to fit passively into the buccal attachments on these bands. This wire extended mesial of the first premolar to permit attachment of the Class III ICS. Note the bonding of the remaining teeth on the same appointment and the initial round nickel–titanium arch wires.

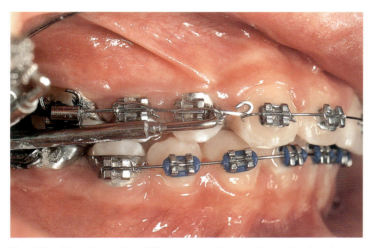

Fig. 8.6.**5** **After 5.5 months of ICS treatment.** The posterior sectional can be seen clearly, as can the maxillary round wire which ends at the canine.

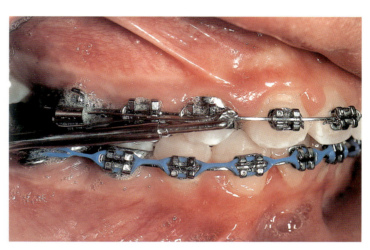

Fig. 8.6.**6** **A lesser Class III ICS force of 90 g, calculated from the free distance of the push rod, continued for another six months.**

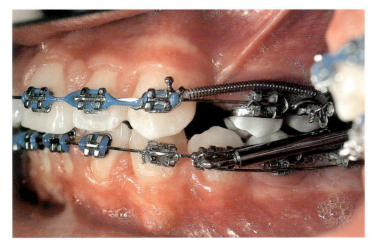

Fig. 8.6.**7** **Left buccal occlusion six months later.** Since the extraction space diminished more from mesial migration of the posterior dentition (see [3]) than from distal migration of the anterior teeth, a Class II ICS was then placed to support the molar anchorage. This also permitted an increase in the Class I force.

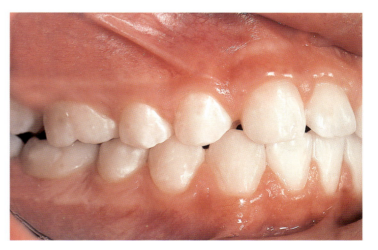

Fig. 8.6.**8** **Buccal occlusion at debanding with the right maxillary canine in the lateral location and the first premolar functioning as the right canine.**

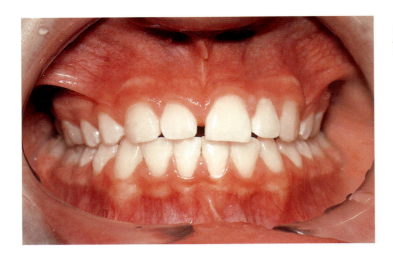

Fig. 8.6.9 **Frontal view at debonding with the "central" incisor positioned for an eventual veneer.** Note the midline correction. Active treatment time was 19 months.

The illustrations in Example 8.7 were selected from the files of a 43-year-old woman to illustrate a treatment plan utilizing a Class III ICS. She presented with a deep overbite with a cant and mandibular mid-line shift to the left [1], a missing left first premolar [2], and mandibular posterior crowding more pronounced on the left [3]. A unilateral Class III ICS could help correct all these conditions. The intrusive component of this Class III vector would contribute to the correction of the asymmetrical and excessive overbite, while the horizontal force component would be used to distalize the left mandibular molars, developing much needed space for future correction of anterior crowding. The slight Class I molar and partial Class III canine would be protracted by the horizontal force component of the ICS, which would help correct the midline and obtain Class II molar and Class I cuspid relationships.

Example 8.7: Treatment plan utilizing Class III ICS

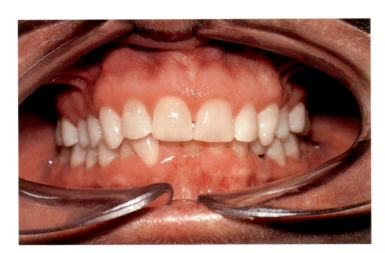

Fig. 8.7.1 Frontal view of a 43-year-old woman with an excessive overbite, a missing maxillary left first premolar, and a pronounced maxillary midline shift.

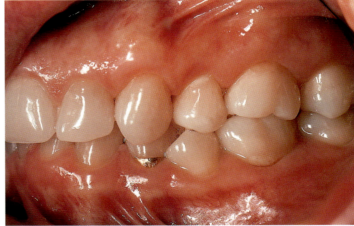

Fig. 8.7.2 Buccal occlusion showing an excessive overbite, a missing premolar, a partial Class II molar relationship, and mandibular crowding.

Clinical Case Studies

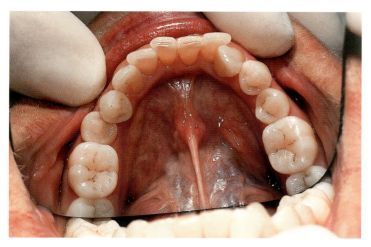

Fig. 8.7.**3** **Occlusal view of mandibular crowding.** The use of a unilateral Class III ICS to the left side would distalize the left mandibular molars, protract the maxillary posterior teeth into a complete Class II relationship, shift the maxillary midline to the right, and deliver an intrusive component of force to the maxillary anterior teeth.

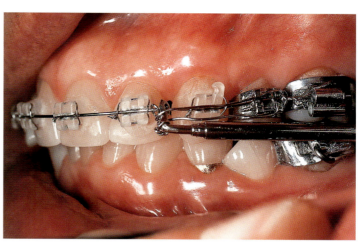

Fig. 8.7.**4** **Buccal occlusion at initial bonding, insertion of a nickel–titanium leveling wire, and delivery of a unilateral class III ICS.** The two left mandibular molars were soldered together for increased anchorage against the intrusive component of the force that will be delivered, but a lingual arch was not used. The lingual arch would have had adverse effects on the opposite molars and retarded the distalization of the left molars. The remainder of the mandibular dentition will not be bonded until sufficient space has been obtained. A 0.016 in. stainless wire was used in the maxillary arch because the intrusive component of the force to the maxillary anterior teeth can be more quickly expressed. The larger the wire, the less intrusion from the ICS.

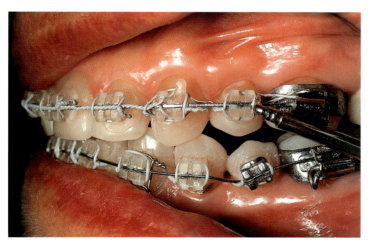

Fig. 8.7.**5** **Eight months and four appointments later, at bonding/banding of the mandibular dentition.** Note the complete Class I canine, the reduced overbite, and the change in the attachment of the ICS from mesial of canine for four months (Ex8.8–04) to distal of canine for four months (Ex8.8–05) to distal of premolar at this appointment.

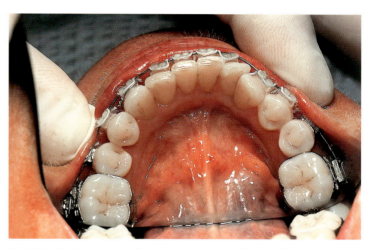

Fig. 8.7.**6** Occlusal view at the same appointment showing the decrease in crowding (compare to [3]) at the time of complete mandibular arch bonding/banding.

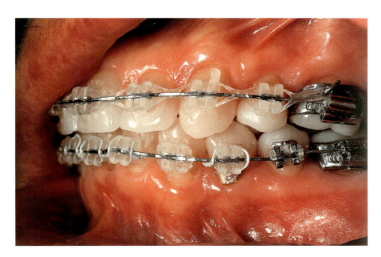

Fig. 8.7.**7** **Left buccal view four months later after two more appointments.** A mandibular 16 × 22 arch wire was placed at this time, and the ICS was removed.

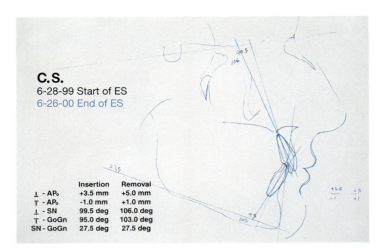

Fig. 8.7.8 Cephalometric changes during the Class III ICS force. Black represents the beginning cephalogram two months prior to the initial bonding/banding and ICS placement. Blue represents the progress cephalogram at the time of ICS removal. Note that there was no change in the mandibular plane angle, a slight intrusion of the maxillary incisors, mesial tipping of mandibular incisors, and a decrease in the interincisal angle. A decrease in this angle is considered important in helping to prevent a return of the original deep overbite.

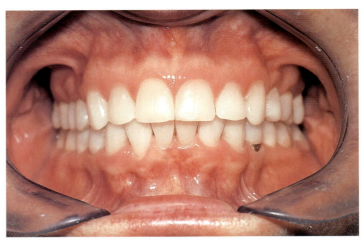

Fig. 8.7.9 At bond/band removal five months later. Compared to the original frontal view Fig. 8.7.1, overbite and midline corrections are evident. Active treatment time was 17 months.

The patient lived over 300 kilometers away, was seen every two months while the ICS was in place, and completed the active phase of treatment in 17 months. This could not have been accomplished with Class III elastics, because they would tend to increase the overbite. Unilateral Class III Herbst treatment is not possible, while Class III correction with a Jasper Jumper would enhance the possibility of appliance breakage. What could have treated this patient faster, easier, and better than an ICS?

It is hoped that these examples of treatment planning with the ICS will encourage the clinician to consider a greater variety of options when designing individualized treatments. For those clinicians who master the art of using the ICS, greater variety in planning and more flexibility in treatment will be the reward.

Relapse Following Rapid Tooth Movement Utilizing the ICS

Clinical tools, like the ICS, that enhance the rate of tooth movement will increase the amount of relapse if not accompanied by supporting-tissue remodeling (Reitan 1969). An excellent review by Thilander (2000) will sensitize the clinician to the importance of and reasons for this relapse. Immediate posterior relapse is a much more important concern when utilizing the ICS than when employing older techniques such as elastics, lip bumpers, extraoral anchorage, and functional appliances worn for an extended period. It is my own clinical observation that the more rapid and extensive the correction, the more pronounced the ensuing relapse.

The findings of a study evaluating the contributing factors in the return of overjet following ICS treatment have been reported (DeVincenzo and Smith 2001) and are presented in Table 8.7. Clinical steps can be taken either to avoid this short-term relapse completely or, at least, to greatly reduce it.

Most importantly, the ICS force vector should be maintained for an extended period after the desired correction has been obtained. This can be accomplished by reducing the ICS-generated force by approximately 50 g, an effect obtained by increasing the free distance (Fig. 8.9, see **d**; Ex. 8.6, Figs. 8.6.5 and 8.6.6). After removal of the ICS, interarch elastics should be prescribed for several months (Ex. 8.2, Fig. 8.2.3).

Table 8.7 Return of overjet following rapid (0.8 mm per month) Class II correction using ICS*.

Of the observed return:

- 58% due to maxillary incisor anterior movement (1.5 mm)
- 42% due to mandibular incisor posterior movement (1.1 mm)
  - 4.4° forward tipping of maxillary incisor
  - 4.3° backward tipping of mandibular incisor
  - 0.7 mm of maxillary incisor intrusion
  - 0.8 mm of mandibular incisor extrusion
  - 1.0 mm of maxillary molar extrusion
  - No changes in anteroposterior molar positions, anterior face height, and mandibular plane angle
  - This degree of relapse occurred in 28 of 115 consecutively treated adolescents, or nearly 25%

* Cephalometric evaluation of 28 patients in whom there occurred a return of at least 2 mm of overjet within four months after Eureka Spring therapy (DeVincenzo 2001).

The prevention of this immediate relapse by overcorrecting initially has not been satisfactory. Overcorrection occurs very rapidly, usually in one to two additional appointments, but the undesirable intrusion force and moments also continue to be expressed. By decreasing the force, sometimes even before the goal is achieved, and extending the treatment time with the ICS, this type of relapse and undesirable movements can be minimized. Reduction in relapse can also be obtained by incorporating 4–5 months of cervical or occipital anchorage as part of the initial retention program (Ex. 8.**2**, Fig. 8.2.**5**).

The Use of the ICS with Removable Appliances

With transpalatal stabilization and incorporation of the four maxillary molars with Class II ICS force in the range of 150 g, molar stability is good. However, spaces mesial to the molars will tend to appear (Fig. 8.7; Ex. 8.**4**, Fig. 8.4.**4**; Ex. 8.**5**, Fig. 8.5.**3**) unless all the anterior teeth are bonded or tied back to the molars. This also occurs in the mandibular dentition (Ex. 8.**4**, Fig. 8.4.**4**). The use of vacuum-formed thermolabile retainers is becoming more popular. Mild to moderate Class II conditions in which some excess overbite is available lend themselves to correction using these two appliances in concert.

The adult patient illustrated in Figure 8.**15** had a Class II tendency and accompanying overjet with some maxillary anterior rotations. She wanted the overjet and rotations corrected but was unwilling to wear bonded appliances. She had to be able to remove the appliances for some of her daily activities.

An ICS was fixed, but the maxillary and mandibular retainers were removable. During the 10-month treatment interval, no interproximal spaces appeared, the anterior rotations were corrected, and the overjet was reduced.

Of the three ICSs available today, only the Eureka Spring lends itself to adaptation for removable retainers during treatment in the early mixed dentition. This occurs because the spring module (Fig. 8.**9**, see **a**) can be completely disengaged from the molar attachment tube (Fig. 8.**9**, see **b**). In the past, this offered significant financial savings, as the components can be purchased separately. Now, with adaptation to removable appliances, shown in Figure 8.**16**, another use for an ICS is available.

Although it requires some initial dexterity, the young patient quickly learns how to insert, connect, and remove the ICS. The type and rate of tooth movement are similar to those obtained from more conventional ICS applications, but the force required to achieve correction is less.

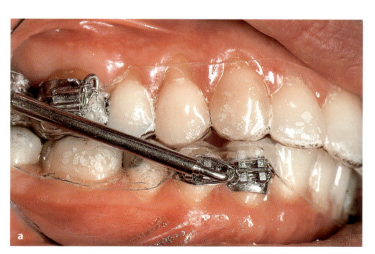
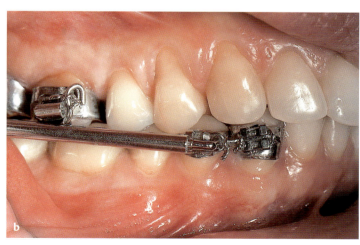

Fig. 8.**15** **An adult patient with some anterior irregularities, excessive overjet, and a moderate bilateral Class II malocclusion.**

a **Initial view.** Note that the four maxillary molars are joined together by a transpalatal bar, the mandibular first premolars and canines are banded, and a lingual bar is soldered to the premolars and canines in the lower arch, with the lingual bar closely adapted to the incisal surfaces. Vacuum-formed clear retainers are worn as much as possible while the ICSs are permanently attached.

b **After 10 months in treatment.** The molar and canine relationships are improved, and the overjet and anterior irregularities resolved. Note the gingival stripping in the maxillary premolars and canines. The retainer had been made so that it did not contact these areas by waxing out on the models before construction.

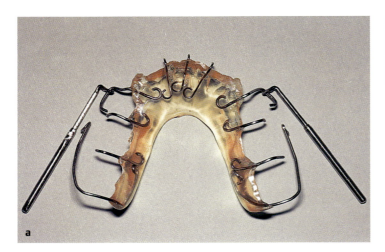
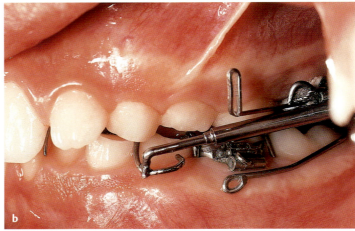
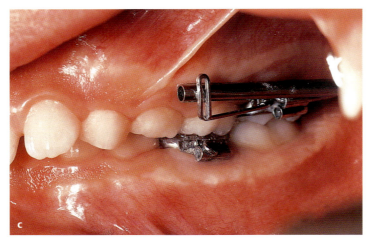

Fig. 8.**16** **Use of the ICS with removable appliances.**
a The removable appliance with spring modules (see Fig. 8.**9**a) attached.
b The removable appliance in place. Note the extent of the free distance (see Fig. 8.**9**d), indicating a force of approximately 80 g. Higher forces are not needed at this age.
c On removal—during eating and brushing, for example—the molar attachment tube (see Fig. 8.**9**b) is placed in the buccal sling.

The Use of the ICS with Orthognathic Surgery

Of the three ICSs available, the Eureka Spring permits the greatest flexibility in varying the magnitude of the force. This ICS has been placed numerous times on surgical cases, generally within one to two weeks after surgery. It is particularly valuable in LeForte procedures because of the intrusive force component of the ICS and its versatility, permitting use in both Class III and Class II situations. All of the ICSs work equally well in mandibular advancement surgery. The intrusive force vector probably makes a contribution, as downward and backward rotation does not occur during treatment. Contrast this with the use of Class II elastics. This advantage of ICS over elastics can be particularly important in dolichofacial patients.

In Example 8.**8**, Fig. 8.8.**1**, we can see the occlusal results following mandibular advancement surgery and previous removal of mandibular first premolars. This patient had an extreme dolichofacial pattern with an original sella–nasion to mandibular plane angle (SN–GoGn) of 54°. The surgeon recommended a second operation. A unilateral ICS was used instead (Fig. 8.8.**2**). Ex. 8.**8**, Figs. 8.8.**3** to 8.8.**6** indicate an acceptable occlusion and profile change.

Example 8.8: Occlusal results after mandibular advancement surgery and previous removal of mandibular first premolars

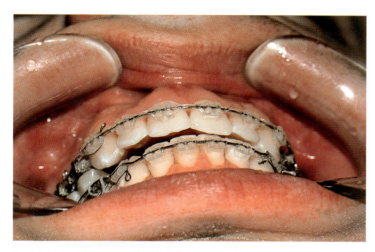

Fig. 8.8.1 Occlusion immediately following mandibular advancement surgery. The surgeon recommended a second operation.

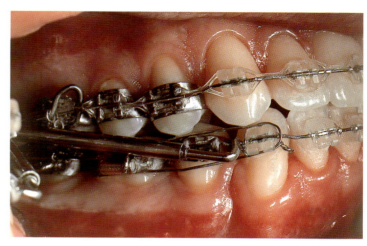

Fig. 8.8.2 **Buccal occlusion on the affected side.** Rather than having the patient undergo further surgery, a unilateral ICS was placed.

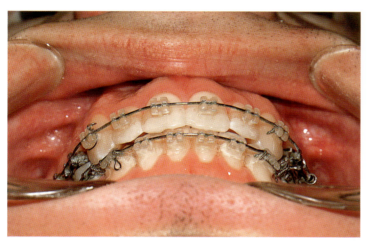

Fig. 8.8.3 Six months later, the anterior occlusion was acceptable.

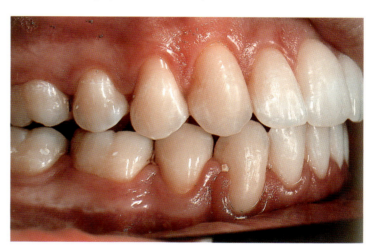

Fig. 8.8.4 At bond/band removal seven months after placing the ICS.

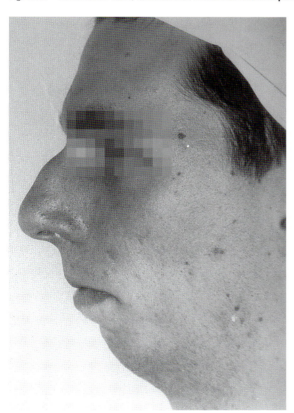

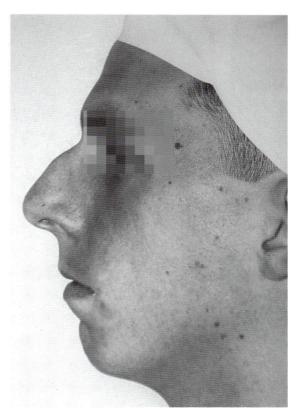

Fig. 8.8.5 **Initial photograph of this dolichofacial patient.** The use of Class II elastics in this facial type, particularly immediately following surgery, is not recommended.

Fig. 8.8.6 **Facial photograph at the time of bond/band removal.** The extraction of only the mandibular first premolars permitted a larger mandibular advancement. The removal of two maxillary premolars would have decreased dental support to the superior labialis.

Disadvantages of the ICS

The ICS is not without disadvantages. As with any new technique, a learning period is necessary. The integration of the ICS into a busy clinical practice will create additional stress. It is certainly easier to hook up a Class II elastic than a Class II ICS, and the pressures of the moment often influence decisions of this kind.

All inter-arch systems are prone to more breakage than any intra-arch appliance. This is more than an annoyance as it disrupts the flow of an office and requires staff time for repairs and because the ICS is expensive, particularly when compared with elastics. Tissue irritation can be significant for some patients, sometimes so severe that it necessitates removal.

There are orthodontic reasons not to use the ICS. In severe brachyfacial patients, extrusion of maxillary incisors and downward and backward mandibular rotation may be desired. Class II elastics and cervical anchorage are better choices for these patients. There is a current trend in orthodontics to treat more patients by nonextraction. This results in protrusion of the lower incisors. An ICS treatment accentuates this condition. If the initial lower incisor to the APo plane is greater than 2 mm, long-term ICS treatment may be contraindicated for nonextraction treatment plans.

Summary

The ICS offers so many advantages and opportunities that it should be a part of every clinician's armamentarium. The clinical limitations of using Herbst or Jasper Jumper appliances, compared with the ICS's wider range of applications, should be considered. If there is no lasting, long-term benefit to using a Herbst appliance, it is difficult to understand why they remain so popular among clinicians.

The predictable and rapid tooth movement afforded by the ICS requires an appreciation of moments, vectors, and differential forces. This rapid movement also requires heightened awareness of subsequent immediate relapse, along with knowledge of clinical approaches to its prevention. When the clinician masters the technique of the ICS, a whole array of new treatment options become available. The ICS is becoming firmly entrenched in the clinical practices of an increasing number of orthodontists. Dependable results, versatility, patient acceptance, reduced need for compliance, and rapid tooth movement make the ICS an attractive new addition to the orthodontist's armamentarium for the correction of sagittal discrepancies.

References

Braga GC. Eureka Spring for finishing correction of class II and improving anchorage. R Dental Press Orthodon Orthop Facial. 2002; 6: 51–60.

DeVincenzo JP. Changes in mandibular length before, during and after successful orthopedic correction of class II malocclusion, using a functional appliance. Am J Orthod Dentofacial Orthop. 1991; 99: 241–257.

DeVincenzo JP. The Eureka Spring: a new interarch force delivery system. J Clin Orthod. 1997; 31: 454–467.

DeVincenzo JP. Treatment options for sagittal corrections in noncompliant patients. In: Graber TM, Vanarsdall RL Jr., eds. Orthodontics: current principles and techniques. St. Louis: Mosby; 2000: 779–800.

DeVincenzo JP, Smith KD. Analysis of relapse following rapid class II correction utilizing Eureka Springs. Eur J Orthod. 2001; 23: 449.

DeVincenzo JP, Winn MW. Maxillary incisor intrusion and facial growth. Angle Orthod. 1987; 57: 279–289.

Graber TM, Vanarsdall RL Jr, eds. Orthodontics: current principles and techniques. St. Louis: Mosby; 2000: 794–795.

Jasper JS, McNamara JA. The correction of interarch malocclusions using a fixed force module. Am J Orthod Dentofacial Orthop. 1995; 108: 641–658.

Pancherz H. Treatment of class II malocclusion by jumping the bite with the Herbst appliance. A cephalometric investigation. Am J Orthod. 1979; 76: 423–442.

Pancherz H. The effects, limitations, and long-term dentofacial adaptations to treatment with the Herbst appliance. Semin Orthod. 1997; 3: 232–346.

Reitan K. Principles of retention and avoidance of post-treatment relapse. Am J Orthod. 1969; 55: 776–790.

Stromeyer EL, Caruso JM, DeVincenzo JP. A cephalometric study of the class II correction effects of the Eureka Spring. Angle Orthod. 2002; 72: 203–210.

Thilander B. Biological basis for orthodontic relapse. Semin Orthod. 2000; 6: 195–205.

Waters D, Harris EF. Cephalometric comparison of maxillary second molar extraction and non-extraction treatments in patients with class II malocclusions. Am J Orthod Dentofacial Orthop. 2001; 120: 608–613.

Wieslander L. Long-term effects of treatment with the headgear–Herbst appliance in the early mixed dentition. Stability or relapse? Am J Orthod Dentofacial Orthop. 1993; 104: 319–329.

9 Anchorage Control in Orthodontic Extraction Therapy

Michael Marcotte

In most malocclusions, extraction of teeth is required to solve the crowding of teeth and/or to produce a desired lip profile. When teeth are removed (usually the first or second premolars), the posterior teeth are typically moved mesially in varying amounts to close the extraction sites. The amount that the posterior teeth are moved mesially (the anchorage) can be graded: i.e., in Group A anchorage, for example, the posterior teeth are essentially stationary (i.e., moved between 0.0 and 0.5 mm). In Group B anchorage, the posterior teeth can be moved up to half the extraction site (i.e., < 3.5 mm) and, in Group C anchorage, the posterior teeth are moved more than half the extraction site (i.e., > 3.5 mm).

In a 15.5-year-old girl, it was decided to retract her lower incisors 2.0 mm to reduce her lower lip protrusion by the same amount. The lower arch form was constructed over the lower occlusogram tracing (Marcotte 1976) and, when the upper arch form was folded over the lower arch form, the upper arch form could likewise be drawn (Fig. 9.1). Starting at the treatment midline, the mesiodistal widths of the teeth can be placed on the arch form with a set of dividers. [See Box. 9.1 for definitions of the notations used.] In Figure 9.1, it is seen that arch length inadequacies were present in all quadrants: the upper right (−5.5 mm), the upper left (−4.0 mm), the lower left (−6.0 mm) and the lower right (−2.5 mm). These arch length inadequacies were solved by the removal of the upper right first premolar and the upper left primary second molar (the patient had a congenitally missing upper left second premolar) as well as the removal of the lower left first and lower right second premolars The anchorage in each quadrant could be graded: Upper right = Group B, Upper left = Group B, Lower left = Group B; and Lower right = Group C.

The manner of extraction site closure is based on the anchorage classification, i.e., rigid anchorage requirements exist in Group A anchorage, moderate anchorage requirements exist in Group B anchorage, and relaxed anchorage requirements exist in Group C anchorage.

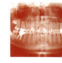

Closure of Extraction Sites with Group B Anchorage

The discussion of extraction site closure will begin with Group B anchorage, since it is more straightforward than either Group A or C anchorage. The upper arch will be used as an example, but exactly the same principles hold true for the lower arch. In Group B anchorage, approximately half the extraction site will be filled by

Box 9.1	Glossary of Notations and Abbreviations
C_{Res}	Center of resistance
C_{Rot}	Center of rotation
A	Upper arch–maxillary arch
/A	Lower arch–mandibular arch
BS	Upper buccal segment
/BS	Lower buccal segment
/SAS	Lower anterior segment
SAS/c T & E	Upper steel anterior segment with tubes and eyelets
NOP_U	The upper natural plane of occlusion; the plane of occlusion of the upper posterior teeth
NOP_L	The lower natural plane of occlusion; the plane of occlusion of the lower posterior teeth
A	Activation
IBD	Distance between the molar auxiliary tube and the crimpable crisscross tube
LA	Lingual arch
SAS	Steel anterior segment wire
SAW	Steel archwire
SBS	Steel buccal segment wire
T & E	Tubes and eyelets formed
TMA	Titanium–molybdenum alloy
TPA	Transpalatal arch
TTLRS	Titanium T-loop retraction spring

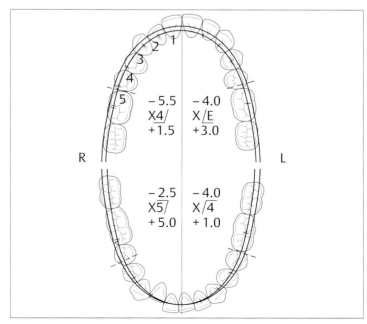

Fig. 9.1 An occlusogram tracing.

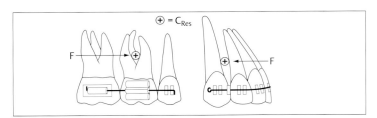

Fig. 9.2 For translation, a single force is needed through the Center of Resistance of each segment.

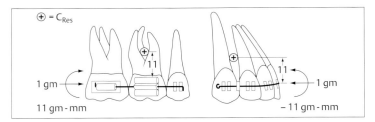

Fig. 9.3 For a single force at the C_{Res}, an equivalent force system must be placed at the level of the bracket.

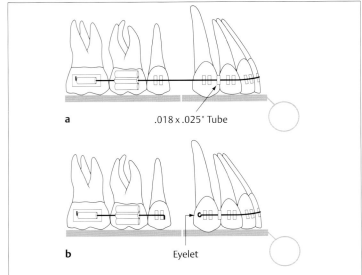

Fig. 9.5 Upper arch at end of the initial stage of treatment.
a 0.018 × 0.025 in. upper steel archwire (SAW) from 7–7. 0.018 in. × 025 in. crisscross tubes have been crimped onto the archwire between the canines and lateral incisors.
b 0.018 × 025 in. upper SAW has been cut into three wire segments: a right (SBS|) and a left (|SBS) and an SAS with T&E (tubes and eyelets).

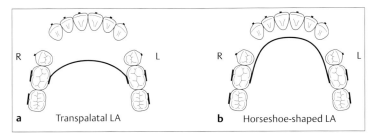

Fig. 9.4 Upper lingual arches (LA).
a Upper transpalatal arch.
b Horseshoe-shaped upper lingual arch.

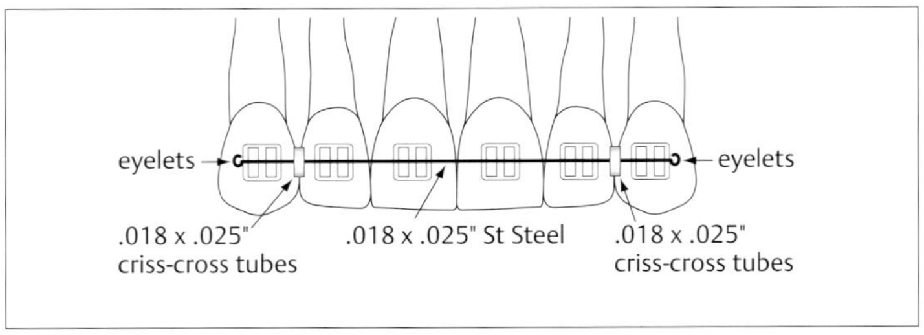

Fig. 9.6 Upper steel anterior segment with tubes and eyelets (SAS/c T&E).

anterior retraction and the remaining half will be filled by posterior protraction. Both anterior and posterior segments can usually be approximated by "translation" for this translation, a single force is needed through the center of resistance (C_{Res}) of the anterior and posterior segments (Fig. 9.2). Since forces and moments are applied at the bracket level, which is about 11 mm away from the C_{Res} of each segment, an equivalent force system at the bracket level must have a moment-to-force ratio (M/F) of 11/1 (Fig. 9.3).

Upper and lower 0.036 in. lingual arches (LA) should be in place before space closure begins (in the upper arch, either a transpalatal or a horseshoe-shaped lingual arch) (Fig. 9.4). These require horizontal lingual arch sheaths (ORMCO 673-3672) to be welded to the molar bands. One could also use the 0.032 in. × 0.032 in. precision lingual arches (available preformed), which also require precision lingual arch brackets (ORMCO 134-0001 [upper] and 134-0010 [lower]) to be welded to the molar bands.

At the end of the initial stage of treatment, the upper arch should look like Figure 9.5a, i.e., each segment of teeth should be consolidated. 0.018 in. × 0.025 in. crisscross tubes (ORMCO 624-1825) can be crimped onto the archwire between the cuspid and lateral incisors. The upper 0.018 in. × 0.025 in. steel archwire (SAW) can then be cut into three sections (Fig. 9.5b): a right and left steel buccal segment wire (SBS) connecting the second premolar, first and second molars and an anterior segment of wire (SAS) with tubes crimped and eyelets formed (T&E).

Eyelets are formed at the end of the anterior segment, flush-up against the distal of the canine bracket (Fig. 9.6). These eyelets serve to contain the canine-to-canine segment and also act as a "point restraint" if needed later during the process of root retraction.

The exact location of the titanium T-loop retraction spring (TTLRS; see below) in the distance between the crimpable vertical tube and the mesial of the molar auxiliary tube varies according to the anchorage classification. One can position the spring where the teeth are "to move the most." In Group A anchorage, for instance, the anterior teeth will be moved more than the posterior teeth. Thus, the TTLRS is best positioned closer to anterior teeth, i.e., in the "alpha" (α) position. In Group C anchorage, the posterior teeth will be moved more than the anterior teeth. Thus, the spring is best positioned close to the posterior teeth, in the "beta" (β) position. In Group B anchorage, the segments will be moved equally, so the spring is best placed midway between the two segments, in the "mu" (μ) position.

For extraction site closure by translation, a moment and a force are required to the anterior and posterior segments in a ratio of 11/1. A 0.017 in. × 0.025 in. titanium molybdenum alloy (TMA)

T-loop is also preactivated and will be positioned in the mu position. For this mu position, the length of the alpha leg [Lα] can be calculated by the formula: Lα = (IBD−A)/2, where IBD is the distance between the molar auxiliary tube and the crimpable crisscross tube and A is the activation (7 mm for 350 g).

Fabrication and Preactivation of the Titanium T-Loop Retraction Spring

0.017 in. × 0.025 in. TMA wire is used to fabricate the titanium T-loop retraction spring (TTLRS) approximately 10 mm long and 6 mm high. The beta leg is slid into the molar auxiliary tube and the alpha leg is bent 90° to fit into the crimped crisscross tube on the anterior segment of wire (Fig. 9.7a). As always, all bends are "overbent and adjusted by bending back." The loop-forming plier (Hu-Friedy 678–316) is especially well-suited for this procedure, because it consists of two round turrets: a graduated turret and an opposing turret (Fig. 9.7b). There are no rectangular edges present, so no sharp, easily-deformable bends can be produced. Six bends (actually, two sets of three identical bends) are made. The T-loop has two short vertical legs and two longer horizontal legs (Fig. 9.7c).

Bend #1: The opposing barrel of the loop-forming plier is placed into corner 1 of the passive TTLRS (Fig. 9.7c,d). The corner is "opened" until the short alpha leg is about 45° from its original position (Fig. 9.7d).

Bend #2: The opposing barrel of the plier is then placed into corner 2, and the pliers are again squeezed until the alpha leg is preactivated 90°. The spring can be placed on a tabletop to see that each leg has been preactivated about 45° (Fig. 9.7e,f).

Bend #3: With the smallest turret of the loop-forming plier held at the foot of the T-loop (position 3), finger pressure is used to bend the beta leg until it contacts the corner of the T-loop (Fig. 9.7g). The beta leg is then released and it will spring back slightly (Fig. 9.7h).

Bend #4: The same small turret is then placed at the other foot of the "T" (position 4) and, again with finger pressure, the beta leg is made to contact corner 2 (Fig. 9.7h). The alpha leg is released and springs back slightly (Fig. 9.7i).

Bend #5: On the beta leg, the smallest turret of the loop-forming plier is placed about 2 mm from the foot of the "T" (Fig. 9.7j). Using finger pressure, the beta leg is made to contact corner 1 and, once contact is made, heavy finger pressure is used to "overbend" the beta leg into corner 1. When released, the beta leg will still be in contact with corner 1 (Fig. 9.7k).

Bend #6: On the alpha leg, the smallest turret of the loop-forming plier is again placed about 2 mm from the foot of the "T" (position 6) and, again with heavy finger pressure, the alpha leg is "overbent" into corner 2. When released, the alpha leg will still be in contact with corner 2 (Fig. 9.7l). The short alpha leg will now be preactivated about 200–210°.

In summary: Bends #1 and #2 opened the corner of the T-loop (for about 90°). Bends #3 and #4 were done at the foot of the "T," essentially making each leg contact the corner of the T-loop, and then released (for about 135–140°). Bends #5 and #6 "overbent" each leg into the corner so that contact was maintained when the spring leg was released (the short alpha leg is now preactivated about 200–210° from its original position).

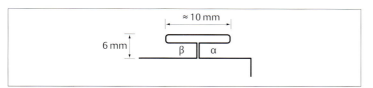

Fig. 9.7a **Fabrication and preactivation of the TTLRS. a Passive TTLRS (.017 × .025 in. TMA).** The short vertical legs should contact each other.

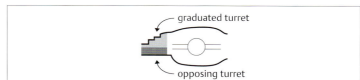

Fig. 9.7b **Loop-forming plier.** Two round turrets: a graduated turret and an opposing turret.

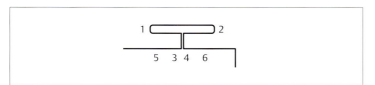

Fig. 9.7c Passive TTLRS with the location and sequence of the preactivation bends.

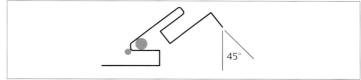

Fig. 9.7d The large barrel of the loop-forming plier is used to open position 1 so that the alpha leg is preactivated about 45°.

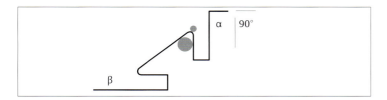

Fig. 9.7e **The large barrel opens position 2 another 45°.** The alpha leg is now about 90° from its original vertical position.

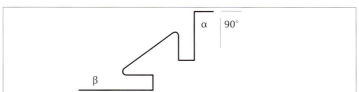

Fig. 9.7f **The spring should look like this with both alpha and beta legs preactivated about 45° for a total of about 90°.**

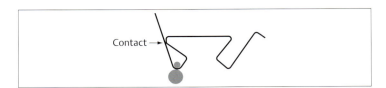

Fig. 9.7 g Position 3 is preactivated using the small turret. Contact is made and then released.

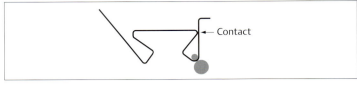

Fig. 9.7 h Position 4 is preactivated in the same manner. Contact made and released.

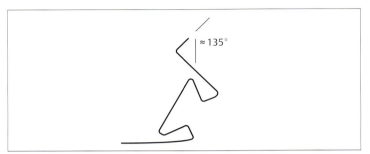

Fig. 9.7 i When placed on the beta leg, the alpha leg should show about 135–145° of preactivation with these four preactivation bends.

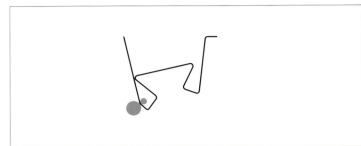

Fig. 9.7 j About 2 mm from the foot of the "T," the beta leg is overbent into the corner of the T-loop, wire contact is maintained after being released.

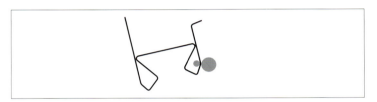

Fig. 9.7 k The same overbending is done on the alpha leg 2 mm from the foot of the "T", again wire contact is maintained after being released.

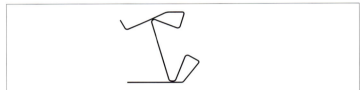

Fig. 9.7 l When released and placed on the beta leg, the alpha leg should show about 200–210° of preactivation.

The Trial Activation

A trial activation should be done on any orthodontic spring before it is placed into the mouth. The trial activation mimics the actual use of the spring, and one can see the activation remaining *after* the trial activation, for this is what is actually present to move the teeth. Experience and laboratory testing have shown that a 4000 gm-mm moment and a 350 g distal force can be used to approximate the B anchorage segments by translation (M/F ~ 11/1). With the 0.017 in. × 0.025 in. TTLRS, 180° of moment preactivation will produce about a 4000 gm-mm moment, and 7 mm of distal activation will produce about a 350 gm distal force.

For the trial activation, the legs of the preactivated TTLRS are grasped with flat-beaked pliers such as the Howe Pliers (Fig. 9.8 a a1). For this first part of the trial activation, only the activation moments are applied to the legs of the TTLRS. When the activation moments are placed, the short vertical legs of the TTLRS will be seen to cross 2 mm. This is called the neutral position of this TTLRS and is said to be –2 mm, minus because the short legs cross each other.

The second part of the trial activation is the distal activation (Fig. 9.8 a a2). For 350 g of force, the legs of the TTLRS will need to be separated 7 mm but, since the neutral position was –2 mm, the short legs of the TTLRS will be separated only 5 mm (7 – 2 = 5).

After the trial activation, the TTLRS is released. It will spring back to about 180° from the original vertical position (Fig. 9.8 b). This procedure can be done repeatedly, and it will always spring back the same amount. This moment preactivation (180°) and the 7 mm of distal activation will produce the necessary M/F ratio for translation. The neutral position can always be checked using two pairs of flat-beaked pliers, like the Howe pliers (Fig. 9.8 c).

After the trial activation, the beta leg of the spring is first slid into the molar auxiliary tube and the alpha leg can then be slid into the crisscross tube and cinched (Fig. 9.8 d).

The beta leg is pulled out of the molar auxiliary tube with a pair of straight Howe pliers until 5 mm is seen between the short vertical legs of the TTLRS. The beta leg is then "cinched," i.e., bent gingivally and cut with the distal end cutters (Fig. 9.8 e). Space closure can be monitored by measuring the distance between the short vertical legs of the TTLRS (Fig. 9.8 f). Ideally, about 1–1.5 mm occurs monthly and, after 2–3 mm of space closure has occurred, the TTLRS can be reactivated until there is again 5 mm between its short vertical legs (Fig. 9.8 g). If necessary, further reactivation can be done on the alpha leg to regain the 5 mm between the TTLRS's short vertical legs.

During the entire space closing procedure, a mirror handle can be used to monitor the translation (Fig. 9.8 h). The segments should be seen to approximate each other without any tipping, and the cusp tips should be in the same relationship as when the procedure commenced (Fig. 9.5 b).

Space closure by translation is graphically summarized in Figure 9.9.

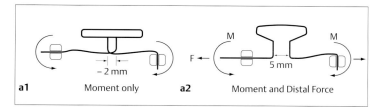

Fig. 9.8 a 1 Howe pliers grasping the legs of the TTLRS. The Neutral Position.
2 The Trial Activation: Moments and Distal Force

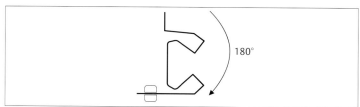

Fig. 9.8 b After trial activation, the alpha leg is released: 180° of moment pre-activation should remain.

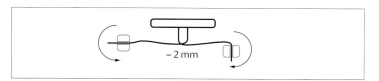

Fig. 9.8 c Two Howe pliers are used to check the neutral position.

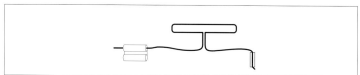

Fig. 9.8 d The TTLRS is now placed into the tubes. First into the molar auxiliary tube and then into the soldered or crimped tube.

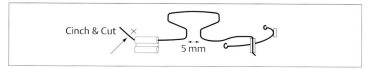

Fig. 9.8 e A 7 mm activation is made by cinching distally.

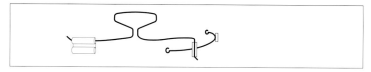

Fig. 9.8 f Space closure is ideally about 1–1.5 mm per month. After about eight weeks, 2–3 mm of space closure should have occurred, and the spring can be reactivated.

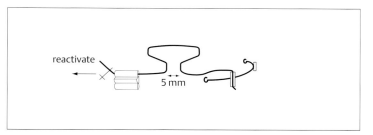

Fig. 9.8 g The TTLRS can be reactivated. To reactivate, cinch distally to regain 7 mm (5 mm between the vertical legs). The next reactivation can be made intra-orally on the alpha leg in order to maintain the μ position of the TTLRS.

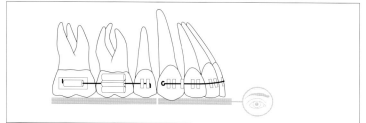

Fig. 9.8 h Space closure is completed by translation. All during the translation, the anterior segment should ideally remain on the Natural Plane of Occlusion (NOP).

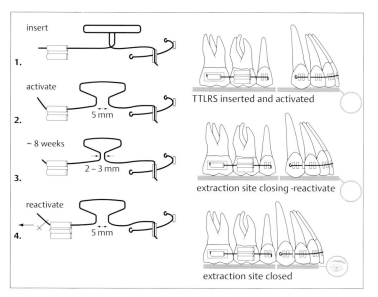

Fig. 9.9 **Summary of translation.**

Extraction Site Closure with Group A Anchorage

In Group A anchorage, the buccal segments are essentially "ankylosed"(stationary), i.e., moved mesially between 0.0 and 0.5 mm. There are two possible scenarios that need to be considered: patients who will provide good headgear cooperation and patients who will *not*.

First Scenario: Patients Who Will Provide Good Headgear Cooperation

One-stage extraction site closure will be done, i.e., the translation of the anterior teeth and the pull of the headgear being distal through the C_{Res} of the upper jaw. In Group A anchorage, little or no slippage of the posterior teeth (0.0–0.5 mm) is desired, and the extraction sites are closed by distal translation of the anterior teeth. Translation will again be done using the 0.017 in. × 0.025 in. TTLRS (Fig. 9.10) preactivated with 180° of moment preactivation and 7 mm of distal activation (Fig. 9.11) and placed midway between the molar auxiliary tube and the crisscross tube on the anterior segment (Fig. 9.12).

The anteroposterior (AP) position of the anchorage will be maintained by the use of a distal headgear pull, through the C_{Res} of the upper jaw (as with an Interlandi or Combination type of headgear) (Fig. 9.13).

Location of the C_{Res} of the Upper Arch

To ensure that there is no change (steepening or flattening of the occlusal plane), the distal pull of the combination headgear should be through the C_{Res} of the maxilla. One might reasonably ask, "Where is this C_{Res}?" The location of the C_{Res} depends on two factors: the number of teeth within the segment and/or the number of teeth in the arch. With the teeth aligned in the pre-retraction stage and a continuous arch wire cinched from the second molar to the second molar (Fig. 9.5a), a combination headgear can be placed with the distal pull being about 5 mm superior to the roots of the upper molar teeth. The overbite is carefully measured, e.g., "Upper incisal edges are at the level of the lower incisor bracket slot."

At the next appointment, assuming that the patient has been cooperative in his or her headgear use (one can check the color and appearance of the neck strap, the appearance of the hair, contiguous skin, mobility of the teeth, etc.), the orthodontist can again examine the overbite relationship. If the pull is below the C_{Res} of the maxilla and the upper incisal edges are inferior to the lower bracket slot, the present distal pull of the headgear is inferior to the C_{Res} and needs to be raised. If the incisal edges of the upper incisors are superior to the lower bracket slots, the distal pull of the headgear is superior to the C_{Res} of the maxilla and needs to be lowered. Obviously, if the overbite is exactly the same as it was at the last appointment, then the distal pull is through the C_{Res}.

Of course, if the treatment occlusal plane is to be flatter than the cant of the original occlusal plane, the distal pull of the Combee headgear must be superior to the C_{Res} of the upper jaw. The opposite is true if the treatment occlusal plane is to be steeper than the cant of the original occlusal plane, i.e., the distal pull of the Combee headgear should be below the C_{Res} of the upper jaw.

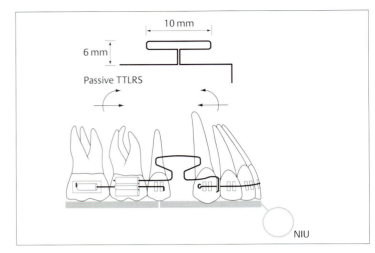

Fig. 9.10   .017 × .025 in. TMA T-loop retraction spring (TTLRS).

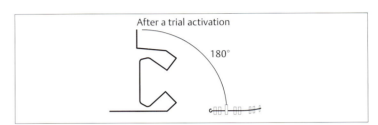

Fig. 9.11   After a trial activation, 180° of moment preactivation should still remain in the TTLRS.

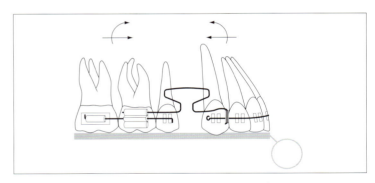

Fig. 9.12   TTLRS placed in the mu position and activated.

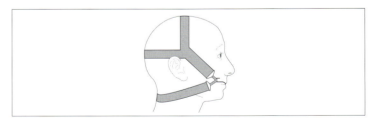

Fig. 9.13   Combination-type headgear with the pull distal through the C_{Res} of the maxilla.

With the corrections made, the overbite is again recorded in detail, and the patient is allowed to use the headgear for another appointment. The overbite relationship is examined again at the next appointment to confirm where the distal pull is in relation to the C_{Res} of the maxilla.

As with segmental translation, the TTLRS should be reactivated every 2–3 mm of space closure by cinching distally out of the molar auxiliary tube (Fig. 9.**14**). A mirror handle can be used to monitor the space closure; i.e., to check that the anterior segment is being translated on the natural plane of occlusion (Fig. 9.**15**). With the distal pull of the headgear being through the C_{Res} of the maxilla, there should not be any change in the cant of the natural plane of occlusion. The extraction site should close at about 1–1.5 mm per month.

Second Scenario: Patients Who Will Not Provide Good Headgear Cooperation

In the second scenario, where no headgear cooperation can be anticipated, anchorage preservation is accomplished by resolving the retraction procedure into two separate procedures: a first-stage of en-masse, controlled tipping of the anterior teeth, and a second stage of en-masse root retraction of these same teeth. Success with this procedure hinges on the distal force in both procedures remaining at 300 g or less.

In the first stage of this two-stage procedure, the anterior teeth are tipped distally with a center of rotation (C_{Rot}) at the apices of the incisors. In the second stage, the roots are uprighted with a C_{Rot} at the incisal edge (or brackets) of the incisors.

First Stage: Controlled Tipping of the Six Anterior Teeth

Either a 0.036 in. transpalatal lingual or a horseshoe-shaped upper lingual arch is required for this procedure (Fig. 9.**16a**). The lingual arch does not influence the AP anchorage, only the rotational integrity of the buccal teeth. At the end of the initial stage of treatment, a mirror handle is placed across the level of the natural plane of occlusion (Fig. 9.**16b**). The segments should be level. A 0.017 × 0.025 in. TTLRS is placed in the alpha position (closer to the crisscross vertical tube). The short alpha leg is bent right under the anterior corner of the TTLRS. Only a 45° beta preactivation bend is placed (Fig. 9.**16c**).

There are no preactivation bends made on the T-loop itself. The spring will be used passively, and the activation moment that develops as the spring is activated provides a M/F ratio of about 8/1 anteriorly. The 45° beta bend provides a M/F ratio of about 11/1 posteriorly (Fig. 9.**16d**). Since the load–deflection rate of the TTLRS is about 50 g/mm, 5 mm of distal activation will provide a distal force of about 250 g. Controlled tipping of the anterior segment will be pitted against the translation of the posterior segment; i.e., the controlled tipping distally should be completed before the posterior teeth are significantly translated mesially. With the C_{Rot} being at the incisor apices, the canines are seen to lift up off the monitoring mirror handle (Fig. 9.**16e,f**) while the incisal

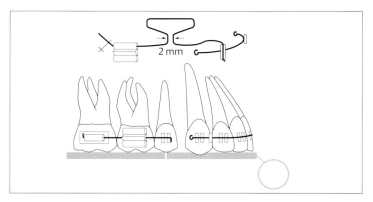

Fig. 9.**14** The TTLRS should be reactivated every 2–3 mm of closure by cinching out of the auxiliary tube.

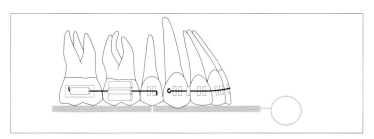

Fig. 9.**15** The anterior segment should translate distally along the plane of occlusion. A mirror handle can be used to monitor the translation.

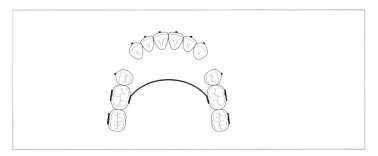

Fig. 9.**16a** Controlled tipping of the six anterior teeth.

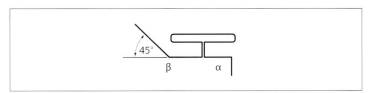

Fig. 9.**16c** Preactivated .017 × .025 in. TTLRS in the alpha position with only a beta preactivation (45°).

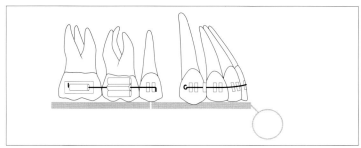

Fig. 9.**16b** .018 × .025 in. steel anterior and buccal segments. Upper anterior segment is level with the Natural Plane of Occlusion.

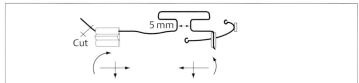

Fig. 9.**16d** TTLRS activated 5 mm for 250 g distal activation.

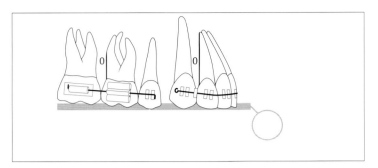

Fig. 9.**16e** Anterior segment is seen to tip distally, canines lifting up slightly.

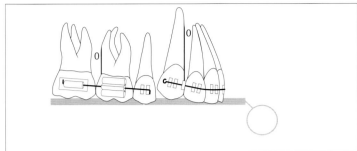

Fig. 9.**16f** Note position of incisal edges on NOP. The canines are up, off the NOP. Note space distal to the canine.

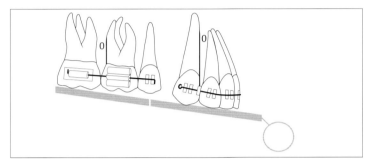

Fig. 9.**16g** Anterior segment dropping below the NOP.

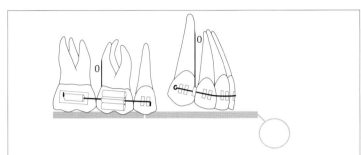

Fig. 9.**16h** Upper anterior segment lifting up off the NOP.

edges stay in contact with the mirror handle. The extraction site should not be completely closed. Rather, about 0.5–1.0 mm is left so that the canines can be brought down during the stage of root retraction (Fig. 9.**15**).

If the incisal edges of the incisors are dropping below the NOP_U (Fig. 9.**16g**), the beta bend must be increased. If the incisors are lifting up off the NOP_U (Fig. 9.**16h**), the beta bend must be decreased.

Thus, the beta bend is adjusted so that the incisors stay on the NOP_U during the retraction procedure. Research has shown that this two-stage retraction procedure maintains the anchorage if the mesial force is kept below 300 g; the tendency for protraction of the buccal teeth is significantly reduced.

Second Stage: En-Masse Root Retraction

Root retraction should commence when the space is almost closed, i.e., with about 0.5–1.0 mm remaining (Fig. 9.**17a**), just to ensure that the distal cusp of the canine is not caught under the mesial cusp of the second premolar (Fig. 9.**17b**). The C_{Rot} during this stage of root retraction of the anterior teeth is the incisal edges or brackets of the incisal teeth. A heavy ligature tie (0.012 in. or, if unavailable, two strands of 0.009 in. wound together) is needed to prevent the crowns of the anterior teeth from flaring forward during the root retraction procedure. This heavy ligature tie can be "figure-eight" tied from the second molar, first molar, and second premolar and twisted forward to the eyelet of the anterior segment or to the vertical tube on the anterior segment (Fig. 9.**17c**). This tie-back should not be made excessively firm for fear of catching the distal cusp of the canine below the mesial cusp of the second premolar (Fig. 9.**17b**).

The force system required to produce a C_{Rot} at the incisal edges or brackets of the anterior segment is shown in Figure 9.**17d**. Specifically, the alpha moment must be greater than the beta moment. This results in an eruptive force on the anterior segment which, together with the alpha moment, produces a C_{Rot} at the incisal edges or brackets of the anterior teeth. When a mirror handle can be held contacting the incisal edges of the incisors and the cusp tips of the second bicuspids with the canines slightly below the mirror handle, root movement is complete (Fig. 9.**17e**).

Fabrication and Preactivation of the Double Helix Spring

The opposing beak of the loop-forming plier is used to form the helices of the double helix spring. One-and-a-half helices are used for both the anterior (alpha) and posterior (beta) helices. For patient comfort, as one proceeds anteriorly from the molar auxiliary tube, the spring is wound toward the buccal. At the alpha position, the spring is then wound toward the lingual (Fig. 9.**18c**). The spring is first made passively (Fig. 9.**18a–c**). The opposing beak of the loop-forming plier can then be used to preactivate the helices (Fig. 9.**18d**). As always, the preactivation bends are "overbent" and adjusted by bending back (Fig. 9.**18e**).

Assume, for example, that both helices are preactivated 45° (Fig. 9.**19a**). As both helices are activated, the wire between the helices takes the form of a segment of a circle (Fig. 9.**19b**). The fact that the wire takes the form of a segment of a circle when moments are placed is due to its elastic properties. The farther apart the helices and/or the more elastic the wire, the greater this curvature will be. Relative to the bracket or tube, this wire curvature reduces the activation to each helix and so the curvature must be removed. It can be removed by placing a "compensatory bend" or "reverse curve" between the helices (Fig. 9.**19c**) so that, when the helices are fully activated, the wire section between the helices

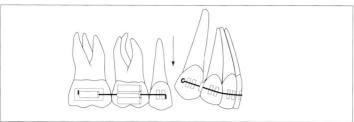

Fig. 9.**17a** En-masse root retraction.

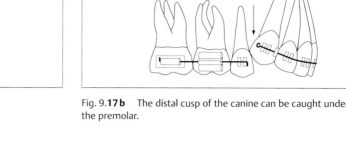

Fig. 9.**17b** The distal cusp of the canine can be caught under the mesial cusp of the premolar.

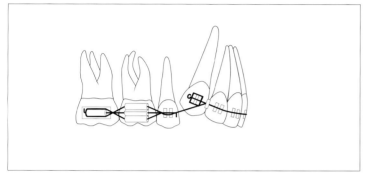

Fig. 9.**17c** The buccal segment of teeth is "figure-eight" tied and the tie is extended to the vertical tube of the anterior segment.

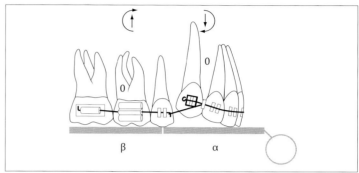

Fig. 9.**17d** A C_{Rot} at the incisal edge or brackets of the incisors requires an alpha moment greater than the beta moment.

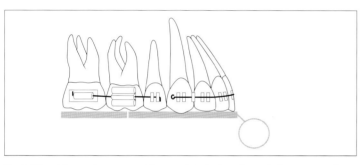

Fig. 9.**17e** The root movement is completed when the anterior segment is on the NOP.

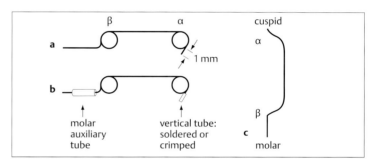

Fig. 9.**18a–c** .018 × .025 in. passive stainless-steel double helix spring.
a Upper right double helix spring.
b Lateral view of the double helix spring. Helices are formed with opposing beak of the loop-forming plier.
c Upper right root spring viewed from above.

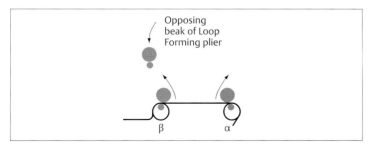

Fig. 9.**18d** The opposing beak of the loop-forming plier is also used to preactivate the helices.

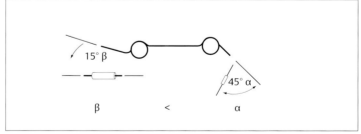

Fig. 9.**18e** Preactivation bends: alpha helix = 45°, beta helix = 15°.

will be "noncurved" or straight (Fig. 9.**19d**). Since, however, the beta helix will be preactivated with only 15° (Fig. 9.**19e**), the beta section of wire between the helices can receive less anticurvature bend (Fig. 9.**19f**) than the alpha section.

With α = 45° and β = 15°, the activation force system is diagrammed as in Fig. 9.**20a**, and the deactivation force system as in Figure 09.**20b** (equal and opposite). This force system will produce a C_{Rot} at the incisal edges or brackets of the anterior teeth.

Root movement is continued until it looks as though a straight wire can be placed from second molar to second molar (Fig. 9.**21**).

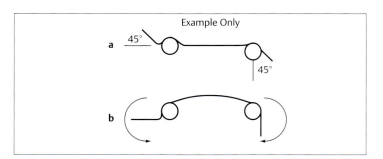

Fig. 9.**19 a, b** Double helix spring preactivated with 45° at the alpha and beta helices.

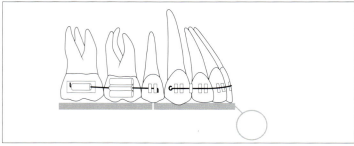

Fig. 9.**21** Root movement is complete when a straight wire can be placed 7–7.

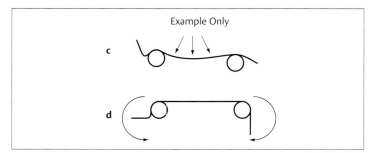

Fig. 9.**19 c, d** Compensation curves are necessary.
c A compensation curve placed.
d When the helices are activated, the section of wire between the helices is straight.

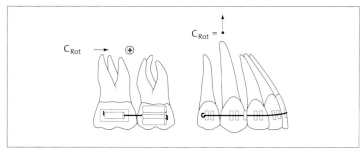

Fig. 9.**22** Desired C_{Rot}. Anterior segment: translation. Buccal segment: controlled tipping.

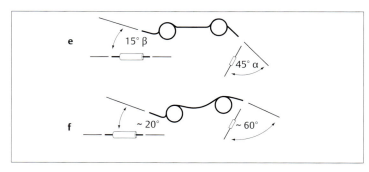

Fig. 9.**19 e, f**   α > β preactivation bends.
e 45° alpha and 15° beta preactivation bend is needed.
f More compensation curve placed in the alpha section than in the beta section.

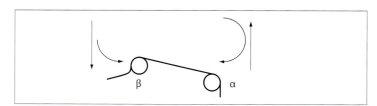

Fig. 9.**20 a**   Activation force system: α > β.

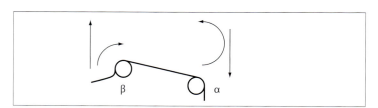

Fig. 9.**20 b**   Deactivation force system. "High alphas always erupt."

Closure of Extraction Sites with Group C Anchorage

When buccal segment protraction is needed, Group C mechanics are employed. In Group C anchorage situations, extraction of the second bicuspids is preferred over extraction of the first bicuspids. This alone helps with buccal segment protraction, as it is much easier to protract two molars than two molars and one premolar. The objective is, then, to protract the buccal segment of teeth more than half the extraction site while maintaining the position of the anterior segment of teeth. The rationale is that an eight-tooth anterior segment (first premolar to first premolar) can be made to translate, while the two two-tooth posterior segments can be made, first, to tip about their apices (controlled tipping) and, second, to undergo root uprighting (Fig. 9.**22**).

The necessary M/F ratio delivered to the anterior teeth is 11/1 (for translation), while, on the posterior teeth, it is 8/1 (for controlled tipping) (Fig. 9.**23 a**). Because the alpha moment is greater than the beta moment, vertical forces exist for equilibrium (Fig. 9.**23 b**). The eruptive force on the anterior segment is spread out over eight teeth while the intrusive force on the buccal segment places the center of rotation at the apices of the first and second molars.

The appliance of choice is the 0.017 in. × 0.025 in. titanium T-loop retraction spring (TTLRS), which will be placed in the beta position (5 mm anterior to the molar auxiliary tube). The TTLRS will first be made to fit passively (Fig. 9.**24 a**) in the molar auxiliary tube and the crisscross tube crimped onto the anterior segment of wire. A 45° preactivation bend is placed in the alpha leg (Fig. 9.**24 b**). When activated, the passive TTLRS to the molar segment will deliver a force system with a M/F ratio of 8/1 (controlled tipping). When activated, the preactivated alpha leg of the TTLRS

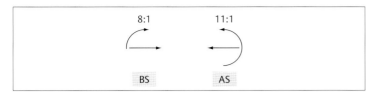

Fig. 9.23 a Necessary moment/force ratios for buccal protraction.

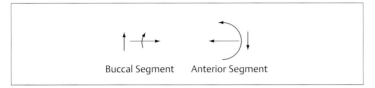

Fig. 9.23 b Equilibrium diagram.

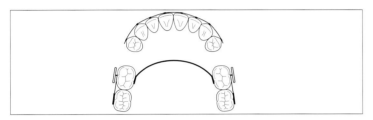

Fig. 9.25 a Controlled tipping of the buccal segments.

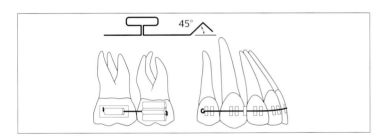

Fig. 9.25 c Preactivated .017 × .025 in. TTLRS positioned in the beta position with only a 45° alpha preactivation bend.

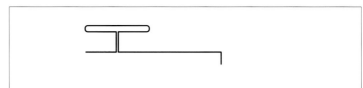

Fig. 9.24 a Appliance of choice: .017 × .025 in. TTLRS.

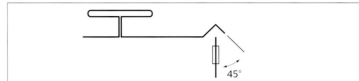

Fig. 9.24 b 45° alpha preactivation bend.

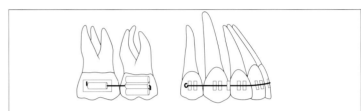

Fig. 9.25 b .018 × .025 in. steel buccal-segment wire and steel anterior-segment wire with tubes and eyelets.

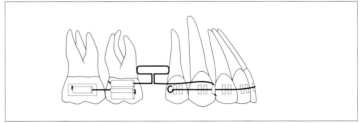

Fig. 9.25 d **The preactivated TTLRS is placed into the molar tube first and then into the crimpable vertical tube.** The TTLRS gives about a 1500 g-mm activation moment, with 4–5 mm of distal activation.

will deliver a force system with a M/F ratio of 11/1 (for translation) to the anterior segment of teeth.

First Stage: Controlled Tipping

A upper transpalatal lingual arch is placed into the lingual sheaths of the permanent first molars (Fig. 9.25 a) to control the widths of the buccal segments of teeth during their protraction. As the segments are protracted, they will come to occupy a narrower position on the arch form so the intermolar widths must be constricted with this transpalatal lingual arch. 0.018 in. × 0.025 in. stainless-steel wire segments are placed posteriorly between the first and second molars and anteriorly from the first premolar around to the other first premolar (Fig. 9.25 b). 0.018 × 0.025 in. tubes (ORMCO 624-1825) are crimped onto the anterior segment of wire between the canine and lateral incisor brackets. The alpha leg of the TTLRS is held over the vertical tube until the T-loop is 5 mm anterior to the molar auxiliary tube. The position of the vertical tube is marked on the alpha leg, and the vertical leg is bent at this position.

The alpha leg of the TTLRS is then preactivated with a 45° bend (Fig. 9.25 c); TTLRS is inserted into the molar auxiliary tube (Fig. 9.25 d), and the alpha leg is inserted into the vertical tube and cinched (Fig. 9.25 e, f). The TTLRS is activated by cinching the spring distally out of the molar auxiliary tube until 4–5 mm exists between the vertical legs of the TTLRS (~ 200 g) (Fig. 9.25 g).

Class III elastics can also be used as desired. Once the extraction site has closed 2–3 mm, the TTLRS can be reactivated either distally out of the molar auxiliary tube or anteriorly in the alpha position. If the TTLRS is reactivated in the alpha position, the alpha leg must be uncrimped and removed from the vertical tube. It is then straightened, and a mark is made 4 mm distal from the vertical tube. The new alpha leg can be formed at this mark.

One will see that the mesiobuccal cusp of the permanent first molar will start to lift up off the plane of occlusion (mirror handle) (Fig. 9.25 h). 1–2 mm of the extraction site will be closed, and one will notice further elevation of the mesiobuccal cusp of the permanent first molar as the extraction site closes (Fig. 9.25 i). The distal cusp of the second molar should remain on the plane of occlusion (mirror handle) during this retraction.

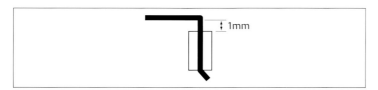

Fig. 9.25e Allow about 1 mm between the horizontal part of the T-loop and the edge of the tube to facilitate its removal.

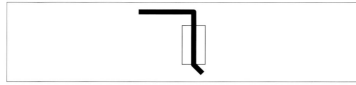

Fig. 9.25f With a green stone in the handpiece, ensure that all cut edges are smoothed.

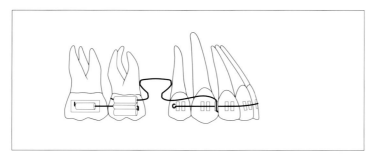

Fig. 9.25g Activation of the TTLRS.

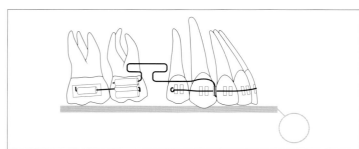

Fig. 9.25h Early buccal segment protraction.

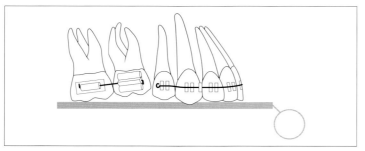

Fig. 9.25i Controlled tipping of buccal segments completed.

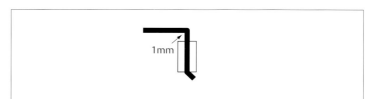

Fig. 9.25j 1 mm space is needed.

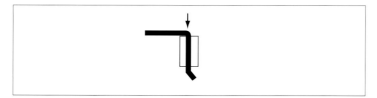

Fig. 9.25k Free end sticks out ~ 1 mm.

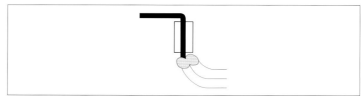

Fig. 9.25l Free end is straightened.

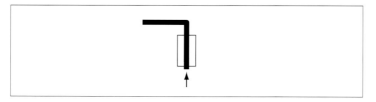

Fig. 9.25m The free end can now be pushed/pulled out of the vertical tube.

The buccal segment of teeth continues to protract, rotating about its apices. When the distance between the vertical legs of the TTLRS has decreased 2–3 mm, reactivation is necessary (Fig. 9.25h). This can be done by using a band pusher to push the alpha leg down in the vertical tube until the free end is sticking out about a millimeter (Fig. 9.25j, k). Using flat-beaked pliers, like the Howe pliers, the bent end is straightened (Fig. 9.25l) so that it can be pushed or pulled out of the vertical tube (Fig. 9.25m).

Intraoral Reactivation of TTLRS

When the alpha leg is out of the vertical tube, it can be straightened out by using the loop-forming plier and finger pressure to remove the 45° bend in the wire (Fig. 9.26a). Then the 90° bend for the alpha leg is "unbent" in the same manner (Fig. 9.26b).

The alpha leg of the TTLRS looks like Figure 9.26c. A mark is placed 4 mm distal to the vertical tube, and a 90° bend can be made at that mark using a small, round beak of the loop-forming plier (Fig. 9.26d).

Again using the opposing turret of the loop-forming plier (for a large-diameter bend), the alpha leg can be preactivated approximately 45° (Fig. 9.26e). The TTLRS is re-activated when placing the alpha leg back into the crimpable vertical tube and cinched (Fig. 9.26f).

Class III elastics can be used on the buccal segments in the upper jaw (Class II elastics if in the lower jaw) to increase the mesial

Second Stage: Uprighting Buccal Segment

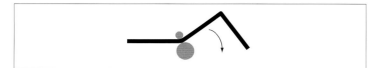

Fig. 9.**26 a** Intraoral reactivation of TTLRS.

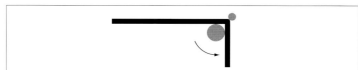

Fig. 9.**26 b** 90° alpha bend is also "unbent."

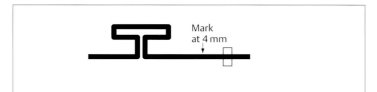

Fig. 9.**26 c** The alpha leg is marked.

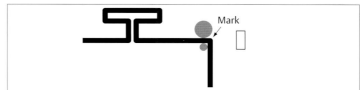

Fig. 9.**26 d** 90° bend is made at the mark.

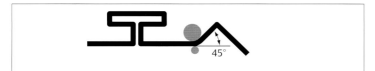

Fig. 9.**26 e** Alpha leg is preactivated ~ 45°.

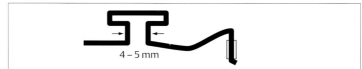

Fig. 9.**26 f** The alpha leg is re-inserted into the vertical tube and cinched.

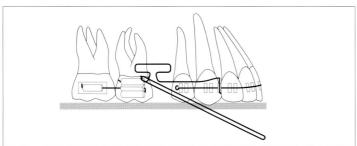

Fig. 9.**26 g** Intermaxillary elastics, if needed.

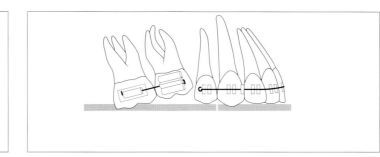

Fig. 9.**26 h** Possible problem: increasing mesial force to the buccal segments.

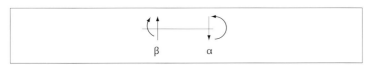

Fig. 9.**26 i** By increasing the alpha moment, one can increase the intrusive force to the posterior teeth.

force for buccal protraction (Fig. 9.**26 g**). Sometimes, the distobuccal cusp tip of the upper second molar falls below the plane of occlusion and a prematurity develops (Fig. 9.**26 h**) with subsequent potential TMJ pain and dysfunction. Of course, this happens only on Saturday nights, just before the theater. In this case, the alpha leg must be removed, and the alpha moment preactivation bend must be increased to increase the intrusive force to the posterior teeth (Fig. 9.**26 i**), just the opposite of what one might naturally think.

While the buccal teeth are tipping about their apices, the extraction site should not be closed completely. About 0.5 mm of the extraction site should left open, which will allow the mesial aspect of the first molar to descend during the stage of root uprighting (Fig. 9.**26 h**).

Second Stage: Uprighting Buccal Segment

One will need:
1. 0.018 in. × 0.025 in. SAS with T&E tied in (SAS usually from 4–4) (Fig. 9.**27 a**)
2. 0.0018 in. × 025 in. SBS (Fig. 9.**27 b**)
3. A heavy (> 0.012 in.) ligature tie from the buccal segment (molar hook) to the eyelet of the SAS
4. A passive 0.018 in. × 0.025 in. stainless-steel double helix spring

After the posterior teeth have been protracted by controlled tipping, the teeth must undergo root uprighting (Fig. 9.**28 a,b**). The necessary force system is a crown distal–root mesial moment (positive) and an eruptive force for a C_{Rot} at the distal marginal ridge of the second molar. In order to prevent the segment from moving distally, a mesial force is also necessary. The equilibrium diagram of this force system is seen in Fig. 9.**28 c**. This force system can be delivered by an 0.018 × 0.025 in. stainless steel double helix spring (Fig. 9.**28 d,e**) with a heavy ligature tie (0.012 in.) providing the necessary mesial force (Fig. 9.**28 f**). The double helix spring fits into the molar auxiliary tube and the crisscross vertical tube crimped onto the 0.018 in. × 0.025 in. steel anterior segment (Fig. 9.**28 g**). The double helix spring receives an asymmetric pre-

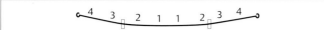

Fig. 9.27a 18 × 25 SAS from 4–4 with T&E.

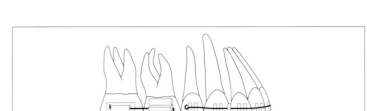

Fig. 9.27b 18 × 25 SBS from 6–7.

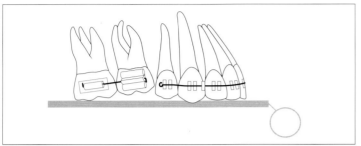

Fig. 9.28a Uprighting buccal segment. Posterior segment mesially tipped.

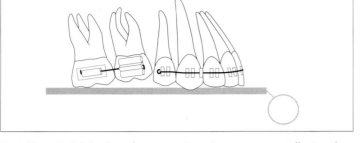

Fig. 9.28b Posterior segment uprighted.

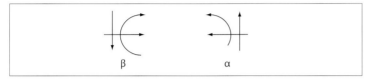

Fig. 9.28c Equilibrium diagram for uprighting posterior teeth in (a).

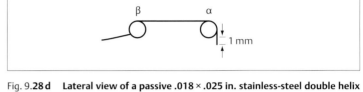

Fig. 9.28d Lateral view of a passive .018 × .025 in. stainless-steel double helix spring.

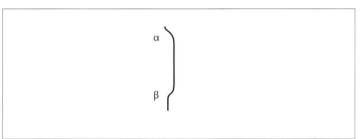

Fig. 9.28e Looking down on a .018 × .025 in. stainless-steel double helix spring for the upper right side.

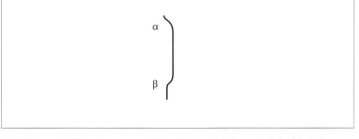

Fig. 9.28f Mesially-tipped buccal segments tied with a double strand of ligature wire (at arrow) to the eyelet of the anterior segment.

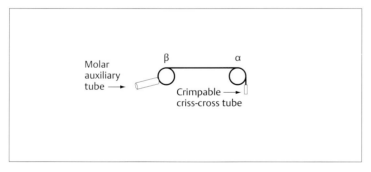

Fig. 9.28g Double helix spring inserted passively into the molar auxiliary tube and into the soldered vertical tube.

Fig. 9.28h Preactivation bends. Each helix is bent against the large turret.

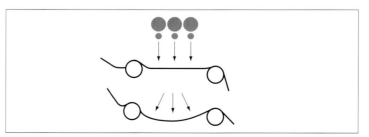

Fig. 9.28i Beta anticurvature is greater than alpha anticurvature.

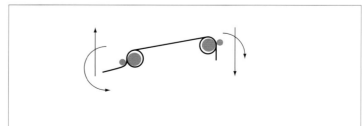

Fig. 9.28j An activation force system is placed. The center portion is straight, i.e., β is 45° and α is 15°.

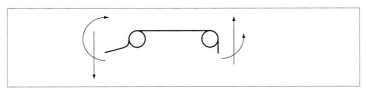

Fig. 9.**28k** Deactivation force system. High β intrudes anteriors and extrudes posteriors.

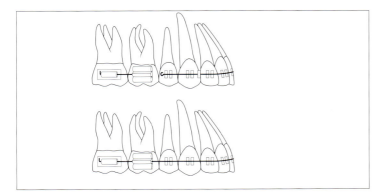

Fig. 9.**28 l, m** Wire segments are replaced with a straight, continuous archwire from second molar around to second molar.
l Posterior segment is uprighted. Wire segments are still in place.
m Wire segments have been replaced with a continuous wire.

activation: a high beta–low alpha or about a 45° beta preactivation and a 15° alpha preactivation (Fig. 9.**28h**).

Anticurvature bends are also placed in the straight wire portion between the helices to negate the curvature of the wire due to the activation of the helices. More curvature is placed in the beta section than in the alpha section (Fig. 9.**27i**). Typically, when beta is greater than alpha or when alpha is greater than beta, 45° and 15° are used. So, here, β = 45° and α = 15°.

When sufficient anticurvature bends are placed, the wire section between the helices is seen to be straight during activation of the helices (Fig. 9.**28j**). One can now have confidence that, indeed, 45° of beta activation and 15° of alpha activation are being delivered. The activation force system will produce an eruptive tendency in the alpha position and an intrusive tendency in the beta position (Fig. 9.**28j**). In the deactivation force system, just the reverse is seen: the alpha position tends to intrude while the beta position tends to extrude (Fig. 9.**28k**).

Once the segment has been uprighted (Fig. 9.**28l**), a continuous wire can be placed from second molar to second molar (Fig. 9.**28m**) and finishing procedures can be initiated; i.e., small tooth-to-tooth adjustments.

Asymmetric Space Closure

Most instances of extraction therapy involve symmetrical extractions: i.e., first premolars or second premolars. Sometimes, however, an extraction will be required on only one side, and the extraction site must be closed according to the same requirements as before. When the anchorage must be maintained, Group A mechanics are employed. When the anchorage must be displaced mesially as much as the anterior segment must be retracted, Group B mechanics can be employed. When the anchorage must be displaced mesially more than anterior segment needs to be displaced distally, Group C mechanics can be employed. The only caveat in all instances is that the lingual arch cannot be used, and antirotation twists must be placed into the TTLRS.

In Group B anchorage, the extraction site will be closed by equal retraction of the anterior teeth and protraction of the posterior teeth. In the example given in Figure 9.**29**, an upper right first premolar was removed for orthodontic treatment (Fig. 9.**29a**). Since the extraction site was to be closed by equal retraction of the anterior teeth as well as protraction of the posterior teeth, the left anterior segment must be allowed to rotate in the first-order plane. Allowances for this rotation were made by connecting the upper left anterior segment to the upper left buccal segment with a ligature tie (Fig. 9.**29b**).

Since in Group B anchorage, the TTLRS is positioned midway in the extraction site, the first-order anti-rotation bends will be symmetrical in both the alpha and beta positions. After the trial activation (Fig. 9.**29c**), two pairs of flat-beaked pliers (e.g., Howe pliers) are used to twist the short vertical legs of the TTLRS. Each leg is grasped in the corner, and 80–85° of torsional twists are placed in the full length of each vertical leg (Fig. 9.**29d**). As usual, the "twists" are overtorqued and adjusted by "torquing back." Looking down on the upper right TTLRS after the first-order anti-rotational "twists" are placed, the TTLRS will look like the one shown in Figure 9.**29e**. The body of the upper right T-loop will next be made slightly concave lingually by using a three-prong plier (Fig. 9.**29f**) and will look like Figure 9.**29g**.

For patient comfort, a cotton roll is can be placed in the mucobuccal fold during insertion of the preactivated TTLRS. The beta leg is first inserted into the molar auxiliary tube, and the alpha leg can then be placed on the cotton roll temporarily. The alpha leg is then rotated around and placed into the crisscross tube on the anterior segment and cinched. The beta leg is then extended out of the molar auxiliary tube until 5 mm exists between the vertical legs of the TTLRS and is cinched in this position (Fig. 9.**29h**). In the first-order plane, the antirotation moments will prevent the molar segment from rotating mesial in and the anterior segment from rotating distal in (Fig. 9.**29i**). The first reactivation occurs after the space has closed by 2–3 mm. This is usually done by extending the beta leg out of the molar auxiliary tube until 5 mm exists between the vertical legs of the TTLRS. A subsequent reactivation may have to be done in the alpha position in order to maintain the mu position of the TTLRS. The alpha leg is uncinched and removed from the crisscross tube. The 90° bend is removed and, 2–3 mm distal to the crisscross tube, a mark is placed on the wire. The 90° bend is made at this mark and the alpha leg is re-inserted with 5 mm between the vertical legs of the TTLRS.

When the buccal segment must be protracted more than half the extraction site (Group C anchorage), the TTLRS is positioned in the beta position. When this is done unilaterally, some problems may be experienced with the buccolingual position of the buccal segment as it is protracted. Hence, extraction site closure that follows translation is often used, and an intermaxillary elastic is used to augment the distal force of the TTLRS. This means that the TTLRS would be placed in the mu position with 180° of anti-rotation moment, and a Class III elastic would be used to augment the buccal protraction.

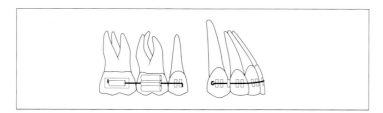

Fig. 9.**29** Asymmetric space closure in group B anchorage.
a Group B anchorage in a unilateral extraction sight (upper right).

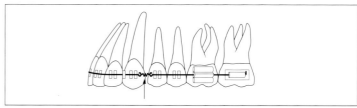

Fig. 9.**29 b** Two eyelets on the proximal ends of each segment are connected with a heavy ligature tie.

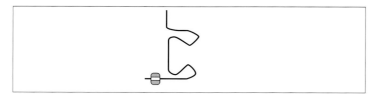

Fig. 9.**29 c** The TTLRS preactivated 180° for translation.

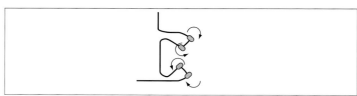

Fig. 9.**29 d** The two pairs of flat-beaked pliers are used to "twist" the vertical legs of the TTLRS.

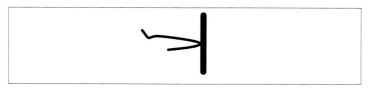

Fig. 9.**29 e** With ~ 170° of antirotational twist, the TTLRS will look like this.

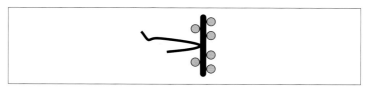

Fig. 9.**29 f** The body of the TTLRS is made slightly concave lingually with a three-prong plier.

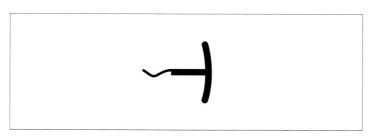

Fig. 9.**29 g** The upper right TTLRS preactivated with antirotational bends and twists for unilateral space closure (translation).

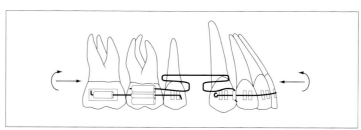

Fig. 9.**29 h** TTLRS is placed first into the crisscross vertical tube and then into the molar auxiliary tube and is activated distally out of the molar tube and cinched.

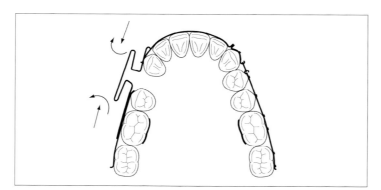

Fig. 9.**29 i** In the X–Z plane, antirotational moments prevent rotation of the segments during extraction site closure.

Finishing Procedures

The finishing procedures are relatively short-lived, since ideal tooth alignment was produced in the initial stage of treatment, and the intermediate stage merely brought these idealized segments together. At this time, ideal arch wires are placed in both dental arches, and the upper and lower lingual arch wires are removed to allow each arch to assume the nice arch forms now available in modern archwires. These ideal wires can remain in place for two or three appointments and the patient can then be "debanded."

At the time ideal arch wires are placed, we make an impression of the patient's bracketed teeth in the centric relation position and send the casts to the laboratory to have a tooth positioner fabricated. In the laboratory, the brackets are carved away from the plaster teeth, and the teeth are cut from the model and ideally reset in wax. From this ideal setup, a polyurethane tooth positioner is made.

At the end of two or three months with the ideal arch wires in place, the patient is "debanded" and is given a tooth positioner to use starting immediately. The patient is asked to use the tooth positioner "26 hours a day," hoping to elicit a small laugh from the patient, and pressing the point: "Well, you know what we mean … as much as possible, OK? It's really crucial to producing nice teeth."

We go on to explain, "This is because your teeth are now 'loose' from the braces and they'll continue to be loose for about two to three weeks. We want to take advantage of this 'looseness' by wearing the tooth positioner as much as possible to get your teeth to look just like these [the ideal set-up is shown]. Can do? Great!"

Two weeks after this "deband" appointment, the patient returns to have deband records made; their teeth will be nearly ideal (usually), and the gingivæ will have good color and tone. The deband records are made in this ideal condition, and the patient is then instructed to use the tooth positioner for 2–3 hours/day "minimum" plus during sleep for the next six weeks. They are usually elated at the time reduction. In six weeks, the patient returns to have impressions made for their upper and lower Hawley retainers. The Hawley retainers are then used for six months for 24 hours a day. Then, for next six months, they are used only during sleeping hours. If ever the Hawley retainers are lost or deformed, the tooth positioner is usually available to carry the patient over until new retainers can be made.

Conclusion

Different retraction procedures are available to manage different anchorage situations:
- In Group A anchorage, the first premolar extraction sites are closed, first, by the en-masse controlled tipping of the anterior segments and, second, by the en-masse root retraction of the anterior segment, both procedures being accomplished with a mesial force of 300 g. or less. If good headgear cooperation can be expected, translation of the anterior segment can be done.
- In Group B anchorage, the first premolar extraction sites are closed by equal anterior segment retraction and buccal segment protraction, with both segments translating en masse toward each other with a mesial force of 350 g.
- In Group C anchorage, the second premolar extraction sites are closed, first, by the en-masse controlled tipping of the buccal segments and, second, by the en-masse uprighting of the buccal segment of teeth, both procedures being accomplished with a mesial force of 350 g or more (with intermaxillary elastics, if desired).

The preactivation of the titanium T-loop retraction spring varies according to the anchorage requirements. In the event of asymmetrical extractions or unilateral space closure, the TTLRS must also be preactivated with antirotational twists since the lingual arch is not in place during the extraction site closure.

Finishing procedures are usually short-lived since ideal tooth position has been produced early in treatment. The use of a tooth positioner is optional but, with good patient compliance, it has been used to produce nearly ideal tooth positioning with normal gingival tone and contours.

References

Burstone CJ. The rationale of the segmented arch. Am J Orthod. 1962; 48(11): 805–821.

Burstone CJ. Mechanics of the segmented arch technique. Angle Orthod. 1966; 36(2): 99–120.

Burstone CJ, Koenig, HA. Force systems from an ideal arch. Am J Orthod. 1974; 65(3): 270–289.

Burstone CJ, Marcotte MR. Problem solving in orthodontics. Chicago: Quintessence; 2000.

Marcotte, MR. The use of the occlusogram in planning orthodontic treatment. Am J Orthod. 1976; 69(6): 655–667.

Marcotte MR. Biomechanics in orthodontics. Philadelphia: B. D. Decker; 1990.

10 Segmented Arch Mechanics

Andrew Kuhlberg

Segmented arch mechanics uses specific problem-oriented appliances to facilitate goal-oriented orthodontic treatment. Not an explicit technique or treatment protocol, segmented arch mechanics includes spring designs and treatment strategies that can be incorporated into almost any orthodontic treatment technique. Many initially find segmental mechanics complicated, but its major foundational principles are not difficult. Burstone (1966), Marcotte (1990), and Mulligan (1982) have all provided substantial contributions to the development and advancement of these techniques. Isaacson, Lindauer, and their colleagues succinctly summarize the themes that prevail throughout the basis of design and utilization of these springs (Isaacson 1995).

The segmented arch technique as developed by Burstone emphasized three major biomechanical principles of orthodontic treatment (Burstone 1966): force constancy, force magnitude, and moment-to-force ratio. Force magnitude and force constancy are related conceptually. Efficient tooth movement is best achieved with constant, optimal force magnitudes acting throughout the range of desired movement. This principle aims at achieving a more constant force stimulus to the teeth to obtain the tooth movement we want. The moment-to-force ratio determines the specific type of tooth movement as defined by the movement's center of rotation. Low moment-to-force ratios (~7:1) produce tipping movements; moderate M/F ratios (~10:1) produce translation or bodily movement; and high M/F ratios (~12:1) produce root movement.

Additionally, a key concept in this approach to orthodontic treatment is based on understanding the characteristics of the force vectors that the springs exert on the teeth. In addition to magnitude, the point of origin (or the point of force application), the line of action, and the sense (direction) also specifically describe vectors. These characteristics define the reactions of a body to the applied force vector. The *moment* of a force is its tendency to produce rotational movement. With segmented arch mechanics, one frequently exploits these fundamental principles of mechanics.

Another feature of segmented springs is their use of increased interbracket distances between attachment points. By increasing the interbracket distance, the appliances are activated depending on the nature of the necessary tooth movement. Generally, this means that the springs are used and adjusted on the basis of response to treatment, not simply the deactivation of wires within any given wire sequence. These comparatively large activations improve the force constancy with lower magnitudes throughout the treatment stage.

Because segmented arch techniques are force-oriented appliances, they can be used with any type of orthodontic bracket system. The sole requirement for their use is that the orthodontic attachments permit the use of auxiliary springs. Generally, this necessitates the use of "triple" or "double" tube molar attachments. Otherwise, these spring designs can be used with any bracket prescription or slot dimensions. The segmented arch technique divides each arch into an anterior and posterior unit. Anterior wire segments join either two or four incisors, or all six anterior teeth (incisors and canines). In most cases, a passive rectangular wire provides the optimal segment. The posterior teeth are similarly joined from premolars through second molars, depending on the specific needs of the individual patient. A lingual arch or transpalatal arch (TPA) unites the left and right buccal segments

The primary spring designs aim to achieve precise movements of these segments along the vertical and horizontal axes. These movements are deep overbite correction (anterior intrusion), space closure/anchorage control, and root correction.

Intrusion Arches and Deep Overbite Correction

Perhaps the signature mechanism of the segmented arch technique is the intrusion arch. Burstone pioneered the development of segmented arch techniques for deep overbite correction by intrusion (Burstone 1977). Intrusion mechanics feature a statically determinate force system, meaning that the magnitudes and directions of the active forces are all measurable. Figure 10.1a diagrams the treatment objectives of incisor intrusion. Figure 10.1b shows the biomechanical force system of an intrusion arch. The forces and moments exerted by an intrusion arch will promote anterior intrusion, posterior extrusion, and molar distal "tipback." The intrusion arch is a cantilevered spring designed to produce low continuous intrusive forces on the anterior teeth. One of the principal features of this approach to deep overbite correction is the ability to carefully control the magnitude and direction of the applied forces. Intrusion arches can be fabricated from stainless steel, beta-titanium, or nickel–titanium wires. The spring is inserted into the auxiliary tube on the molar, bypasses the premolars and canines, and is tied to the anterior segment, not into the anterior bracket slots (Figs. 10.2, 10.3). Although simple in design, this spring affords the adept clinician a huge variety of controlled therapeutic applications (Schroff et al. 1995; Nanda et al. 1998) (see Figs. 10.4 to 10.9). Because the intrusion arch is a cantilever-type spring, a single force is applied to the anterior teeth to

Intrusion Arches and Deep Overbite Correction

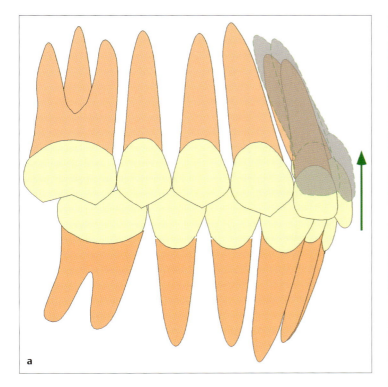

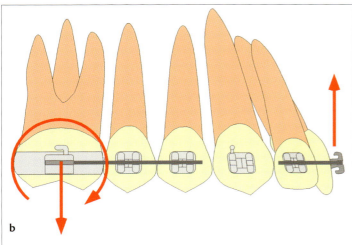

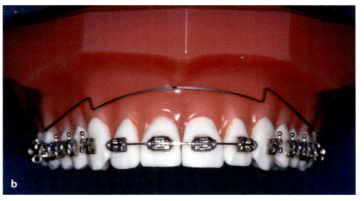

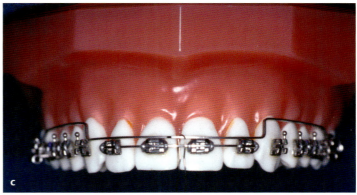

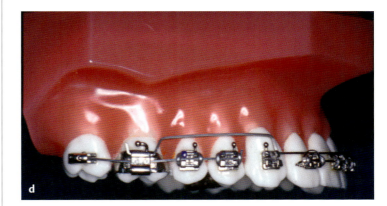

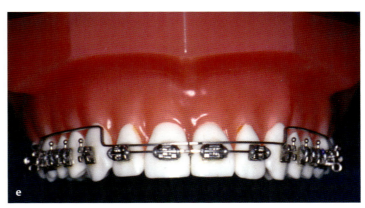

Fig. 10.**1** **The objectives of deep overbite correction by intrusion.**
a The incisor teeth are moved apically or vertically to resolve the malocclusion. The gray-shaded teeth, outlined in green, represent the treatment objective.
b The force system delivered by an intrusion arch. An active intrusion arch applies a vertical force to the anterior teeth with the reactive vertical, extrusive force on the molar and/or posterior teeth as well as a "tip-back" moment on the posterior.

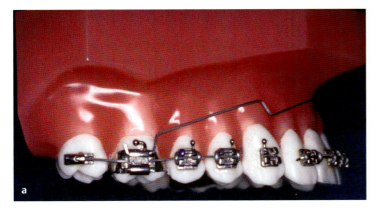

Fig. 10.**2** **Intrusion arch design. a, b** An intrusion arch fabricated from 0.017 in. × 0.025 in. beta-titanium inserted passively into the molar auxiliary tube. The steps in the archwire allow the spring to bypass the premolar and canine brackets without interference.
a Buccal view.
b Frontal view.
c Tying the intrusion arch to the anterior segment. Ligature wire is looped around the intrusion arch as well as the anterior segment.
d Activated intrusion arch, buccal view.
e Activated intrusion arch, frontal view

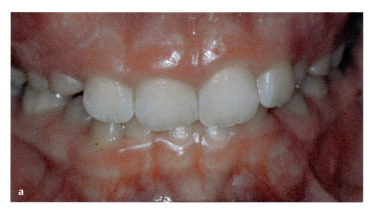
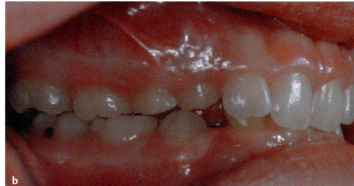
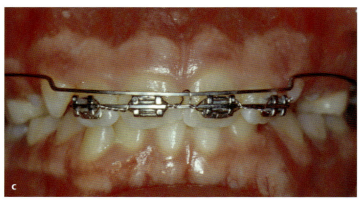
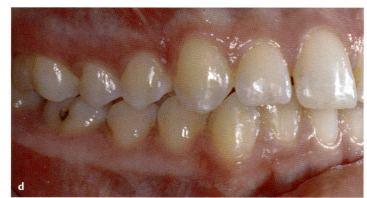

Fig. 10.**3** **Clinical example of deep overbite correction by intrusion.**
a Anterior view of deep overbite, before treatment.
b Buccal view, before treatment.
c Anterior incisor intrusion.
d Buccal view, after treatment.

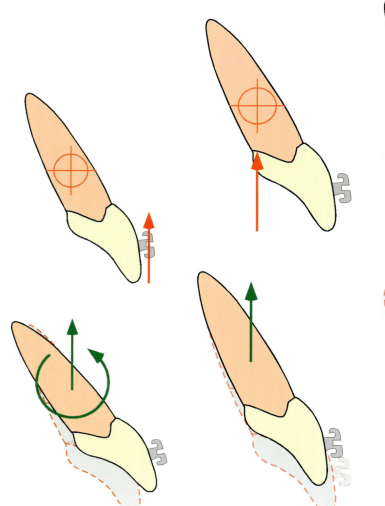
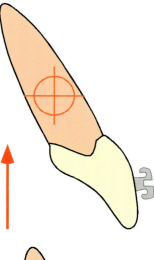
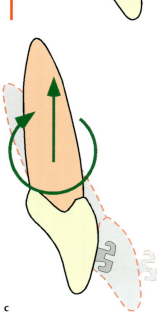

Fig. 10.**4** **The effect of alternative points of force application on tooth movement.** Note: Cross-hair represents the tooth's center of resistance (CR).
a A force labial or anterior to the center of resistance will result in intrusion and crown-labial/root-lingual rotation.
b The same force applied slightly more posteriorly with a line of action passing through CR will produce only a linear, upward movement.
c Applying the force further posteriorly produces a rotation in the opposite direction; the incisor will move upward and rotate crown-lingual/root-labial.

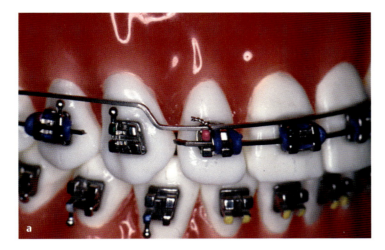
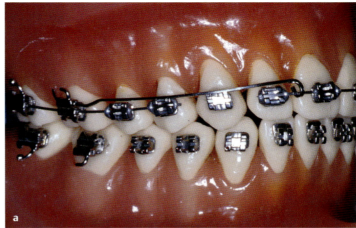
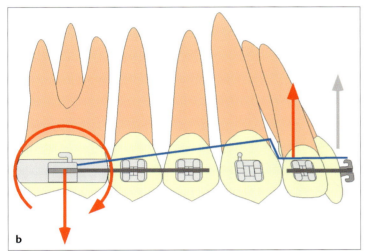
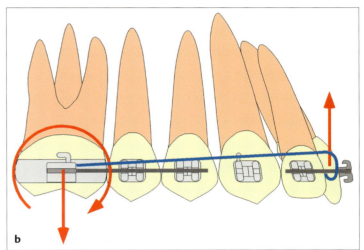

Fig. 10.**5** **To produce alternative points of force application, the intrusion arch can be tied to different points on the anterior segment.**
a Here the intrusion arch is tied at the distal wing of the lateral incisor.
b The line of force passes through the incisor(s) center of resistance, eliminating the tipping effect caused by the moment of the applied force.

Fig. 10.**6** **Three-piece intrusion arch.**
a Another design for anterior intrusion utilizes separate cantilever springs on the left and right sides. This approach allows the orthodontist tremendous control of the point of force application.
b Force system from three-piece intrusion arch. The cantilever spring segment allows precise positioning of the point of force application by locating the hook attachment where desired.

produce different tooth movements (Figs. 10.4, 10.5). Placing the line of force through the center of resistance of the tooth causes bodily movement. Otherwise, the moment of the force results in various combinations of translation and rotation. Variations of the intrusion spring design further expand the clinical applications. The hook attachment style of separate spring segments on the left and right increase the precision of point force application (Fig. 10.6). Also, this design increases the freedom of movement of the incisor versus the molar teeth by allowing the hook to slide freely along the anterior segment. This is especially beneficial when substantial molar "tip-back" is needed (Fig. 10.7). The intrusion arch may be combined with the retraction forces to achieve simultaneous deep overbite correction and anterior retraction (Fig. 10.8). The "tip-back" moment enhances posterior anchorage, while the intrusion-retraction assembly addresses both overjet and overbite correction. The intrusion of single teeth can also be obtained by applying the force to an individual tooth, as in separate canine intrusion (Fig. 10.9). The simple design of the intrusion arch and with its many clinical uses make it a valuable item in the orthodontist's toolbox. An important consideration for the orthodontist is that anchorage control, headgear, and multitooth anchor units may be necessary to restrain the reactive movements (molar extrusion, "tip-back") when they are undesirable.

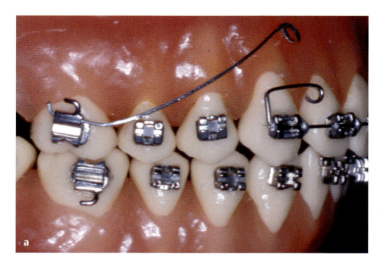
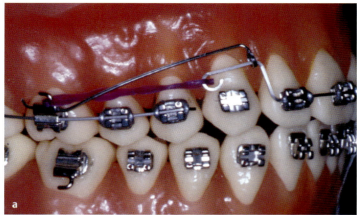
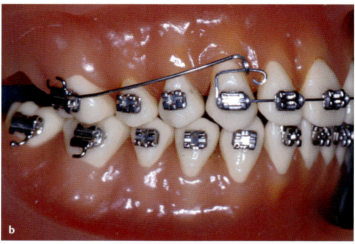
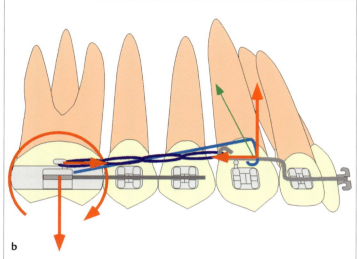

Fig. 10.7 **A three-piece intrusion arch designed to emphasize molar "tip-back."** The anterior segment incorporates the canine, providing more teeth in the anterior anchorage unit.
a The cantilever spring inserts into the molar auxiliary tube without any posterior buccal segments.
b The activated spring; the spring's hook is free to slide distally as molar "tip-back" movement occurs.

Fig. 10.8 **Simultaneous incisor intrusion and retraction with the three-piece intrusion arch.**
a A light retraction force is applied by either chain elastic or coil springs. With control of the magnitude of the intrusive and distal forces, the resultant force can produce intrusion along the long axis of the incisors.
b Force system from simultaneous intrusion and retraction. The green arrow represents the resultant force acting on the anterior teeth. Controlling the magnitude of the intrusive versus the retraction force allows one to control the nature of the tooth movement.

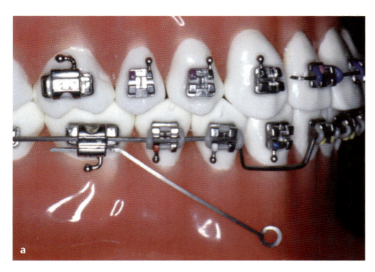
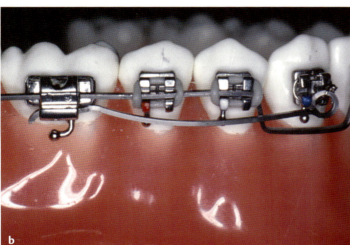
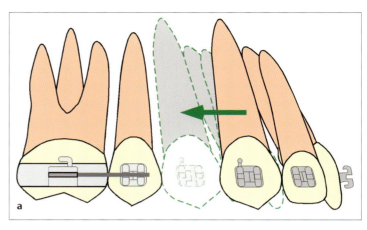
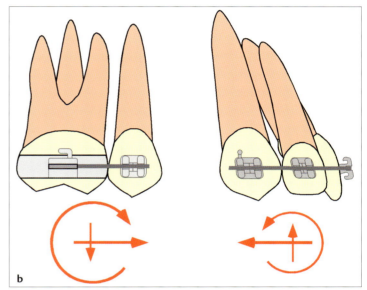

Fig. 10.**9** **Separate canine intrusion by a segmented spring.**
a The base archwire provides anchorage by joining the majority of the teeth while the spring exerts a point force on the canine, passive intrusion spring.
b Note that the intrusion spring is not engaged in the canine bracket slot.

Fig. 10.**10** **Objectives of maximum posterior anchorage.**
a With maximum anchorage control, treatment aims to retract the anterior teeth without any mesial movement of the posterior teeth. The gray-shaded green-outlined teeth represent the treatment goal.
b The force system delivered by segmental springs for anterior retraction. These springs emphasize the principle of differential moment force systems to achieve the anchorage objectives.

Space Closure and Anchorage Control

One of the great challenges of orthodontic therapy is controlled, differential tooth movement during extraction space closure, diagrammed in Fig. 10.**10a**. The segmented arch approach to anchorage control during space closure employs a strategy of differential moment force systems (Burstone and Koenig1976; Kuhlberg and Priebe. 2001) (Fig. 10.**10b**). The essence of this method is the delivery of different force systems to the anterior and posterior teeth by varying the magnitude of the applied moments on each segment of teeth. The "T-loop" spring has been developed for this purpose (Figs. 10.**11**, 10.**12**). Several alternative T-loop spring designs incorporate features that produce this differential force system (Burstone and Koenig 1976; Burstone 1982; Manhartsberger C et al. 1989; Kuhlberg et al 1997). Due to the force stimuli of these mechanics, tooth movement occurs very differently from that observed in "conventional" sliding-type styles of space closure. The expected movement of the teeth passes from tipping, through translation, and ends with root correction (Fig. 10.**11**). Insertion and activation of segmented closing loops/T-loops appears somewhat different from that of common continuous wire loops (Fig. 10.**12**). Clinical control comes from proper activation and monitoring of the springs during space closure (Fig. 10.**13**).

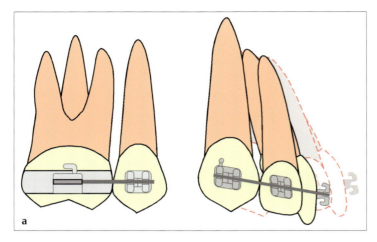
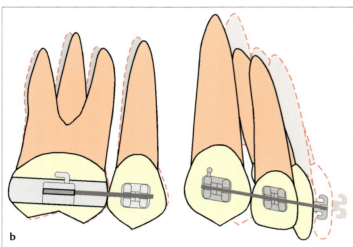
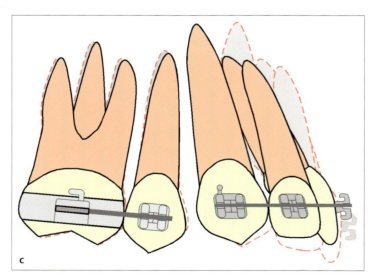

Fig. 10.**11** **Stages of tooth movement with single spring activation.**
a Controlled tipping is the initial movement.
b As the spring deactivates and the teeth are retracted, the moment-to-force ratio increases, resulting in anterior translation.
c Reductions in the spring's activation force allow the springs potential to deliver root movement with the further increase in the M/F ratio. At this stage, the spring requires reactivation.

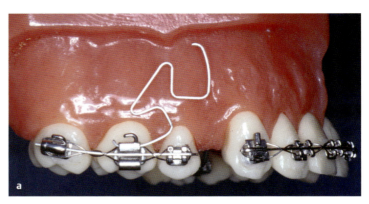
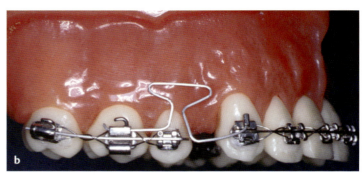

Fig. 10.**12** **Insertion and activation of the segmented T-loop, fabricated from 0.017 in × 0.025 beta-titanium wire.**
a The spring is inserted in the auxiliary tube of the molar.
b The spring must be activated horizontally to engage the anterior segment.

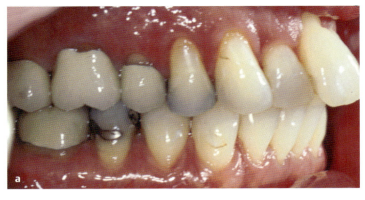
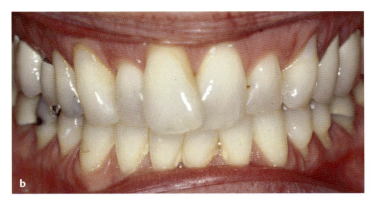
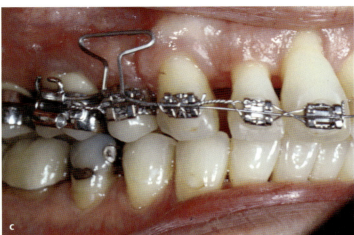
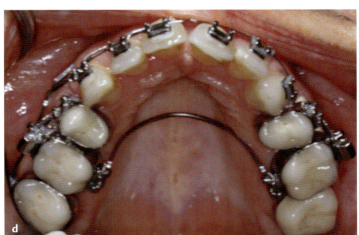
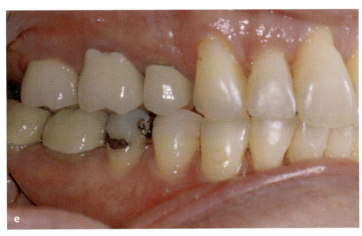
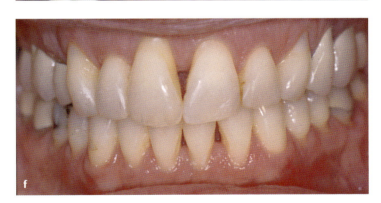

Fig. 10.**13** **Clinical example of a treatment requiring maximum anchorage control and anterior retraction.**

a Initial buccal view; this is an adult patient with a history of periodontal disease and reduced dentoalveolar support of several teeth. The canine must be fully retraced to achieve a Class I relationship.
b Front view. Notice the significant incisor overlap.
c Treatment progress with segmented T-loop, buccal view.
d Treatment progress with segmented T-loop, occlusal view. A transpalatal arch supplements the posterior anchorage.
e Post treatment, buccal view.
f Post treatment, frontal view.

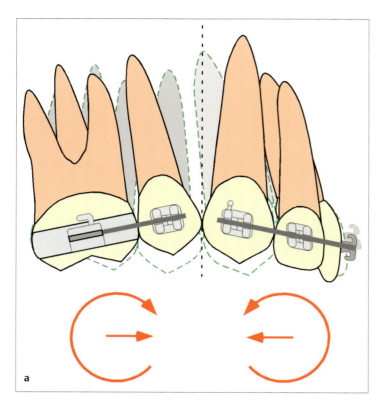
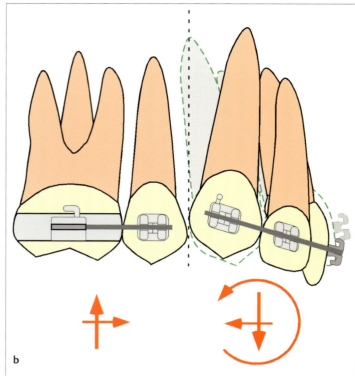
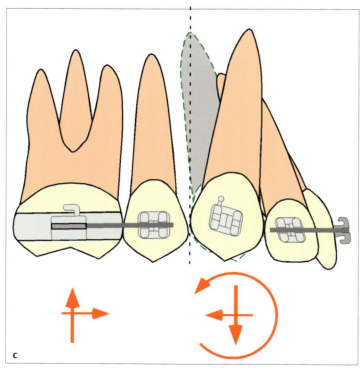

Fig. 10.**14** Common presentations of anterior and posterior segments following space closure.
a Symmetrical tipping of each segment toward the extraction space results in root divergence at the apices, requiring equal and opposite moments to obtain root correction.
b Following anterior retraction, the anterior teeth require more root movement than the posterior teeth.
c Separate canine root correction. The force system for this movement is similar to the incisor root correction.

Fig. 10.**15** Symmetrical helical spring for root correction.
a Spring fabricated from 0.017 in. × 0.025 in. stainless steel and inserted into auxiliary tubes.
b,c Evaluating the activation helical root springs, inserted into the molar tube. Assess the spring activation by creating equal distances between the free end of the spring to its tube when inserted only at one end.

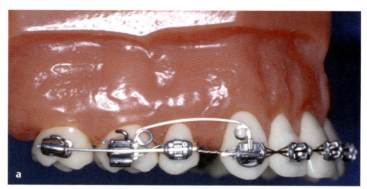
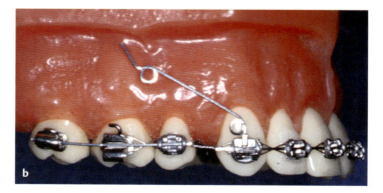
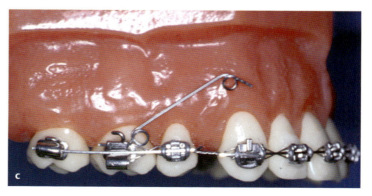

Root Correction

Segmented spring mechanics emphasize the use of biomechanical concepts in the development and action of the appliances. The resulting tooth movements often leave the appearance of poor clinical control, when in fact the clinical responses may be entirely predictable on the basis of treatment stage and goals (Fig. 10.14). Tipping movements aid in anchorage preservation but create concerns about occlusal plane leveling and root parallelism. This is especially true with extraction space closure, where the differential force system results in specific differences in the types and amounts of tooth movement of the anterior versus posterior teeth. This demands a distinct stage of root correction following space closure in order to obtain root parallelism and occlusal plane leveling. Most commonly, one of three types of root correction is needed. First, when the anterior and posterior teeth have been equally tipped into the extraction space, symmetrical root correction is needed (Fig. 10.15). Second, excessive incisal uprighting following anterior retraction may require only incisor root correction (Figs. 10.16, 10.17). Third, separate canine retrac-

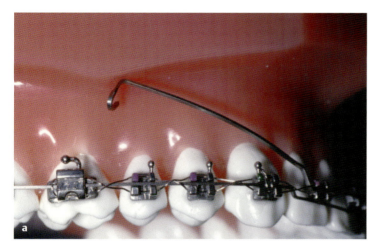
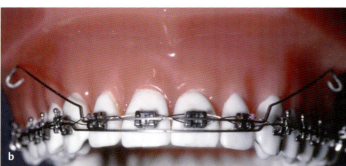
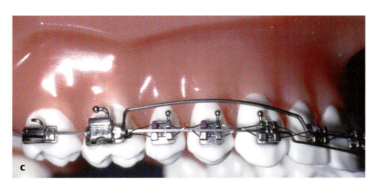

Fig. 10.16 **Incisor lingual root correction spring.**
a Spring fabricated from 0.021 in. × 0.025 in. beta-titanium wire in a 0.022 in. bracket slot, buccal view. Full bracket engagement is important for efficient spring activation.
b Incisor lingual root correction spring, frontal view. The base wire steps incisal to the anterior brackets to inhibit the extrusive side effect. Additionally, the arch is "figure-eight" tied throughout to restrict incisor flaring.
c Activated incisor lingual root correction spring, buccal view.

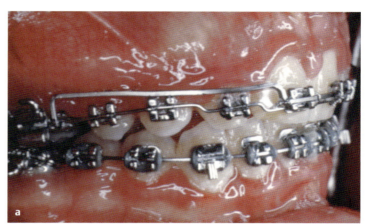
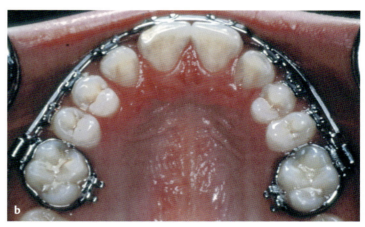
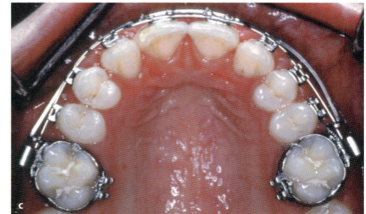

Fig. 10.17 **Clinical example requiring incisor lingual root correction.**
a Buccal view. Note the upright facial surfaces of the incisors. The spring is fabricated from full slot thickness beta-titanium wire.
b Occlusal view before treatment.
c Occlusal view following treatment. Note the increased visibility of the lingual surfaces of the central incisors (compare with b).

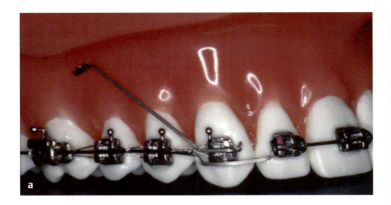
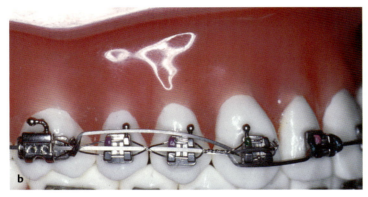

Fig. 10.**18** **Separate canine root spring.**
a Passive, buccal view. A base wire steps occlusal to the canine to prevent extrusion.
b Separate canine root spring, active, buccal view. The canine is "figure-eight" tied to the posterior teeth to prevent space opening between the canine and premolar.

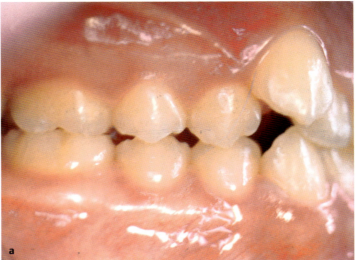
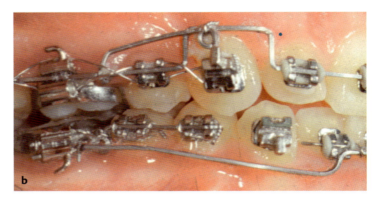
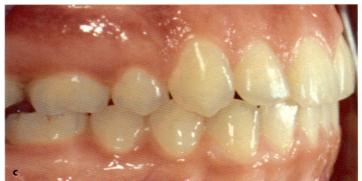

Fig. 10.**19** **Clinical example of canine root correction.**
a Initial buccal view.
b Active root spring. In this case, the root spring was ligated to an apically step base wire to avoid the extrusive side effect. Also, notice the incisor intrusion spring in the mandibular arch.
c Buccal view, post treatment.

tion may simply require canine root correction (Figs. 10.**18**, 10.**19**). There are two major segmented spring designs used for this treatment stage: (1) double helical root springs, which are particularly useful for symmetrical root correction; and (2) cantilever root springs for incisor and/or canine root correction.

Transpalatal and Lingual Arches

Transpalatal arches (TPAs) and lingual arches play an integral role in the segmented arch technique (Burstone and Manhartsberger 1988; Burstone 1989). Passively, TPAs and lingual arches join the left and right buccal segments (Fig. 10.**20**). Uniting the left and right sides allows arch width maintenance and rotational control during mesial–distal movements, and aids in establishing anchorage units. TPAs and lingual arches can be used for a variety of active tooth movements. Two common uses of these wires are molar rotation, especially mesial-out rotation (Fig. 10.**21**), and unilateral tip-back mechanics (Fig. 10.**22**).

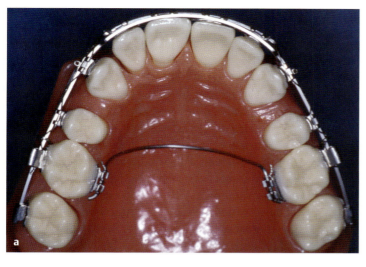
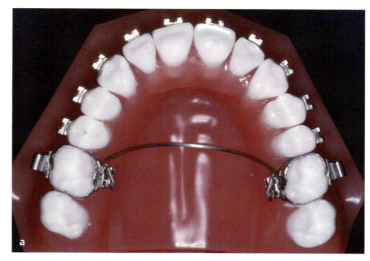
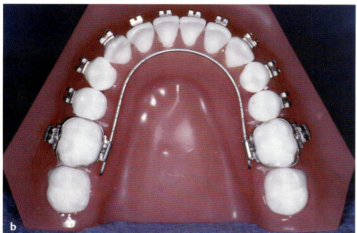
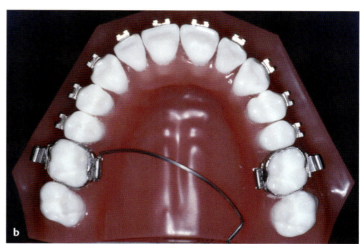
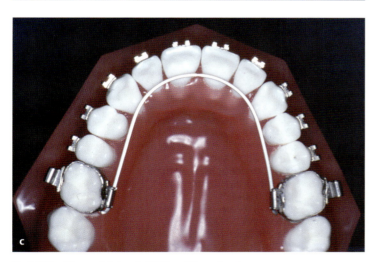
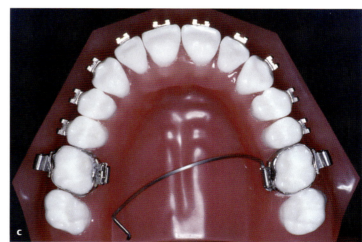

Fig. 10.**20** Transpalatal arch (TPA) and lingual arch.
a TPAs have many passive and active applications in segmented arch mechanics. They may be made from round or rectangular wire depending on the specific treatment needs and appliance attachments utilized.
b Round mandibular lingual arch.
c Rectangular mandibular arch

Fig. 10.**21** Bilateral, "mesial-out" activation of a TPA. The distances of the free end of the TPA inserted unilaterally to its attachment demonstrates the wire's activation. Equal distances on the left and right sides indicate symmetrical activation as is shown when the wire is inserted separately into each side (**b**) and (**c**).

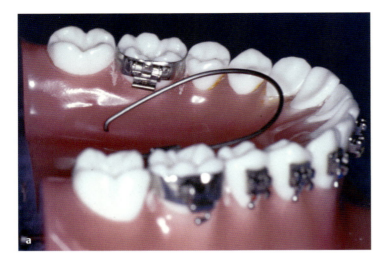

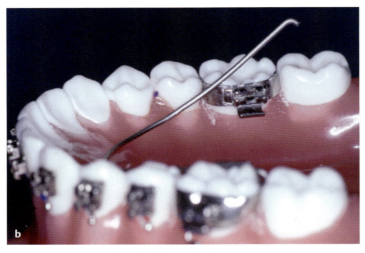

Fig. 10.22 **"Tip-forward tip-back" lingual arch activation.**
a The "tip-back" activation of the lingual arch; inserting the wire into the lingual attachment will result in a crown-distal–root-mesial tipping movement of the molar.
b The "tip-forward" activation of the lingual opposing the "tip-back" side. Unilateral "tip-back" can be useful for asymmetrical molar correction; combined with an intrusion arch (see Fig. 10.**7**), this mechanism is capable of significant resolution of occlusal asymmetries.

Summary

Segmented arch orthodontic springs permit the orthodontist to have a high level of control of the force systems used to meet individual patient treatment goals. Unlike techniques following archwire sequences, these techniques are aimed at reaching specific objectives of tooth movement to correct a patient's problems. Development of the spring designs used in the segmented arch technique was based on application of the principles of biomechanics. The emphasis on biomechanical considerations focuses the treatment on selecting the best force system for a clinical situation, to be used as necessary within any patients needs. The major components include intrusion mechanics, extraction space closure and anchorage control, and root movement. Intrusion arches are routinely used for deep overbite correction, but their simple design offers many other refinements and adaptations to clinical orthodontics. Segmented space closing springs rely heavily on the biomechanical force system for anchorage control, making these springs helpful in cases of limited compliance. The root correction spring designs are helpful in efficiently correcting those problems that arise following previous treatment stages. Additionally, the mechanisms described for these treatment elements may be applied creatively to resolve those unique problems and challenges that occasionally defy conventional therapies (Kuhlberg 2001). Innovative uses of the segmented spring designs can be helpful in addressing difficult stages of treatment. The key is to identify the problems one faces and select the best mechanics to effectively achieve the desired results.

References

Burstone CJ. The mechanics of the segmented arch techniques. Angle Orthod. 1966; 36(2): 99–120.
Burstone CR. Deep overbite correction by intrusion. Am J Orthod. 1977; 72(1): 1–22.
Burstone CJ. The segmented arch approach to space closure. Am J Orthod. 1982; 82(5): 361–378.
Burstone CJ. Precision lingual arches. Active applications. J Clin Orthod. 1989; 23(2): 101–109.
Burstone CJ, Koenig HA. Optimizing anterior and canine retraction. Am J Orthod. 1976; 70(1): 1–19.
Burstone CJ, Manhartsberger C. Precision lingual arches. Passive applications. J Clin Orthod. 1988; 22(7): 444–451.
Isaacson RJ. Biomechanics and appliance design. Semin Orthod. 1995; 1(1).
Kuhlberg AJ. Cantilever springs: force system and clinical applications. Semin Orthod. 2001; 7(3): 150–159.
Kuhlberg AJ, Burstone CJ. T-loop position and anchorage control. Am J Orthod Dentofacial Orthop. 1997; 112(1): 12–18.
Kuhlberg AJ, Priebe DN. Space closure and anchorage control. Semin Orthod. 2001; 7(1): 42–49.
Manhartsberger C, Morton JY, Burstone CJ. Space closure in adult patients using the segmented arch technique. Angle Orthod. 1989; 59: 205–210.
Marcotte MR. Biomechanics in orthodontics. Philadelphia, PA: BC Decker; 1990.
Mulligan TF. Common sense mechanics. Phoenix, AZ: CSM; 1982.
Nanda R, Marzban R, Kuhlberg A. The Connecticut intrusion arch. J Clin Orthod. 1998; 32(12): 708–715.
Schroff B, Lindauer SJ, Burstone CJ, Leiss JB. Segmented approach to simultaneous intrusion and space closure: biomechanics of the three-piece base arch appliance. Am J Orthod Dentofacial Orthop. 1995; 107(2): 136–143.

11 The Alexander Discipline

R. G. Wick Alexander

The Alexander Discipline (Alexander RG 1983, 1986a, 1986b, 2001) grew out of the Tweed technique, and today maintains many of Tweed's principles. The present technique incorporates ideas found in other teachings and techniques, but much of it was gained empirically from trial and error. Its originality is the result of proven ideas and concepts put together to create a unique package.

Four specific factors make the Alexander Discipline different from others: unique bracket selection and prescription; unique arch form; the treatment mechanics; and evidence-based studies.

Unique Bracket Selection and Prescription

(Alexander RG 1986b, 2001)

1. Specific bracket designs are created for specific teeth. (Bagden 2001) (Fig. 11.**1a–c**).
2. Single brackets create increased interbracket space, as compared to twin brackets, which will allow more flexibility with stiffer archwires, resulting in easier engagement and fewer archwire changes (Fig. 11.**2**).
3. Rotational wings give controlled guidance and direction to the teeth. Wings can be activated or deactivated for increased rotation (Fig. 11.**3a**). Interfering wings can be removed for better bracket placement (Fig. 11.**3b**). The advantage of rotation wings is that the force is exerted on the "active" wing (Fig. 11.**3c**). Since the "active" wing holds the rotation, there is no need to replace the bracket (Fig. 11.**3d**). If the bracket is placed off-center, the remaining wing creates a greater rotational lever (Fig. 11.**3e, f**).
4. The special prescription of torques and angulations (Fig. 11.**4a–d**) in the Alexander discipline makes the resulting straightwire appliance unique. If one believes that control of intercanine width and mandibular incisor flaring is important, as shown in the literature (Glenn et al. 1987; Elms et al. 1996a,b; Frasch 2002) maximum effort should be made to control this area. Possibly the most significant and important

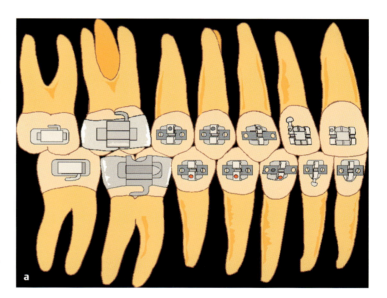

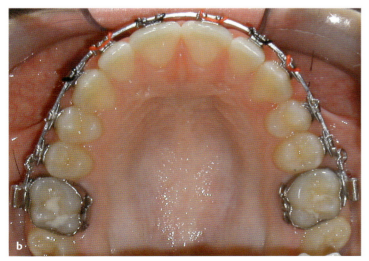

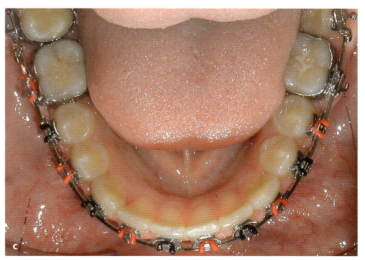

Fig. 11.**1 Bracket and wing design.**

a Specific bracket design for specific teeth.

b, c Wing design, bracket position (occlusal views).

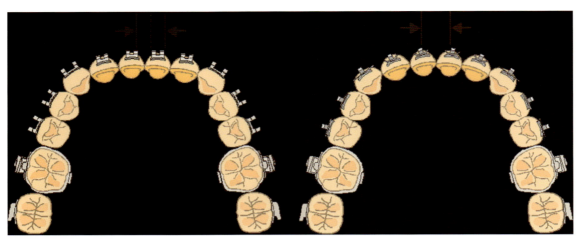

Fig. 11.2 **Forty-eight percent increased interbracket space compared to twin brackets.**
Left: Twin brackets
Right: Alexander bracket with wings

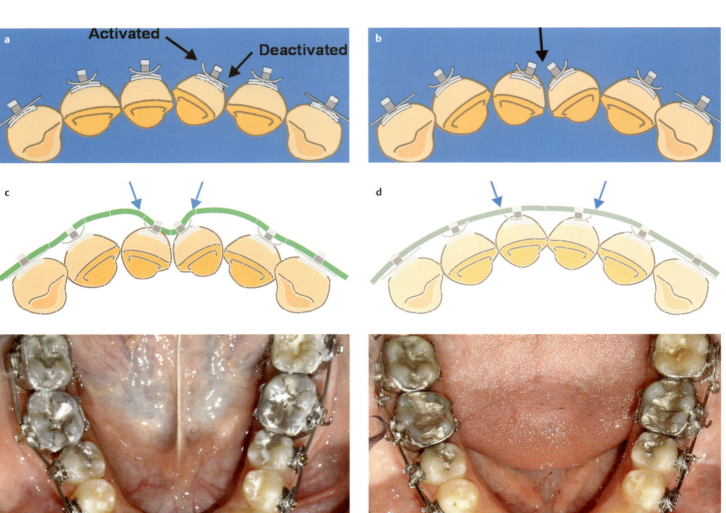

Fig. 11.3 **Rotational wings.**

a Wing activation. Wings can be activated or deactivated for increased rotation.
b Interfering wings removed for better bracket placement.
c Archwire engagement demonstrates force on active wings.
d After correction no need to replace brackets.
e When the bracket is placed off center on the rotated tooth, it creates a better rotational lever. Initial occlusal view.
f Progress occlusal view showing rotational correction.

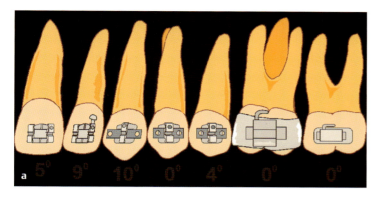
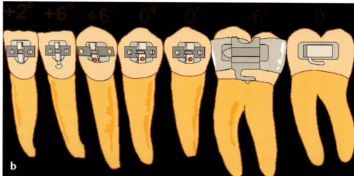
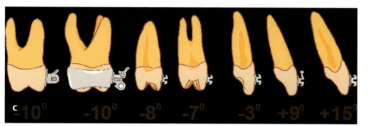
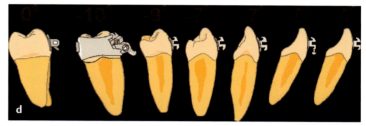
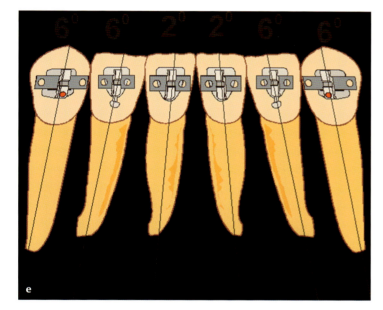

Fig. 11.**4 Torques and angulations.**
a Maxillary angulations: notice 2nd bicuspid.
b Mandibular angulations: notice centrals, laterals and 1st molars.
c Maxillary torques.
d Mandibular torques: notice 5° torque on incisors.
e Mandibular anterior bracket placement – spreading the roots apart for long term stability.
f Initial flexible rectangular archwire helps control mandibular incisor torque.
g Automatic uprighting of 1st molars.

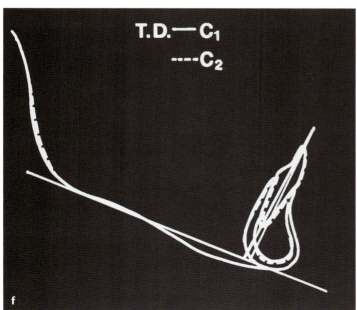
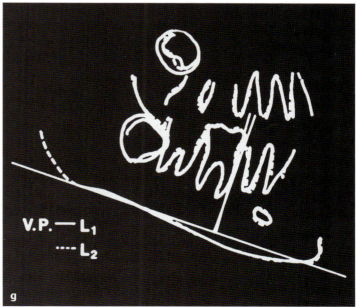

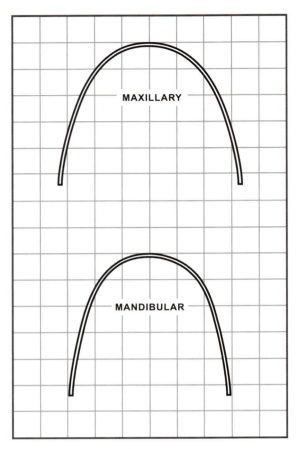

Fig. 11.5 **Archform template.**

of the unique design elements of this bracket system is expressed in the lower mandibular anterior brackets (Fig. 11.**4e**). Using single brackets with wings creates an advantage that is not possible with twin brackets. The prescription allows for controlled and effective mandibular arch leveling, especially in nonextraction cases. This is accomplished by first placing the brackets and ligating each tooth with a rectangular wire. The incisors' resistance to tipping labially, caused by the −5° torque, places a distal force on the first molars angulated at −6°, causing them to upright (Trammell 1980). This can gain 2–3 mm of arch length without flaring the incisors (Fig. 11.**4f, g**). The unique biomechanical principles of actively tying back a heat-treated, curved, rectangular stainless-steel archwire contributes to successful and stable arch leveling (Bernstein 2007; Carcara 2001).

Unique Arch Form

(McKelvain 1982; Alexander RG 1992a)

The arch form used in the Alexander Discipline was developed as a result of the compilation of hand-bent archwires that provide individualized archforms (Fig. 11.5) that will fit most patients within one standard deviation. This arch form has been compared to other commercially available arch forms and found to be more stable (Felton et al. 1987).

Through the history of orthodontics, archwire design has been connected to a specific technique. Every guru has their own archform. Throughout my years in practice, I too feel there is one arch-

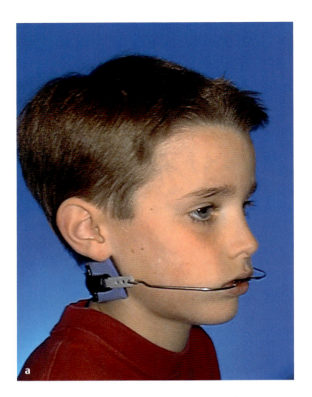

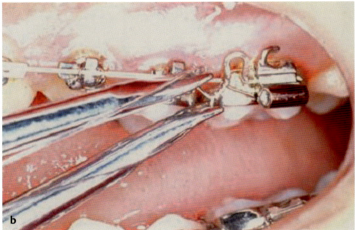

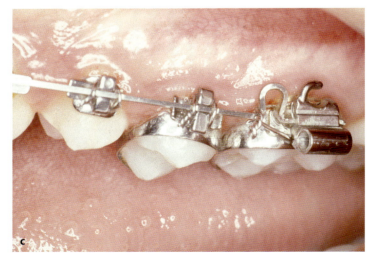

Fig. 11.**6**
a Patient wearing cervical facebow.
b Tying back the archwire with ligature tying plier.
c The archwire tied back.

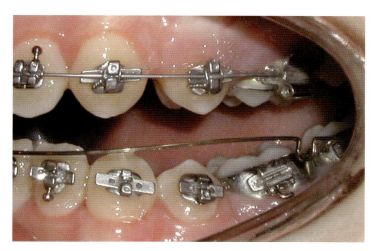

Fig. 11.7 Reverse curve bent in archwire.

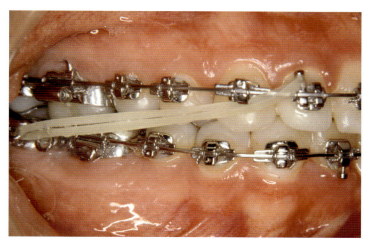

Fig. 11.8 Class II elastics creating more horizontal face vector when attached to maxillary lateral brackets.

form that can generally be used within on standard deviation on most cases. One must ask why is this so? The following is my reasoning.

For long term stability in orthodontic treatment the mandibular anterior teeth positions are vitally important. With rare exceptions, inter-canine width must stay within 1 mm of its original position. Mandibular incisors can be advanced not more than 2 mm if long term stability is the goal. Exceptions exist but this is the general rule. Therefore, it makes sense that the anterior portion of the maxillary and mandibular archforms should be built around the mandibular six anterior teeth.

Regarding the posterior teeth, it is well know that an intermolar width of ± 36 mm is stable in the long term.

When combining these goals, the resulting archform will be ovoid, regardless of the patient's beginning archform.

Treatment Mechanics

The Alexander Discipline, however, is much more than a bracket system or arch form. Certain specific mechanics were first created or popularized by this technique. Among them:

1. One arch is treated at a time, beginning with the maxillary arch.
2. Driftodontics: In extraction cases, the maxillary arch is treated while allowing the crowded mandibular arch to "drift" before placing brackets (Papandreas 1993).
3. A cervical facebow (Fig. 11.6a) is attached to a tied-back arch wire (Fig. 11.6b,c) to create an orthopedic correction in low and average angle skeletal Class II cases (Glenn et al. 1987; Elms et al. 1996a, b; Romine 1982; Plunk 1985; Guymon 1990; Alexander CD and Alexander JM 2001).
4. Borderline cases can often be treated without extraction by using RPE (rapid palatal expansion) (Alexander RG 2000a; Buschang et al. 2001) and lip bumpers for gaining space (Nevant et al. 1991; Alexander RG 1992b; Buschang et al. 2001). The long-term stability of this technique has been verified (Ferris 2005).
5. Mandibular incisor flaring is controlled by −5° torque in the bracket and the initial rectangular flexible archwire (Glenn et al. 1987; Elms et al. 1996a, b; Bernstein 1999; Carcara 2001; Frasch 2002).
6. Mandibular first molars are uprighted with a −6° tip (Trammell 1980).
7. Mandibular anterior roots are spread with specific angulated brackets (see Fig. 11.4e) (Buschang et al. 2001).
8. Mandibular arches are leveled by a reverse curve in the archwire (Fig. 11.7), using a specific prescription for each patient (Carcara 2001; Bernstein 1999).
9. Ball hooks are placed on the lateral brackets for elastic attachment (Bagden 2001).
10. Class II elastics are attached on lateral incisors (Fig. 11.8) rather than canines in order to produce a more horizontal vector of force on the arches (Alexander RG 1986b).
11. Maxillary canines are retracted on 0.016 in. stainless-steel archwire with power chains (see Case Study 11.1 [15–18]).
12. Specific archwire sectioning and elastic attachments are used to finalize posterior occlusion (see Case Study 11.1 [31–34]) (Alexander RG 1987, 1997; Haltom 2001).
13. The unique maxillary wrap-around retainer wire design controls posttreatment settling (see Case Study 11.1 [41,42]) (Alexander RG 1987, 1997; Haltom 2001). A maxillary retainer is worn at night only (Alexander RG 1997; Haltom 2001).

Clinical Case Studies

Maximum Anchorage: Extraction Case Demonstrating Typical Extraction Mechanics

Case Study 11.1   J.S.K.: Class I Bi-Maxillary Protrusion Extraction Case

This 23 year-old woman presented with Class I occlusion (Fig. 11.1.**3, 4**) with the chief concern of anterior crowding in both arches (Fig. 11.1.**5, 6**) and some concern with her protrusive profile (Fig. 11.1.**1, 2**).

Evaluating the panoramic radiograph (Fig. 11.1.**7**) and cephalometric tracing (Fig. 11.1.**8**) and noting protrusion of the maxillary and mandibular incisors, in addition to the moderate crowding and the convex profile, the decision was made to extract four first premolars.

The treatment plan was to use maximum anchorage mechanics, which included a combination high-pull facebow and Class III elastics. (This case was treated before implant anchorage was an option.)

The maxillary arch was bracketed first with the typical initial flexible 0.016 in. NiTi wire (Fig. 11.1.**9–12**). Since this patient had a cephalometrically low-angle mandibular plane, a cervical headgear would normally be used. However, since Class III elastics would be necessary during lower anterior retraction, a combination facebow (Fig. 11.1.**13, 14**) was needed to prevent any extrusion of the maxillary molars resulting from the use of the Class III elastics. The facebow was conscientiously worn nightly during retraction of the incisors. A 0.016 in. stainless-steel (SS) archwire was placed the second month and power chains were used to begin retraction of the maxillary cuspids (Fig. 11.1.**15–18**). After three months, the mandibular arch was bracketed using a 16 × 22 SS multistranded archwire as the first wire.

At six months, while the maxillary canines were being retracted on a 0.016 in. SS archwire, a 16 × 22 SS closing loop archwire was placed in the mandibular arch. When the archwire was activated Class III elastics were used to maximize the retraction of the mandibular anterior teeth. The patient was instructed to wear these elastics for 72 hours initially, then at night only with the facebow (Fig. 11.1.**19–22**).

The mandibular closing arch was activated monthly with the same instructions for elastic use.

During this time the maxillary canines continued to be retracted. In this adult patient, the canines did not move as rapidly as usual. So, at 13 months, the third maxillary archwire, a 0.018 in. × 0.025 in. losing loop reduced to 16 × 23 distal to the loops, was placed (Fig. 11.1.**23–26**) This archwire was also activated monthly.

At 12 months of treatment—nine months of treating the mandibular arch—the lower spaces had been closed, so the third and final archwire was placed. This finishing wire is a 17 × 25 SS archwire bent with omega loops and a reverse curve of Spee. This SS wire is heat treated before being tied in and tied back with steel ligatures. At this appointment, the Class III elastics were discontinued. The facebow was continued until the maxillary anterior teeth had been retracted. At this point, 19 months into treatment, the maxillary finishing archwire (17 × 25 SS) was bent similarly to the mandibular wire, except with slightly less accentuated curve of Spee. Note how the overbite was corrected and the arches were leveled with the finishing archwires – a good example of "let it cook" (Fig. 11.1.**27–30**).

During the last three months Class II elastics were used to achieve maximum interdigitation/centric relation balance. Finishing elastics then finalized the posterior occlusion (Fig. 11.1.**31–34**).

Total active treatment time was 24 months (Fig. 11.1.**35–40**). The patient was given a maxillary circumferential retainer (Fig. 11.1.**41, 42**), to be worn at night only, and a mandibular bonded cuspid-to-cuspid fixed retainer. After three years of nighttime wear, the patient was instructed to wear the maxillary retainer once a week to maintain the positions.

Maxillary and mandibular archwire sequences and individualized forces are listed in Boxes 11.**1**–11.**3**. Final panoramic (Fig. 11.1.**43**) and cephalometric (Fig. 11.1.**44**) radiographs show the results, together with the composite tracings (Fig. 11.1.**45**). Five-year post-treatment intraoral (Fig. 11.1.**46–49**) and facial photographs (Fig. 11.1.**50, 51**) show good stability.

Box 11.**1**   J.S.K. – Maxillary Archwire Sequence.

1. 0.016 in. NiTi	2 months
2. 0.016 in. SS (Retract 3's)	9 months
3. 18 × 25 closing loops SS	8 months
4. 17 × 25 finishing SS	5 months
Active treatment time	**24 months**

Box 11.**2**   J.S.K. – Mandibular Archwire Sequence.

None	3 months
1. 6 × 22 D-Rect	3 months
2. 16 × 22 closing loops SS	6 months
3. 17 × 25 SS	12 months
Active treatment time	**21 months**

Box 11.**3**   J.S.K. – Individualized Forces.

Combination facebow	16 months
Elastics	
*Class III	6 months
*Class II	1 month
*Finishing	2 months
CSF maxillary and mandibular	
Anterior teeth 3 months before RB	

Clinical Case Studies 241

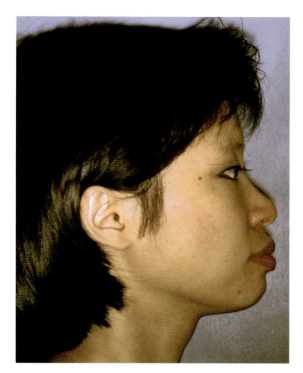
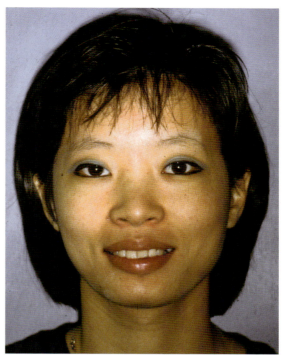

Fig. 11.1.**1, 2** **Patient J. S. K.**
Age 23 years 11 months. Patient treated before mini-implant anchorage available.

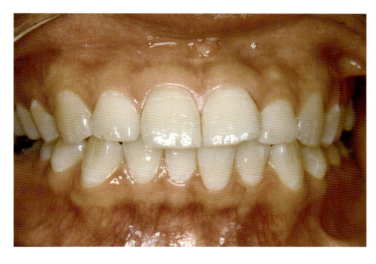
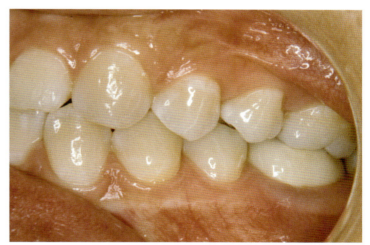

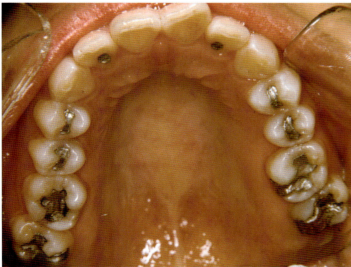
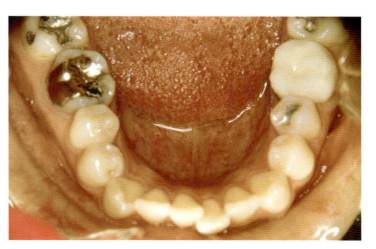

Fig. 11.1.**3–6** **Class I, overbite 1 mm, overjet 4 mm, maxillary discrepancy 3 mm, mandibular discrepancy 5 mm.**

3, 4 Labial and buccal views.   **5, 6** Occlusal views.

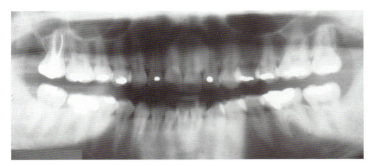

Fig. 11.1.7 **Pretreatment panoramic radiograph.**

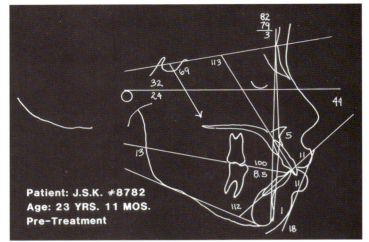

Fig. 11.1.8 **Pretreatment cephalometric radiograph.**

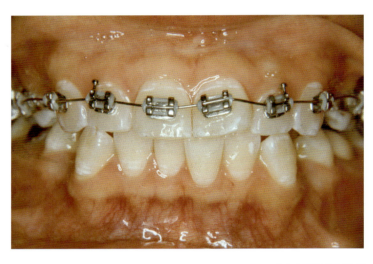

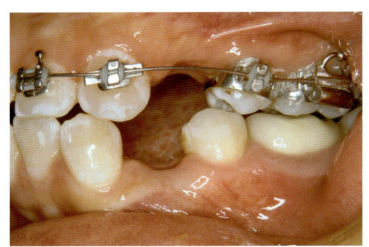

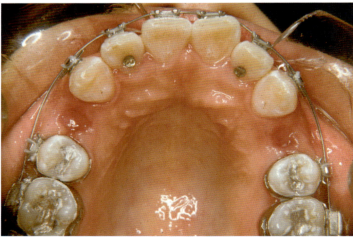

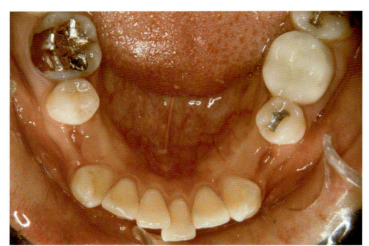

Fig. 11.1.**9–12 Maxillary bracket placement, 0.016 in. NiTi archwire.**

9, 10 Labial and buccal views.

11, 12 Occlusal views.

Clinical Case Studies 243

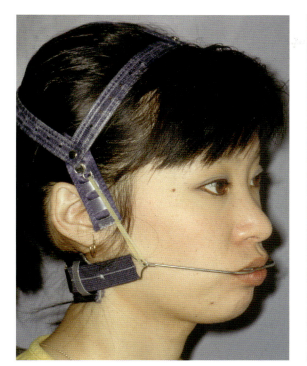
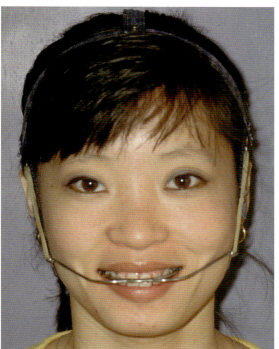

Fig. 11.1.**13, 14** Combination facebow placed one month later.

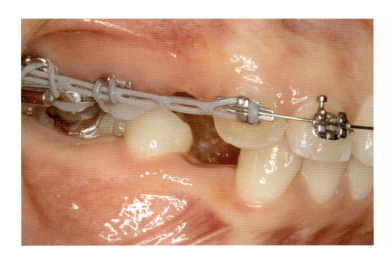
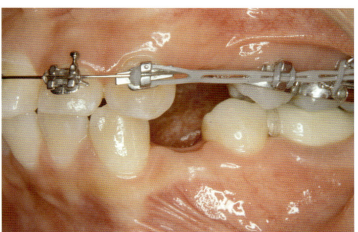
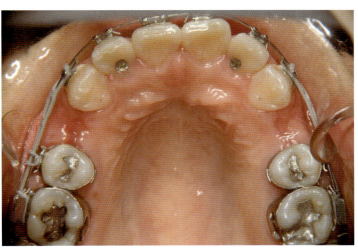
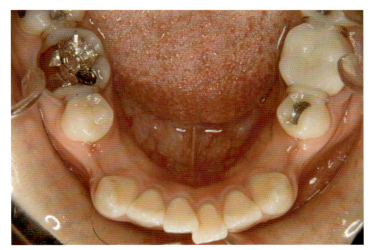

Fig. 11.1.**15–18**   Two months. 0.016 archwire. Initiate canine retraction with elastic chains.

15, 16 Labial and buccal views.   **17, 18** Occlusal views.

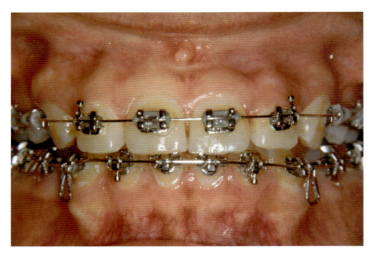
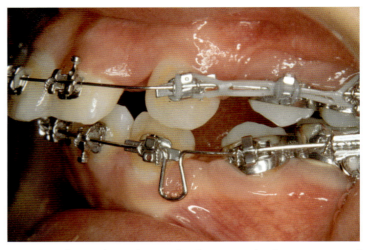

Fig. 11.1.**19, 20 Mandibular bracket placement at three months.** At six months, 16 × 22 SS closing loops archwire. Photographs taken at 9 months, showing retraction of mandibular anterior teeth.

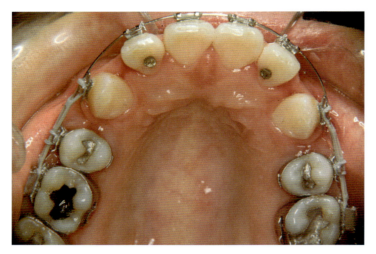
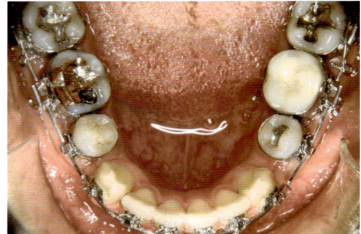

Fig. 11.1.**21, 22 Class III elastics worn 72 hours, then at night only with headgear.** Occlusal views.

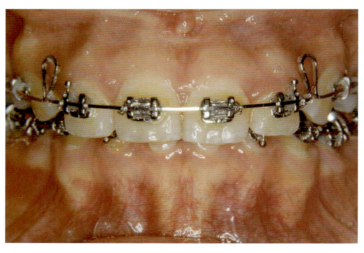
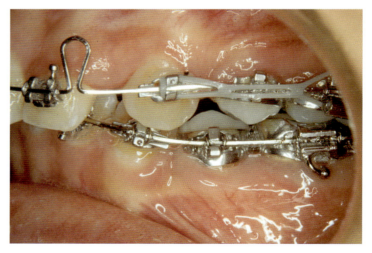

Fig. 11.1.**23, 24 Thirteen months of treatment.** Maxillary archwire is 18 × 25 SS with closing loops. Mandibular archwire is 17 × 25 SS with reverse curve of Spee. Labial and buccal views.

Clinical Case Studies

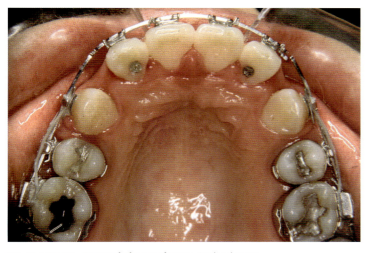
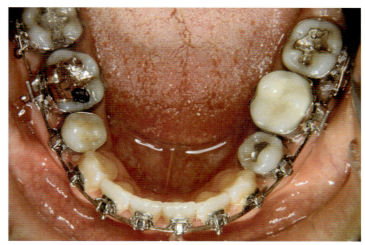

Fig. 11.1.**25, 26** **Stopped Class III elastics.** Occlusal views.

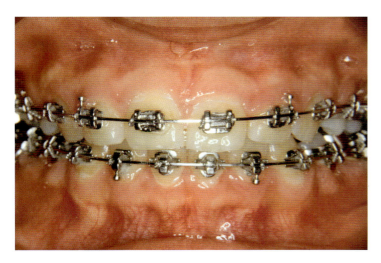
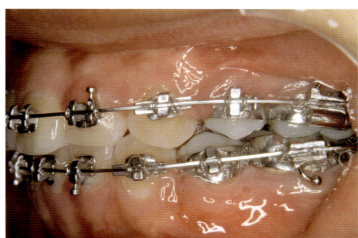

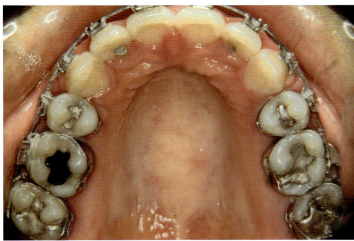
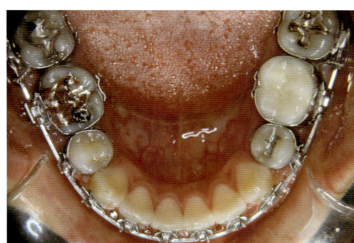

Fig. 11.1.**27–30** **Twenty months into treatment.**

27, 28 17 × 25 stainless steel finishing archwire. Labial and buccal views.

29, 30 Occlusal views.

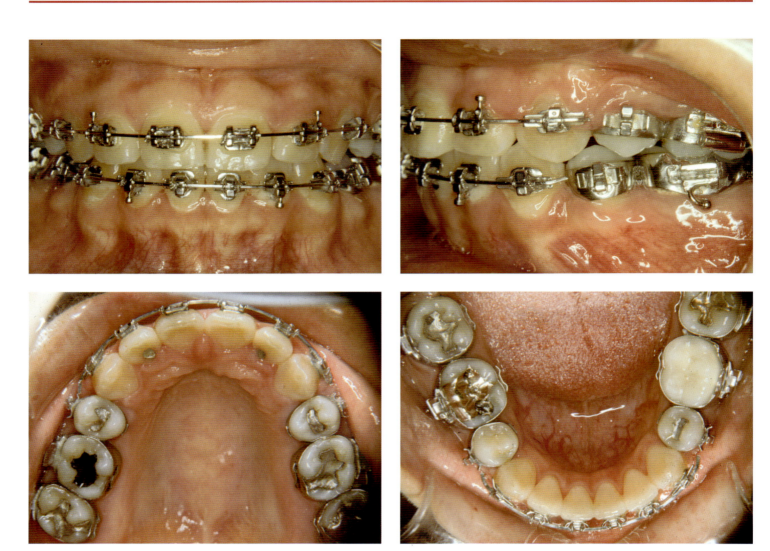

Fig. 11.1.**31–34** Twenty-three months, archwires sectioned for finishing elastics.

31, 32 Labial and buccal views.

33, 34 Occlusal views.

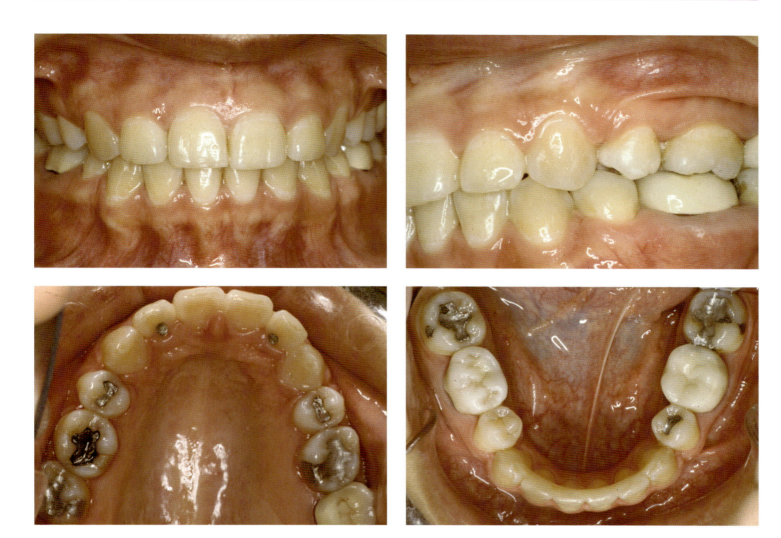
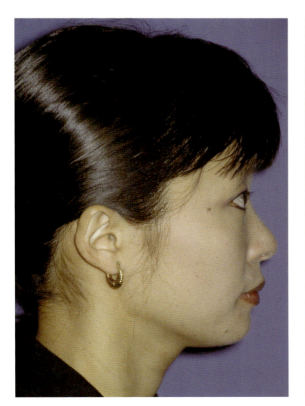
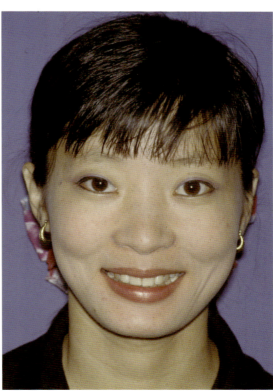

Fig. 11.1.**35 – 40 Twenty-four months, final results.**
35, 36 Labial and buccal views.
37, 38 Maxillary and mandibular arches, occlusal views.
39, 40 Facial photographs.

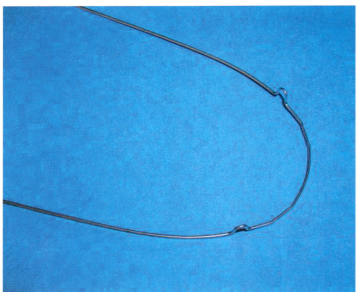

Fig. 11.1.**41** Wire for the retainer.

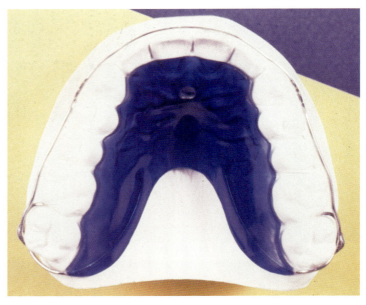

Fig. 11.1.**42** Retainer.

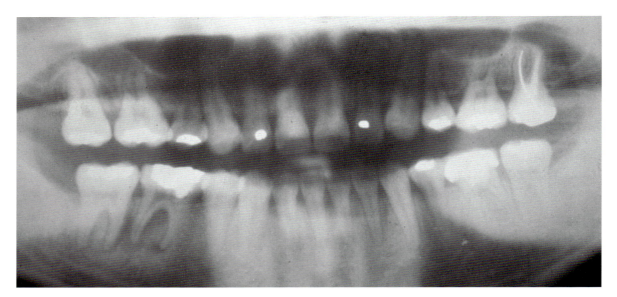

Fig. 11.1.**43** Posttreatment panoramic radiograph.

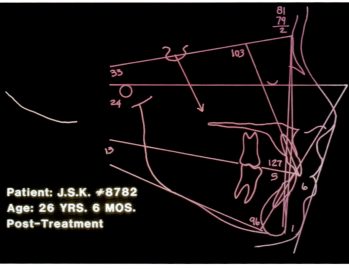

Fig. 11.1.**44** Posttreatment cephalometric radiograph.

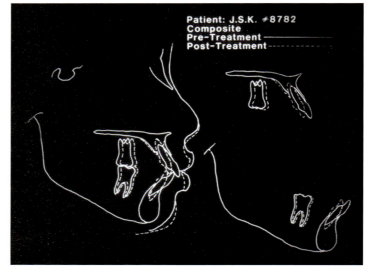

Fig. 11.1.**45** Composite tracings.

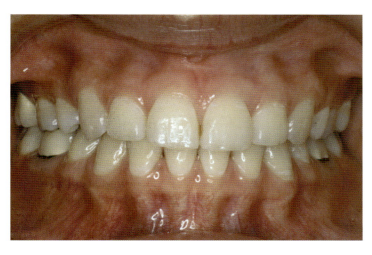
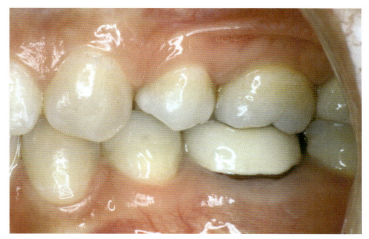
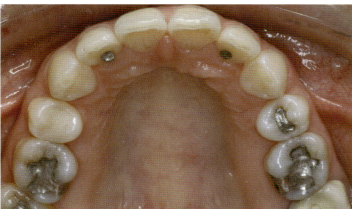
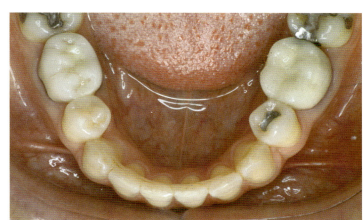
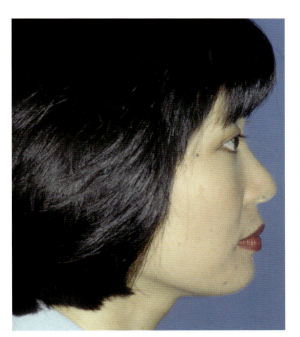
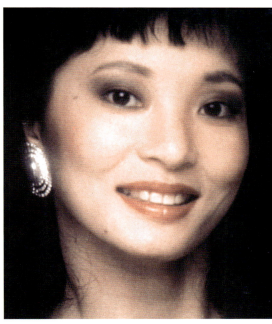

Fig. 11.1.**46–51**
Five years post treatment.
46, 47 Labial and buccal views.
48, 49 Maxillary and mandibular arches, occlusal views.
50, 51 Facial photographs.

Class II Division 2: Nonextraction Case Demonstrating Typical Nonextraction Mechanics

Case Study 11.2   D.P.: Class II Div. II Nonextraction Case
(Treated by Dr. Charles D. Alexander)

A male patient, 15 years 3 months old (Fig. 11.2.**1, 2**), presented with a severe class II Division 2 malocclusion (Fig. 11.2.**3–6**). His overbite was 13 mm, and overjet was 2 mm. To complicate the problem, the mandibular right central incisor was missing. His chief concern was the appearance of his anterior teeth. The panoramic radiograph demonstrated healthy bone support (Fig. 11.2.**7**). Cephalometrically, he presented with a very low mandibular plane angle (Fig. 11.2.**8**). The maxillary and mandibular incisors were excessively tipped lingually. His soft-tissue profile was slightly concave, as demonstrated with most Division 2 cases.

In determining the treatment plan, the major concerns were whether this patient had completed growth and his determination to follow instructions. He was presented with three treatment options. (1) Attempt to treat nonextraction, using a cervical facebow and Class II elastics; (2) extract maxillary first premolars and finish in a Class II molar relationship; (3) surgical mandibular advancement.

Addressing the missing mandibular incisor because of the small maxillary lateral incisors, the decision was made to treat the mandibular arch nonextraction and place the remaining central incisor in the middle of the arch.

The decision was made to begin treatment using the facebow for six months and then reevaluate the progress to see whether options (2) or (3) might be necessary. Because of the patient's excellent compliance and growth that occured, the patient was successfully treated with option 1: nonextraction, cervical facebow.

The maxillary arch was first bracketed, and a 0.016 in. NiTi archwire was placed. Note the unusual bracket placement on the anterior teeth (Fig. 11.2.**9, 10**). Because of the excessive overbite, the decision was made to place the incisor and canine brackets more incisally to help correct the overbite. The incredible flexibility of this archwire was demonstrated in the ligation of the anterior teeth. The cervical facebow was placed one month later.

At four months, note how the anterior teeth have leveled and flared (Fig. 11.2.**11–14**). The second archwire, a 0.016 in. SS wire with accentuated curve of Spee in the archwire, was placed. Because of the spaces that had been created with the initial wire, an elastic power chain was placed to close all spaces in the maxillary arch. Also at this time, the mandibular arch was bracketed, and a 0.016 in. NiTi wire was placed.

Normally, much focus is placed on *not* flaring the mandibular incisors. This type of case, however, is the exception to the rule because these teeth have been tipped abnormally lingually.

To verify the efficiency of this technique, note that in six months the maxillary arch is ready for its finishing archwire (Fig. 11.2.**15–18**). This 17 × 25 SS wire is bent with omega loops and a slight curve of Spee. After being heat treated, it is tied in with steel ligature wire and tied back. Again, breaking away from normal sequence Class II elastics were initiated at this time. Its purpose was to advance the mandibular incisors while helping hold the maxillary incisors.

At 11 months, a 16 × 22 NiTi with accentuated reverse curve of Spee was placed to help level the mandibular arch (Fig. 11.2.**19–22**). The cervical facebow and Class II elastics were continued.

The 14-month photographs show how both arches are leveling and the overbite is improving (Fig. 11.2.**23–26**). At this time, the 17 × 25 SS finishing archwire was placed in the mandibular arch.

At 24 months, the arches had been leveled by the stainless-steel wires to an overcorrected position. The remainder of the treatment was devoted to obtaining a concentric CR–CO relationship with Class II elastics, then finishing elastics for posterior settling.

Final results show a slight overcorrection of the overbite and the Class I posterior occlusion with the mandibular central incisor being placed in the center of the mandibular arch (Fig. 11.2.**27–30**). The patient's final photographs (Fig. 11.2.**31, 32**) show a balanced facial profile and an ideal smile.

The final panoramic (Fig. 11.2.**33**) and cephalometric (Fig. 11.2.**34**) radiographs show results together with the composite tracing (Fig. 11.2.**35**). The maxillary and mandibular archwire sequences are listed in Boxes 12.4 and 12.5. Intraoral (Fig. 11.2.**36–39**) and facial photographs (Fig. 11.2.**40, 41**) show the patient two years post treatment.

Box 11.4   D.P. – Maxillary Archwire Sequence.

1. 0.016 in. NiTi	4 months
2. 0.016 in. SS	2 months
3. 17 × 25 SS	18 months
Active treatment time	**24 months**

Box 11.5   D.P. – Mandibular Archwire Sequence.

None	4 months
1. 16 × 22 NiTi	2 months
2. 16 × 22 NiTi	7 months
3. 17 × 25 SS	12 months
Active treatment time	**21 months**

Clinical Case Studies 251

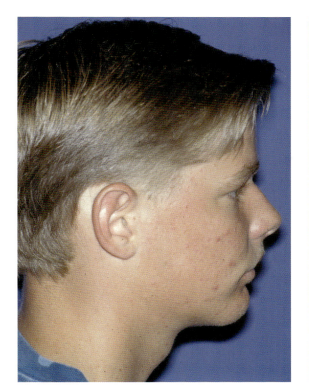
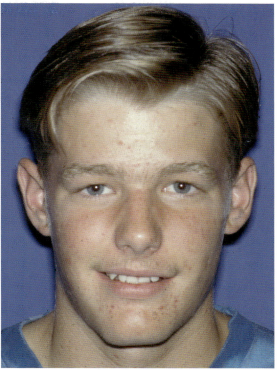

Fig. 11.2.**1,2** **Patient D.P.**
Age 15 years 3 months.

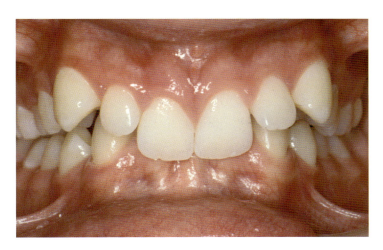
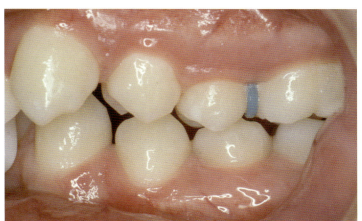

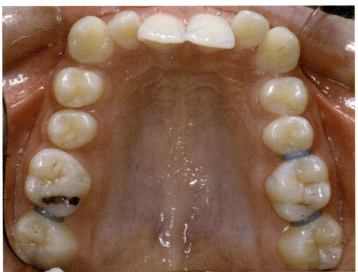
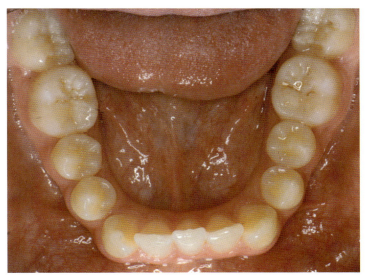

Fig. 11.2.**3–6** Class II Div. II, overbite 13 mm, overjet 2 mm. Missing mandibular central incisor.

3,4 Labial and buccal views. **5,6** Occlusal views.

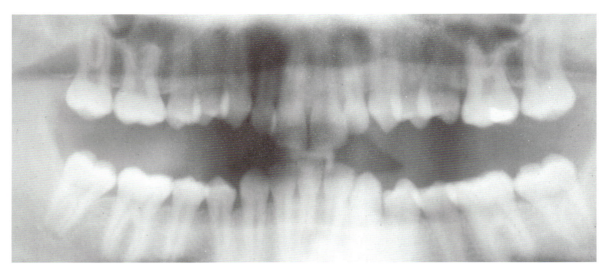

Fig. 11.2.**7** **Pretreatment panoramic radiograph.**

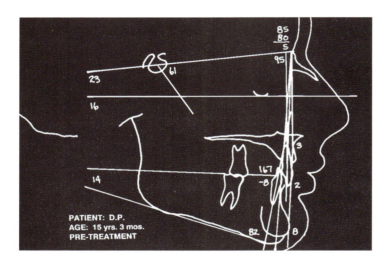

Fig. 11.2.**8** **Pretreatment cephalometric radiograph.**

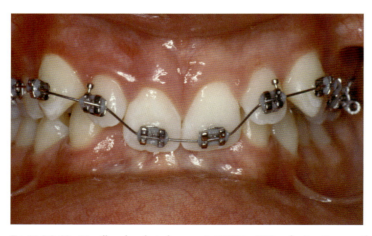 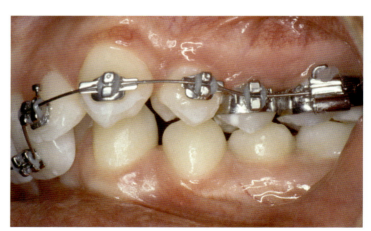

Fig. 11.2.**9, 10** **Maxillary bracket placement: 0.016 in. NiTi archwire.** One month: seated cervical facebow (labial and buccal views).

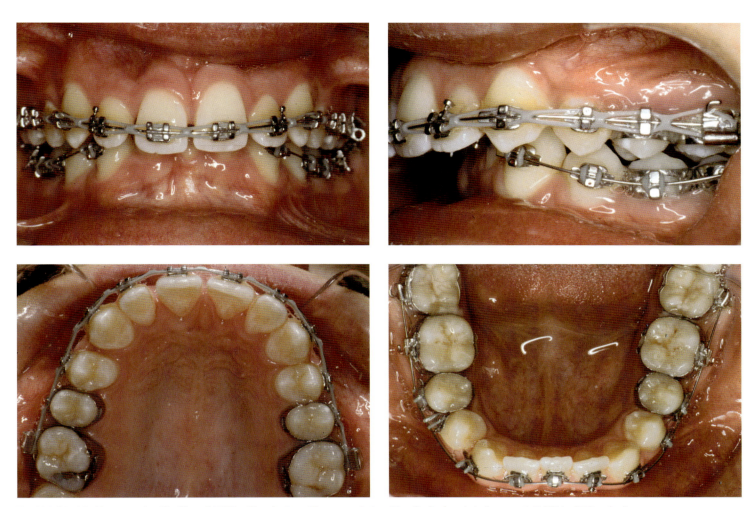

Fig. 11.2.**11–14** Four months. Maxillary 0.016 in. SS archwire with power chains. Mandibular bracket placement: 0.016 in. NiTi archwire.

11, 12 Labial and buccal views.

13, 14 Maxillary and mandibular arches (occlusal views).

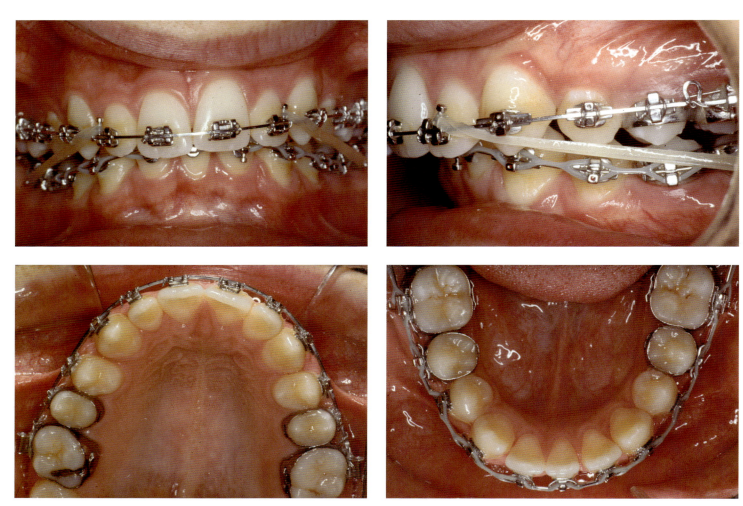

Fig. 11.2.**15–18** Six months. Maxillary **17×25 SS archwire. Mandibular 0.016 in. SS archwire. Begin Class 2 elastics.**

15, 16 Labial and buccal views.

17, 18 Maxillary and mandibular arches (occlusal views).

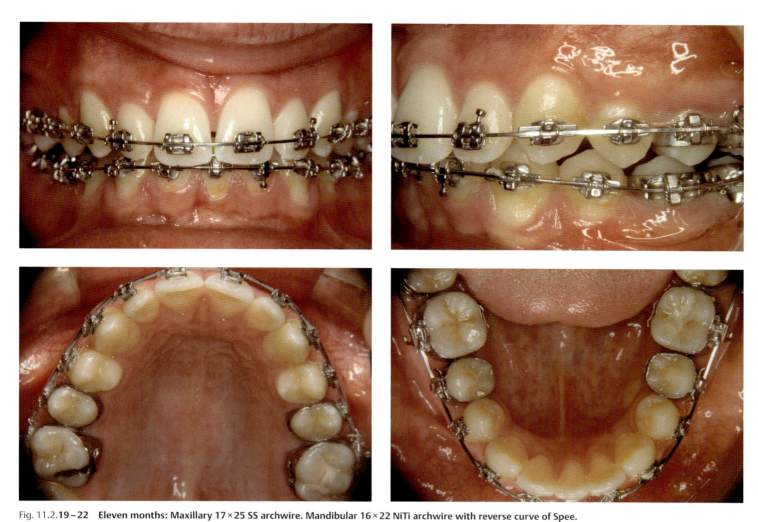

Fig. 11.2.**19 – 22** **Eleven months: Maxillary 17 × 25 SS archwire. Mandibular 16 × 22 NiTi archwire with reverse curve of Spee.**

19, 20 Labial and buccal views.

21, 22 Maxillary and mandibular arches (occlusal views).

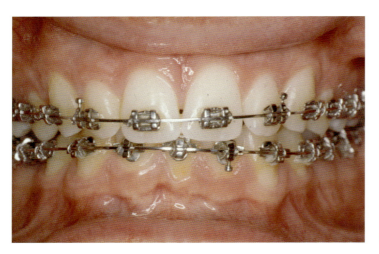
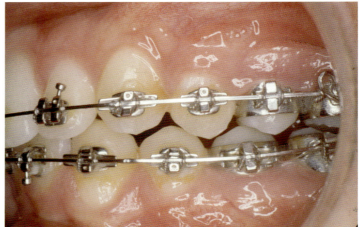
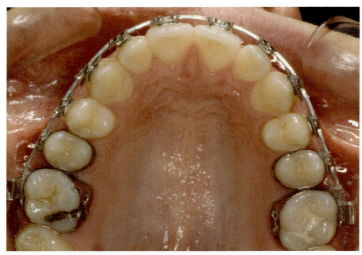
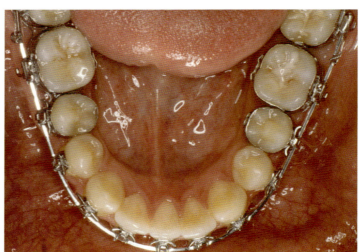

Fig. 11.2.**23–26** **Fourteen months: Maxillary and mandibular 17×25 SS archwires.**

23, 24 Labial and buccal views.

25, 26 Maxillary and mandibular arches (occlusal views).

Clinical Case Studies

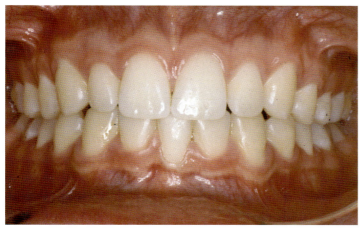
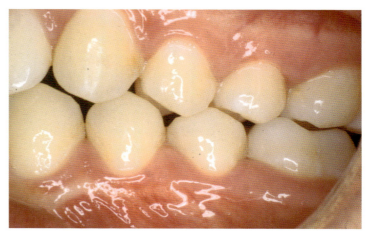
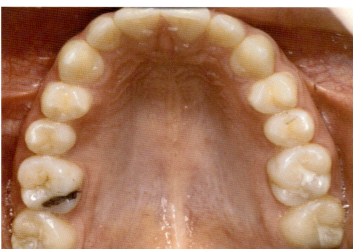
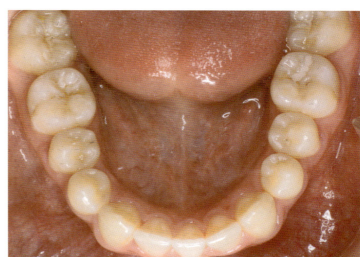
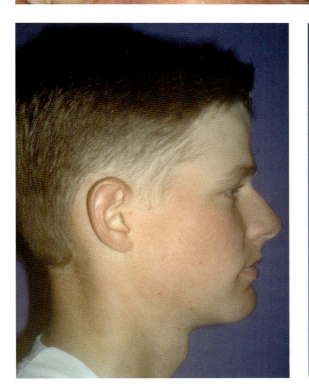
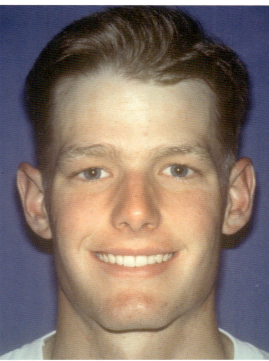

Fig. 11.2.**27 – 32 Twenty-four months, final results.**
27, 28 Labial and buccal views.
29, 30 Maxillary and mandibular arches (occlusal views).
31, 32 Facial photographs.

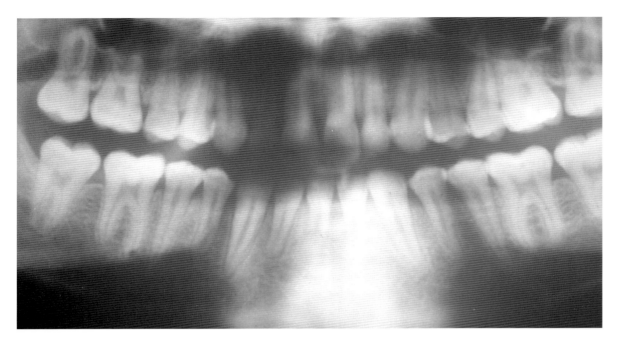

Fig. 11.2.33 Posttreatment panoramic radiograph.

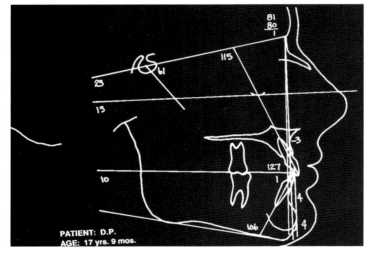

Fig. 11.2.34 Posttreatment cephalometric radiograph.

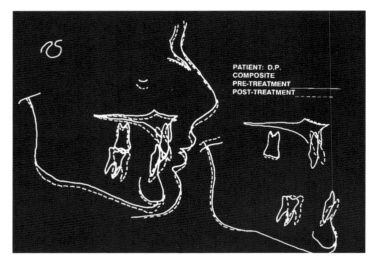

Fig. 11.2.35 Composite tracings.

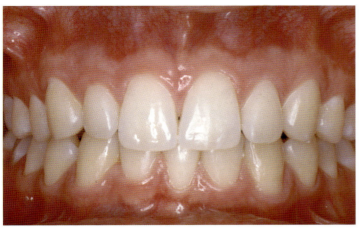
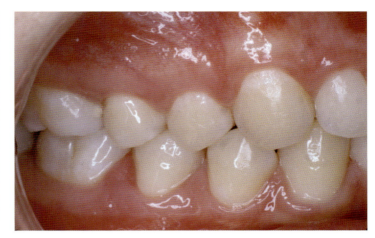
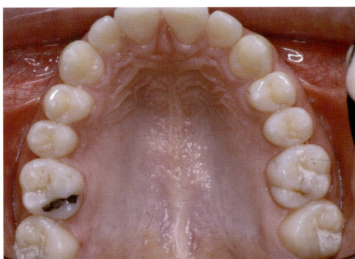
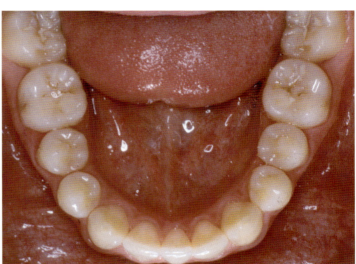
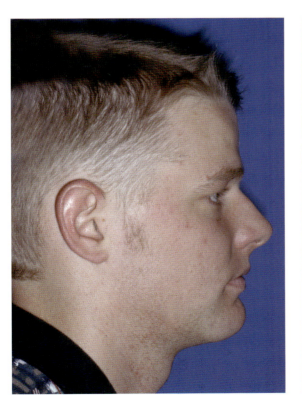
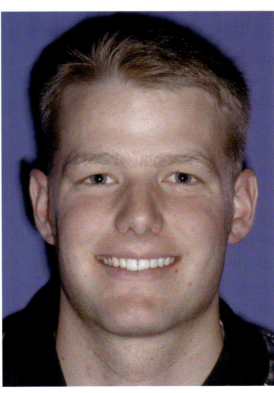

Fig. 11.2.**36–41** **Two years posttreatment.**
36, 37 Labial and buccal views.
38, 39 Maxillary and mandibular arches (occlusal views).
40, 41 Facial photographs.

Evidence-Based Studies

Having been privileged to teach in the Baylor Orthodontic Department over 40 years I have made a concerted effort to take beginning and final diagnostic records on most cases treated in my private office. Today, many new patients are the offspring of those treated years ago. This situation has allowed the taking of long-term records on a good number of patients. This library of potential knowledge has allowed many graduate students to investigate particular questions in orthodontics. To date, over 30 research studies have been done by Baylor graduate students, and additional research has been performed by students from the Universities of Texas, Tennessee, Alabama, Buffalo, Southern California, St. Louis, Juarez, Mexico, Manitoba, Canada and Munich, Germany.

As a result, it may be that no technique has been investigated using its creator's cases as thoroughly as the Alexander discipline. And the good news is that the results of these studies have changed many anecdotal clinical observations into evidence-based facts. The long-term stability of these cases has been reported (Glenn et al. 1987; Alexander JM 1995; Elms et al. 1996a,b; Bernstein 1999; Carcara 2001; Frasch 2002), and book chapters have been written to document the results (Alexander RG 1993; Alexander et al. 1997).

In addition, clinical observations on the technique have been published regarding patient compliance (Alexander RG 1996), vertical growth (Alexander RG 1966, 2000b) and nonsurgical adult rapid palatal expander (Alexander RG 2000a). My second book detailing this technique is titled "The 20 Principles of the Alexander Discipline". If the reader wants greater knowledge, details and explanations, this book will be beneficial and educational (Alexander RG 2008).

Box 11.6   D. P. – Individualized Forces.

Cervical facebow	15 months
Elastics:	
Class 2	16 months
Lateral Box	3 months
Finishing	2 months

References

Alexander CD, Alexander JM. Facebow correction of skeletal Class II discrepancies in the Alexander Discipline. Semin Orthod. 2001; 7(2): 80–84.

Alexander JM. A comparative study of orthodontic stability in Class I extraction cases. [Master's thesis]. Waco TX: Baylor University Department of Orthodontics; 1995.

Alexander RG. The effects on tooth position and maxillofacial vertical growth during scoliosis treatment with the Milwaukee Brace: an initial study. Am J Orthod. 1966; 52(3): 161–189.

Alexander RG. The Vari-Simplex Discipline. J Clin Orthod. 1983; 17(6): 380–392.

Alexander RG. Vari-Simplex Discipline orthodontic technique. In: Graber LW, ed. Orthodontics: state of the art, essence of the science. St. Louis: Mosby; 1986a: 222–232.

Alexander RG. The Alexander discipline, contemporary concepts and philosophies. Ormco Corp, Orange, CA; 1986b.

Alexander RG. Countdown to retention. J Clin Orthod. 1987; 21(8): 526–527.

Alexander RG. A practical approach to arch form. Clinical Impressions. 1992a; 1(3): 2–5.

Alexander RG. The lip bumper alternative.... Clinical Impressions. 1992b; 1(1): 6–9.

Alexander RG. Treatment and retention for long-term stability. In: Retention and stability in orthodontics. Philadelphia: WB Saunders; 1993: 115–134.

Alexander RG. Retention, a practical approach to that critical last step to stability. Clinical Impressions. 1997; 6(3): 14–17.

Alexander RG. Adult rapid palatal expansion. World J Orthod. 2000a; 1(2): 157–163.

Alexander RG. The role of occlusal forces in open-bite treatment. J Clin Orthod. 2000b; 34(1): 23–29.

Alexander RG. The Principles of the Alexander Discipline. Semin Orthod. 2001; 7(2): 62–66.

Alexander RG. THe 20 Principles of the Alexander Discipline. Hanover Park: Quintessence; 2008.

Alexander RG, Alexander CM, Alexander CD, Alexander JM. Creating the compliant patient. J Clin Orthod. 1996; 30(9): 493–497.

Alexander RG. Glenn G, Alexander JM. The quest for long term stability. In: Orthodontics for the next millennium. Ormco, Orange, CA; 1997: 425–441.

Bagden MA. The Alexander Discipline, appliance design and construction. Semin Orthod. 2001; 7(2): 74–79.

Bernstein RI. Leveling the curve of Spee with a continuous archwire technique—a long-term cephalometric analysis. Am J Ortho 2007; 131(3), 363–371.

Buschang PH, Horton-Reuland SJ, Legler L, Nevant C. Nonextraction approach to tooth size arch length discrepancies with the Alexander Discipline. Semin Orthod. 2001; 7(2): 117–131.

Carcara SJ. Leveling the curve of Spee with a continuous archwire technique—a long-term study cast analysis. The Alexander Discipline. Semin Orthod. 2001; 7(2): 90–99.

Elms TN, Buschang PH, Alexander RG. Long-term stability of Class II Division 2 non-extraction cervical facebow therapy: I. Model analysis. Am J Orthod Dentofacial Orthop. 1996a; 109: 271–276.

Elms TN, Buschang PH, Alexander RG. Long-term stability of Class II Division 2 non-extraction cervical facebow therapy: II. Cephalometric analysis. Am J Orthod Dentofacial Orthop. 1996b; 109: 386–392.

Felton JM, Sinclair PM, Jones DL, Alexander RG. A computerized analysis of the shape and stability of mandibular arch form. Am J Orthod. 1987; 92: 478–483.

Ferris T, Buschang P, Alexander RG, Boley J. Long-term stability of combined rapid palatal expansion–lip bumper therapy followed by full fixed appliances. Am J Orthod. 2005; 128(3): 310–325.

Frasch I. Comparison of bionator and cervical facebow: skeletal and dental long term results. Germany: University of Munich; 2002. [Unpublished].

Glenn G, Sinclair PM, Alexander RG. Non-extraction orthodontic therapy: post-treatment dental and skeletal stability. Am J Orthod. 1987; 92(4): 321–328.

Guymon M. A cephalometric evaluation of two-phase treatment of Class II Division I malocclusion. [Master's thesis]. Waco TX: Baylor University Department of Orthodontics; 1990.

Haltom T. Finishing and retention procedures in the Alexander Discipline. Semin Orthod. 2001; 7(2): 132–137.

McKelvain GD. An arch form designed for use with a specific straight wire orthodontic appliance. [Master's thesis]. Waco TX: Baylor University Department of Orthodontics; 1982.

Nevant C, Buschang PH, Alexander RG, Steffen JM. Lip bumper therapy for gaining arch length. Am J Orthod. 1991; 100: 330–336.

Papandreas S. Physiologic drift of the mandibular dentition following first premolar extractions. Angle Orthod. 1993; 63(2): 127–134.

Plunk MD. A cephalometric evaluation of the effects of early headgear therapy. [Master's thesis]. Waco TX: Baylor University Department of Orthodontics; 1985.

Romine L. A cephalometric evaluation of the effects of cervical facebow on the craniofacial complex. [Master's thesis]. Waco TX: Baylor University Department of Orthodontics; 1982.

Trammell CD. The combined application of negative torque and angulation in the mandibular arch to improve control and increase non-extraction therapy. [Master's thesis]. Waco TX: Baylor University Department of Orthodontics; 1980.

Williams R. Eliminating lower retention. J Clin Orthod. 1985; 19(5): 342–349.

12 Implants and Orthodontics

Magdalena Kotova

Anchorage is a fundamental problem in the treatment of malocclusions. The loading of the anchorage unit is based on the condition of static balance defined by Newton. Newton's Third Law outlined in 1687 (action and reaction are equal and opposite) applies to the forces affecting tissues during orthodontic treatment. The force of orthodontic or orthopedic appliances changes the position of individual teeth and their groups as well as the shape and position of the dental arches. To make this force work in the planned direction, with the planned size, and for the planned time, it is necessary to reduce or completely eliminate unwanted reciprocal effects by a reliable anchorage and to respect the principles of orthodontic biomechanics at the same time. A reliable anchorage of orthodontic appliances influences the result of orthodontic treatment significantly. Anchorage can be classified in many ways: intraoral and extraoral anchorage, dental and extradental anchorage, and so on. The simplest way to classify orthodontic anchorage is as dental and skeletal.

Dental Anchorage

When an orthodontic force is applied, individual teeth or their groups are used for the reduction of unwanted reactive forces. In reality, absolute dental anchorage does not practically exist; with the help of dental anchorage we only reduce the movement of specific teeth to achieve the desired movement of others. Dental anchorage depends on the number and quality of the teeth that can be used, and on the state of their periodontium and the alveolar process bone. The morphology of tooth roots that are used as dental anchorage differs from person to person as well as the surface of the periodontal ligament that can be used. Jarabak and Fizzel wished to express the force of dental anchorage, so in 1972 they created a table of anchorage values for the permanent dentition (Jarabak and Fizzel, 1972). For dental anchorage, the lower central incisor has the lowest value (1 unit), the first permanent molar has the highest (10 units). If the anchorage is lost during orthodontic treatment, the planned correction of the malocclusion anomaly will not be achieved. Headgear, intermaxillary elastics, or the Nance appliance can be used together with dental anchorage, but a great disadvantage of these complementary appliances is the fact that the disciplined and reliable cooperation of the patient is needed.

Skeletal Anchorage

An anchorage device inserted into the bone can be used to block unwanted effects of orthodontic forces. Skeletal anchorage can be used as a separate anchorage unit or in combination with teeth.

Skeletal anchorage is based on the principle of *osseointegration* as described in 1977 by Brånemark. His 10-year experience with osseointegration of dental implants meant a radical turning point that enlarged the treatment possibilities in orthodontics (Brånemark et al. 1977). Brånemark started his research in the 1950's. While studying the intravascular dynamics of blood circulation in bone marrow, he found that it is difficult to remove a residue of bone tissue from repeatedly used titanium chambers because it adheres very tightly. Brånemark and colleagues published a study in 1964 in which they confirmed that it is possible to have a stable anchorage of titanium in the vital bone without negative side-effects (Cope, 2005).

Osseointegration was first characterized as integration of inert alloplastic material into the bone; nowadays it implies direct contact between the bone and an inserted implant. Roberts expanded the concept of osseointegration to include no fibrous tissue between the implant and the bone, high tone on percussion, absence of physiological drift, no movement under orthodontic load, and the functional equivalent of a dental ankylosis. An implant fulfilling these criteria represents the dream of an ideal absolute anchorage that resists the force of both orthodontic and orthopedic loads, stays stable, and has no influence on the teeth.

The first attempt to use orthodontic skeletal anchorage dates back to 1945. Gainsforth and Highley (1945) worked with six dogs. They inserted screws made of Vitallium into a hole created in the mandibular ramus, and moved maxillary canines distally. However, all the screws were lost within 16–31 days. This experiment was not successful, but studies continued.

In 1969, Linkow advised the use of an endosseal blade implant placed in the area of the first permanent molar that could be used for both prosthetic rehabilitation and temporary orthodontic anchorage (Linkow, 1970).

In 1980, Creekmore and Eklund were probably the first to use a temporarily inserted surgical bone screw made of Vitallium in a patient for orthodontic anchorage only. They inserted it below the spina nasalis anterior and intruded upper incisors to it; the result was an intrusion of 6 mm (Creekmore and Eklund 1983).

Block and Hoffman used an onplant as orthodontic anchorage in 1989, and Wehrbein and Merz introduced palatal implants that were used for the retraction of the upper front segment in 1996 (Wehrbein, Merz et al, 1996).

Nowadays we can use a large group of temporary anchorage devices that originated in the direct modification of orthopedic osseosynthetic methods, in addition to implants that can be used

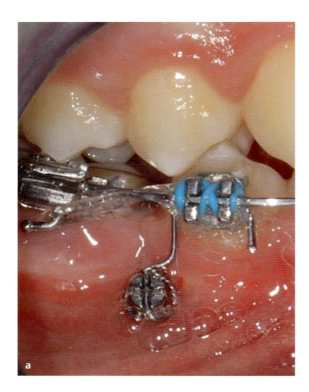
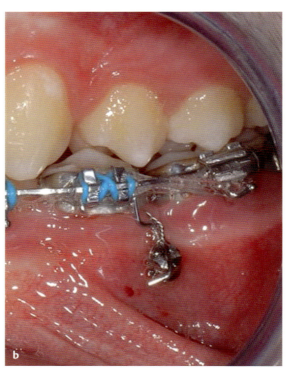

Fig. 12.**1** Bilateral mesial movement of the first molars with vestibular miniscrew anchorage, to hold the bicuspids.

as orthodontic anchorage based on osseointegration. These include wire ligature anchorage and skeletal anchorage systems with bone plates and miniscrews. Melsen and colleagues introduced wire orthodontic anchorage ligatures in 1998 (Melsen et al. 1988); Sugawara presented a skeletal anchorage system with bone plates and screws in 1992 (Sugawara, 2000). Kanomi inserted a modified bone screw between the roots of lower incisors and intruded them by 6 mm (Kanomi 1997). The term "mini-implant" appeared in the literature for the first time. The search for the simplest and the least invasive methods of inserting orthodontic anchorage implants that would be least trouble for the patient lasted until the middle of the 1990.

Temporary anchorage devices include all kinds of implants, screws, pins, and onplants, inserted solely to serve as orthodontic anchorage. They are removed after use. Prosthetic endosseal implants are also used when they are no longer needed as orthodontic anchorage; their function is prosthetic reconstruction.

In the literature, temporary anchorage devices have been classified according to the prevailing type of anchorage in bone either as osseointegration anchorage (retromolar implant, palatal implant, onplant) or as systems with mechanical retention (wire ligatures, bone plates, miniscrews, and mini-implants). This classification is now largely of didactic use and is valid to only a limited degree; osseointegration is even in systems with mechanical retention.

Temporary skeletal anchorage can be used in two ways: direct or indirect. *Direct* anchorage means that the system is loaded with orthodontic force directly—e.g., by means of a coil spring tightened between a miniscrew and a distalized tooth. *Indirect* anchorage means that the system is fixed in a block together with one or more teeth or with the intraoral arch of a fixed appliance; the orthodontic force works through these linked anchorage devices and affects a target tooth or teeth.

The **applications** of skeletal anchorage in orthodontics are:

- Orthodontic anchorage by temporarily inserted special screws: miniscrew implant, palatal implant
- Dental implant used temporarily as orthodontic anchorage
- Skeletal anchorage for orthodontic use (nonpalatal, out of the alveolar process bone)

The following **anatomical regions** are suited for application of skeletal anchorage:

- The interradicular septum of the alveolar process (Fig. 12.**1**)
- The supra-apical area
- The infrazygomatic area
- The retromolar areas
- The anterior palate (median or paramedian depending on the age of the patient)

The **indications** for skeletal orthodontic anchorage are generally:

- Distal or mesial movements of teeth or space closure from distal or mesial. The space closure can be achieved, for example, with coil springs anchored on vestibularly inserted miniscrews (Figs. 12.**2**, 12.**3**).
- Intrusion of incisors or elongated molars disturbing the occlusion as premature contact teeth (Fig. 12.**4**). Intrusion can also be necessary in cases of elongated molars because of loss of antagonists, or even in skeletal open-bite cases.
- Extrusion of teeth, especially of impacted canines or molars (Fig. 12.**5**).
- Uprighting of tipped molars, especially after loss of neighboring teeth, before prosthetic reconstruction.
- Midline correction in cases of dental midline shift.

At present, endosseus implants are predominantly used for skeletal anchorage purposes. The osseointegrated implants remain stable under orthodontic and orthopedic load conditions. They can be used as skeletal anchorage elements for orthodontic and orthopedic treatment purposes.

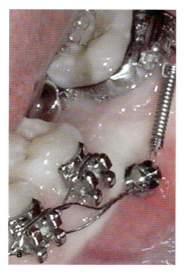 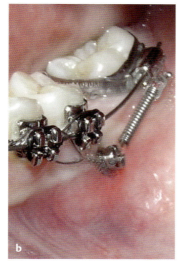 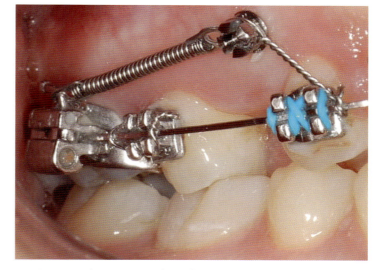

Fig. 12.**2** Mesial movement of the second molar with coil spring anchorage to miniscrew.
a Before treatment.
b After space closing.

Fig. 12.**3** Mesial movement with vestibular anchored coil spring.

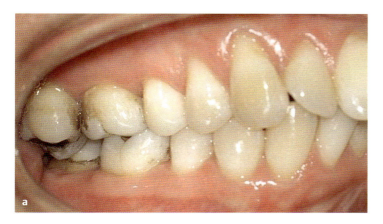 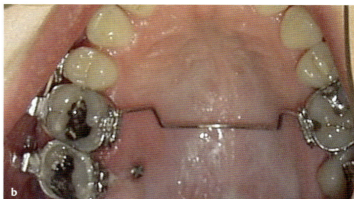

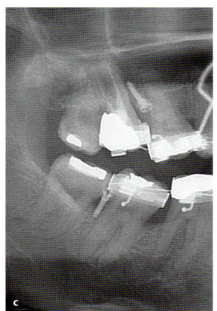

Fig. 12.**4** Intrusion of extruded upper second molar.
a Extruded second molar.
b Space after extraction of first bicuspids is closed and the second molar is intruded.
c Radiograph shows the interradicular upper and lower miniscrews used to intrude the upper molar and upright the lower second molar.
d After finishing the treatment.

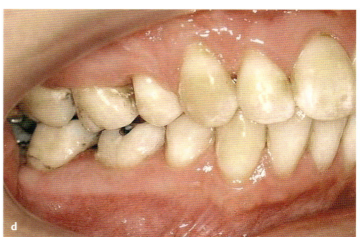

264 Implants and Orthodontics

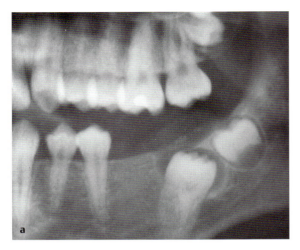
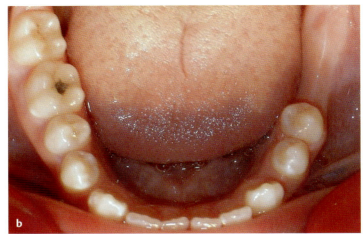
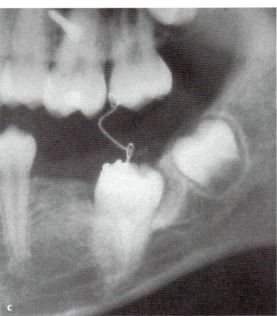
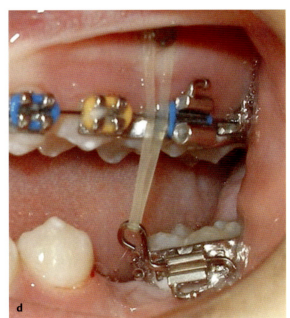
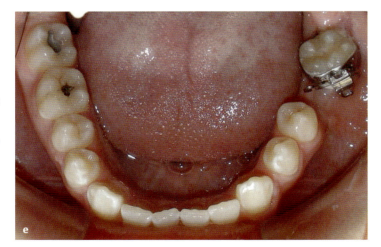

Fig. 12.**5 Extrusion of impacted molar with miniscrew anchorage.**
a Radiograph shows agenesis of the tooth −6, impaction of −7, and a supernumerary molar.
b Lower dental arch before treatment.
c After bonding a bracket onto the impacted tooth and insertion of a miniscrew interradicularly between +5 and +6, and traction on −7.
d Extrusion of −7.
e Before treatment with multibracket appliance in the lower arch.

Miniscrew Implant

We encounter various terms for skeletal cortical anchorage with miniscrews in the literature: microimplant, microimplant anchorage, microscrews, mini-implants for orthodontic anchorage, mini-implant system, mini-implant, minipin, miniscrew, miniscrew anchorage system, miniscrew implant, ortho-implant, orthodontic anchorage implant, orthodontic implants, orthodontic miniscrews, ortho TAD (Temporary anchorage device), small titanium screws, titanium implant anchorage, and many others. In this chapter we will uniformly use the term *miniscrew*. Miniscrews are largely a product of osteosynthesis technology (Fig. 12.**6**).

Miniscrews are most widely used for skeletal orthodontic anchorage. They represent a single-phase (unburrowed) temporarily inserted implant system. In 2007, Lietz indicated that he was using more than 30 systems of miniscrews. Their use is very easy, incurring only the minimum of trouble for patients. Miniscrews have the great advantage that they can be used in the full dentition because they are small and can easily be inserted between teeth roots. They can be loaded immediately after insertion.

Miniscrews offer a great advantage for orthodontic treatment, but it must be recognized that the basic mechanical principles still apply. The easier the use of reliable stationary anchorage is, the more cautious the active orthodontic movement must be. Practically all of the applied force anchored on a stably inserted miniscrew is transferred to the periodontal ligament. On the other hand, we cannot rely on absolute anchorage when using miniscrews. Kinzinger et al. (2008) reported that miniscrews inserted into the palate and used as a combined anchorage for distalization of molars with the Distal Jet appliance do not provide a stationary anchorage. The combination of dental anchorage created by two premolars and two miniscrews inserted into the palate is sufficient in clinical use for distalizing molars, but miniscrews have a tendency to lean back and extrude slightly. Liou and colleagues described the same result; in 2004 he pointed out that when miniscrews are continuously loaded by orthodontic force, the anchorage in not stable at all (Liou et al. 2004).

What Are the Requirements of Orthodontic Anchorage with Miniscrews?

When choosing miniscrews we must take into consideration their length, their diameter, the shape of the head, the material, and the shape of threads and their height; we must also consider whether they are self-tapping (ST) or self-drilling (SD) and whether it is necessary to predrill. Another important consideration is how technically complicated the method of inserting a miniscrew and the economic indications are. Miniscrews must be made of biocompatible materials. Their reduced size is a great advantage for safe interradicular insertion.

Primary stability should be established after insertion, and immediate loading with forces up to 0,5–1 N is optimal. When a miniscrew is used, clinical results must be the same as or better than with other types of anchorage. The *removal* of a miniscrew should be a simple process. When choosing orthodontic anchorage miniscrews, we have to consider whether the system is known and well established, whether its structural elements have been further developed, and whether we can find references to its use

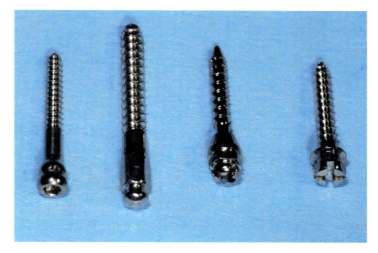

Fig. 12.**6** **Miniscrews with various bodies and various heads.** On the right a head with a slot.

in the literature. One must choose a system that has after-sales service and back-up. Systems without an EU certificate (CE) cannot be used in EU countries; an FDA certificate is required in the United States. We need long-term quality at the required level.

The application of a miniscrew is considered to be the least invasive method; the insertion itself is short-term. Nevertheless, we can face complications leading to loss of the miniscrew, which necessitates modification of the orthodontic treatment plan. Valid indications and recommendations for implant insertion in prosthetic dentistry must be respected and one must not underestimate the potential risk of TAD peri-implantitis because of microbial infection. Care is needed with the initial loading of a miniscrew, especially in the first 6 weeks after insertion: during this period the miniscrew can be easily overloaded and become unstable.

Considerations in the Use of Miniscrews

1. Material
2. Surface of the implant
3. Shape and length (head, neck, platform, body)
4. Accessories (e.g., tools for inserting miniscrews)
5. Factors influencing the clinical success of miniscrews.

Material

At present miniscrews are made of titanium or surgical steel. The first screws used for skeletal anchorage in the middle of the twentieth century were made of Vitallium, a biocompatible alloy of cobalt, chromium and molybdenum (CoCrMo) that was used for the reinforcement of partial dentures. The alloy did not stand the test of time and it is no longer used.

Another material that appeared in implantology is surgical steel. This is biocompatible but in terms of the formation of connective tissue between the bone and the surface of steel implant, this also is not recommended for dental implants. Steel is recommended for the anchorage of orthodontic systems as it has a higher elastic modulus than titanium; when bent, a steel miniscrew does not break easily. It is also reported that steel miniscrews are easily removed from the bone because they are not osseointegrated; this is probably the reason why there is a high rate of failure.

In some cases it is possible to accept surgical steel for temporary skeletal anchorage, but its use is not preferred.

Titanium and its alloys do not have any side-effects on vital cells and are the best materials for making various types of implants and miniscrews. Titanium alloys (for instance, Ti-6Al-4V, Ti 5) are said to have more advantageous characteristics than commercial pure titanium (solidity, tensility, wear hardness, resistance to corrosion, better surface). Screws made of pure titanium (Ti 1, Ti 4) break more often during insertion or removal (Müller-Hartwich et al. 2006). In contrast even very small parts of implants made of titanium alloys (e.g., threads) are strong and resilient.

Surface of Implant

The success of implant insertion has been evaluated mainly in prosthetic patients, but this information can help us to understand problems connected with temporarily inserted orthodontic anchorage devices. The result of an implant treatment depends on careful work, on the quality and quantity of the bone, and on the type, shape, and surface of the intraosseal part of the implant. A rough surface and a larger surface of the implant help osseointegration. The moment during the removal of such an implant is higher than that of an implant with smooth surface. The **modification** of an implant surface can be additive, as when a coating is added, or subtractive, as when microscopic particles are removed from the surface of an implant by etching or sandblasting.

The reaction of the bone after insertion of an implant depends on the physical characteristics and morphology of the implant surface. The adhesion of blood coagulum that occurs after insertion of an implant depends on the wettability of its surface; with titanium the wettability can be markedly increased by subtractive modification.

A rough and rugged surface of an implant makes adhesion of the bone cells easier (the rough surface of titanium alloy T 5 is connected with the activity of osteoblasts), but it can cause inflammation of the surrounding soft tissues. For this reason, new implants were developed whose apical part is modified by etching while the rest of the surface is smooth (a so-called *hybrid* design).

Immediately after the insertion of a miniscrew implant, its **retention** is purely mechanical and depends on how the threads cut into the bone, which is compressed by the miniscrew. Primary stability of an implant is achieved in bone of good quality. In this phase the stability depends on its shape and not on the material of which the miniscrew is made. In 3–6 weeks from insertion, the surrounding bone is **remodeled**. This interval is critical for its possible loss of the miniscrew/implant. The least direct contact between the bone and the implant surface is available in this period.

During healing, osteoblasts form fibrous and lamellar bone around the inserted implant, and so-called *secondary stability* is achieved. This is highly dependent on the implant material and the modification of its surface.

The results of studies on the **healing** of dental implants can be assumed valid for orthodontic anchorage miniscrews. However, because their function differs from the function of dental implants, their shapes and surface modifications will differ as well. When inserting miniscrews, the effect of an orthodontic force on remodeling of the surrounding bone and their limited use as anchorage devices must be taken into account.

As the interpretation of the concept of "osseointegration" develops, it is noted that with miniscrews inorganic material is firmly fixed into the living bone when it is functionally loaded, and we can also remove it easily. Histological studies demonstrate that direct contact is formed between bone and a miniscrew made of titanium and titanium alloys, and that the bone is retained on the surface of the miniscrew (Berens et al. 2006; Büchter 2006; Melsen and Costa 2000).

In contrast to present dental implants, the surface of a miniscrew is more or less polished and no further special modification is recommended because it would reduce the amount of direct contact between the newly formed bone and the surface of the miniscrew. With miniscrews the achievement of reliable *primary* stability is a must (macroretention); there is no requirement for long-term stability of orthodontic miniscrews.

Shape and Length of Miniscrews

A miniscrew consists of a head, a gingival neck, and a body with threads. The structure and size of miniscrews was the subject of a long development process seeking the optimal shape. The **length** of the whole implant is the sum of the lengths of the head, the neck, and the body, though in practice when we speak of the length of a miniscrew we refer to the length of the body only. A single system usually offers miniscrews of different lengths or of different body diameters, but the shape and size of the head and the gingival part of the neck remain the same.

At present three lengths of miniscrews are recommended: 6, 8, and 10 mm with one body diameter of 1.6 mm. Because the quality of insertion of a miniscrew is determined by the layer of cortical bone, miniscrews longer than 10 mm are not needed. On the other hand, miniscrews shorter than 6 mm do not guarantee firm fixation in the bone.

The Head of a Miniscrew

The head of a miniscrew is made in a way that enables the fixation of elastics and ligatures, attachment of a partial intraoral arch of a fixed appliance, and so on. To accommodate this there are special head **variations** for every potential orthodontic application, including hook tops, ball-shaped heads, heads with a hole or eyelet, simple slots, or cross-shaped slots. When we choose the shape of a miniscrew head, it must be clear what the future use of the miniscrew will be. We need to specify whether it will be used for direct or indirect anchorage and gauge how difficult the indirect anchorage will be. Ideally the head enables the fixation of a simple active force as well as of a round or a square wire. Miniscrews with simple slot or cross-shaped slot heads are probably the most often used.

A miniscrew with a *ball-shaped* head is suitable for a simple direct anchorage for mesial movement and distal moment or intrusion. The ability to attach a chain or a ligature from different directions is a great advantage of this type of head. If we use a head with a *hook*, the attachment of traction is easy, but if the miniscrew turns it can easily slip. Traction can move or slip down during later adjustments of the miniscrew by turning or tightening. With a complicated design of a miniscrew head, the risk of cracking or breaking a part of the head while changing orthodontic traction is higher.

Miniscrews with cross-shaped *slots* or simple slots are optimal for a simple or a combined indirect anchorage. The presence of the slot makes insertion easier and this modification enables a combination of attachment of simple elastics together with a round or a square wire. A square wire should be attached in such a way that it does not cause torque; if it does, the miniscrew will start to move.

The most advantageous head modification is therefore a *cross-shaped* slot. This has the widest use and the risk of head damage is low. If the square wire is suitably modified, the square slot enables better control of orthodontic tooth movement as well as providing a skeletal anchorage unit. When choosing a miniscrew with a cross-shaped or a simple slot, attention must be paid to the size of the slot. Apart from other considerations, a wire inserted into the slot should not overtop the surface of the head.

The **size** of miniscrews with various head shapes should be reduced as much as possible so as to cause the least trouble for the patient. The simultaneous attachment of an active force needs to be easy and reliable. The tools necessary for inserting miniscrews differ with the shape of the head, and reliable insertion is a prerequisite for successful function. Repeatable tool sterilization is an absolutely necessary feature. Tools have to be simple, easy to work with, and available on the dental market, and during manipulation they must fix the miniscrew reliably.

Transgingival (Transmucosal) Portion

The transgingival portion, also known as the gingival *neck,* is a critical part of a miniscrew as it has to prevent microorganisms from penetrating into the bone and causing inflammation. After insertion of a miniscrew, the mucosa should adapt as closely as possible to the miniscrew to seal the area.

The shape of the neck of miniscrews in use is either conical or cylindrical (square, hexagonal, or octagonal), or there may be no neck between the threads and the head part. When a miniscrew is inserted with angulation toward the surface of the cortical bone, the miniscrew neck part should not compress the mucosa, which should heal around the neck part as closely as possible. The thickness of the mucosa varies from 1.5 to 4.0 mm; the height of a miniscrew neck part is usually between 1.0 and 3.0 mm. We often insert a miniscrew in the maxilla and mandible between the roots of the first and second premolars, where the average thickness of soft tissues is usually 2.0 mm. If we insert a miniscrew in some other area, we should first examine the thickness of the soft tissues at the site of insertion. For economic reasons, we usually do not have many types of miniscrews in stock, so it is not possible to choose a miniscrew according to the actual clinical finding. In practice, the most advantageous neck shape seems to be a cone with height of 2.0 mm. If the diameter of the head is larger than that of the neck, a void results between the miniscrew and the soft tissue that could provide a site for inflammation. For hygienic reasons, therefore, it is appropriate for the head and the gingival neck of the miniscrew to be the same size or for the diameter of the head to be smaller.

Platform

There may be a platform between the head and the neck of a miniscrew. The main purpose of the platform is to prevent irritation of the surrounding gingival tissues from the attached elastic or coil springs with resultant overgrowth.

The Body with Threads (Intraosseal Part)

The thickness of the cortical bone at the site of insertion is critical for stability of a miniscrew. We choose the length of a miniscrew according to the amount of bone, the thickness of the soft tissues, and the required height of the miniscrew head. It is recommended that the length of the miniscrew part inside the bone should be the same as the part outside the bone. The length of a miniscrew body for the mandible is usually 6.0 mm, for the maxilla it is 8.0 or 10.0 mm. Miniscrews shorter than 6.0 mm do not usually provide sufficient anchorage. A diameter of 1.6 mm is considered optimal for cylindrical miniscrews.

A certain span of screw threads is needed for screwing a miniscrew firmly into the bone. A span of 0.8–0.9 mm is considered optimal for bone screws; the thread depth should be between 0.4 and 0.6 mm.

The layout of the threads and the shape of a miniscrew tip differ between *self-drilling* and *self-tapping* miniscrews. If one needs to use great force for insertion of the miniscrew, it is difficult to maintain the required direction or the miniscrew may even break.

For insertion of a self-tapping miniscrew, a *pilot drill* and noninvasive preparation are necessary, together with effective cooling of the bone.

Self-drilling miniscrews do not need predrilling, but many authors recommend at least partial perforation of the cortical bone, otherwise excessive force is needed when screwing the miniscrew into the bone, which causes heating. Furthermore, the body of the miniscrew can easily bend or break when larger force has to be applied. According to some studies, self-drilling miniscrews seem to be more stable after insertion and they have better contact with the bone. No definite preferences have emerged yet. When the layer of cortical bone is thin, self-drilling miniscrews are recommended; when it is thick and compact, self-tapping miniscrews are recommended. If one has chosen one's assortment and does not want to change it, it is better to opt for the self-drilling type. A hole can be predrilled in the desired direction in the case of thick cortical bone.

The body of a miniscrew has either a cylindrical or a conical shape. Its diameter should be smaller than the gingival part of the neck. The gingival neck merges with the body either directly or with a step. The advantage of the *cylindrical* shape of the body is that it presses on the surrounding bone tissue over its whole length; as a result, the primary stability of the miniscrew is better and it can be loaded immediately. Disadvantages of the cylindrical body are the higher risk of breaking the miniscrew and the fact that its removal is usually more difficult. A *conical* body is screwed firmly into the bone only in the thicker part under the neck; the apical part is anchored into the bone more loosely. A miniscrew with a conical body is easier to remove and the risk of breakage is smaller, but it also can loosen more easily when loaded.

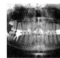

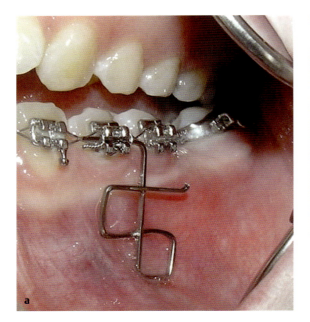
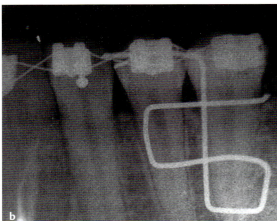

Fig. 12.**7 a** Appliance made of wire to determine the site of insertion of the miniscrew. **b** Intraoral radiograph of the same tool.

Accessories

Instruments for Miniscrew Insertion

The instruments that enable reliable insertion of a miniscrew comprise a tool that helps to specify the place for insertion of the miniscrew, a punch instrument, a pilot drill, and a tool for screwing the miniscrew into the bone. Their repeatable sterilization is an absolute prerequisite.

Tools That Help to Specify the Site of Insertion of a Miniscrew (Figs. 12.**7**, 12.**8**)

The wire element that can be seen on the radiograph in Fig. 12.**8** can help those who are less experienced to determine the exact insertion site. We use this tool and make an intraoral radiogram of the area in which we want to insert a miniscrew to determine the exact insertion site. We use it especially in anatomically more complicated interradicular parts of the alveolar process bone. With this tool one can simulate the whole process on plaster models of the dentition.

The Punch Instrument for Perforation of the Gingiva (Mucosa)

It is possible to insert a miniscrew directly through the gingiva or mucosa. Disadvantages of this method are the rough edge at the site of perforation and the possibility of trauma if one inserts a miniscrew through a thicker layer of mobile mucosa. Another possibility is a small incision in the insertion site or removal of soft tissue with a so-called *mucotome*, which easily makes a small hole with a smooth edge in soft tissue. The size of the hole must correspond with the system of miniscrews used. With miniscrews that have a place for fastening a screwdriver on the transgingival portion, we also prefer perforation of the gingiva.

The Pilot Drill

Although the majority of today's miniscrews are self-drilling, pilot drills are supplied with them. The drill diameter must correspond with the size and the type of the miniscrews and should be a little smaller than that of the miniscrews so that they are firmly screwed into the compact layer of bone. A pilot drill diameter 20–30% less than the diameter of the miniscrew body is recommended. The length of a pilot drill is determined by the length of the miniscrew used. A color symbol or a stop-part (a wider part on the end of the working part) indicates the depth of the hole. Before using a pilot drill, it is useful to make a starter hole on the surface of the bone with a ball-point bone drill. This helps to determine the direction of insertion of the pilot drill during perforation of the compact bone.

With this procedure the risk of breaking a miniscrew is minimal. The orthodontist also has better tactile control of insertion of the miniscrew into the bone.

The Screwdriver

Careful preparation and the correct method of miniscrew insertion using proper tools are the prerequisites for a good result—primary stability of the miniscrew. Attention should be paid to the quality of the screwdriver, which has to be a part of the selected miniscrew system. Any kind of improvization leads to failure.

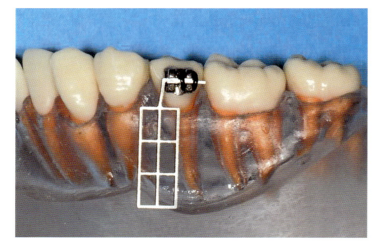

Fig. 12.**8** Plastic frame to determine the site of insertion of miniscrews.

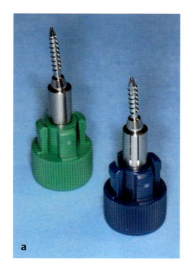 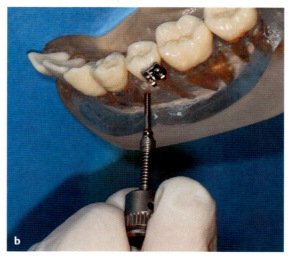

Fig. 12.**9 a** Screwdrivers used by hand for insertion of miniscrews. **b** Interradicular insertion of a miniscrew.

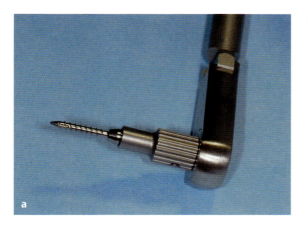 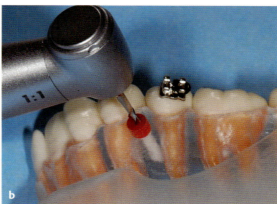

Fig. 12.**10 a** Machine screwdriver. **b** Insertion of a miniscrew with machine screwdriver.

The screwdriver has to fit perfectly into a miniscrew head. It should not loosen at any time during the manipulation and the maximum moment should be applied. Miniscrew heads or the transgingival portions have hexagonal or octagonal systems for fixing the screwdriver in, or there may be a simple or cross-shaped slot in the head. A slot system requires larger force during insertion and the risk of mechanical damage to a miniscrew during insertion is higher. It is also possible to fix a miniscrew into the screwdriver by slot or spring systems. Apart from screwdrivers designed for insertion by hand (Fig. 12.**9**), preferred in the majority of studies, some systems also have screwdrivers for machine insertion (Fig. 12.**10**).

The *length* and the *diameter* of the miniscrew body and the length of the screwdriver are important during insertion of a miniscrew. Using a long screwdriver with a large diameter, screwing the miniscrew into the bone is easy; with a short screwdriver with a small diameter, we have to use greater force to achieve the same effect. The same force with a big screwdriver produces a greater moment than with a small one, which can lead to faster, "smoother" screwing, but it should be realized that it leads to higher resistance of the bone and higher loading of the miniscrew material, so that it can easily break. Screwing should be even and gentle. There is not just the question of damaging the miniscrew, we also have to avoid the bone overheating and cracking, which leads to poor healing and reduced primary stability of the miniscrew. We must also keep in mind the possibility of damaging anatomical structures that surround the miniscrew.

If we use a *short* screwdriver, the control of the moment is better and we also feel better the resistance of the bone and the presence of any obstacle, though we have to work with greater force. Some manufacturers mount a wheel on their screwdrivers for easier screwing by hand. Even with miniscrews we can also use a ratchet, the use of which is common for insertion of dental implants.

Machine insertion of miniscrews requires rather expensive equipment. The advantage of this method is the ability to set and control the number of turns and the moment, as well as easier insertion into less-accessible places. With machine insertion, the bone and the miniscrew are loaded steadily. Disadvantages are poorer estimation and appreciation of the bone resistance and the possibility of over-screwing, with attendant higher risk of breaking the miniscrew.

Factors Influencing the Clinical Success of a Miniscrew

The basic condition for clinical success with a miniscrew is choice of the correct type of orthodontic anchorage with respect to anatomical conditions at the insertion site, the quality and the layer of the bone, and the biomechanics of the orthodontic system of which the miniscrew is a part.

It has to be appreciated that insertion of a miniscrew is a more or less invasive procedure, so we have to prepare it and perform it in accordance with standard hygienic practices for surgical procedures. A miniscrew and the accessories must meet the requirement of the ability for repeated sterilization. One must use only miniscrews that are delivered in sterile packing. Some tools are disposable, for example the mucotome.

Fixation of traction to the miniscrew head should be easy and reliable with both orthodontic wire and elastics.

Apart from correct miniscrew insertion, the success of treatment is based on regular monitoring and adjustment of the miniscrew after loading and detailed instruction of the patient about hygiene of the oral cavity in particular.

Insertion of a Miniscrew

Any evaluation of factors that influence the success of insertion of miniscrews is more or less subjective. It is difficult to compare different studies because usually different types of implants from different orthodontic systems are used. In addition to detailed knowledge of anatomy, a good practical know-how of insertion of implants and good work with the selected system are basic conditions for successful orthodontic treatment with implants used as an anchorage. More important than the selection of the type of miniscrew is the orthodontist's knowledge and experience deriving from continual comparison of results achieved and analysis of the possible causes of complications.

Behrens and colleagues published the results of an interesting experiment evaluating the success of treatment with 239 miniscrews that were inserted for skeletal orthodontic anchorage purposes. Two specialists worked with two different types of miniscrews. After insertion of 133 miniscrews into different sites in the maxilla and mandible, a detailed analysis was made of treatment and the results achieved with the aim of identifying possible causes of failure and complications. The data were later used for insertion of the other 106 miniscrews. The team was able to reduce the loss rate from 23% to 5% (Behrens et al. 2006)!

The authors stated that the higher success rate was achieved mainly because they observed the following principles: in the lower jaw do not insert miniscrews into the lingual side of the alveolar process bone; use miniscrews 2 mm in diameter in the vestibular slope of the alveolar process bone in the lower jaw. In the palate use miniscrews with a diameter of at least 1.5 mm; in the vestibular slope of the alveolar process bone in the upper jaw, we use a maximum diameter of 1.5 mm.

The study confirmed that the anatomical conditions of the selected site are important in the selection of the type, length, and diameter of miniscrews. More importantly, it showed that by the continual analysis of completed work it is possible to reduce failure rates significantly.

Preparation

In the following we will consider examples from routine orthodontic practice dealing with insertion of miniscrews into the alveolar process bone in the lower and upper jaws and into the palate.

The type and size of the miniscrew are selected according to the quality of the hard and soft tissues. Anatomical conditions at the site of insertion have to be respected, but the placement of the miniscrew is also determined by its role as anchorage and its attachment to an orthodontic appliance. The optimal anatomical site does not have to correspond with the planned layout of the anchorage unit. The miniscrew must not be placed in such a way as to block the planned movement of teeth during treatment. The application of orthodontic traction has to be simple and it must not traumatize soft tissues. This means, for example, that there should not be close contact between the coil spring and the mucosa of the alveolar process bone and that traction should not be closed by mucosa.

If the procedure for insertion of an implant for skeletal anchorage and the method of attachment to an orthodontic appliance are not planned in detail, we are forced to improvise, and this greatly increases the risk of failure.

For insertion of a miniscrew, we should have, in addition to routine data for preparing an orthodontic treatment plan (models, dental cast, panoramic radiograph, cephalometric radiograph, photographic documentation), a high-quality cast of the jaw where we are going to insert the implant, and intraoral photographs of the site of insertion, including anatomical structures in the surrounding areas. As the miniscrew is loaded by an orthodontic force just after insertion or after healing, it is good to plan and to simulate individual clinical situations on a model. Detailed preparation of the procedure on a model should be a standard part of a treatment plan, especially in those cases where it is necessary to prepare parts of the orthodontic appliance in a laboratory.

Evaluation of the Anatomical Situation (Imaging Methods, Dental Cast)

A miniscrew is selected according to the quality and thickness of the tissues. Detailed information is needed about the amount of bone tissue and the thickness of cortical bone; these are the most important data for reliable insertion of a miniscrew and its use. One needs to know the amount of trabecular bone and the character of the soft tissues at the site of insertion.

Miniscrews used as skeletal anchorage are most often inserted interdentally and interradicularly on the vestibular slope of the alveolar cortical bone in the upper and lower jaws. In the upper jaw we can also use sites in the palatal slope of the alveolar process bone and the palatal vault. We pay attention to roots, permanent tooth germs, the proximity of the antrum of Highmore, nerves, and blood vessels, and the anatomy of the mandibular canal mandibulae. One must also consider the state of the bone and its healing processes after extraction of teeth.

The thicker the layer of *cortical* bone, the better and more reliable is the primary stability of a miniscrew—when the miniscrew does not move, surrounding tissues heal better. To ensure maximum contact between the miniscrew and the bone, it is recommended to insert the miniscrew with angulation toward the bone. In the upper jaw, the miniscrew is inserted monocortically; in the lower jaw it is possible to use the bicortical insert.

To determine the size and the shape of the area where we need to insert a miniscrew, draw the line of attached gingiva, the axis of the teeth and the edge of the mobile gingiva. We want the head of the miniscrew to be placed in the zone of attached gingiva. The layer of the intact bone around the miniscrew should be at least 1–2 mm.

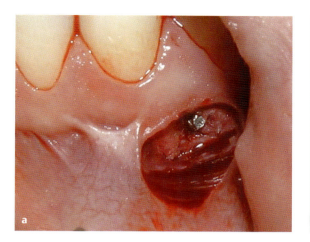
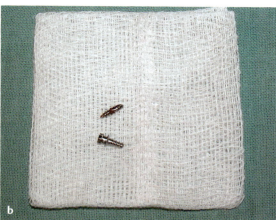

Fig. 12.11 **a** Breakage of a miniscrew because of too rapid screwing. **b** Removed fragments; the removal took 20 minutes.

We determine the exact insertion site of the miniscrew with a tool fixed onto the teeth with resin and make an intraoral radiograph. If cooperation with a dental technician is necessary, we mark the site of the miniscrew insertion on a dental cast with the tool. Using the same tool we mark the site of the miniscrew insertion in the mouth of the patient. We also can use radiographic-contrast pins and marks that can be pinned into the mucosa after application of topical anesthesia at the site of the planned procedure. The exact insertion site can be determined according to the situation as visualized on the radiograph.

The site of the miniscrew insertion on the *palatal* vault is prepared in a similar way. In these cases it is good to evaluate the anatomical situation on a lateral skull radiograph. The diameter and the length of the miniscrew are selected according to the results of these findings. Miniscrews of diameter 1.6 mm and length of 6–10 mm are generally recommended. Apart from anatomical conditions, successful use of a miniscrew is determined by the quality and the means of attachment between the miniscrew and an orthodontic appliance. The shape of the miniscrew head should allow simple changing of an orthodontic traction or attachment of a square wire, and so on.

Miniscrew Insertion

Although the insertion of a miniscrew is a planned nonacute and minimally invasive procedure, the same conditions apply as for all other surgical procedures in the oral cavity.

Prior to insertion, the patient rinses his or her mouth with a disinfectant solution containing 0.1% chlorhexidine gluconate. Topical anesthesia of mucosa and periosteum at the site of insertion should ensure painless screwing-in of the miniscrew and should also enable the patient to feel any possible contact of the miniscrew with the periodontal ligament of the neighboring tooth. For palatal insertion of a miniscrew, local terminal anesthesia is more productive.

Punch mucosa with a standard tool; make a shallow hole on the surface of the bone, insert the pilot drill into it, and drill the hole in the desired direction. The diameter of the pilot drill must be smaller than that of the inserted miniscrew. When drilling the bone, we must apply effective cooling to limit overheating.

The miniscrew is usually inserted by hand as the procedure is simple and reliable. Self-drilling miniscrews usually require a larger moment than self-tapping ones. Screwing should be uninterrupted, without pressure or torque. Atkin-Nergiz et al. (1998) recommend a screwing speed of 30 rpm; one full turn of the head should last 2 seconds. Too fast screwing and excessive pressure usually lead to breakage of the miniscrew (Fig. 12.11) and trauma to the bone tissue. The conditions are less favorable for screwing by hand when inserting a miniscrew into the *palate*. It is a good idea to fail-safe a short screwdriver with a fiber. One can use mechanical screwing, for which special equipment is needed. Tactile control is worse when using machine insertion; if the miniscrew is overscrewed, it can easily break.

After finishing the screwing, one must check the correct positioning of the transgingival neck of the miniscrew; the mucosa must not be pressurized. The neck of the miniscrew must be in contact with the bone. If one does not move the inserted miniscrew firmly, it may lead to poor healing and reduced primary stability. Some degree of mobility is present after loading of miniscrews, but they can still be used for clinical purposes.

Miniscrews can be loaded with a force immediately after insertion, which is their great advantage (Melsen and Costa 2000). According to the literature, the loading force varies from 30 to 500 g. If a miniscrew is sufficiently firm, the applied force does not compromise successful use.

A miniscrew is usually used for 2–3 months; use for as long as 12 months and more is reported in the literature. The length of time depends on the requirements of the orthodontic treatment.

Miniscrew Removal

Removal of a miniscrew is a simple and a quick procedure. In many cases no application of anesthetic is necessary. Long and well-healed miniscrews can break if one attempts to remove them quickly. If a miniscrew is firmly in the bone, it should be turned a little before the planned removal to break the connection between the bone and the surface of the miniscrew; the subsequent removal will be easier. It has to be accepted that unscrewing is more difficult than screwing-in because in most cases a hole was made into the bone for insertion. Before unscrewing, the screwdriver has to be properly fitted into the head of the miniscrew – we do not want the miniscrew to fall into the patient's mouth. After removal of the miniscrew, the small wound usually heals completely within a few days.

Disadvantages of Miniscrews

- There may be insufficient stability after insertion, resulting in subtle movement. A site of insertion must be chosen with sufficient amount of compact bone. "High-angle" patients have thinner cortical bone.
- Delayed mobility of miniscrews may appear days or months after insertion, caused by overloading or insufficient loading. The initial loading should not exceed 0.5 N.
- Anatomical structures may be damaged during insertion; there may be lesions or infection of soft tissues during insertion.
- Miniscrews may have been inserted into the antrum.
- Peri-implantitis may occur with osseointegrated prosthetic implants; the cause is usually anaerobic infection.
- Miniscrews may fracture during removal.

Palatal Implant

Palatal implants are extradental orthodontic anchorages that have been used in orthodontics for more than 20 years. They are bone anchored. They are substitutes for orthodontic anchorage by the Nance appliance and extraoral traction. The Nance appliance has disadvantages of difficult hygiene, the possibility of a bruised palate, and uncertain results, together with an undesirable effect on the dentition. When extraoral traction is used, the full cooperation of the patient is needed, which represents another disadvantage.

The palatal implant derives from the standard principles of dental implantology. It is a length-reduced screw with a low head, a rough surface on the body, and a smooth, polished transmucosal neck.

A palatal implant is inserted into the palate near the palatal suture. This is an advantageous site: it has good bone quality; the access is easy; and the soft tissues are thin and keratinized and are fixed in the central part of the palate. One must appreciate and respect that the vertical bone layer in the palatal arch is not thick (as seen on the lateral skull radiograph) and most orthodontic patients are still growing. This is why it is not recommended to insert a palatal implant directly into the palatal suture but rather beside it to prevent damage to skeletal tissues that are still growing. Melsen states that transversal growth in a palatal suture can be demonstrated up to the age of 16 years in girls and 18 years in boys (Melsen 1975; Wehrbein and Göllner 2008). For this reason, palatal implants were initially recommended only for adult patients, again to prevent damage to still-growing skeletal tissue. Present clinical practice shows that a palatal implant inserted beside the palatal suture in patients who are still growing poses no problem and can be used with patients over the age of 12 years.

Keith and colleagues evaluated the layer of vertical bone in the area of the palatal arch. On the basis of CT results they stated that the optimal site for implants of body length 3 mm is a region 4 mm distal and 3 mm lateral from the foramen incisivum. According to their results, more than 90% of adolescents have an adequate layer of vertical bone at this site (Keith et al. 2007). Some authors tend to prefer more distal sites for insertion of a palatal implant, behind the level of the line connecting the first premolars. Their reasons are better access and easier work with tools since they do not have to angle them so much. These authors also take into account damage to the canalis incisivus and nervus incisivus.

Yildizhan states that the average thickness of the bone in the central palate is 8.08 mm, but 3 mm laterally the thickness is only 3.34 mm. In adult patients with closed palatal suture he recommends insertion of anchorage implants into the center of the front part of the palate. In patients who are still growing, he recommends a paramedian location 1–2 mm away from the palatal suture (Yildizhan 2004).

At present miniscrews are used in various parts of the palate for palatal anchorage. Miniscrews, unlike palatal implants, can become unstable and they carry a higher risk of penetration into the nasal cavity during insertion.

A palatal implant can be used independently or may be firmly fixed with a modified palatal arch into an anchorage unit together with molars or premolars. Protruded upper incisors and canines are moved distally to this anchorage unit in a block. A similar anchorage system—a palatal implant or miniscrews linked together with a pendulum appliance—can be used for distal or mesial movement of lateral teeth or as a reliable anchorage for moving teeth on only one side of the dental arch.

We anchor orthodontic appliances to a palatal implant mainly because of the lack of space at the sagittal level in the upper dental arch, especially in the area of the upper canines. We gain needed space for them in the upper dental arch by successive *distal movement* of premolars and molars; in some patients we can avoid the usually recommended extraction of premolars (Fig. 12.**12**).

Other indications for use of an implant for palatal anchorage are distal driving of molars with a palatally anchored distal jet appliance (Fig. 12.**13**), or transversal palatal expansion. With skeletal anchorage expansion is achieved without undesirable buccal leaning of lateral teeth; this usually happens with a dentally anchored orthodontic appliance when the lean of teeth is greater than that of the alveolar process bone.

Skeletal anchorage with a palatal implant is advantageous in the case of protraction of the maxilla with the face mask. The advantage of a palatal implant is that with one implant we can successively deal with more tasks. For this purpose we change only the shape and the length of the palatal arches. When using palatal implants in the paramedian area, there is no undesirable interference with tooth roots.

Loss of a palatal implant, if it occurs, is usually in the phase of healing; miniscrews can loosen at any time during treatment.

Advantages of palatal implants over other skeletal anchorage include:
- Multifunction anchorage
- Rigid anchorage control
- Rotational stability
- Standardized insertion site
- No danger of injury to roots

Admitted **disadvantages** of palatal implants in comparison with miniscrews are their more demanding insertion and removal, which usually requires separation of the bone from the implant with a trephine drill, the necessity of cooperation with a dental technician, and the requirement for precise work when making and adapting extraosseal elements of the anchorage unit.

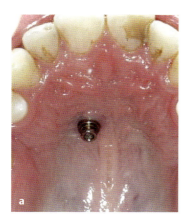 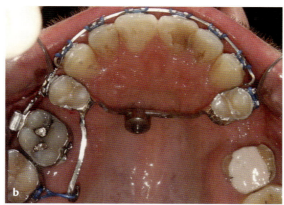

Fig. 12.**12** **a** Paramedian location of a palatal implant. **b** Palatal appliance anchored on a palatal implant.

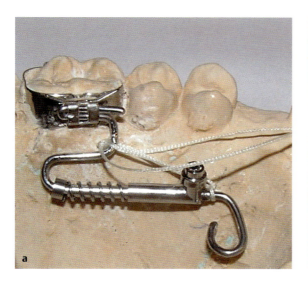 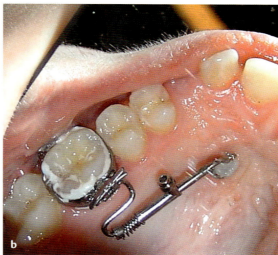

Fig. 12.**13** **a** Distal jet appliance on the cast. **b** Palatally anchored distal jet appliance activated for distal driving of the first molar.

Comparison of the stability of inserted palatal implants that were loaded with orthodontic force 3 days and 3 months after insertion shows that after attaining the primary stability of the palatal implant there is no significant difference in final results of the treatment.

Insertion of Palatal Implants

Under local anesthesia, remove gingiva on the selected site, perforate the cortical bone, and prepare a 4 mm implant bed using a standardized drill. The bed is prepared at an angle of 60° ventrally in the sagittal plane. Use a probe to ensure that the nasal floor is not penetrated. The implant is screwed in manually; we try to avoid lateral excursion of the screwdriver and fix the implant in its final position using a ratchet wrench so that the lower surface of the implant neck rests on the bone surface. After healing, required parts are prepared from the plaster model and we load the implant by a transpalatal arch or other constructional modifications of the anchorage unit.

Once the orthodontic treatment phase is completed, the palatal implant is removed using a standard trephine drill whose internal diameter has to correspond with the external diameter of the transgingival portion of the implant.

Dental Implant Used Temporarily as Orthodontic Anchorage

Dental implants are a good alternative in a partially edentulous patient needing orthodontic treatment. They are less often used as anchorage for an orthodontic appliance than are miniscrews. One reason for this is the considerably higher cost connected with prosthetic reconstruction of the dentition using dental implants; another reason may be that the implant may be lost after loading with an orthodontic force, which means the loss of an important prosthetic abutment. Considering orthodontic requirements, a prosthetic implant is not the ideal type of anchorage because its siting is dictated by the needs of the prosthetic treatment and not by those of the layout of an orthodontic anchorage. The orthodontic use of prosthetic implants can sometimes seem a forced improvization, but it can be very useful. Anchorage with a dental implant placed in a dental arch is simple and can be well arranged, especially in a dentition with a weak periodontal ligament and in edentulous patients. Another advantage is the reduction of treatment time. From the biomechanical point of view, the question is that of direct orthodontic loading of an implant. The use of anchorage with a dental implant is indicated in dentitions with tooth loss on one or both sides and for correction of malposed teeth near the implant. Patients must be adults, although a dental implant in the alveolar process bone is slowly burrowed.

The issue is how to make a plan of complex dental treatment in a case where dental implants should replace missing teeth. The basic principle of preparing a treatment plan involves not only a detailed diagnosis of the state of the teeth and periodontal ligament, but also an analysis of orthodontic irregularities that very often complicate a professional prosthetic reconstruction of the dentition. It is essential to determine priorities in the individual phases of treatment, especially if some kind of orthodontic treatment will be necessary before the prosthetic treatment. Diagnostic data will indicate whether orthodontic treatment must be finished before insertion of dental implants or whether it is possible to achieve the required orthodontic changes after the insertion of implants and use the implants as a reliable skeletal anchorage. The results of many studies show that we need not be afraid to load dental implants with orthodontic or orthopedic forces. Occlusal forces that affect the healed dental implant are much higher (20–200 N) than the force of orthodontic loading, but they affect it for at most 20 minutes a day and are oriented mainly in the axial direction (Skalak 1983). Orthodontic loading is low; it acts continuously, and horizontal forces and moments predominate. If the implant heals steadily there are no undesirable side-effects of its use for orthodontic needs (Douglas and Killinay 1988; Higuchi 2000). Nevertheless, it is important to keep in mind that the change of mechanical qualities of the bone after insertion of an implant and the relations between temporary orthodontic loading and establishing of primary and secondary stability with different types of implants are not the same. We load a miniscrew with an orthodontic force immediately after insertion or 2 weeks later. This is possible thanks to primary stability provided by the shape of the miniscrew and its mechanical anchorage in the bone. The dental implant we can load with a temporary orthodontic force after a period necessary for its healing, which should be at least 2 months (Ohashi et al 2006).

According to present experience, dental implants with immediate prosthetic loading are not suitable for orthodontic purposes.

When an implant is inserted, necrotic changes start in the thin layer of bone that surrounds its intraosseal portion. The bone that is in connection with the surface of the implant has to remodel; new bone tissue has to be built (contact osteogenesis). The activity of osteoblasts and osteoclasts is demonstrable a week after insertion of an implant. The 6–8 weeks following insertion of a dental implant are critical and decisive in establishing secondary stability, which depends especially on the material of the implant and the nature of its surface (Slaets et al. 2006).

Odman and colleagues published a study evaluating the loading of dental implants used as orthodontic anchorage by different orthodontic movements (tipping, torquing, rotation, intrusion, extrusion). They studied 23 dental implants and stated that after orthodontic treatment that lasted from 4 to 33 months it was possible to use all of the inserted implants as abutments for prosthetic replacement (Odman et al. 1994).

Rugani and Ibañez emphasized the great importance of the surface of the endosseous implant. They studied 93 dental implants with special surfacing, which were loaded with an orthodontic anchorage of 100–200 g for a period of 2–9 months. On radiographs they did not find any unfavorable changes in bone tissue and all the implants were still used for prosthetic replacement. In the maxilla, implants were allowed to heal for 6 months, in the mandible for 5 months, before loading (Rugani and Ibañez 2008).

Wehrbein and colleagues published results of a pilot study in dogs in which they studied changes in bone tissue surrounding implants (length 6 mm, diameter 4 mm). Implants healed for 16 weeks and then were loaded with an orthodontic force in the vertical direction toward the long line of the implants for 26 weeks. The authors confirmed increased remodeling activity of the bone surrounding the implants loaded with an orthodontic force ($n = 4$) in comparison with nonloaded implants ($n = 4$). Although the number of implants studied was small, the results drew attention to an interesting finding. As there is no "periodontal slit" around the implant, the force that works in the horizontal direction is transferred directly onto the bone and causes remodeling activity. The reaction of the bone surrounding the root of a tooth loaded with an orthodontic force depends on the reaction of the bone surrounding the loaded implant. The reaction of the bone surrounding the implant is similar on the "side of traction" and on the "side of pressure." The authors did not find loss of or damage to bone, and they formulated a hypothesis that it may be possible to evaluate the loading of an implant by the extent of remodeling activity of the bone. The experiment proved that loading of an implant is advantageous for remodeling and strengthening the surrounding bone and that the orthodontic force does not damage a healed implant (Wehrbein et al. 1999).

The layout of an orthodontic appliance has to be adapted to the placement of a dental implant that will function as its anchorage. To be able to use a dental implant for prosthetic purposes, we put a temporary resin cap on it; then we can easily fix an orthodontic bracket, band, button, or hook onto it, or we can use a special orthodontic abutment that can be screwed into the fixture. The abutment has either a built-in retention for attachment of an orthodontic traction or we can put an orthodontic band in it, and so on.

We use a dental implant as a temporary orthodontic anchorage mainly in an intramaxillary fashion for changing the vertical or horizontal position of a tooth or a group of teeth. According to Kokich, one third of dental implants used as orthodontic anchorage are used for simple mesial or distal movement of teeth in nearby space (Kokich 2000). Besides correction of spaces and positioning of teeth that are next to them, we use dental implants as an anchorage for other corrections in the dental arch, especially in the frontal part of the dentition.

When planning treatment that combines orthodontics with prosthetic implantology, repeated changes of dental casts are necessary as it is not possible to determine where to insert dental implants into the dental arch in which orthodontic changes have not yet occurred. Simulation of the planned result of the treatment on the original dental cast, gives an exact idea of the extent of set-up and the placement of dental implants. Accordingly, an implant placement guide is made (Smalley 2006). In skeletal orthodontic–prosthetic anchorage, the prosthetic implants are initially used as orthodontic anchorage and later as abutments upon which to attach a fixed prosthetic replacement. In combined treatment, for example, the upper molars can be intruded prior to prosthetic reconstruction in the lower arch (Fig. 12.**14**) or to enable insertion of an implant (Fig. 12.**15**).

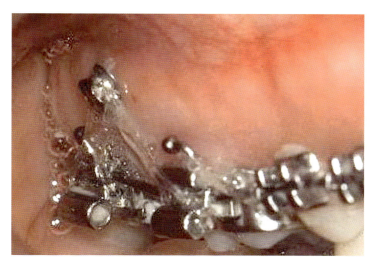

Fig. 12.**14** **Intrusion of the upper first molar with vestibular interradicularly inserted miniscrew**; preparation for a prosthetic reconstruction in the lower arch.

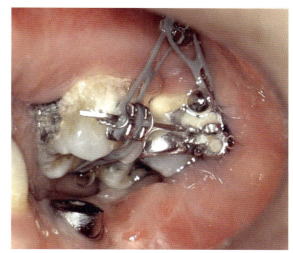

Fig. 12.**15** **Intrusion of + 67 with a miniscrew**, to enable insertion of a dental implant in the space after − 6.

Conclusion

In this chapter we have dealt with miniscrews, dental implants, and palatal implants, which are the most used types of skeletal orthodontic anchorage. In a short time, implants have become a common part of orthodontic treatment. They have brought new dynamics into orthodontics and have enriched this discipline with new possibilities of interdisciplinary cooperation.

Acknowledgment

I express my thanks to my colleagues I. Marek, M. Starosta, J. Petr, and O. Hajnik for allowing me to use photographs from their collections.

References

Atkin-Nergiz N, Nergiz I, Schulz A, Arpak N, Niedermeier W. Reaction of peri-implant tissues to continuous loading of osseointegrated implants. Am J Orthod Dentofacial Orthop. 1998; 114: 292–298.

Behrens A. Wiechmann D. Dempf R. Mini- und Mikroschrauben zur temporären skelettalen Verankerung in der Kieferorthopädie. J Orofac Orthop. 2006; 67: 450–458.

Borsos G, Rudzki-Janson I, Stockmann P, Schlegel KA, Végh András. Immediate Loading of palatal implants in still-growing patients: a prospective, comparative, clinical pilot study. J Orofac Orthop. 2008; 69: 297–308.

Brånemark PI, Hansson B, Adell R, et al. Osseointegrated Implants in the Treatment of the Edentulous Jaw. Experience from a 10-year Period. Stockholm: Almquist and Wiksell; 1977.

Büchter A, Wiechmann D, Meyer U, Wiesmann H-P, Joos U. Tierexperimentelle Untersuchung von sofort belasteten Mikroimplantaten. Z Zahnärztl Impl. 2006; 22(3): 238–250.

Creekmore TD, Eklund MK. The possibility of skeletal anchorage. J Clin Orthod. 1983; 17(4): 266–269.

Douglas J, Killinay D. Dental implants used as orthodontic anchorage. J Oral Implantol. 1988; 13: 28–38.

Gainsforth BL, Higley LB. A study of orthodontic anchorage possibility in basal bone. Am J Orthod Oral Surg. 1945; 31: 406–417.

Higuchi K W. Orthodontic applications of osseointegrated implants. Chicago: Quintessenz; 2000.

Kanomi R. Mini-implant for orthodontic anchorage. J Clin Orthod. 1997; 31: 763–767.

King KS, Lam EW, Faulkner MG, Heo G, Major PW. Vertical bone volume in the paramedian palate of adolescents: a computed tomography study. Am J Orthod Dentofacial Orthop. 2007; 132: 783–788.

Kinzinger G, Gülden N, Yildizhan F, Hermanns-Sachweh, Diedrich P. Anchorage efficacy of palatally-inserted miniscrews in molar distalisation with a periodontally/miniscrew-anchored distal jet. J Orofac Orthop. 2008; 69: 110–119.

Kokich VG. Implantate zur orthodontischen Verankerung und prothetischen Versorgung – Aspekte der interdisziplinären Zusammenarbeit. Kieferorthop. 2000; 14: 279–290.

Liou EJW, Pai BCJ, Lin JCY. Do miniscrews remain stationary under orthodontic forces? Am J Orthod Dentofacial Orthop. 2004; 126: 42–47.

Melsen B. Palatal growth studied on human autopsy material. A histologic microradiographic study. Am J Orthod. 1975; 68: 42–54.

Melsen B, Costa A. Immediate loading of implants used for orthodontic anchorage. Clin Orthod Res. 2000; 3: 23–28.

Melsen B, Petersen JK, Costa A. Zygoma ligatures: an alternative form of maxillary anchorage. J Clin Orthod. 1998; 32(3): 154–158.

Müller-Hartwich R, Präger T, Park J-A. Kieferorthopädische Verankerung mit Minischrauben – Auswahl geeigneter Insertionsorte und Mechaniken. Kieferorthop. 2006; 20(3): 195–202.

Odman J, Lekholm U, Jemt T, Thilander B. Osseointegrated implants as orthodontic anchorage in the treatment of partially edentulous adult patients. Eur J Orthod. 1994; 16(3): 187–201.

Ohashi E, Pecho OE, Moron M, Lagravere MO. Implant vs. screw loading protocols in orthodontics. A systematic review. Angle Orthod. 2006; 76: 721–727.

Rugani de CM, Ibañez JC. Assessing double acid-etched implants submitted to orthodontic forces and used as prosthetic anchorages in partially edentulous patients. Open Dent J. 2008; 2: 30–37.

Schlegel KA, Kinner F, Schlegel KD. The anatomic basis for palatal implants in orthodontics. Int J Adult Orthod Orthognath Surg. 2002; 17: 133–139.

Skalak R: Biomechanical considerations in osseointegrated prostheses. J Prosthet Dent 1983; 49: 843–848.

Slaets E, Carmeliet G, Naert I, Duyck J. Early cellular responses in cortical bone healing around unloaded titanium implants: an animal study. J Periodontol. 2006; 77(6): 1015–1024.

Smalley WM. Zahnimplantate zur Abstützung von orthodontischen Zahnbewegungen: Bestimmung der Insertionstelle und der Insertionsrichtung. Inf Orthod Kieferorthop. 2006; 38: 83–90.

Wehrbein H, Göllner P. Miniscrews or palatal implants for skeletal anchorage in the maxilla: comparative aspects for decision making. World J Orthod. 2008; 9: 63–73.

Wehrbein H, Yildirim M, Diedrich P. Osteodynamics around orthodontically loaded short maxillary implants an experimental pilot study. J Orofac Orthop. 1999; 60: 409–415.

Yildizhan F. Strukturparameter des medianen Gaumens und orthodontische Verankerungsimplantate. Eine radiologische, histologische und histomorphometrische Studie. Med. Diss. Aachen 2; 2004.

13 Treatment with the Invisalign System

Rainer-Reginald Miethke

Kesling's positioner can be seen as a kind of predecessor of an aligner of the present day. As early as 1945 Kesling foresaw the development when he stated that "Major tooth movements could be accomplished with a series of positioners by changing the teeth on the setup slightly as treatment progresses. At present this type of treatment does not seem to be practical. It remains a possibility, however, and the technique for its practical application might be developed in the future" (Kesling 1945).

The decades after 1945 were characterized by positioner-like thermoformed splints that covered all teeth and the marginal parts of the alveolus and were fabricated from various acrylics. The basis of the manufacturing process was a set-up working model. The disadvantage of this process is that it is labor-intensive and thus cost-intensive. Also, the amount of tooth movement had to be very limited because it was restricted by the physiological, or at most the orthodontically induced, somewhat increased tooth mobility. Any violation of this limit would harm the entire periodontal ligament and jeopardize the fit of the appliance. Because of these two restrictions, it was generally agreed by experienced clinicians that during the set-up the position of only very few teeth should be changed (McNamara and Brudon 2001).

In spite of the system's limitations, such splint aligners became quite popular through Sheridan, who broadened their use by the introduction of his air-rotor stripping, by blocking out or grinding off areas on the working cast, cutting windows in the appliance, thermoforming the material with special pliers (Fig. 13.**1**), placing composite mounds on the teeth, attaching elastic tractions, and so on (Sheridan et al. 1993).

In 1997, Align Technology was founded. This company approached the solution of moving teeth with series of aligners by combining 3D imaging technology and mass customization.

The Principles of the Invisalign System

It is not appropriate to expend too many words on this aspect because clinicians and orthodontists-to-be are much more interested in the practical features. Apart from this, Align is a highly innovative company that constantly releases new developments of the total CAD-CAM process. Accordingly, the following text reflects the situation only at the time when it was written (October 2008).

Basically, a patient's maxillary and mandibular impressions and the respective bite registration are CT scanned while rotating in front of an amorphous silicon x-ray sensor (Fig. 13.**2a,b**). Since the captured data originate from the impression, they are inverted to allow the creation of a virtual model. The precision of the scanning process is around 100 μm (Lee et al. 2002).

Next, the proprietary Align software ToothShaper is used to define the facial axis of the clinical crown, color-code all teeth, and separate them from each other as is done on a real cast with a jig saw. The individual teeth receive a rudimentary root and then are worked over so they will be free of any imperfections and artifacts. At the same time, the gingival margin is defined, which will later delineate the extension of the aligner onto the marginal areas of the alveolus. The intraoral photographs submitted from the orthodontists are also often used for this purpose. A virtual gingiva is then draped over the alveolar processes, which improves the visual presentation (Fig. 13.**3a,b**) (Beers et al. 2003).

Finally, the models of both jaws are aligned with each other in centric occlusion by another tool of ToothShaper suite named AutoBite, which basically maximizes the tooth–tooth interarch contacts using algorithms by matching corresponding occlusal contact points. Because this bite orientation is highly successful, the scanned bite registration is only exceptionally used, for instance, in patients with a Class III malocclusion or an open bite that extends over many teeth. In these situations, the maxillary and mandibular virtual models are placed within the virtual bite registration, which is very time-consuming. Alternatively, the intraoral photographs might be used to verify a patient's centric occlusion.

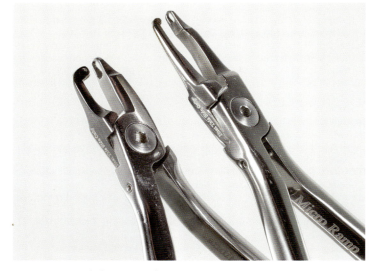

Fig. 13.**1** **Special pliers** are available to form the splint aligner material for activation.

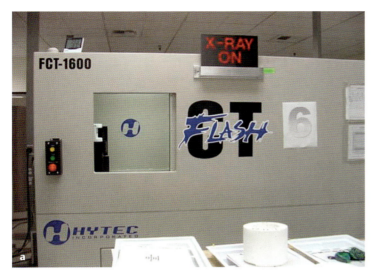 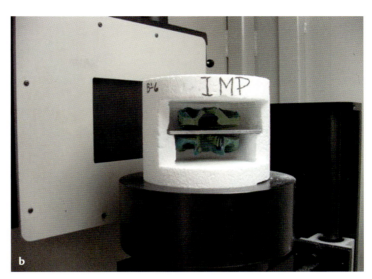

Fig. 13.2 The impressions are scanned by a CT-scanner (a) as they rotate in a styrofoam holder in front of an amorphous silicon x-ray sensor (b).

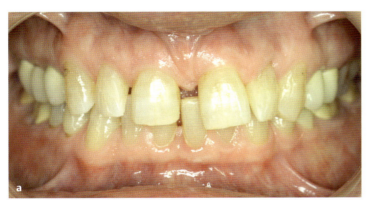 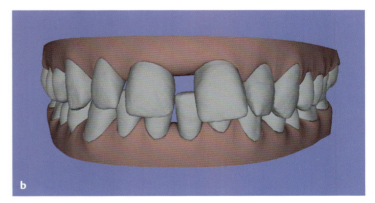

Fig. 13.3 A patient's intraoral photograph (a) and corresponding virtual 3D-model (b).

Subsequently, the individual teeth will be aligned by the Align software Treat to the orthodontist's prescription, while at the same time the path and speed of movement (i.e., the number of aligners that will each move specific teeth or one tooth by ~0.2 mm) of separate teeth is calculated. This manipulation is accomplished with a widget that allows movements of any tooth in all three planes of space. Initially, it was mainly the orthodontist who defined which teeth would move in what sequence. This repeatedly led to the use of an unacceptable number of aligners. For this reason, the so-called best practice protocol was recently introduced. In this, all teeth to have their position changed will move at the same time, though at different speeds (i.e., through different distances). The tooth to be moved over the longest distance – the so-called lead tooth – will define the maximum number of aligners required for the complete treatment. The remaining teeth will move simultaneously, but in much smaller increments. During these movements the program automatically detects overlaps between neighboring or antagonistic teeth. In this case either the path of movement has to be adjusted or, especially in the case of neighboring teeth, the collision has to be eliminated by removal of some enamel (interproximal enamel reduction, IPR, see Chapter 14, Stripping).

Finally, the definitively programmed virtual therapy will be sent to the orthodontist, who will evaluate it on computer using the Align software ClinCheck. If satisfied, the orthodontist will accept it and then Align Technology prepares the virtual models with the Fab software for manufacture. The next step is to produce a physical model of each treatment stage. This is done with stereolithography (Fig. 13.4a,b). On every model, an aligner is thermoformed, marked, robotically cut, removed from the model, tumbled, polished, disinfected, and packaged. More details on the highly complex process are to be found elsewhere (Kaza 2006; Kuo and Miller 2003; Wong 2002).

Aligners (Fig. 13.5) are made from 0.75 mm thick foils of polyurethane with methylene diphenyl diisocyanate and 1,6-hexanediol (Ex 40). Its stress-strain curve is extremely steep, which means that a minor deformation of the material leads to a major increase in force delivery (Tricca and Chunha 2006). This might be one reason why not all Invisalign treatments are successful. Also, due to its limited viscoelasticity the aligner material might not contact the whole crown surface of a tooth but only certain areas of it. This can be followed by an intrusion of the respective tooth. This unfavorable material property is partially compensated by the fact that most Invisalign treatments will not lead to any root resorptions.

Overall, Align Technology holds more than 60 patents for all the procedures involved.

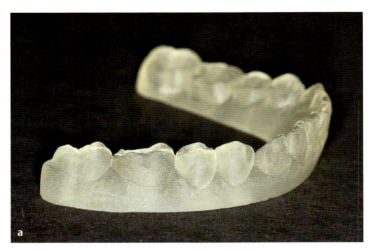
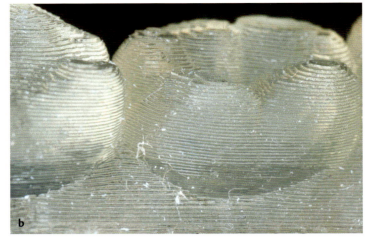

Fig. 13.**4** **Stereolithography.** An acrylic model made by stereolithography (**a**). A detail view shows the individual acrylic layers produced by laser polymerization (**b**).

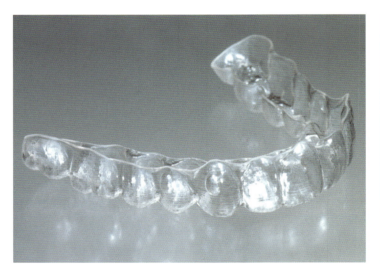

Fig. 13.**5** An aligner made of clear polyurethane (Ex 40).

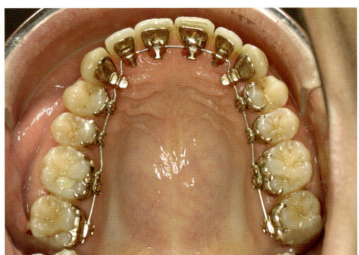

Fig. 13.**6** **In comparison with a lingual appliance like this**, an aligner does not limit oral hygiene, speech, and tongue functions.

The Clinical Approach

When a patient is interested in orthodontic treatment, the conscientious specialist should counsel the patient as to the treatment options. This includes various treatment goals as well as treatment methods. In every case the orthodontist should fairly describe the advantages and disadvantages of each option. If the patient wants to be treated with an invisible appliance, he or she has basically a choice between lingual appliances (Fig. 13.**6**), the Invisalign system, or possibly a Crozat appliance, including variations of these three.

Compared with a lingual appliance, the Invisalign system allows unhindered oral hygiene, it interferes barely, if at all, with speech and with other tongue functions, and it can be used even in patients with multiple artificial tooth surfaces where bonding imposes a severe problem. Also, because aligners are temporarily removed (for eating, cleaning of the teeth and the appliance, and sometimes for drinking), the periodontal ligament has a chance to recover; they provoke less discomfort or pain; chair time is reduced; emergencies are rare; the armamentarium is very sparing;

and finally because of a kind of bite block effect there is good vertical control. A Crozat appliance shares many of these advantages but, compared with an aligner, is much more susceptible to damage. Of the two alternatives, only the Invisalign system protects the dentition from bruxism; but most of all it allows visualization of the treatment outcome, which can even be modified until patient and orthodontist are satisfied. Nevertheless, there are limitations to this system, which will be discussed later.

After an evaluation of all the pros and cons, and assuming that the patient's malocclusion can be well corrected with the Invisalign system, the standard procedure of anamnesis and clinical and radiological examination should be initiated. At the request of Align Technology the records have to comprise photographs (extraoral: frontal [at rest/smiling] and profile; intraoral: frontal, left/right lateral, maxillary/mandibular occlusal) (Fig. 13.**7 a–h**), and radiographs (panorex; optional cephalogram) for every patient. Align Technology will further require vinyl polysiloxane impressions (maxillary, mandibular) and a bite registration.

Irrespective of the regular treatment plan, the orthodontist must submit a specific plan that consists of a form in which cells

The Clinical Approach 279

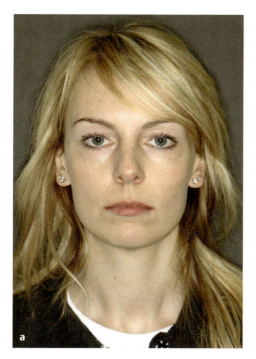
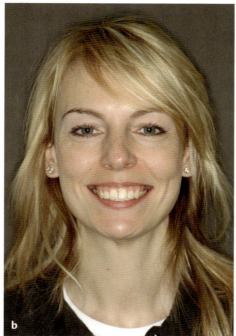
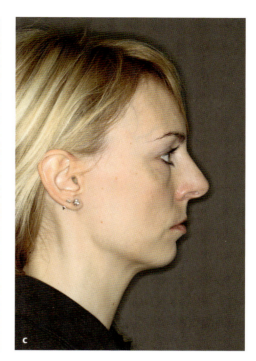
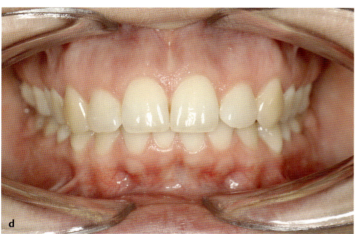
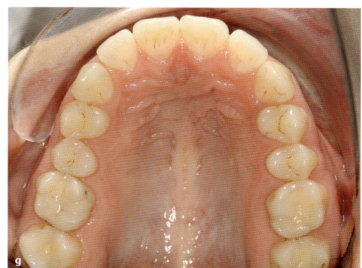
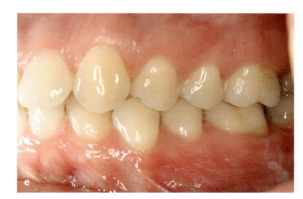
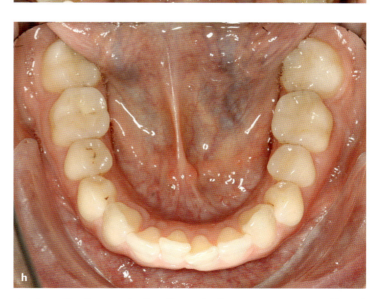
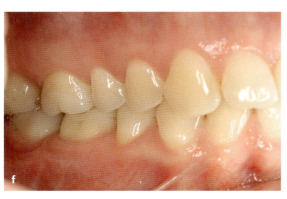

Fig. 13.7 **The photographs that Align Technology requests. a** *Extraoral* frontal at rest; **b** smiling; **c** profile. **d** *Intraoral* frontal; **e** left; **f** right; **g** maxillary; **h** mandibular occlusal.

have to be ticked and one section in which free text can be entered. Both parts are equally important because the executive software laboratory technician is not an orthodontist, although all of these specialists undergo rigorous training in orthodontics. To properly complete the orthodontist's vision of the outcome of therapy, the technician needs as much detailed instruction as possible. One must be aware that working with the Invisalign system implies planning the total treatment sequence right at the start from the very first to the very last movement in every possible detail. While other treatment modalities might allow continual changes of the sequence, the direction, and the amount of tooth movements, during Invisalign therapy this would be feasible only by a midcourse correction (see below). At first sight, this might be perceived as detrimental. However, the development of a complete problem list that must be dealt with should be looked on as an intellectual challenge and an education. At this stage, the visualization of the treatment in the form of ClinCheck is a great support.

All records can be submitted via e-mail; only the impressions still need to be sent by express mail service.

Since Invisalign treatment is most often requested by adult patients who have already had various tooth restorations, the orthodontist has to stress that it is important that before impression-taking all teeth should be thoroughly checked and if necessary treated. All fillings should be high-quality provisionals; high-quality restorations would be at risk because the final treatment outcome can never be predicted with absolute certainty, whereas any restoration should fit the final occlusion perfectly. What has been said about fillings is even more important for crowns and bridges, which should be repaired to last to the end of Invisalign therapy to be replaced afterward in accordance with the outcome of therapy.

As mentioned previously, ClinCheck is the complete virtual treatment that is sent to the VIP (Virtual Invisalign Practice) site of the orthodontist, whose task it is to scrutinize it. The first step should be verification of the correct morphology of all teeth and whether the occlusion is accurate. Any inaccuracy can be an indication of an impression failure and in such a case the ClinCheck should not be accepted because the related aligners might not fit from the beginning. Subsequently, the operator should compare the submitted treatment plan and special remarks with the virtual treatment. If they do not match, the ClinCheck also has to be rejected and the discrepancy must be discussed with someone from the clinical support staff. The importance of a detailed ClinCheck evaluation cannot be overstressed because any imprudent acceptance of a ClinCheck will lead immediately to the production of all aligners with the related charges. Only if everything is flawless should a ClinCheck be accepted.

Every ClinCheck is accompanied by a reproximation chart (Fig. 13.**8**) and an attachment form (Fig. 13.**9**). The former indicates that the Treat software has recognized a collision at some point that requires IPR, whereas the latter shows which teeth should receive composite shapes to improve the aligner performance. The next section will deal with the attachments just mentioned.

Attachments

Teeth per se have no effective purchase points. For Invisalign treatment they are therefore provided with so-called attachments that are equivalent to the brackets of a fixed appliance. Like brackets, these small custom-made composite shapes are bonded onto certain teeth. They serve three main purposes: assistance with movements, augmentation of retention, and support for auxiliary functions. In ClinCheck they are indicated as red geometric structures. They routinely come in ellipsoidal and rectangular shapes in various lengths and thicknesses, and they can be orientated parallel or perpendicular to the long axis of the crown on the vestibular and/or on the oral side (Fig. 13.**10a,b**) The standard thickness is 1.0 mm, whereas with the latest protocol the length is automatically adjusted to the height of the clinical crown. Further, rectangular attachments can be beveled, which means that one flange of the body is virtually buried into the crown. Better appliance performance is expected because of increased engagement.

Although it might seem complicated to decide which attachment of which size should be attached to which teeth, a beginner can rely on the suggestions of the experienced Align laboratory technicians. In any case, it would be wrong to assume that many attachments are better than only a few, because each one will increase the appliance retention significantly, making it difficult for the patient to disengage or insert the aligner without breaking it. In general, patients whose teeth have long clinical crowns need only few attachments; those with short clinical crowns definitively require a good number of them. Attachments are almost mandatory during intrusion (on the "anchor teeth" to withstand dislodgement), rotations, and changes in angulation and inclination.

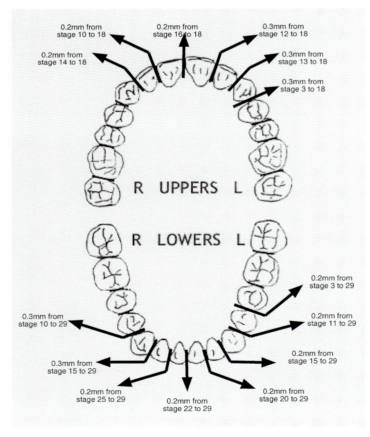

Fig. 13.**8** **Reproximation chart** gives the information about the amount of enamel reduction at a given stage.

Enclosed you will find the following:
- One thin shell template aligner for each arch that requires attachments.

Directions for: Tooth preparation and attachment placement

1. Rinse the thin shell template aligner in cold water.
2. Snap the aligner onto the patient's teeth to check for gingival impingement. if necessary, trim the aligner using scissors, an acrylic bur or a stone in a slow speed.
3. Isolate the arch with cheek retractors and cotton triangles, making sure to leave room for aligner insertion.
4. Each tooth that will receive an attachment should be pumiced, etched, rinsed, dried and sealed as is traditionally done for bonding.
5. Match the tooth shade and load a small amount of restorative composite into each attachment well of the thin shell template aligner (indicated on the schematic below). Use a plastic instrument to adapt the composite into the well, so that the well is slightly overfilled.
6. Fully seat the loaded aligner onto the teeth, visually confirming the composite-tooth adaptation.
7. Use a plastic instrument to maintain gentle pressure on the aligner area adjacent to the attachment. Light cure each attachment for 30 seconds.
8. Remove the template aligner by peeling the edges away from the teeth.
9. Remove any composite flash from the teeth using a 12 fluted finished bur
10. Deliver the stage 01 aligner and review the patient instructions on the General Instructions Sheet.

Note: The retention will increase greatly when the stage 01 aligner is inserted. Evaluate and adjust attachments prior to insertion of stage 01 aligners as necessary.

Fig. 13.**9 Attachment form** shows which teeth receive composite shapes.

Attachments are indicated below by black squares on the teeth (which are represented by circles). The view is occlusal.

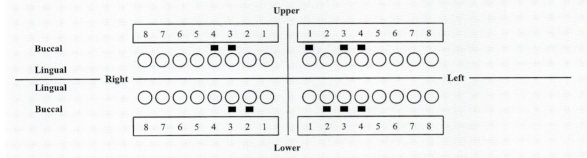

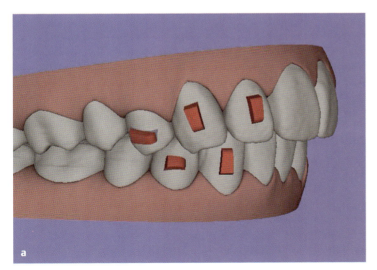
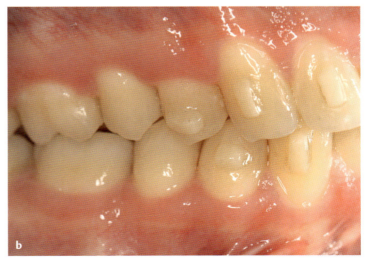

Fig. 13.**10 Attachments are ellipsoidal or rectangular in shape.**

a In the ClinCheck, attachments are visible as red structures.

b They can be oriented perpendicular (teeth 14 and 44) or parallel to the long axis of the crown (teeth 12, 13, 43).

Attachments are fabricated in the mouth with so-called thin-shell templates, which are 0.25 mm thick aligners with concavities that are filled with a strong micro-filled composite to resist abrasion due to eating, brushing, and insertion or removal of the appliance. Preferably, the composite should be light-curing and its color should match that of the crown. Basically, all procedures are almost identical to indirect bonding and do not need to be described in more detail. To accomplish a definite shape, the tray has to be firmly adapted with a ball-end burnisher or similar. After curing, the template is removed and all excess composite has to be removed with finishing burs. The final result of the clean-up should be an attachment with a defined shape (Fig. 13.**11 a–d**).

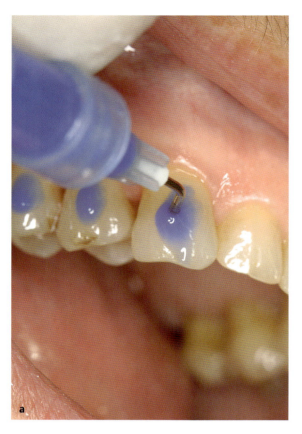
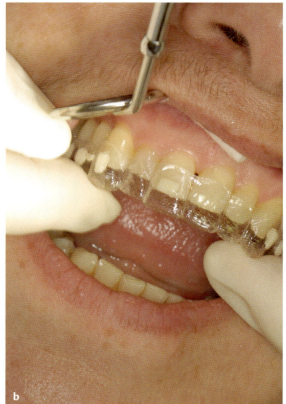
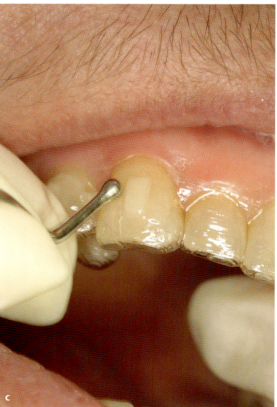
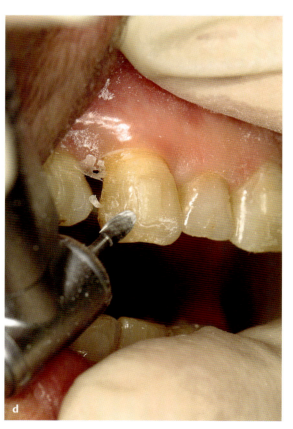

Fig. 13.**11 Fixation of attachments.** Etch gel (**a**) and adhesive agent are applied to the tooth surfaces. **b,c** The attachment template (**b**) is carefully placed onto the dentition and adapted with a ball-end burnisher (**c**). **d** After light curing, all excess composite material has to be removed with finishing burs.

Experience shows that attachments are most favorably bonded after the first aligner has been worn for a week. The teeth are then slightly mobile, improving the adaptation of the template. Lost or damaged attachments can be rebonded. This can be done with the best-fitting aligner or by cutting out the respective part of the original thin-shell template, which always matches the original tooth surface.

The last remark necessary in this context is that attachments undergo constant experimentation to upgrade aligner action (Durrett 2004). Experiments have included preformed attach-

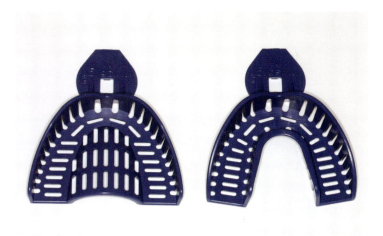

Fig. 13.**12** **Perforated plastic impressions trays**, which do not interfere with scanning, are provided by Align.

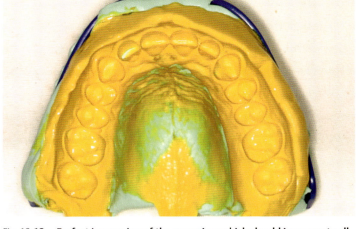

Fig. 13.**13** **Perfect impression of the upper jaw which should incorporate all teeth and their adjacent alveolar process.**

ments and geometric variations. All of these failed to prove their superiority, however: if they were successful, a highly competitive company such as Align Technology would have initiated them immediately.

Impression-taking for the Invisalign System

For the scanning process Align Technology accepts only impressions taken with vinyl polysiloxane (so-called a-silicone). This material has adequate detail reproduction (< 3 µm) and shows a high elastic recovery (< 98%) as well as long-term dimensional stability (~ 3 months) (Lu et al. 2004). It is advisable to choose a quality product and use it to the manufacturer's specification. Normally, a two-step application seems appropriate, which means that a first impression with the heavy-body component precedes a second with the light-bodied corrective material. Care has to be taken that there is enough room for the second step; this can be achieved by placing a plastic foil spacer on top of the heavy component and moving the tray slightly while the material sets. Ideally, the heavy-body material will then be visible nowhere on inspection of the impression from above. Most important is to avoid direct or indirect contact of the silicone material with latex gloves because these contain sulfur compounds that affect the setting reaction negatively (Baumann 1995). It should be kept in mind that the heavy-body impression could be taken on a study model, which would help to save chair time.

Since metal would interfere with the scan, perforated plastic trays (Fig. 13.**12**) are provided by Align, which should be individualized like any others. Before impression taking, distinct undercuts such as spaces gingival to bridges or sagittally tipped teeth must be blocked out to avoid distortion or tearing. The impression should incorporate all teeth with the adjacent alveolar process (Fig. 13.**13**). An exception might be the most terminal teeth. If they are not fully captured, the Align technicians can virtually cut parts of these teeth or even whole teeth out of the virtual model so that the aligner will just extend to the teeth that were completely and correctly caught within the impression.

No virtual model or aligner can be more precise than the impression from which it derives. Therefore, it cannot be overemphasized that the impression must be as perfect as possible. To accomplish this, all teeth should initially be well dried; the impression material should be dispensed free of air bubbles into the tray; and the tray should be taken out of the mouth with a rapid uniform motion to avoid permanent distortion. Before the impression is sent away, it should be carefully examined. No tears, voids, or bubbles should be visible. After all, it seems much more reasonable to repeat an impression rather than risk treatment failure.

Together with the impression, Align requests as mentioned a bite registration, which also should be made with a fast-setting (40–60 seconds) vinyl polysiloxane.

Clinical Aspects of an Invisalign Treatment

All aligners, together with an attachment bonding tray, are sent by express mail to the orthodontist's office. Before the doctor inserts the first aligner, it should be rinsed because the material is hydrophilic and would otherwise unpleasantly dry the patient's gingiva. A check of the appliance's fit will reveal whether the gingiva is compressed in a particular area, which would call for a local shortening of the aligner. The patient should be instructed in how to take the aligner out, always with two hands, and to put it in without damaging force. After this, the patient should practice insertion and removal of the appliance and its fit should be explained.

If occasionally small voids are present between the aligner and teeth, these will almost always disappear if the appliance is subsequently worn extensively. A considerable discrepancy between a patient's teeth and the aligner might indicate an impression flaw, which likely will necessitate a restart.

The patient should also be instructed to wear the aligners continuously except when brushing, eating, and drinking staining or sugar-containing liquids; to store them when they are removed in the containers supplied by Align; to clean them thoroughly at least once a day; and to eliminate minor rough or otherwise irritating margins by covering them temporarily with dispensed protection wax or even by removing such areas with a nail file. Cleaning the aligners is also necessary to avoid discoloration. A slight loss of gleam is unimportant as aligners are usually replaced every other week.

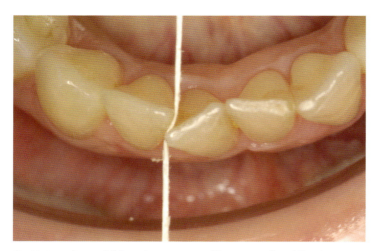

Fig. 13.**14** **The availability of space is tested by moving dental floss between two adjacent teeth.** In this clinical situation the bend in the dental floss indicates that the movement of 41 and 42 is impeded. IPR should be performed.

On balance, the advantage of the Invisalign system—removability of the appliance for unhindered oral hygiene and intermittent recovery of the periodontal ligaments—is at the same time its biggest shortcoming, since therapeutic success requires total cooperation.

Since most patients need some kind of attachments, they should return after wearing their aligners for a week. This time is optimal for bonding of the attachments. This bonding appointment is then considered as the start of treatment proper.

Since generally aligners are changed every 2 weeks (Clements et al. 2003; Owen 2001), patients should return after 14 days. They are asked how they have got along with their aligners and the fit is assessed. Also, the patient's ClinCheck should be reviewed, which will indicate which teeth will move into which plane of space with the successive aligners. If any of these movements could be stalled by neighboring teeth, slight IPR should be performed, especially if this is required according to the reproximation chart. The availability of space is tested by moving dental floss between two adjacent teeth (Fig. 13.14). Since floss is very flexible, it might be bent slightly. Teeth, however, move straight (if they do not rotate) and thus there is sufficient room only if the thread goes straight through the contact area. This modus operandi should be repeated at all subsequent appointments.

If the first aligners fit very well after 2 weeks, this signals that treatment is "on track." Patients can receive the second and the third aligners. This will allow patients to change to the third aligners on their own, thus saving an extra appointment. If patients return after about 4 weeks with properly fitting aligners, they can receive the fourth ones with two extra ones that they can change themselves. Although it is advantageous for patient as well as orthodontist to not to have to see each other too frequently, it is not advisable to give more than two extra aligners as minor adjustments (IPR) are often necessary and no treatment should ever go "off track" because any recovery is questionable.

An "off track" treatment is indicated by ill-fitting aligners, as becomes obvious through mainly occlusal/incisal void spaces, saliva bubbles under the aligners, and discrepancies between attachments and the respective concavities of the aligners (Fig. 13.**15 a, b**). The three most likely causes for such a deviation from the regular course of therapy are lack of cooperation, lack of space, or lack of tooth movement.

If the reason for the malfunction is a lack of cooperation, the aligners could be worn for an extra week or two while the patient tries at this time to gently force the appliances into place by biting on them. This approach is only partially promising because the aligner material ages and loses its original physical properties (Schuster et al. 2004). If lack of space is the likely cause of improper aligner fit, IPR is performed and the last aligners have to be worn for another week or 2 weeks. An omitted tooth movement would be the consequence of trying, for instance, to extrude teeth, to translate them, to change their inclination, or to rotate cylindrical teeth, since all these are less predictable movements within the Invisalign system (Joffe 2003).

If such less predictable movements were included in the treatment but do not occur, two alternatives must be considered. The first could be to resort to a so-called midcourse correction, a procedure that will be described in detail later. This midcourse correction might exclude less-predictable movements, that is, it will modify the original treatment goals. The second alternative tries to resolve the lagging tooth movement with adjuncts (such as

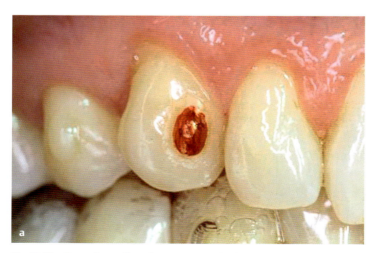
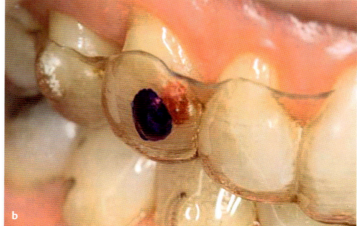

Fig. 13.**15** **Detecting "off-track" treatment.** The discrepancy between the red marked attachment (**a**) and the respective blue marked concavity of the aligner (**b**) indicates poor fit of the aligner.

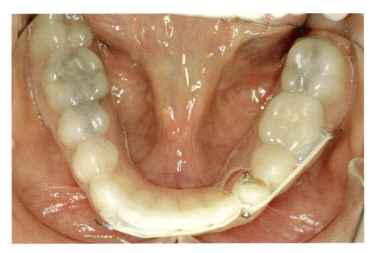
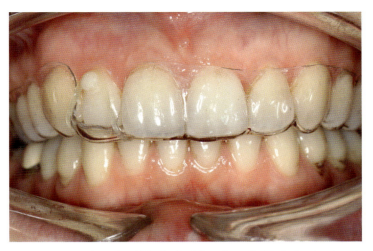

Fig. 13.**16** In such a situation tooth 34 should be rotated with Class I elastics before Invisalign treatment.

Fig. 13.**17** **Extrusions should be dealt with at the end of Invisalign treatment.** Tooth 12 should be extruded with a button on the buccal surface and an elastic.

buttons plus elastics or power-chains) (Fig. 13.**16**) until the tooth position coincides perfectly with the actual aligner.

Another problem that arises occasionally during treatment is the loss of aligners. The action required depends on how soon the patient sees the doctor after such a loss and how long the aligners have been worn up to that time. If the loss occurred late during a 2-week aligner interval, most likely all programmed movements will have taken place. In this case the patient can insert the next aligner, which might fit more tightly and thus should be worn for a slightly extended time.

If the loss happens early during a specific treatment stage, the patient should wear the previous aligner if it is available. Availability is guaranteed if all worn aligners are retained either by the orthodontist or by the patient. If this aligner is not on hand, a retainer made ad hoc could be inserted. While the patient is wearing either of these appliances, a replacement aligner can be ordered from Align Technology; this is a simple process because all required data are stored in the Treat software.

If the time lapse between the loss of the aligner and a visit to the orthodontist is long, it can be assumed that a partial relapse will be manifested. Then the doctor and the patient should try to find the best-fitting of the aligners worn so far. From there on the patient will wear all the aligners in sequence until arriving again at the stage at which the specific aligner was lost. In the meantime, this aligner is reordered or the patient tries to bypass this stage and insert the aligner that was supposed to follow the lost one. A second alternative would be to start a midcourse correction.

A *midcourse correction* is similar to the start of treatment in a new patient. This implies that all the previously mentioned records must be re-taken and re-submitted simultaneously with a new treatment plan. Such a midcourse correction could also become necessary when, for instance, during treatment it is obvious that certain teeth are not moving as planned and that this situation cannot be resolved with any kind of adjunct. It is reasonable that in this situation the new treatment plan should strive for different goals because the original ones could not be attained. Since any midcourse correction will prolong the duration of the therapy, incurs extra effort, and will increase costs, it should be regarded as a last resort.

If at the end of a fairly uneventful treatment the orthodontist might like to add a few extra stages, for instance, to overcorrect some tooth position, a so-called *case refinement* can take place. In contrast to a midcourse correction, a classical case refinement is based on the original data; that is, only the relevant remarks about the desired changes should be submitted but no new impression, photographs, or radiographs.

However, Align Technology even allows hybrids between midcourse corrections and case refinements. Such a hybrid is a case refinement because it is located at the end of treatment, but it is a midcourse correction because new records are submitted together with more specific descriptions of all intended changes.

Indications for Treatment with the Invisalign System

The chief complaints of patients who opt for a treatment with the Invisalign system are predominantly crowding, spacing, incisor flaring, and supra- and infrapositions (Meier et al. 2003; Vlaskalic and Boyd 2001). Apart from extrusions, these movements are achievable without any major problems. However, all these corrections will normally occur as crown and not as root movements. This need not be disadvantageous because crowding, spacing, and flaring are often the consequence of a tipping that will be reversed by the Invisalign therapy. Also, intrusions will pose no problem if the crowns of the anchor teeth are long enough to offer sufficient undercuts. Anchorage could be further increased by providing the anchor teeth with preferably horizontal attachments.

Only extrusions of infrapositioned teeth have to be considered as less predictable movements and thus should be dealt with before or after Invisalign treatment (Fig. 13.**17**). Another less predictable movement is the rotation of cylindrical teeth.

In this context it needs to be discussed whether these two problematic movements should be eliminated before or after proper Invisalign therapy. In the case of extrusion, it seems advisable to delay this movement to the end of treatment because then the necessary elongation can be matched to the vertical position of all other teeth that also change their position in the vertical

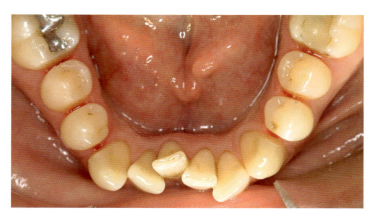

Fig. 13.**18** **Interproximal enamel reduction** (IPR) was performed in the premolar and molar region of both sides in the mandibular arch to align the front.

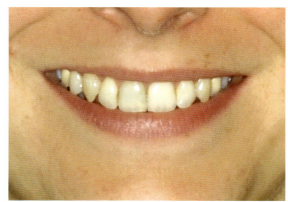

Fig. 13.**20** **Lateral expansion of the dental arch.** This patient shows no buccal corridors while smiling, which is generally considered more attractive.

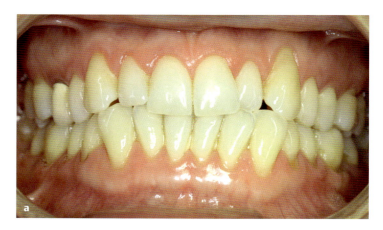

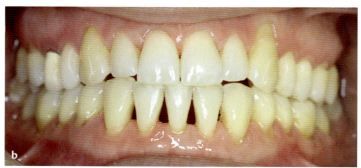

Fig. 13.**19** **Extraction versus IPR. a** This patient with frontal crowding was treated with the extraction of a mandibular incisor to align the front, which leads to open gingival embrasures (**b**). Additionally there is a midline discrepancy. With IPR such problems could be avoided.

plane. Another reason to postpone this movement toward the end of Invisalign therapy is that extrusions are generally very prone to relapse (Malmgren et al. 1991). If extruded at the beginning of treatment, a tooth might slightly intrude again during the Invisalign phase, which might lead to a failure of the whole therapy. The tendency to relapse also needs to be taken into consideration if extrusion takes place at the end of therapy, but this is the same as in any regular orthodontic treatment. It is important, though, to discuss this additional treatment phase before Invisalign therapy because otherwise the patient might get the impression that the treatment failed, at least partially.

Since rotations are almost always connected with a gain or loss of space, it seems preferable to resolve this problem with some kind of adjunct before therapy with the Invisalign system. Of course, the relapse tendency has to be treated at least as seriously as in extrusions, which suggests some overcorrection. Clinical experience shows that with proper cooperation relapse even of teeth with a cylindrical crown shape can be controlled, especially if these teeth are fitted with one or two vertical rectangular attachments.

Although any of the above malocclusion symptoms poses problems, crowding might be the biggest challenge because its correction requires space that can be obtained in different ways. The three most appropriate alternatives are: interproximal enamel reduction (IPR), expansion of the dental arch, or extractions. This order of itemization reflects to some degree the appropriateness of each procedure.

IPR is the first choice because it allows the gain of just as much space as is needed, which is often not very much because Invisalign patients have already been treated and thus the crowding is rarely extreme. In contrast, extractions always provide the space of a given tooth, whether that much room is needed or not. Since with IPR small spaces are created in different areas of the dental arch, all teeth have to move only minimally (Fig. 13.**18**). Another, very serious, consideration is that with extraction in adult patients with a certain amount of attachment loss, open gingival embrasures are almost unavoidable (Atherton 1970; De Harfin 2000; Kurth and Kokich 2001; Zachrisson 2004) (Fig. 13.**19a, b**). With careful IPR the development of such black triangles can be avoided. It should not be overlooked that there are also contraindications for this procedure by which irreplaceable tooth structure is removed (Miethke and Jost-Brinkmann 2006). By and large, IPR is better accepted by most patients than any extraction, especially if the tooth to be extracted is sound. IPR turns every crowding into spacing, which is much easier to deal with. Finally, patients should be convinced that IPR is an essentially physiological process, since extensive attrition occurred regularly before humans' food was refined (Begg 1964).

One alternative to IPR is lateral expansion of the dental arch. However, if posterior teeth are not lingually inclined and expansion is not performed skeletally (rapid maxillary expansion, mandibular symphysis distraction), it is limited to about 2–3 mm per quadrant. Thus, the space gain would be very small (Germane et al. 1991). Also, the risk of producing gingival recessions and an unstable result must be seriously considered (Chenin et al. 2003). The

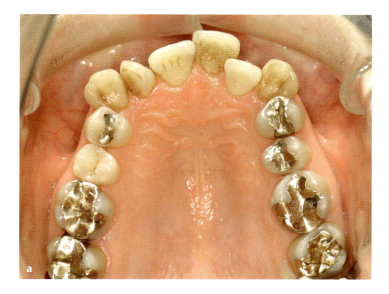
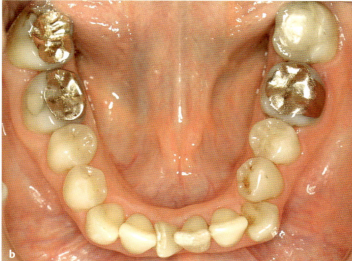
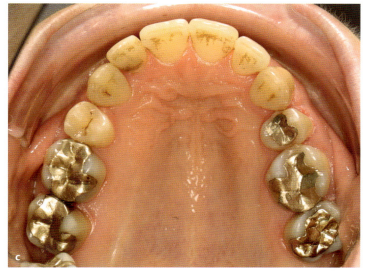
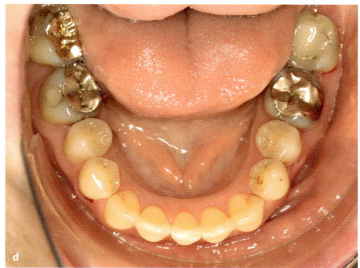

Fig. 13.**21** **Extraction in combination with Invisalign treatment.** This patient with frontal crowding in the upper and lower arches (**a, b**) was treated with the extraction of the teeth 14, 15 and 41. With the help of different invisible auxiliaries, all teeth were aligned (**c, d**).

advantage of lateral expansion is that a wide dental arch helps to eliminate buccal corridors (Moore et al. 2005; Sarver 2001; Sarver and Ackerman 2003; Womack et al. 2002) (Fig. 13.**20**).

Instead of a lateral expansion, a sagittal expansion could be attempted for space creation, likely only in the maxilla. With the Invisalign system this would again be limited to approximately 3 mm per quadrant. To make distal movements more successful, it is advisable to separate the posterior teeth before impression-taking, to provide the posterior teeth with vertical rectangular attachments, and to use Class II elastics. Still, a substantial anchorage loss will occur; that is, not only do the posterior teeth move distally but also the anterior teeth will move mesially.

Clinical experience shows further that the distal movement of posterior teeth is very time-consuming. Thus, a patient who is interested in an alignment of the anterior teeth does not see any progress for a long time, which might compromise the patient's disposition to co-operation.

The last realistic alternative would be tooth extractions, which are still hard to manage uneventfully with the Invisalign system. Because of this, extractions will be discussed in the following section.

Indications for Extraction Therapy in Combination with Invisalign Treatment

Since aligners cannot move teeth bodily over any noteworthy distance, extractions should only be considered as a last resort. As far as basic orthodontic principles apply, all the accepted rules of extraction are also valid in this connection. Generally, extractions (primarily premolars or mandibular incisors) can be considered as another means to resolve crowding or other problems. Because different aspects must be considered subsequently, the extraction of premolars and mandibular incisors are treated separately:

- **Extractions of premolars** (Fig. 13.**21 a, c**)
  Premolar extractions are seldom indicated because the lack of space hardly justifies the extraction of two premolars (with a mesiodistal diameter of about 7.0 mm each). Even if such extraction spaces could be closed with aligners, paralleling the roots of all teeth would be still difficult, especially in a mandibular arch with a deep curve of Spee.
- **Extraction of mandibular incisors**
  Again the lack of space does not often exceed 5.0 mm, above which value such an extraction would be truly justified. Also,

many orthodontists will not find it easy to parallel all incisor roots perfectly even with regular fixed appliances. Finally, there will always remain a midline discrepancy between the two dental arches.

The main objection to extractions is the fact that, especially in adult patients with a certain degree of periodontal destruction (gingival recession), removal of teeth will almost inevitably lead to open gingival embrasures.

There are exceptions, however, where extractions can be managed well provided that the indication is correct, that the patient cooperates well, and that the operator is experienced. Such treatment may also include the use of adequate attachments (see p. 281) and even specific adjuncts (Moore et al. 2005).

References

Atherton JD. The gingival response to orthodontic tooth movement. Am J Orthod. 1970; 58: 179–186.

Baumann MA. The influence of dental gloves on the setting of impression materials. Br Dent J. 1995; 179: 130–135.

Beers AC, Choi W, Pavlovskaia E. Computer-assisted treatment planning and analysis. Orthod Craniofacial Res. 2003; 6 (Suppl. 117): 125.

Begg PR. Stone Age man's dentition. Dent Res. 1954; 40: 298–312, 373–383, 462–475, 517–531.

Chenin DA, Trosien AH, Fong PF, Miller RA, Lee RS. Orthodontic treatment with a series of removable appliances. J Am Dent Assoc. 2003; 134: 1232–1239.

Clements KM, Bollen A-M, Huang G, King G, Hujoel P, Ma T. Activation time and material stiffness of sequential removable orthodontic appliances. Part 2: Dental improvements. Am J Orthod Dentofacial Orthop. 2003; 124: 502–508.

De Harfin JA. Interproximal stripping for the treatment of adult crowding. J Clin Orthod. 2000; 34: 424–433.

Durrett SJ. Efficacy of composite tooth attachments in conjunction with the Invisalign system using three-dimensional digital technology. Masters thesis, University of Florida; 2004.

Germane N, Lindauer SJ, Rubenstein LK, Revere JH, Isaacson RJ. Increase in arch perimeter due to orthodontic expansion. Am J Orthod Dentofacial Orthop. 1991; 100: 421–427.

Joffe L. Invisalign®: early experiences. J Orthod. 2003; 30: 348–352.

Kaza S. Scanning process and stereolithography. In: Tuncay O, ed. The Invisalign system. Chicago: Quintessence; 2006.

Kesling H. The philosophy of the tooth positioning appliance. Am J Orthod. 1945; 31: 297–304.

Kuo E, Miller RJ. Automated custom-manufacturing technology in orthodontics. Am J Orthod Dentofacial Orthop. 2003; 123: 578–581.

Kurth JR, Kokich VG. Open gingival embrasures after orthodontic treatment in adults: prevalence and etiology. Am J Orthod Dentofacial Orthop. 2001; 120: 116–123.

Lee H-F, Wu B, Ting K. Preliminary study on Invisalign tray fabrication. Am J Orthod Dentofacial Orthop. 2002; 122: 678.

Lu H, Nguyen B, Powers JM. Mechanical properties of 3 hydrophylic addition silicone and polyether elastomeric impression materials. J Prosthet Dent. 2004; 92: 151–154.

Malmgren O, Malmgren B, Frykholm A. Rapid orthodontic extrusion of crown root and cervical root fractured teeth. Endod Dent Traumatol. 1991; 7: 49–54.

McNamara J, Brudon W. Orthodontics and dentofacial orthopedics. Ann Arbor: Needham Press; 2001.

Meier B, Wiemer KB, Miethke R-R. Invisalign® – patient profiling. Analysis of a prospective survey. J Orofac Orthop. 2003; 64(5): 352–358.

Miethke R-R, Jost-Brinkmann P-G. Interproximal enamel reduction. In: Tuncay O, ed. The Invisalign system. Chicago: Quintessence; 2006.

Moore T, Southard KA, Casko JS, Qian F, Southard TE. Buccal corridors and smile esthetics. Am J Orthod Dentofacial Orthop. 2005; 127: 208–213.

Owen A H. Accelerated Invisalign treatment. J Clin Orthod. 2001; 35: 381–385.

Sarver D, Ackerman M. Dynamic smile visualization and quantification: part 2. Smile analysis and treatment strategies. Am J Orthod Dentofacial Orthop. 2003; 124: 116–127.

Sarver D. The importance of incisor positioning in the esthetic smile: the smile arc. Am J Orthod Dentofacial Orthop. 2001; 120: 98–111.

Schuster S, Eliades G, Zinelis S, Eliades T, Bradley TG. Structural confirmation and leaching from in vitro aged and retrieved Invisalign appliances. Am J Orthod Dentofacial Orthop. 2004; 126: 725–728.

Sheridan JJ, LeDoux W, McMinn R. Essix retainers: fabrication and supervision for permanent retention. J Clin Orthod. 1993; 27: 37–45.

Tricca R, Li Chunha. Properties of aligner material Ex30. In: Tuncay O, ed. The Invisalign system. Chicago: Quintessence; 2006.

Vlaskalic V, Boyd R. Orthodontic treatment of a mildly crowded malocclusion using the Invisalign system. Aust Orthod J. 2001; 17: 41–46.

Womack WR, Ahn JH, Ammari Z, Castillo A. A new approach to correction of crowding. Am J Orthod Dentofacial Orthop. 2002; 122: 310–316.

Wong BH. Invisalign A to Z. Am J Orthod Dentofacial Orthop. 2002; 121: 540–541.

Zachrisson BU. Actual damage to teeth and periodontal tissues with mesiodistal enamel reduction ("stripping"). World J Orthod. 2004; 5: 178–183.

14 Stripping

Bjørn Zachrisson

Mesiodistal enamel reduction (interdental stripping) is commonly used in orthodontic therapy as a method to provide space, broaden the contact points in the incisor region, and improve areas of interdental gingival recession (Tuverson 1980). This method is most often used in the anterior areas of the dental arches (Keim et al. 2008), especially in the mandibular anterior segment, where development of crowding is a constant threat to the esthetics and stability of orthodontic treatment results. Stripping offers an attractive alternative to extraction therapy, since it significantly reduces treatment time and allows pretreatment transverse arch dimensions and incisor inclinations to be maintained.

Stripping is generally done (1) by hand with various kinds of abrasive strips, (2) by rotating abrasive disks mounted on a contra-angle handpiece, or (3) by use of a turbine with tungsten-carbide (TC) or diamond burs (for review, see Pinheiro 2000). None of these techniques is universally accepted by the profession as the method of choice (Keim et al. 2008; Harfin 2000; Pinheiro 2000). Despite the extensive use of stripping, few studies have been carried out to reveal possible iatrogenic effects, such as increased sensitivity of the ground teeth, potential reduction of interproximal bone, and predisposition to caries and/or periodontal disease.

The purposes of this chapter are:
- To evaluate the risks in grinding teeth and consider the amount of tooth substance that can be removed in different clinical situations
- To discuss and recommend an optimal stripping technique and the most useful instruments
- To illustrate the clinical appearance during and after enamel reduction in selected routine and in more difficult cases
- To discuss the risks involved with the stripping procedures.

Risks in Grinding of Teeth

Among the risks involved in extensive remodeling of teeth by grinding are development of increased sensitivity, pulp and dentin reactions, discoloration (due to retention of colored pigments on rough surfaces), and caries (Zachrisson and Mjör 1975). Hence the stripping technique selected for use by a clinician must eliminate these risks.

Zachrisson and Mjör (1975) evaluated the short-term histological reactions to extensive recontouring of teeth by grinding. As an experimental model, they used grinding of canines to lateral incisor shape associated with orthodontic space closure in patients with missing maxillary lateral incisors. Obviously, such grinding is more extensive than interdental stripping. Changes in the dentin and pulp were studied after grinding of 48 premolars with different techniques, with observation periods from 1 week to 5 months. The premolars were ground on the cusp to expose cuspal dentin, on the facial surfaces, and on one interproximal surface to approximately half the mesiodistal enamel thickness (Fig. 14.1). Routine histology was performed with particular attention to alterations in the predentin/odontoblast region and to vascular and cellular changes in the pulp.

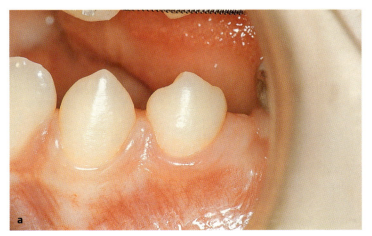
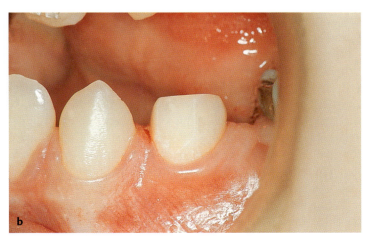

Fig. 14.**1** **Clinical experimental model used for microscopic evaluation of different grinding techniques.** First premolars were reshaped by extensive interproximal (either mesial or distal, at random), labial, and cuspal grinding with diamond instruments (**b**). The amount of enamel removed corresponds to that in clinical recontouring of canines to resemble lateral incisors. (From Zachrisson and Mjör 1975.)

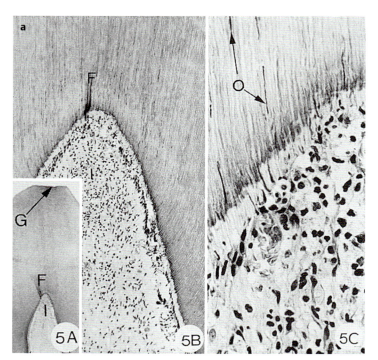
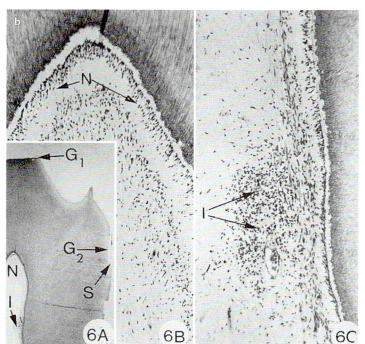

Fig. 14.2 **Histological findings after extensive grinding toward and into dentin.**

a Inadequate cooling. Odontoblast nuclei (O) displaced into the dentinal tubules after dentin exposure at G during remodeling of tooth by grinding three weeks prior to extraction. The cell-free zone in the affected area of the pulp is obscured. This microscopic picture may be seen as an immediate response to grinding if inadequate cooling is used. F = fold in section. (HE stain; original magnifications × 12 × 125 × 540.) (From Zachrisson and Mjör 1975.)

b Unintentional interproximal step. Histological reaction to unintentionally produced interproximal step (S) during grinding three months prior to extraction. Plaque accumulation in step subjacent to mesial grinding (G_2) has resulted in cellular infiltration (I) in an area of pulp tissue corresponding to dentinal canals originating from the step. (HE stain; original magnifications × 12 × 125 × 540.) (From Zachrisson and Mjör 1975.)

The short-term results showed that as long as adequate cooling was employed and the ground facets were smooth and self-cleansing, even extensive grinding of teeth can be done with minor or no pulp and dentin reactions. No significant discomfort was reported by the patients, except for an initial period of a few days during which there was increased sensitivity to temperature changes.

The best results were obtained with abundant water and air cooling. Grinding with no cooling caused marked odontoblast aspiration into the dentinal tubuli, which is an obvious sign of damage (Fig. 14.2a). Also, interdental steps must be avoided during the grinding. Steps can be produced unintentionally and may result in plaque accumulation and development of caries. Histologically, such steps resulted in inflammatory cell infiltration in the pulp (Fig. 14.2b).

The favorable short-term results of careful grinding were confirmed in clinical and radiographic long-term follow-ups 10 to 15 years after the grinding (Thordarson et al. 1991). This material consisted of 37 maxillary canines in 26 patients with agenesis of the lateral incisors. No radiographic pathology, reduction in response to electric pulp vitality testing, color change, temperature sensitivity, reaction to percussion, or other signs of damage were found in the ground teeth when compared with nonground contralateral teeth.

In conclusion, these experiments indicated that adequate cooling is to be recommended during grinding of teeth and that production of retention areas while grinding interdentally must be avoided as they may result in caries and marked alterations in the pulp and dentin.

Since the use of water and air spray is not feasible during stripping, a more practical solution would be to use abundant air cooling by an assistant in a four-handed approach (see Fig. 14.5a). The use of an air coolant during the disking procedure will contribute to patient comfort, making anesthesia unnecessary (Tuverson 1980; Thordarson et al. 1991). The initial increased sensitivity of ground teeth to temperature variations can be handled by twice-daily mouth rinsing with dilute fluoride solutions.

Amount of Enamel Removal in Stripping

The recommendation on how much enamel can be removed from each contact area is controversial and has been debated for the past 45 years (for review, see Pinheiro 2000).

In the 1970's, Peck and Peck (1972a,b) presented a formula and claimed that excess mesiodistal width in relationship to buccolingual diameter would predispose toward incisor irregularity. This theory was later disproved by Smith et al (1982). At present, most authors recommend that a certain amount of enamel can be removed per tooth contact, generally in the neighborhood of 0.3–0.5 mm per tooth contact, up to 50% of the existing enamel (Sheridan 1985), or an amount related to variations in enamel thickness between the different tooth categories (Pinheiro 2000).

There are two reasons why I feel such recommendations are not very useful clinically: (1) The grinding studies quoted above (Zachrisson and Mjör 1975; Thordarson et al. 1991) demonstrated that with proper technique the entire enamel layer can be ground away down to dentin with no untoward side-effects; and (2) there

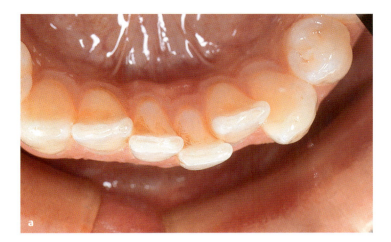
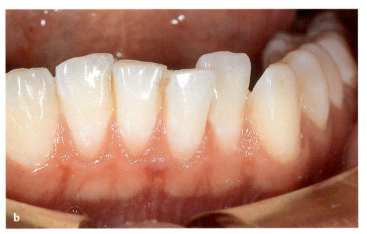

Fig. 14.**3** **Amount of enamel reduction depends on tooth morphology.** The optimal incisor shape for extensive stripping is triangular. An incisor that is wide in the incisal area and narrow gingivally allows considerable mesial and distal enamel removal and still provides a shape that will approach ideal anatomical morphology. Oval first and second mandibular premolars can be rounded and thus provide extra space for incisor leveling (**a**).

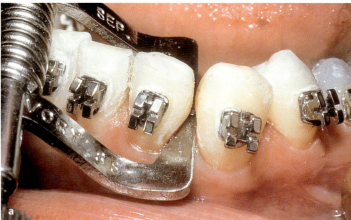
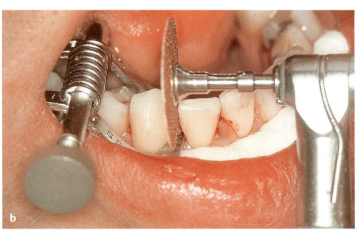

Fig. 14.**4** **Original Tuverson technique for mesiodistal enamel reduction.** Stripping of mandibular incisors is performed by means of a anterior straight Elliot separator (**a**) and a medium garnet disk mounted on a contra-angle handpiece (**b**). The separator permits a controlled reduction of enamel and protects the interdental gingival papilla. Polishing is made with fine sand and cuttle disks.

is a tremendous individual variation in morphology for all tooth categories. A more practical guide, therefore, is to relate the amount of tooth substance that can be removed to the actual shape of the teeth, and fillings and crowns, in each individual case. The principle will therefore be to recontour each individual tooth with a deviating morphology toward a more "ideal" shape for each tooth category. This principle is illustrated by the changes made from the pretreatment appearance of the teeth in the Case Studies presented later.

Reshaping of teeth toward their ideal shape enhances the potential for more individual variation in selecting the amount of enamel removal. The amount can be very substantial on teeth with deviating morphology (Fig. 14.**3**), such as triangular incisors (Case Study 14.1.**4**), oval premolars, teeth with overextended fillings, etc., whereas incisors with parallel proximal surfaces, screwdriver-shaped teeth, and round premolars may not at all be candidates for any stripping.

Other possible contraindications to stripping in selected situations include the crowding being too severe, the teeth being already too small, hypersensitivity to temperature variations, or the oral hygiene and dental awareness of the patient being inadequate for orthodontic treatment (Pinheiro 2000).

Instruments for Enamel Reduction and Polishing

The stripping effect of enamel removal by the various methods is related to several factors, such as the relative hardness of the materials used, the particle size of the abrasive, the pressure exerted, and the effective time used for stripping. Coarser abrasives will inevitably introduce scratches, which must subsequently be reduced by progressively finer abrasives.

Interproximal stripping techniques started with the use of hand-held media and fine metallic strips, as recommended by Hudson in 1956; over time, different techniques have been carefully tested and progressively improved. It was shown that coarse steel or diamond strips are effective (Harfin 2000), but the quality of the remaining enamel is not optimal. Studies by scanning electron microscopy (SEM) and profilometric analyses (Radlanski et al. 1988; Lundgren et al. 1993) have shown that coarse steel strips and diamonds should be avoided, as they may produce marked surface irregularities. The deep scratches and furrows remained to such an extent that they could not be eliminated by subsequent polishing (Lundgren et al. 1993; Piacentini and Sfondrini 1996; Puigdollers 1998).

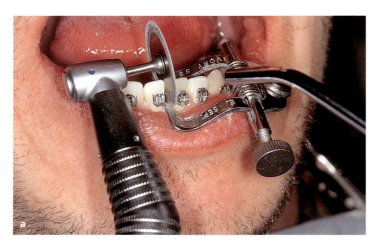
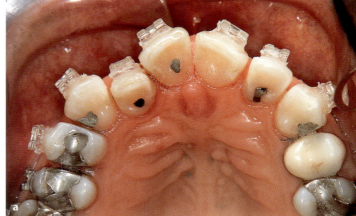
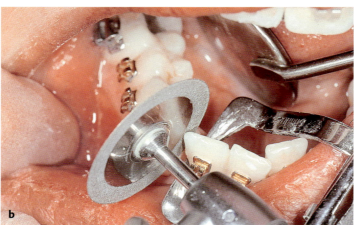
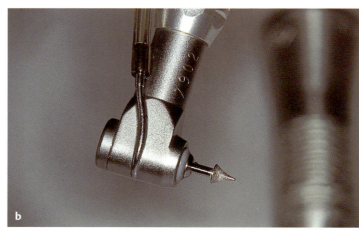

Fig. 14.**5** **Modified Tuverson stripping technique.** Less separation between incisors is needed when an ultrathin (0.1 mm) safe-sided diamond disk rather than the garnet disk is used for enamel stripping. A four-handed approach is recommended, with an assistant shooting a constant stream of air coolant from the three-way syringe. The assistant also uses a mouth mirror to protect the tongue from the disk during stripping (**b**).

Fig. 14.**6** **Need for mesiodistal rounding of interdental enamel subsequent to use of diamond disk.** Due to the hardness of mesial and distal labial and, particularly, lingual enamel, it is necessary to use a tapered diamond bur to round off the interdental "corners" when stripping with diamond disks (**a**). The no. 8833 diamond from Komet (**b**) is ideal for this purpose. This bur is only available as friction-grip, and should be used at around 60 000 rpm.

Later developments for interproximal enamel removal included the use of medium grit garnet disks (Fig. 14.4), ultrathin safe-or double-sided diamond disks (Fig. 14.5), and specially designed triangular diamond burs (Figs. 14.6, 14.7, 14.8) for rounding off the disk-treated enamel (Phillipe 1991). These instruments will be discussed below under Optimal Stripping Technique.

In the mid-1980's, air-rotor stripping (ARS) was introduced by Sheridan (Sheridan 1985; 1987; Sheridan and Hastings 1992) and became popular. ARS is a method of creating space by the removal of interproximal enamel with tungsten-carbide (TC) burs, primarily in the posterior segments of the mouth. By stripping the posterior contact points and working from posterior to anterior, the teeth can be moved distally into the spaces created like beads on a string. Although the technique is effective, the use of TC or diamond burs interdentally (Fig. 14.9) may produce scratches and grooves more easily than when disks are used (Zhong et al. 1999, 2000).

More recent developments are the Ortho-Strips system and the Proxoshape set, and a fine grain diamond-coated perforated disk developed exclusively for enamel stripping (Fig. 14.10).

The Ortho-Strips system is composed of four double-sided diamond-coated flexible metallic strips with grain size between 15 and 90 μm for enamel removal and polishing (Fig. 14.11). The strips can be adapted to the EVA system with oscillating movements of about 0.8 mm. The strips have the advantage of being flexible and adapting well to the shape and convexity of the teeth, especially cervically. However, the present design is not effective compared with other systems for enamel removal.

The Proxoshape set consists of several flexible, safe-sided diamond-coated tips for the EVA system contra-angle handpiece (Fig. 14.12). The grains vary from 15 to 125 μm, and they appear to be useful for interproximal polishing after the use of high-speed burs to reduce or eliminate the incidence of scratches and grooves.

Obviously, the rougher the surface resulting from enamel removal, the more difficult it is to achieve a perfectly smooth surface by polishing. Consequently, the finer the grain size used for enamel stripping, the easier and less time consuming is the subsequent polishing (Hein et al. 1990; Zhong et al. 1999, 2000). The furrows and scratches resulting from grinding are minimized with the recently introduced fine diamond-coated perforated disk that has a grain size of < 30 μm (Fig. 14.10). This diamond disk is very effective in enamel removal and it does not clog, because of to its multiple perforations. According to Zhong et al. (2000), the mean time needed clinically for enamel removal is about 30 seconds per tooth surface, and the mean time required

Instruments for Enamel Reduction and Polishing

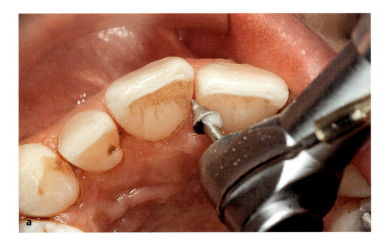
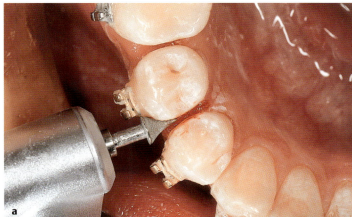
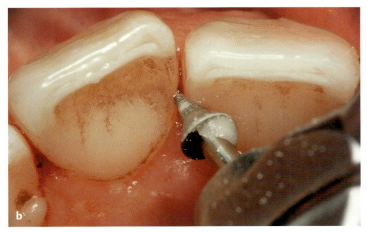
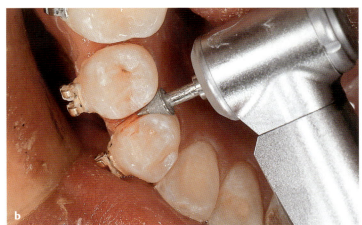

Fig. 14.**7 Recontouring incisors toward ideal shape.** The friction-grip no. 8833 diamond bur (Komet, Gebr. Brasseler) used at around 60 000 rpm in a red ring contra-angle handpiece is excellent for rounding off interproximal tooth surfaces that have been stripped with a diamond-coated disk. The bur can be inserted between two neighboring incisors, and both teeth can be rounded off almost at the same time.

Fig. 14.**8 Recontouring premolars toward ideal shape.** The no. 8833 diamond bur has a shape that makes it optimal for mesial (**a**) and distal (**b**) recontouring of premolars toward their correct anatomical shape. The use of this bur is a necessary step when diamond-coated disks are used for stripping purposes in the premolar regions.

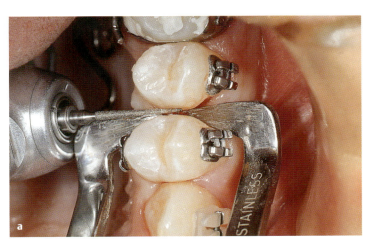
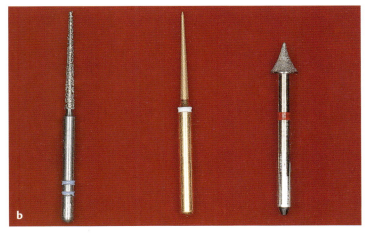

Fig. 14.**9 High-speed posterior stripping and polishing with diamond burs.** Used at high speed, fine-pointed long diamond burs are effective for interdental stripping and polishing in the premolar region (**a**). Length of fine and superfine grit diamond burs are compared with no. 8833 bur in (**b**).

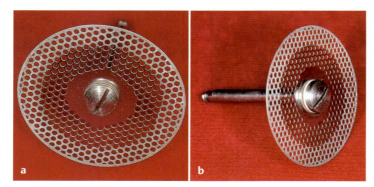

Fig. 14.**10** **New perforated diamond-coated disk developed for stripping purposes.** This diamond disk is the instrument of choice for careful interproximal stripping. Although the diamond particles are fine, the disk is effective and the multiple perforations prevent clogging. There are diamond particles also along the edge, so that it can cut through a noncrowded contact area.

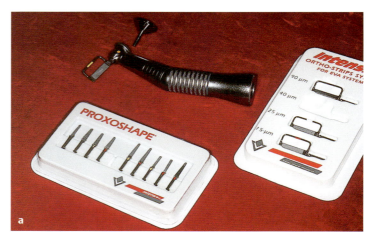

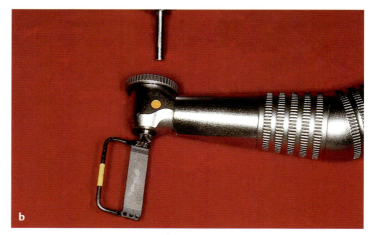

Fig. 14.**11** **Ortho-Strips system and Proxoshape set. a** Flexible diamond-coated strips with grain sizes from 15 to 90 μm (Ortho-Strips) and flexible files (Proxoshape) with grit from 15 μm (superfine) to 125 μm (extra coarse) to be used with KaVo EVA-head (**b**) contra-angle (back-and-forth oscillating motion) have been developed for stripping and prepolishing purposes. The models available at present are helpful for interdental finishing after use of burs in the posterior regions, but not very effective for stripping involving extensive enamel removal, when compared with, e.g., the diamond-coated perforated disk in Fig. 14.**10**.

for the subsequent polishing with fine and ultrafine Sof-Lex (3 M) disks (including disk-changing time) is about 50 seconds per tooth surface. In a clinical study by Zhong et al. (2000), replicas were made of 296 interproximally stripped tooth surfaces in 32 patients (average age 15.5 years) and evaluated by SEM. More than 90% of the stripped surfaces were very well or well polished and, in fact, were smoother than untreated enamel. Even the less perfectly polished tooth surfaces were no more plaque retentive than untreated adult enamel.

Consequently, it appears safer to remove enamel with disks than with TC or diamond burs. Combined mechanical and chemical technique to restore the stripped tooth surfaces, as advocated by Joseph et al. (1992), or the use of a sealant after stripping (Sheridan and Ledoux 1992) appear unnecessary.

Optimal Stripping Technique

The use of abrasive disks mounted on a contra-angle handpiece, which usually requires a mechanical separator, is recommended as the procedure of choice for routine enamel reduction (Figs. 14.**4**, 14.**5**). This procedure was originally described by Tuverson (1980). Although the disk he used (medium-grain garnet disk on snap-on mandrel) may be replaced with ultrathin diamond disks, the principle remains the same. Use of the disks on separated tooth surfaces permits a more controlled reduction of enamel than other methods. As mentioned, it is extremely important to control the amount and area of enamel reduction from each of the tooth surfaces. The contact points of incisors, especially of the lower ones, should be slightly broadened (Tuverson 1980). Small contact points are more susceptible to slippage and rotation of the teeth. One should avoid slice cuts (Fig. 14.**6a**), since they produce nonanatomical morphology and an unstable arch form (Tuverson 1980).

The preferred mechanical separator is a straight anterior Elliot separator (Figs. 14.**4**, 14.**5**). It is placed between the teeth to be separated and carefully tightened short of the amount of space required for the disking process. By allowing 30 seconds for the periodontal membrane fibers to yield to the pressure of the separator and for compression to occur, sufficient disking space is obtained. Since the separation is somewhat painful, it is important when stripping crowded teeth to first separate and reduce the least crowded teeth, which will require less separation. Enamel reduction of these teeth will provide additional space for the more crowded teeth to be moved by the separator with less discomfort to the patient.

As an alternative to the separator, a wooden wedge can be used for the same purpose (Fig. 14.**13**). Like the separator, the wedge will also protect the interdental gingiva from damage during stripping with an abrasive disk.

After diamond disks have been used interproximally, the stripped tooth surfaces are generally too flat and therefore must be rounded off from the labial and lingual sides in both the anterior and posterior regions of the mouth. The triangular diamond bur no. 8833 (Fig. 14.**6b**) is excellent for this purpose (Figs. 14.**7**, 14.**8**).

Rotating versus Oscillating Handpiece

When the diamond-coated perforated disk that is optimal for stripping used rotating in a conventional contra-angle handpiece, there is risk of soft-tissue injury to the lip and tongue. Although disk guards are available (Pinheiro 2000), their use is cumber-

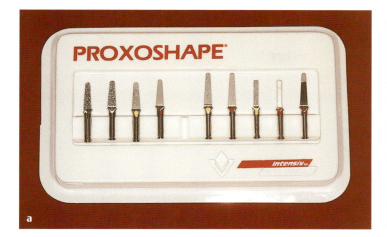
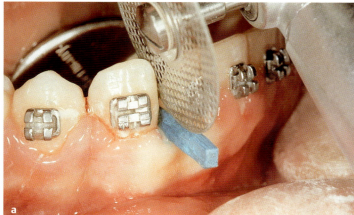
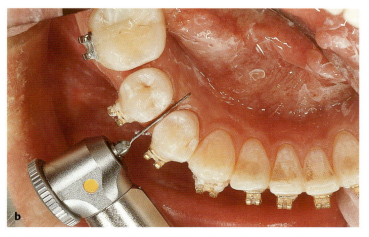
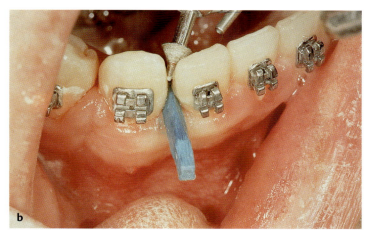

Fig. 14.**12** **Interdental polishing with Proxoshape.** The back-and-forth movement of the Proxoshape diamond-coated tips make them useful for interdental finishing in the premolar areas and allows the practitioner to avoid steps associated with other techniques for enamel removal.

Fig. 14.**13** **"Poor man's" separator.** As an alternative to a mechanical separator, a wooden wedge can also be useful for opening up small spaces between teeth to be stripped with the diamond-coated perforated disk (**a**) and rounded with the no. 8833 diamond bur (**b**). Like the separator, the wooden wedge will protect the interdental gingiva from laceration by the disk.

some. Oscillating handpieces are now manufactured for orthodontic stripping purposes. Zhong et al. (1999, 2000) tested the perforated diamond-coated disk used at moderate speed in a prototype oscillating contra-angle handpiece that rotated about 60 degrees (model no. 962A-H, W&H, Austria). This handpiece made soft-tissue injuries unlikely, and eliminated the need for any lip and tongue protection.

How to Maintain Normal Gingival Papillae during Orthodontic Treatment

The two most important reasons why "black triangles" (interdental gingival recession) develop between neighboring teeth are the location of the contact point and the axial inclination of the teeth (Burke et al. 1994; Kurth and Kokich 2001). According to Tarnow et al. (1992), the decisive factor is the distance between the contact point and the crest of bone. This distance should not exceed 5 mm if an intact gingival papilla is to be maintained. When the distance exceeds 7 mm, an intact interdental gingival papilla is only found in 27% of examined cases. This means that the purpose of the recontouring by stripping is to relocate the contact points as much as required in an apical direction. Such relocation is generally feasible in "normal" adolescent and adult patients (see Case Studies 14.**1**–14.**3**).

In addition, the stripping will increase the connector area between the teeth. There is a distinction between contact point and connector area. The contact points between anterior teeth are generally small areas, whereas the connector is a larger, broader area that is defined as the zone in which two adjacent teeth appear to touch (Morley and Eubank 2001). The ideal connector area between the maxillary central incisors is defined as 50% of the length of the clinical crown of the central incisors (Morley and Eubank 2001). When two central incisors overlap pretreatment in adults (Case Study 14.**3** *[2]*), the gingival papilla generally is lost after initial orthodontic alignment (Kurth and Kokich 2001). This means that the stripping must fulfill the following requirements: (1) Recontour the mesial surfaces to "ideal" shape; (2) relocate the contact point in gingival direction; (3) lengthen the connector area; (4) make the connector area parallel to the facial midline; and (5) eliminate the "black triangle." All these requirements can be met by careful stripping (Case Studies 14.**3** and 14.**4**).

In adults with crowding, large overjet, and triangularly shaped teeth (Case Study 14.**5**), the esthetic problem reaches a magnitude that makes stripping mandatory as part of the orthodontic treatment. During leveling and alignment, the gingival papillae are predictably lost, and extensive recontouring is required to restore normal tooth shape, relocate the contact points, and increase the connector areas (Case Study 14.**5**).

How to Regain Lost Gingival Papillae

In patients with marked periodontal problems, the interdental gingival papillae between maxillary and mandibular incisors are normally lost (Case Studies 14.**6** and 14.**7**). Recontouring tooth shapes by stripping and correcting the axial inclinations of the incisors allows relocation of contact points and lengthening of connector areas so that the gingival papillae may return. In most cases with advanced periodontal tissue break-down, it is not possible to get a complete fill-in of the gingival papillae. However, even in severe periodontal cases (Case Study 14.**7**), it is possible by carefully repeated stripping sequences to reach an esthetic final outcome with almost naturally looking dentitions.

Stripping versus Extraction of a Single Mandibular Incisor

In cases with moderate-to-severe mandibular anterior crowding, the clinician's choice may sometimes be to select between extensive stripping or the extraction of one mandibular incisor.

The single incisor extraction alternative has the advantage of creating space in the area most prone to crowding, but, as discussed elsewhere (Færøvig and Zachrisson 1999; Zachrisson 2001), it may often provide too much space and thus compromise the quality of the anterior tooth relationship, inducing excessive overbite and overjet. The tooth-mass discrepancies between 4 maxillary and 3 mandibular incisors also make it difficult to perform enough stripping of the remaining 3 lower incisors to avoid the development of interdental gingival recession ("black triangles") in the mandibular anterior region (Zachrisson 2001). In contrast, the gingival papillae are more easily maintained intact in the mandible when stripping rather than extraction is performed. This is particularly true when treating adult or elderly adult patients.

Consequently, the one single mandibular extraction alternative should largely be reserved for malocclusions with inadequate overbite and overjet pretreatment, such as cases with Class III + open bite tendencies (Zachrisson 2001).

Predisposition to Caries and Risk of Accelerated Periodontal Tissue Breakdown after Stripping

Unintentionally produced interproximal steps or failure to polish the tooth surfaces after stripping with coarse abrasives may lead to future cavities (Zachrisson and Mjör 1975; Harfin 2000). However, several retrospective studies have shown that carefully performed stripping with optimal techniques will not increase the caries risk for treated patients (Boese 1980; Crain and Sheridan 1990; El-Mangoury et al. 1991; Joseph et al. 1992). A special topical fluoride treatment of the ground and polished tooth surfaces is not necessary, but twice-daily mouth rinsing with weak fluoride solutions is recommended to facilitate the remineralization of the stripped teeth for as long as there are any signs of increased sensitivity to hot and cold.

Some clinicians have expressed the fear that roots might come too close following extensive enamel reduction and that the thin interdental alveolar bone could lead to accelerated periodontal tissue breakdown. However, in a retrospective study 25 years after the orthodontic therapy, no difference in periodontal condition was found between teeth with normally spaced roots and teeth with root proximity and thin bone septa (Årtun et al. 1986, 1987). Apparently, bone quantity is of secondary importance with respect to progression of disease, and a dentogingival unit with a long connective-tissue attachment is not more prone to plaque-induced attachment loss (Brägger and Lang 1996). In fact, very small interroot distances of 0.3–0.5 mm can have a normal periodontal ligament even in the absence of bone (Heins and Wieder 1986). Even theoretically, it is inconceivable that roots of teeth that are recontoured toward ideal shape during stripping should come any closer to one another than they were when the teeth were in a crowded relationship.

A recent follow-up study of a large sample of patients more than 10 years after the stripping in our clinic (Zacharisson et al 2007) substantiate the claims that there is no indication that the enamel reduction has increased the risk for future caries or periodontal problems. Likewise, no patients complained about increased sensitivity to temperature changes in the ground teeth.

Clinical Case Studies

Case Study 14.1 Young adult male patient with Class I malocclusion and mild-to-moderate bimaxillary crowding

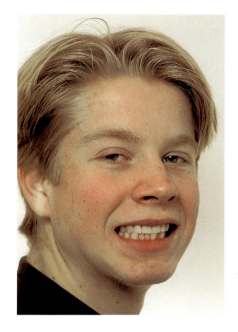

Fig. 14.1.**1**
Pretreatment facial view.

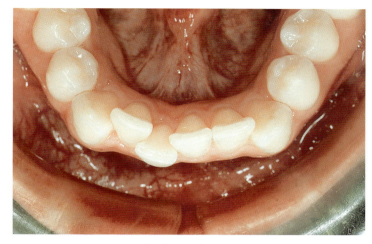

Fig. 14.1.**4** **Pretreatment occlusal view of mandibular anterior region.** Triangular incisors and oval premolars made this case ideal for stripping and leveling with no change of the normal mandibular arch form.

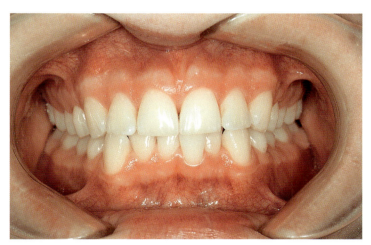

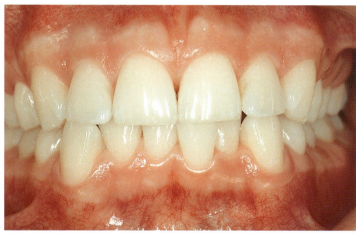

Fig. 14.1.**2,3** **Pretreatment intraoral frontal views.** Nonextraction treatment without lateral expansion or incisor proclination. Treatment time was 7 months.

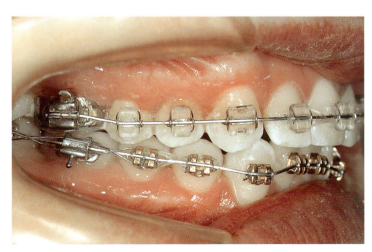

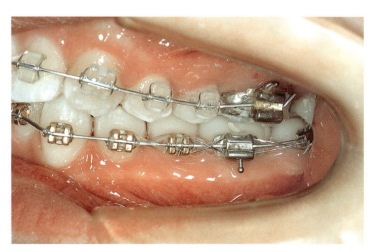

Fig. 14.1.**5,6** **Initial leveling.** After placement of orthodontic esthetic appliances, a 0.016 in. × 0.022 in. Bioforce Sentalloy leveling wire was inserted and maintained for 1–2 months before the stripping was done. The initial period is useful to loosen the teeth, thus facilitating their mechanical separation while stripping.

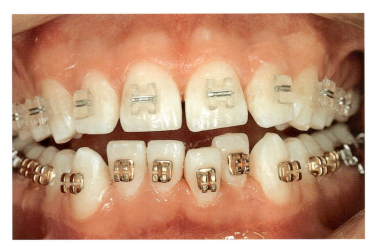
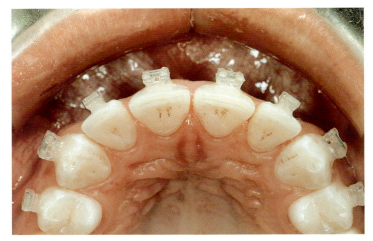

Fig. 14.1.**7, 8 Frontal and maxillary occlusal views after stripping.** The principle in stripping is to recontour each tooth toward its ideal shape. The amount of enamel removal is, of course, also dependent on the degree of malalignment.

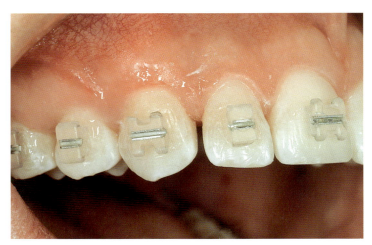
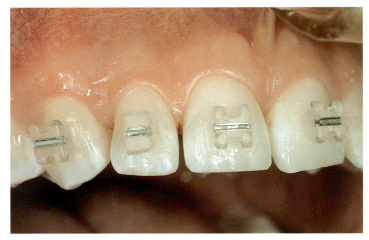

Fig. 14.1.**9, 10 Maxillary stripping—frontal view.** Higher magnification of amount of enamel removed from teeth in maxillary anterior region.

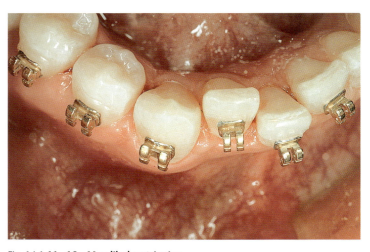
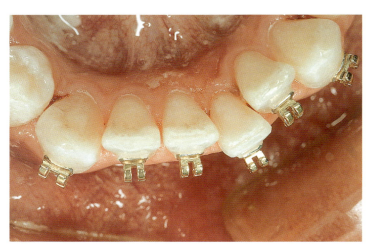

Fig. 14.1.**11–16 Mandibular stripping.**
11, 12 Occlusal views indicate amount of enamel removed from each tooth in the mandibular anterior region.

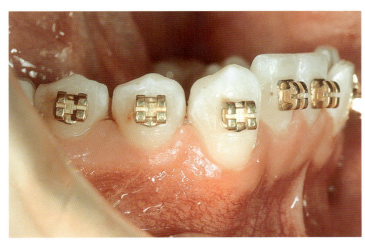
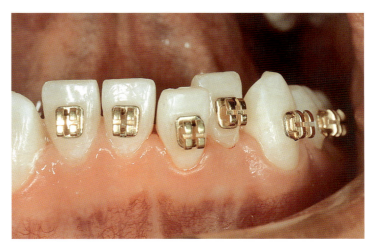

Fig. 14.1.**13, 14** Frontal views indicating amount of enamel removed from each tooth in the right posterior and frontal regions.

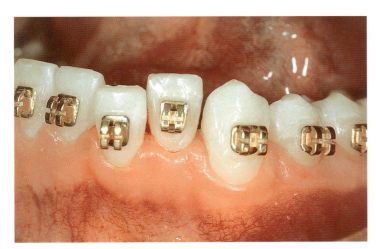
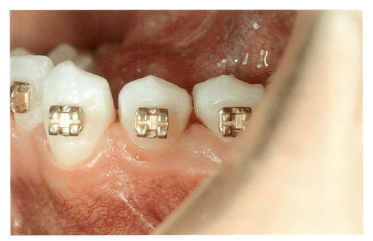

Fig. 14.1.**15, 16** Frontal views indicating amount of enamel removed from each tooth in the left anterior and posterior region.

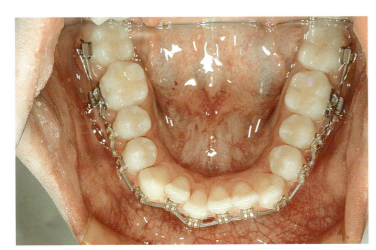
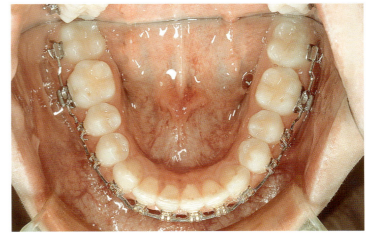

Fig. 14.1.**17, 18 Occlusal views after one month [17] and six months [18] of orthodontic treatment.** Comparison of the occlusal views of the mandibular dental arch before and after treatment. Note that the leveling was done without lateral expansion of the 3–3 distance and with no proclination of the lower incisors.

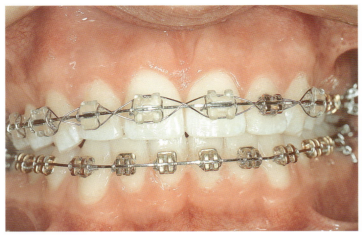

Fig. 14.1.**19, 20 Toward end of seven months' orthodontic nonextraction treatment.** Note intact gingival papillae and teeth with optimal shape. A gold-

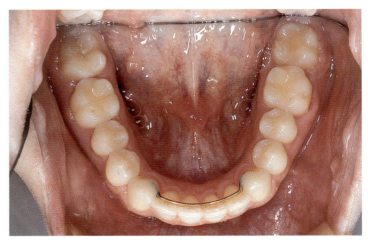

coated mandibular 3–3 retainer was bonded to canines only after completed orthodontic treatment.

Case Study 14.2 Young adult male with bimaxillary crowding

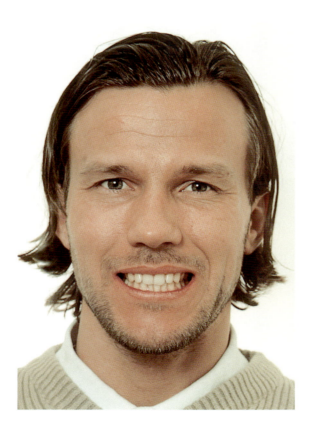

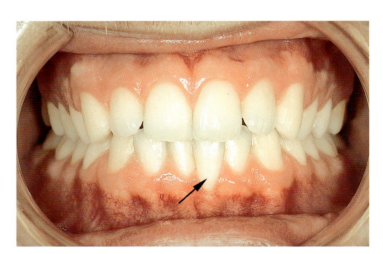

Fig. 14.2.**1, 2 Pretreatment extraoral and intraoral frontal views.** Note labial gingival recession on mandibular left central incisor. Treatment time was 1 year 5 months.

Clinical Case Studies

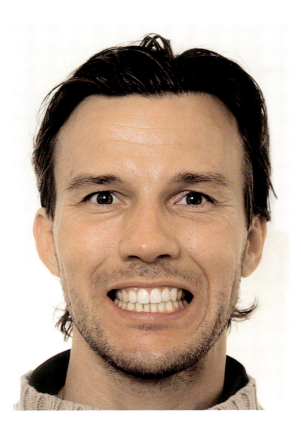

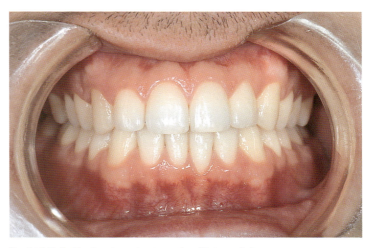

Fig. 14.2.**3, 4** **Posttreatment extraoral and intraoral views.**

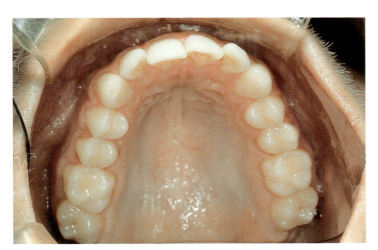

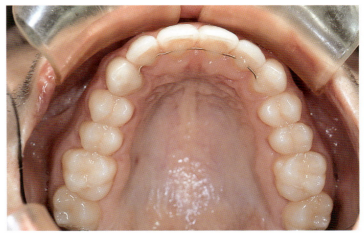

Fig. 14.2.**5, 6** **Pretreatment [5] and posttreatment [6] maxillary occlusal views.** After one month of leveling, stripping was performed on all teeth from the distal aspect of the right first premolar to the distal aspect of the left first premolar. Note the optimal shape of all maxillary teeth post treatment.

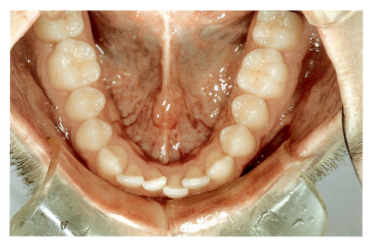
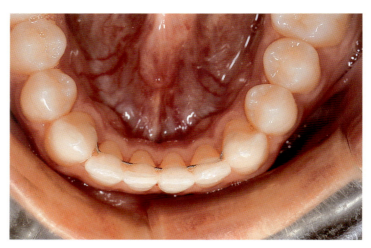

Fig. 14.2.**7, 8** **Pretreatment [7] and posttreatment [8] mandibular occlusal views.** Stripping was done from the distal aspect of mandibular right first premolar to distal aspect of left first premolar, after one month of leveling to loosen the teeth.

However, the stripping between the central incisors was delayed for some further months of leveling to secure optimal tooth shape while disking.

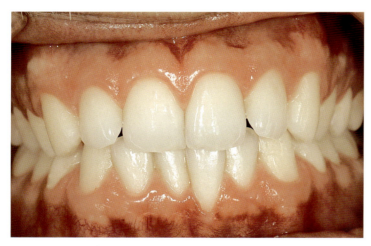
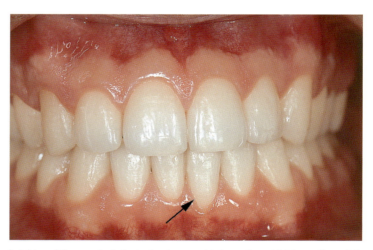

Fig. 14.2.**9, 10** **Higher magnification of intraoral views pretreatment [9] and posttreatment [10]**. Note optimal tooth shapes and intact gingival papillae after treatment. The labial gingival recession on the left central incisor is reduced in height, and the marginal gingiva has increased in buccolingual thickness (from 0.2 to 0.6 mm as determined with ultrasonography) as the stripping has allowed the left central incisor to be moved into the mandibular dental arch form.

Case Study 14.3 Adult female patient with Class III malocclusion and overlapping maxillary central incisors

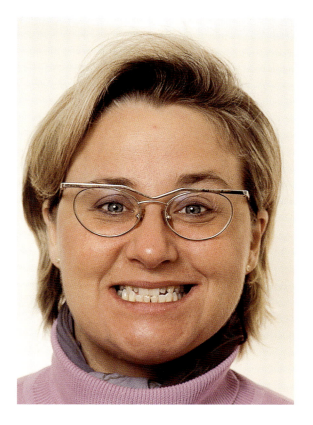

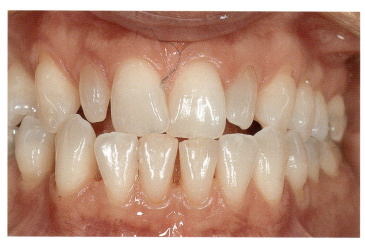

Fig. 14.3.**1, 2** Note intact interdental gingival papilla between the two maxillary central incisors before orthodontic treatment was started.

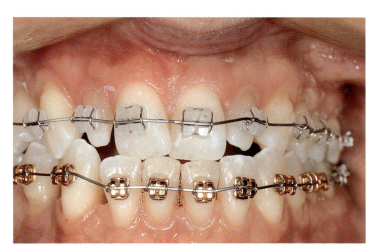

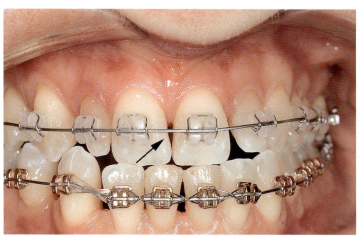

Fig. 14.3.**3, 4 Frontal view at start [3] and after one month of leveling** [4]. As soon as the central incisor overlap was corrected, the interdental gingival papilla was lost. This was predictable.

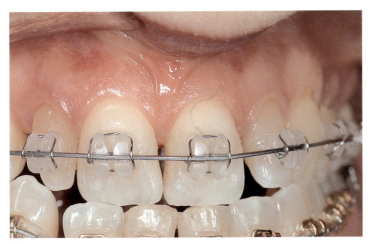
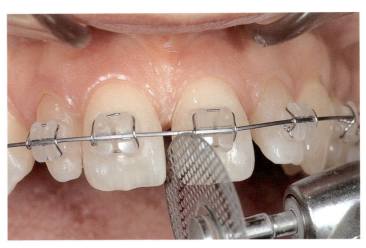

Fig. 14.3.**5, 6** **Higher magnification of maxillary central incisors after initial leveling.** The purpose of the stripping in this case was (1) to relocate the contact point in the gingival direction; (2) to increase the incisal–gingival length of the connector area between the central incisors; (3) to restore the anatomical shape of the mesial surfaces of both central incisors; and (4) to improve the appearance of their interdental gingival papilla. Stripping was initiated with the perforated diamond-coated disk [6]).

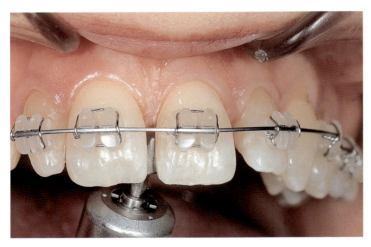
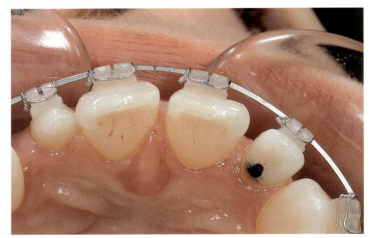

Fig. 14.3.**7, 8** **Rounding and polishing of central incisors.** The mesiolabial and mesiolingual contours of the disk-stripped maxillary central incisors were rounded with the no. 8833 diamond bur [7] to optimal morphology [8].

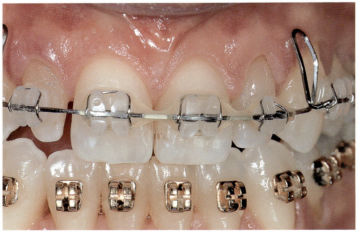
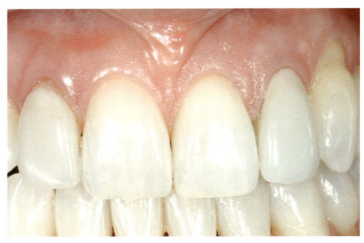

Fig. 14.3.**9, 10** **Improved hard- and soft-tissue esthetics of central incisors.** All four goals mentioned in 14.3.**5, 6** have been reached in that the contact point is relocated gingivally, the connector area is increased, the morphology is optimal, and the interdental gingival papilla is intact. After treatment [10], porcelain laminate veneers were made on the lateral incisors.

Case Study 14.4 Young female patient with Class II: 2 malocclusion, two impacted canines, and bimaxillary crowding after removal of the appliance

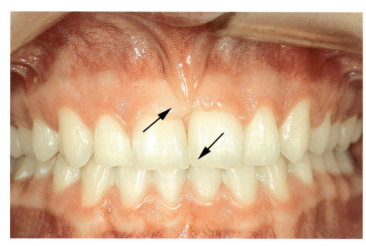 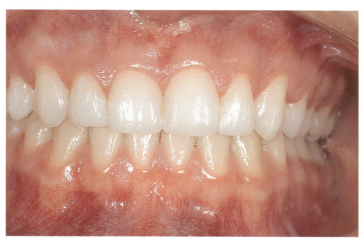

Fig. 14.4.**1, 2** **Esthetic corrections after appliance removal.** Although orthodontic treatment was successful, the esthetic result is not optimal. Contact point between the maxillary central incisors is located too far incisally, the interdental papilla is not filling the area between the central incisors, the marginal gingiva around the central incisors is hyperplastic, and the frenum has a low insertion. Esthetic recontouring, minor surgery (gingivectomy, frenotomy) and stripping between maxillary central incisors has relocated the contact point in a gingival direction and increased the connector area between the two teeth. The connector area was made parallel to the facial midline. The interdental papilla fills the space between the central incisors, and the frenum is relocated apically.

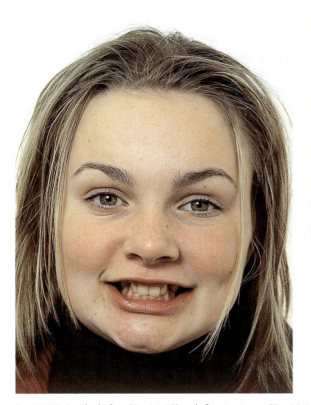 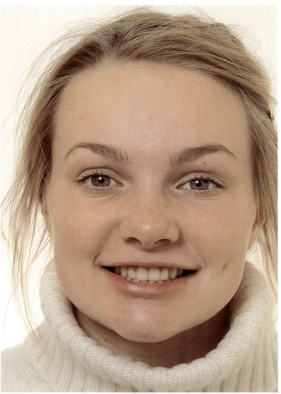

Fig. 14.4.**3, 4** The before (Fig. 14.4.**3**) and after treatment (Fig. 14.4.**4**) facial frontal photographs demonstrate the improved dental and facial appearance with the orthodontic treatment and the esthetic corrections.

Case Study 14.5 Adult female patient with full Class II:1 malocclusion and bimaxillary crowding

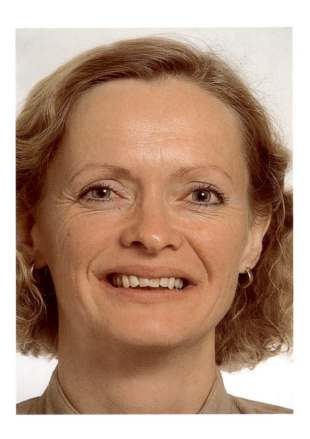

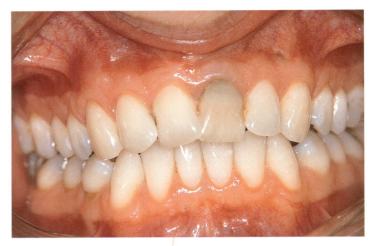

Fig. 14.5.**1, 2** Note intact gingival papillae between all teeth pretreatment. Tooth morphology is triangular.

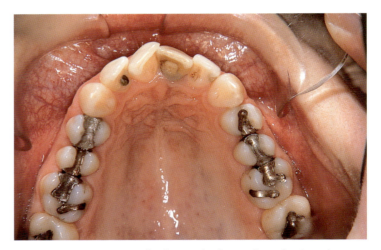

Fig. 14.5.**3** **Pretreatment occlusal view.** The degree of crowding is moderate. The case was treated with extraction of both maxillary first premolars.

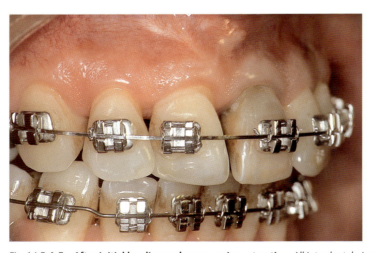

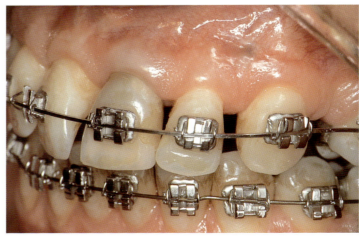

Fig. 14.5.**4, 5** **After initial leveling and some canine retraction.** All interdental gingival papillae between the maxillary incisors have been lost, even though canine retraction is not completed! This tissue response is expected and predictable in adult orthodontics.

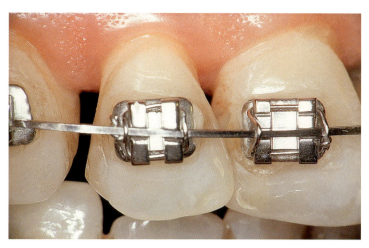 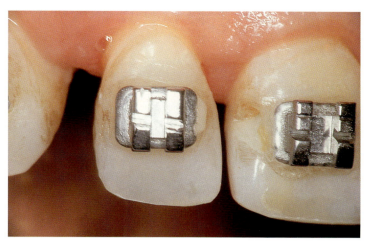

Fig. 14.5.**6, 7** **Higher magnification of maxillary right lateral incisor.** Mesiodistal and incisal recontouring by grinding was performed with diamond instruments, and the surfaces were polished with medium garnet and fine sand and cuttle disks. Compare tooth morphology before [6] and after stripping [7].

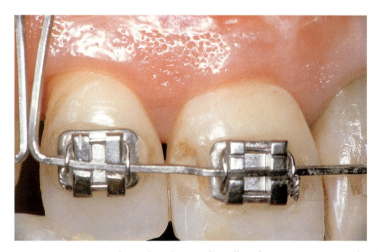 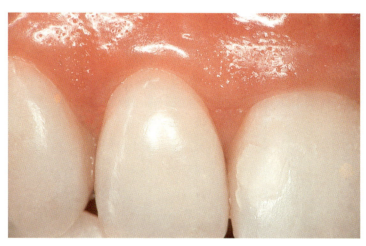

Fig. 14.5.**8, 9** **Return of interdental gingival papillae after stripping.** Due to the relocation of the contact points and recontouring toward ideal shape, the interdental gingival papillae have returned.

Case Study 14.6 Adult female patient with marked periodontal tissue breakdown

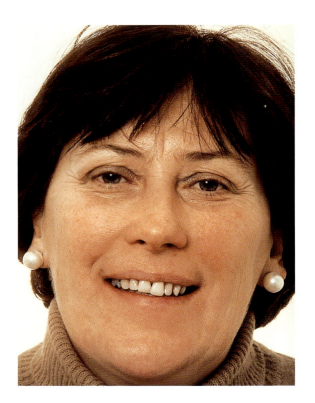

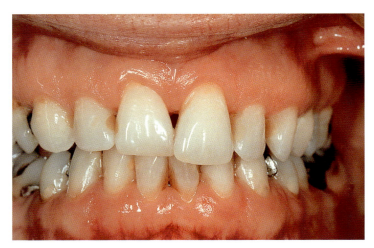

Fig. 14.6.**1, 2** The interdental gingival papilla between the maxillary central incisors is lost pretreatment. The left central incisor is supraerupted.

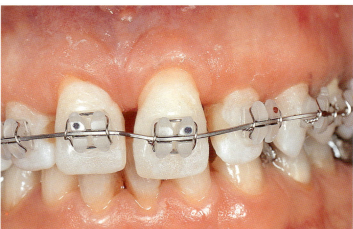

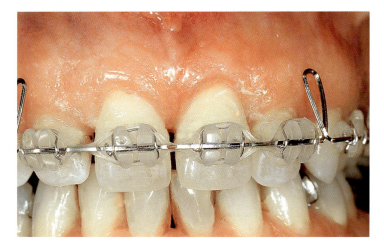

Fig. 14.6.**3, 4** **Recontouring of mesial surfaces of maxillary central incisors.** After marked stripping of the mesial surfaces of the incisors and intrusion of the left central incisor [3], the roots are allowed to come closer to one another [4].

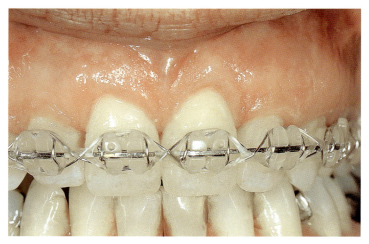

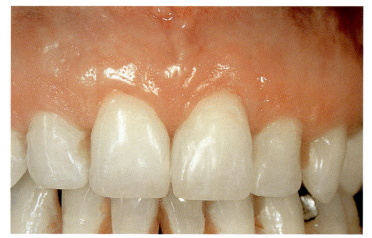

Fig. 14.6.**5, 6** **Return of gingival papilla.** Due to the continued space closure, improved morphology, and relocation of the contact point, the gingival papilla between the maxillary central incisors has returned at the end of the orthodontic treatment.

Case Study 14.7 Advanced periodontal tissue break-down in adult female patient

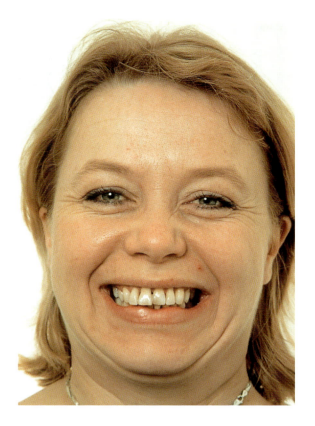

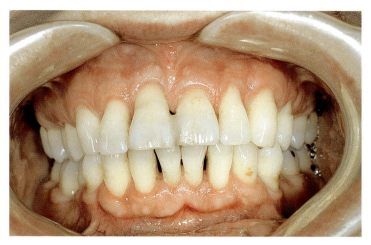

Fig. 14.7.**1,2** **Before orthodontic treatment was started, the patient's periodontist had made an attempt to grind the maxillary right central incisor and contact splint the loose right central incisor to the neighboring teeth.** Note that all interdental gingival papillae between the maxillary and mandibular incisors are retracted.

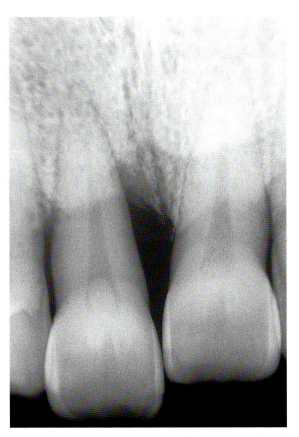

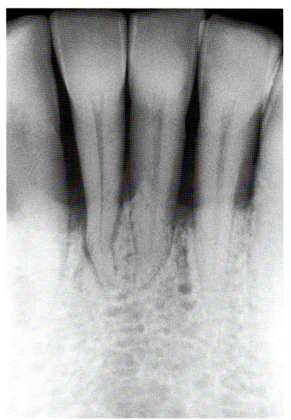

Fig. 14.7.**3,4** **Pretreatment radiographic appearance.** Both the maxillary and the mandibular incisors demonstrate advanced periodontal tissue breakdown before orthodontics was begun.

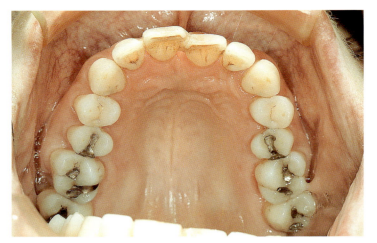
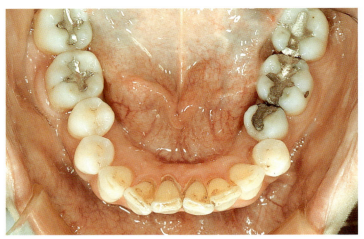

Fig. 14.7.**5, 6** **Pretreatment occlusal views.** Marked anterior and posterior stripping was done in this case for two reasons: (1) to solve the crowding problem without expansion of the dental arches or proclination of the teeth, and (2) to try to reduce the "black triangles" that were present interdentally between all the incisors.

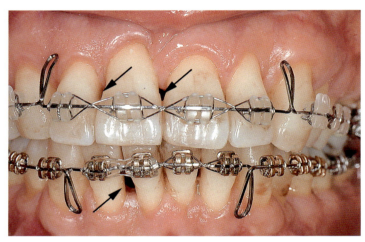
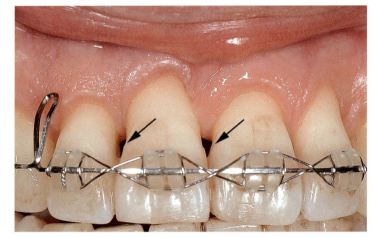

Fig. 14.7.**7, 8** **Clinical appearance after first stripping episode followed by leveling and space closure.** Even after extensive stripping to relocate the contact points and increase the length of the connector area, the interdental papillae remain retracted.

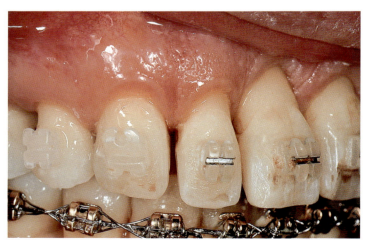
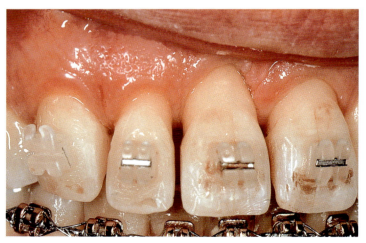

Fig. 14.7.**9–12** **Clinical appearance after second stripping episode.**
9, 10 Higher magnification of the maxillary right front region demonstrates the tooth shapes of the maxillary incisors after the second episode of stripping, the purpose of which was to try to improve the esthetic appearance of the interdental papillae.

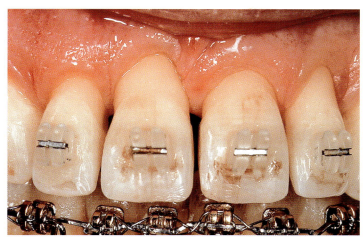
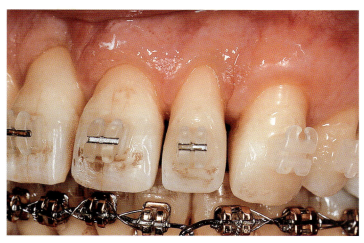

Fig. 14.7.**11, 12** Higher magnification of the maxillary anterior front region and left side demonstrates the tooth shapes of the maxillary incisors after the second episode of stripping.

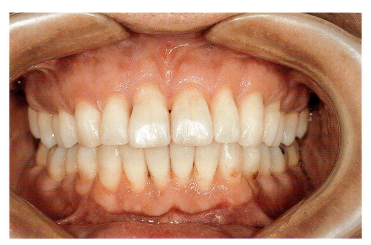
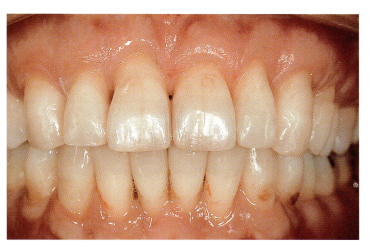

Fig. 14.7.**13, 14 Clinical appearance at end of orthodontic treatment.** Despite the advanced periodontal tissue breakdown, the final esthetic result is satisfactory, with an almost natural-looking dentition. There is little interdental gingival recession in both dental arches. The patient was poorly motivated for connective-tissue grafts and coronally repositioned flaps since she did not show much of the marginal gingival area, even when smiling (cf. 14.7.**1**).

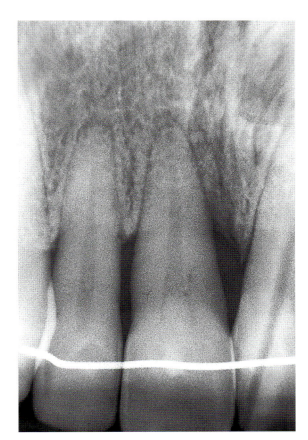

Fig. 14.7.**15 Radiographic appearance post treatment.** Compared with the pretreatment radiograph in 14.7.**3**, there is no further loss of marginal bone level associated with the intrusion and leveling, nor are there any marked signs of apical root resorption. The large crown-to-root ratio makes it prudent to retain the dentition permanently with a fixed bonded retainer.

References

Årtun J, Osterberg SK, Kokich VG. Long-term effect of thin interdental alveolar bone on periodontal health after orthodontic treatment. J Periodontol. 1986; 57: 341–346

Årtun J, Kokich VG, Osterberg SK. Long-term effect of root proximity on periodontal health after orthodontic treatment. Am J Orthod Dentofacial Orthop. 1987; 91: 125–130

Boese LR. Fiberotomy and reproximation without lower retention, nine years in retrospect. Angle Orthod. 1980; 50: 88–97, 169–178

Brägger U, Lang NP. The significance of bone in periodontal disease. Semin Orthod. 1996; 2: 31–38

Burke S, Burch JG, Tetz JA. Incidence and size of pretreatment overlap and post-treatment gingival embrasure space between maxillary central incisors. Am J Orthod Dentofacial Orthop. 1994; 105: 506–511

Crain G, Sheridan JJ. Susceptibility to caries and periodontal disease after posterior air-rotor stripping. J Clin Orthod. 1990; 24: 84–85

El-Mangoury NH, Moussa MM, Mostafa YA, Girgis AS. In-vivo remineralization after air-rotor stripping. J Clin Orthod. 1991; 25: 75–78

Færøvig E, Zachrisson BU. Effects of mandibular incisor extraction on anterior occlusion in adults with Class III malocclusion and reduced overbite. Am J Orthod Dentofacial Orthop. 1999; 115: 113–124

Harfin JF. Interproximal stripping for the treatment of adult crowding. J Clin Orthod. 2000; 34: 424–433

Hein C, Jost-Brinkmann PG, Schillai G. Oberflächenbeschaffenheit des Schmelzes nach approximalen Beschleifen – Rasterelektronmikroskopische Beurteilung unterschiedlicher Polierverfahren. Fortschr Kieferorthop. 1990; 51: 327–335

Heins PJ, Wieder SM. A histological study of the width and nature of inter-radicular spaces in human adult premolars and molars. J Dent Res. 1986; 65: 948–951

Hudson AL. A study of the effects of mesiodistal reduction of mandibular anterior teeth. Am J Orthod. 1956; 42: 615–624

Joseph VP, Rossouw PE, Basson NJ. Orthodontic microabrasive reapproximation. Am J Orthod Dentofacial Orthop. 1992; 102: 351–359

Keim RG, Gottlieb EL, Nelson AH et al. JCO study of orthodontic diagnosis and treatment procedures. Part 1. Results and trends. J Clin Orthod. 2008; 42: 625–640

Kurth JR, Kokich VG. Open gingival embrasures after orthodontic treatment in adults: Prevalence and etiology. Am J Orthod Dentofacial Orthop. 2001; 120: 116–123

Lundgren T, Milleding P, Mohlin B, Nannmark U. Restitution of enamel after interdental stripping. Swed Dent J. 1993; 17: 217–224

Morley J, Eubank J. Macroesthetic elements of smile design. J Am Dent Assoc 2001; 132: 39–45

Peck H, Peck S. An index for assessing tooth shape deviations as applied to the mandibular incisors. Am J Orthod. 1972a; 61: 384–401

Peck H, Peck S. Crown dimensions and mandibular incisor alignment. Angle Orthod. 1972b; 42: 148–153

Philippe J. A method of enamel reduction for correction of adult arch-length discrepancy. J Clin Orthod. 1991; 25: 484–489

Piacentini C, Sfondrini G. A scanning electron microscopy comparison of enamel polishing methods after air-rotor stripping. Am J Orthod Dentofacial Orthop. 1996; 109: 57–63

Pinheiro M. Interproximal enamel reduction. Ortodoncia. 2000; 5: 134–157

Puigdollers A. Rasterelektronmikroskopische in-vitro-Vergleichsstudie der Auswirkungen des Beschleifens (Strippens) des Schmelzes bleibender Zähne von Hand und mit der Luftturbine. Inf Orthod Kieferorthop. 1998; 30: 511–527

Radlanski RJ, Jäger A, Schwestka R, Bertzbach F. Plaque accumulation caused by interdental stripping. Am J Orthod Dentofacial Orthop. 1988; 94: 416–420

Sheridan JJ. Air-rotor stripping. J Clin Orthod. 1985; 19: 43–59

Sheridan JJ. Air-rotor stripping update. J Clin Orthod. 1987; 21: 781–787

Sheridan JJ, Hastings J. Air-rotor stripping and lower incisor extraction treatment. J Clin Orthod. 1992 a; 26: 18–22

Sheridan JJ, Ledoux PM. Air-rotor stripping and proximal sealants. An SEM evaluation. J Clin Orthod. 1989; 23: 790–794

Smith RJ, Davidson WM, Gipe DP. Incisor shape and incisor crowding: A reevaluation of the Peck and Peck ratio. Am J Orthod. 1982; 82: 231–235

Tarnow DP, Magner AW, Fletcher P. The effect of the distance from the contact point to the crest of bone on the presence or absence of the interproximal dental papilla. J Periodontol. 1992; 63: 995–996

Thordarson A, Zachrisson BU, Mjör IA. Remodeling of canines to the shape of lateral incisors by grinding: A long-term clinical and radiographic evaluation. Am J Orthod Dentofacial Orthop. 1991; 100: 123–132

Tuverson DL. Anterior interocclusal relations. Parts I and II. Am J Orthod. 1980; 78: 361–393

Zachrisson BU. Extraction of one single mandibular incisor. World J Orthod. 2001; 2: 190–193

Zachrisson BU, Mjör IA. Remodeling of teeth by grinding. Am J Orthod. 1975; 68: 545–553

Zachrisson BU, Nyøygaard L, Mobarak K. Dental health assessed more than 10 years after interproximal enamel reduction of mandibular anterior teeth. Am J Orthod Dentofacial Orthop 2007; 131: 762–169

Zhong M, Jost-Brinkmann PG, Radlanski RJ, Miethke RR. SEM evaluation of a new technique for interdental stripping. J Clin Orthod. 1999; 33: 286–292

Zhong M, Jost-Brinkmann PG, Zellmann M, Zellmann S, Radlanski RJ. Clinical evaluation of a new technique for interdental enamel reduction. J Orofac Orthop./Fortschr Kieferorthop. 2000; 61: 432–439

15 Active Retention Procedures

John J. Sheridan

The literature indicates that absolute retention of an orthodontic case is not predictable and, in the vast majority of cases, not possible because of the changing physiological dynamics of the stomatognathic system, and that long-term retention is the accepted norm in contemporary retention concepts (Blake and Bibby 1998; Little et al. 1998). Therefore, retention of the finished case is necessary to hold the correction that has been attained. That being the case, how long will the patients have to wear a retention device? For as long as they wish to maintain the finished result.

The primary causes of instability arise because:
- The gingival and periodontal tissues are affected by orthodontic tooth movement and require time to become reorganized when active orthodontic appliances are removed (Reitan 1969).
- The teeth may be in an inherently unstable position because of tissue pressure from the cheeks, lips, and tongue (Proffit 1978).
- The constant changes in oral dynamics due to growth and aging will affect oral tissue tonus and therefore the position of the teeth (Behrents 1984).
- The diagnosis or treatment plan may be faulty.

The following text, photographs, and diagrams will describe the retention devices that are used in contemporary orthodontics for specific retention goals.

Removable Retainers

Removable retainers have the benefit of allowing the patient to remove the appliance in accordance with the clinician's recommendations: i.e., when eating, for more efficient cleaning of the teeth and the appliance, and, in certain instances, on social occasions when the presence of the appliance would make the patient feel self-conscious. For instance, the obvious presence of the labial bow on a Hawley retainer can provide occasion for such removal. For these reasons, removable appliances will be an integral option as a retention device for the foreseeable future.

Hawley Retainers

A Hawley removable retainer is the most commonly used retention device. Its construction and application are usually the first things learned in predoctoral orthodontic laboratory courses. It was first fabricated and described by Dr. Charles Hawley in the 1920 as an active removable appliance to open the bite and retract incisors. Its basic elements—an adjustable outer bow, acrylic base, and retentive clasps—are still essential to this device (Fig. 15.**1**). These basic elements can be held in place by a variety of clasps (Fig. 15.**2**), while the outer bow, constructed of sturdy stainless-steel wire and incorporating adjustment loops spanning from canine to canine, can be activated for adjustment of the anterior teeth if indicated.

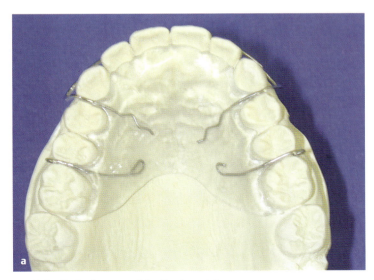
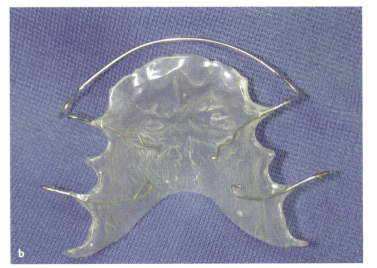

Fig. 15.**1** **Basic elements of the Hawley retainer.**

a The basic elements of a Hawley type retainer (the adjustable outer bow, the acrylic base, and the retentive clasps) on the working cast.

b The basic elements of a Hawley type retainer off the working cast.

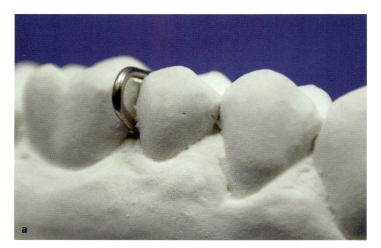
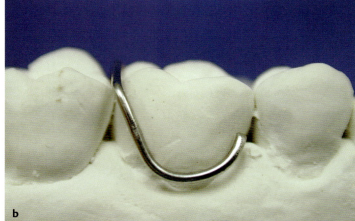
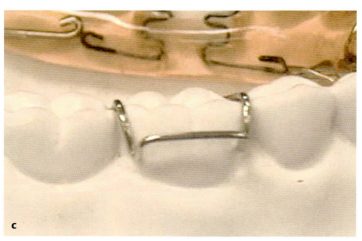

Fig. 15.2 Clasps that can be used to hold the Hawley retainer in place: **a** ball clasp; **b** circumferential clasp; **c** Adams clasp.

Fig. 15.3 Anterior biteplane incorporated into a Hawley retainer to maintain overbite correction.

Because the Hawley retainer covers the palate, it can be easily modified to incorporate an anterior bite plane to control overbite. Further, for relapse prevention of excessive pretreatment overbite, it is prudent to have light contact of the lower incisors against a built-up anterior palatal bite plane (Fig. 15.3).

There are two basic modifications of the Hawley retainer, one for extraction cases, the other for nonextraction cases. In extraction cases, the wire of the labial bow does not cross into the palate distal to the canine (Fig. 15.4). This would cause an interproximal interference and, acting as a wedge, would tend to open the extraction site. A wraparound outer bow is indicated in the extraction case because there would be no transocclusal wire element in the extraction site (Fig. 15.5). One problem with this configuration is that the longer span of unsupported wire is more prone to distortion.

In nonextraction cases, the retentive arm of the adjustment loop can cross into the palate distal to the canine without undue concern about opening space (Fig. 15.6).

Essix Clear Plastic Retainers

Plastic appliances have been used as retainers for decades. In years past, however, they were prone to cracking and distortion due to the inferior quality of the plastic. Such appliances became practical when an extremely durable, thin, clear polymer, such as Essix C+ plastic, became available for intraoral use. With this development, clear plastic appliances became a reasonable alternative to conventional retention devices. The first practical plastic retainer, the Essix appliance, was described be in 1993 (Sheridan et al. 1993). This retainer was inconspicuous and therefore provided an esthetic impetus for the patient to wear the appliance as directed (Fig. 15.7). Additionally, it is inexpensive, quickly fabricated, has minimal bulk and high strength, and does not interfere with speech or function. It is retentive without clasps, usually requires no adjustment, and has little, if any, influence on the efficiency of the occlusion when the patient adheres to the proper schedule of wear, which is only at night.

Data indicate that when worn only at night Essix retainers are as efficient as bonded-wire or Hawley-type appliances (LaBoda et al. 1995; Alexander 1977; Lindauer and Schoff 1998). Additionally, ancillary retention features such as temporary bridges and minor tooth moving can be incorporated into an Essix retainer (Sheridan 1994b; Sheridan et al. 2001). These features will be discussed below.

Impression and Cast Standards

Delivering a satisfactory Essix retainer depends on the attention to arch preparation, impression technique, and cast construction, and requires the same discipline associated with crown-and-bridge standards. A precision impression is necessary for an accu-

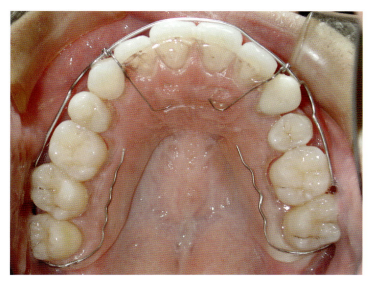

Fig. 15.4 The wire of the labial bow does not cross into the palate distal to the canine in the extraction case because the wedging action in this site could cause the extraction space to reopen.

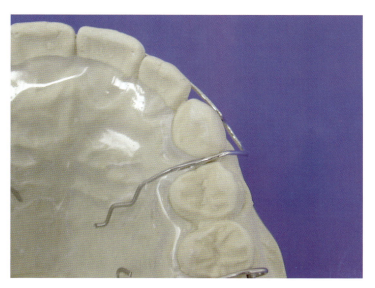

Fig. 15.6 The distal ends of the labial bow crossing into the palate in a nonextraction case will not tend to open space between the canine and the first premolar.

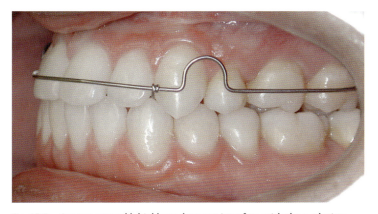

Fig. 15.5 **A wrap-around labial bow does not interfere with the occlusion.** However, the long span of wire is prone to distortion.

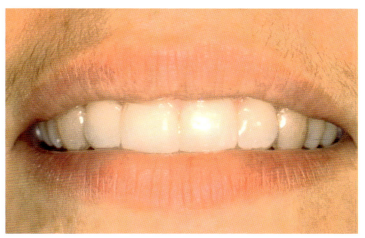

Fig. 15.7 The esthetic appearance of an Essix retainer is a feature appreciated by the patient and an inducement to wear the appliance as directed.

rate cast. The detailed cast is, in turn, necessary to fabricate the appliance. If the clinician is not prepared to follow uncompromising materials and fabrication techniques, a retention device other than an Essix appliance should be considered.

Dimensionally stable materials are mandatory. They are more expensive, but a better-fitting appliance and fewer remakes will more than make up for the cost. The recommended impression material is polyvinyl siloxane. It is an extremely accurate and stable impression material and is usually supplied in a two-phase form with injectable (light-bodied) and puttylike (heavy-bodied) materials. The heavy-bodied material gives the impression stability, while the injectable light-bodied material ensures detail in the retentive interproximals (Fig. 15.**8**). It is essential to pour the impression with a die stone that has very high compression strength with minimal setting expansion. Stone that has been in an open bin, absorbing atmospheric humidity, will develop excessive setting expansion, causing the cast and subsequent appliance to be oversized. Storing the stone in a closed container will eliminate this problem (Fig. 15.**9**). Also, when a quality die stone is used, the extremely small size of the gypsum particles produces a dense, smooth cast that will not require use of a separating medium prior to thermoforming the plastic to the cast.

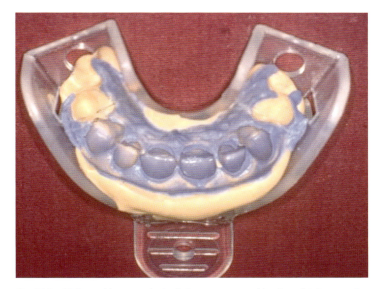

Fig. 15.8 **Light and heavy polyvinyl siloxane are combined to obtain a precision Essix impression.** The lighter-bodied injectable material registers precise detail and the more viscous heavy-bodied material (putty) prevents distortion of the impression.

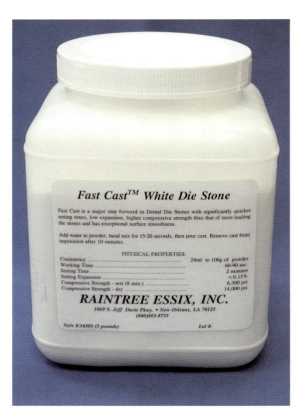

Fig. 15.**9** Storing the stone in a closed container prevents absorption of atmospheric moisture, thereby reducing the setting expansion of the stone and ensuring a more accurate impression of the dentition and supporting tissues.

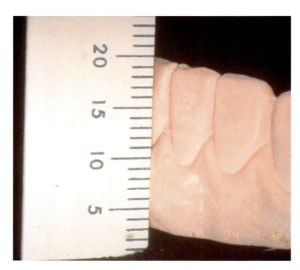

Fig. 15.**10** The height of the cast should be no more than 2.0 cm to ensure a more precise adaptation of the plastic to the cast during thermoforming.

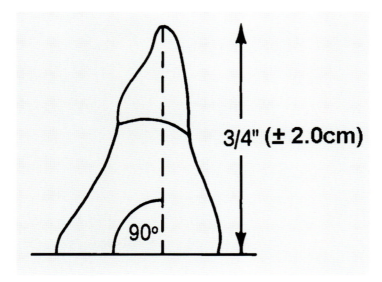

Fig. 15.**11** The base of the cast should be trimmed perpendicular to the long axis of the crown to permit unimpeded adaptation of the plastic to the cast during thermoforming.

When the cast is removed from the impression, it should be trimmed to be relatively short from incisal edges to the base of the cast and not exceed 20 mm (Fig. 15.**10**). The only necessary cast modification is to the base. Trim it perpendicular to the long axis of the incisors (Fig. 15.**11**) and taper the heels of the cast slightly toward the midline for ease in the subsequent removal of the cast from the thermoformed plastic adaptation.

Thermoforming Plastic to the Cast

There are two basic types of devices that adapt heated plastic to a cast: pressure machines and vacuum machines (Figs. 15.**12 a, b**).

The problem with pressure machines is that the process of thermoforming the plastic over a cast takes place in a pressure chamber and the cast cannot be altered immediately afterward. At that critical point, it is not possible to increase the adaptation of the plastic to the retentive undercuts gingival to the contact points, and the thermoformed plastic cannot be brought to ambient temperature immediately. These two steps, immediate retention point amplification and immediate cooling of the plastic, are optimal for plastic adaptation to the cast but not practically possible with pressure machines because the plastic is cooling relatively rapidly within the thermoforming pressure chamber. The reasons for this will be explained in due course.

Alternatively, a vacuum machine adapts heat-softened plastic to a cast by negative pressure, i.e., by sucking the plastic over the cast. Heightening the vacuum amplifies the vacuum force and improves the subsequent adaptation of the plastic to the cast. Amplification is achieved by blocking out the peripheral rings of vacuum holes on the base plate with a gasket and thereby concentrating the power of the vacuum toward the center of the base plate (Fig. 15.**12c**). Since conventional Essix canine-to-canine casts are so small, two can be placed inside the gasket (Fig. 15.**12d**). Some manufacturers provide gaskets for this purpose (e.g., Raintree Essix, Inc. New Orleans, LA, USA). They can also be conveniently fabricated from engine gasket or rubber-dam material.

The holes in the base plate of most vacuum units are too small and there are usually not enough of them. This restricts the vacuum-induced flow of air, choking it down. To compensate for these limitations, enlarge existing holes on the base plate with a 3 mm drill bit and make more of them (Fig. 15.**12e, f**). This feature is supplied by some vendors of vacuum machines (e.g., Raintree Essix).

The heating element of the vacuum unit should be at maximum temperature prior to thermoforming the plastic. It takes about 3–4 minutes after turning on the heat switch to reach this state. The cast is then placed on the base plate of the vacuum machine, and a 1.0 mm sheet of Essix C+ plastic is centered within the holding mechanism and firmly locked in place.

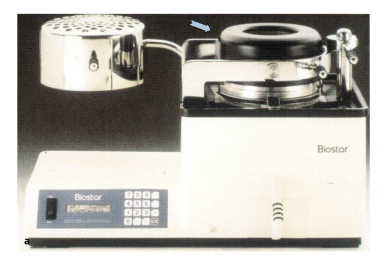
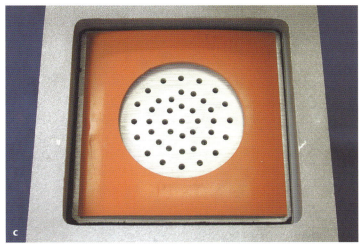
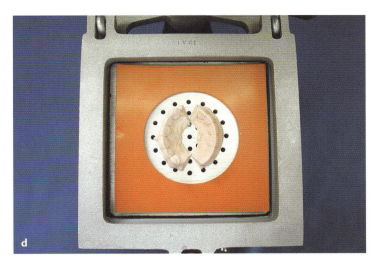
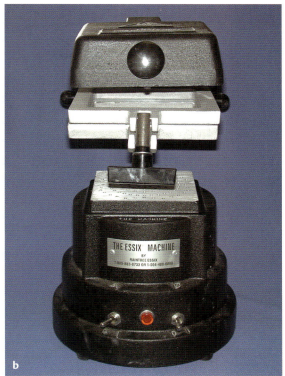
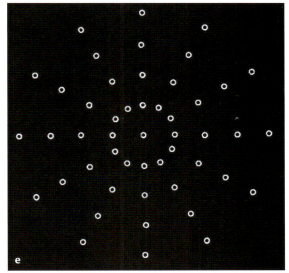
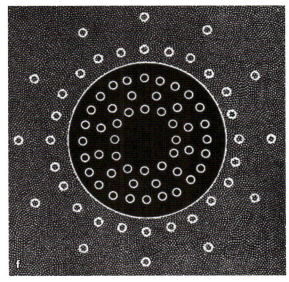

Fig. 15.**12** **Thermoforming plastic to the cast.**
a With pressure thermoforming machines, the adaptation of the plastic to the cast takes place within the pressure chamber (arrow).
b With vacuum thermoforming machines, the adaptation of the plastic to the cast takes place by the vacuum force pulling the heat-softened plastic over the cast.
c Blocking out the peripheral vacuum holes on the base plate with a gasket concentrates the vacuum power toward the center of the base plate. This augmentation will amplify the power of the vacuum force and cause a better adaptation of the plastic to the cast.
d Two Essix canine-to-canine retainers can be positioned inside the vacuum condensing gasket on the base plate.
e, f Amplifying the vacuum power.
e The configuration of this poorly designed base plate on the vacuum machine compromises efficient thermoforming of the plastic to the cast because the power of the vacuum motor cannot be expressed.
f Enlarging the vacuum holes on a contemporary baseplate, coupled with the vacuum condensing gasket, will amplify the vacuum power.

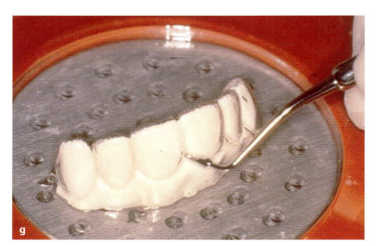
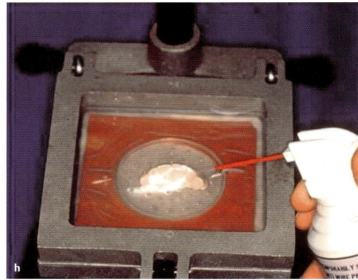

Fig. 15.**12**
g Amplifying the plastic adaptation to the retentive undercuts gingival to contact points with a blunt tapered instrument will significantly increase the retention potential of the retainer.
h Immediately cooling the thermoformed plastic with a compressed coolant spray prevents distortion of the plastic and improves the plastic adaptation to the cast.

When the plastic is pliable enough to be adapted to the cast, usually after 40–45 seconds under the fully activated heat source, push the heating element out of the way immediately and forcefully push a tapered-tip instrument into the retentive undercuts gingival to facial contact points (Fig. 15.**12g**). This should take only a few seconds and amplifies the plastic adaptation where it is most critical – in the retentive undercuts gingival to facial contact points. Forceful hand pressure condensed into the tapered tip of the instrument can generate an adaptation pressure of well over 100 psi. Then immediately spray the still-hot plastic with a compressed refrigerant spray for a few seconds to cool it down as rapidly as possible (Fig. 15.**12h**). This accelerates the final set of the plastic, producing a significant improvement in plastic adaptation to the cast since plastic distorts slightly if allowed to cool slowly to room temperature. Immediate cooling also reduces the possibility of lingual lift-off, i.e., the gingival edge of plastic pulling away from the cast. Alternative but less desirable methods of cooling the plastic are to place it in an ice-water bath or run it under cold water until it reaches room temperature.

Removing the Canine-to-Canine Cast from Essix Plastic and Establishing the Outline

The intact cast can easily be removed from the plastic sheet with the following technique.
1. Cut away the excess plastic sheet with curved Mayo scissors, leaving anterior and posterior tabs (Fig. 15.**13a**).
2. Cut-away the plastic on the heels of the cast with a sharp laboratory knife, acrylic bur, or plastic cutting disk (Fig. 15.**13b**).
3. Pull the facial and lingual tabs 2–3 mm away from the cast (Fig. 15.**13c**) and place a thin-bladed instrument at various points between the plastic and the cast. Then gently pry it out of the plastic with a thin-bladed instrument (Fig. 15.**13d**).
4. Establish the outline with curved Mayo scissors. The scissors' cut produces clean, curved, and smooth edges. It is not necessary or advisable to form the outline of the appliance with a bur, which causes the plastic to fray.

The steps for establishing the outline of the plastic are:
1. Trim the appliance to a gentle curve and extend it 2.0–3.0 mm onto the facial gingiva (Fig. 15.**13e**). Do not scallop the gingival border to conform to the cervical line (Fig. 15.**13f**). This detracts from the esthetic presentation of the appliance and significantly decreases retention because it eliminates the retentive undercuts gingival to contact points.
2. Trim the lingual of the upper and lower appliances in a straight line from canine-to-canine (Fig. 15.**13g**).
3. Trim the plastic to accommodate frenum attachments (Fig. 15.**13e**).
4. Cut away the plastic at the distogingival margin of the canine (Fig. 15.**13h**). Since an Essix appliance cannot be sucked off the teeth (the negative pressure of suction makes it tighter), this modification establishes a fingernail purchase to facilitate removal.

When an Essix appliance is thermoformed on a vacuum machine, the lingual of the cast should face the center point of the baseplate (Fig. 15.**14**). In this configuration, the plastic is pulled slightly thinner on the lingual because of the vacuum differential. This minimizes "tongue awareness" of the lingual plastic edge. To further reduce lingual awareness, the plastic should, if possible, extend below the resting length of the tongue; that is, usually about 5.0 mm onto the lingual alveolus.

The conventional canine-to-canine Essix retainer can be extended to encompass and hold a bicuspid extraction site closed by thermoforming plastic over a cast that has been extended to include the terminal bicuspids (Fig. 15.**15**).

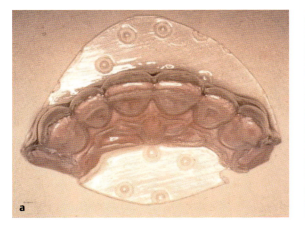
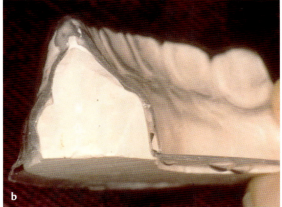
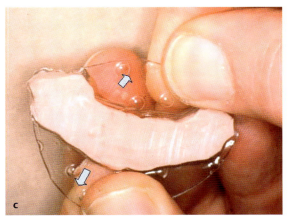
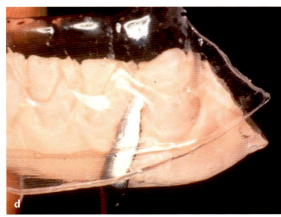
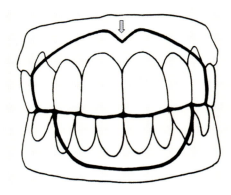
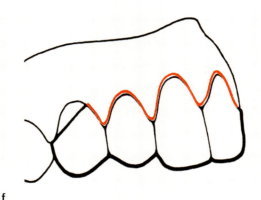
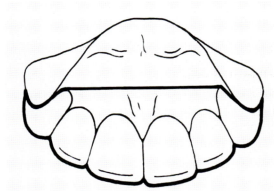
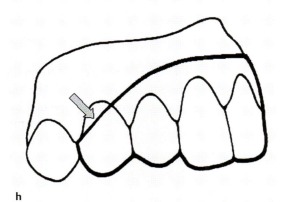

Fig. 15.**13** **Removing the canine-to-canine cast and establishing the outline.**
a Cutting away excess plastic with curved Mayo scissors and leaving anterior and posterior tabs are the preliminary steps to ensure removing an intact cast from the plastic.
b Cutting the plastic that covers the heels of the cast will allow the plastic to be slightly pulled away from the cast.
c Pulling the facial and lingual plastic tabs slightly away from the cast (arrows) will make it easier to remove the cast from the plastic without fracturing the cast.
d Wedging the plastic from the cast with a bladed instrument will ensure a working cast that is not fractured.
e The appliance should be trimmed to a gentle curve and extend 2–3.0 mm onto the facial gingiva. Also, the facial superior border can be notched to avoid impingement on the frenum (arrow).
f Do not follow the curvature of the cervical line when trimming the appliance. This will eliminate the retentive undercuts gingival to contact points.
g The lingual of the appliance is trimmed in a straight line from canine-to-canine.
h Since the appliance cannot be sucked off the teeth, the distogingival margin of the canine (arrow) is cut away to provide a fingernail purchase for removal of the appliance.

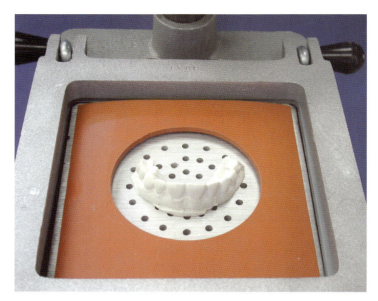

Fig. 15.**14** **The lingual of the cast should face the center of the vacuum machine base plate.** This will cause the lingual plastic to be slightly thinner and thereby reduce tongue awareness.

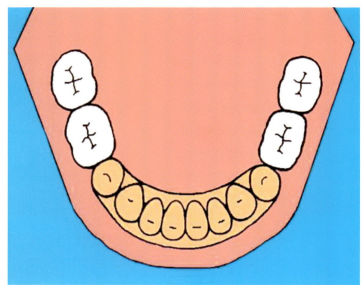

Fig. 15.**15** **Extraction site modification of the appliance involves covering the extraction site with the retainer.** This usually means including the second bicuspid in a first bicuspid extraction case.

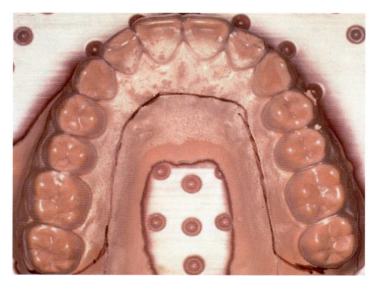

Fig. 15.**16** On the working cast, the height of the palate is trimmed away to allow for vacuum power to be expressed on the lingual of the cast and ensuring efficient plastic adaptation in that area.

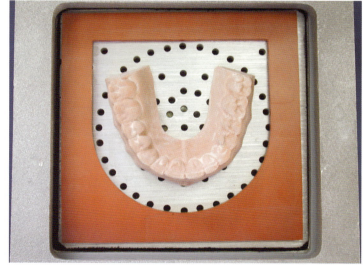

Fig. 15.**17** A larger vacuum condensing gasket necessary to accommodate the increased dimensions of a full-arch cast.

Full-Arch Plastic Retainers: Fabrication, Indications, and Contraindications

As with any Essix plastic appliance, the detail associated with full-arch retainer construction must be associated with crown and bridge standards. Therefore, as stated previously, a stable impression tray, quality impression material, and dimensionally stable die stone are mandatory. All the thermoforming essentials used in the fabrication of the canine-to-canine appliance are employed in the fabrication of the full-arch appliance. There are, however, some differences. The maxillary cast must be modified to allow uniform plastic adaptation to all dental and soft-tissue surfaces of the cast. Therefore, the height of the palatal vault should be trimmed away to allow vacuum adaptation on the lingual aspect of the cast. (Fig. 15.16).

Since the full-coverage cast is larger than a canine-to-canine cast, the vacuum-concentrating gasket must have a larger aperture to accommodate the posterior part of the cast (Fig. 15.17).

The form of the appliance will be U-shaped, covering all teeth, including the terminal molars, and extending 2–3 mm onto the gingiva. To establish this outline:
1. Cut away extraneous plastic from the cast with a plastic trimming disk mounted in a low-speed handpiece (Fig. 15.**18a**).
2. In Class I cases, finished with a Class I molar relationship, the distal of the upper terminal molar is not occluding in the lower arch. Therefore, the plastic covering the distal of the upper terminal molar can be cut away to make it easier to remove the plastic from the cast (Fig. 15.**18b**).
3. To remove the thermoformed appliance from the cast, use a thin-bladed instrument as a lever between the plastic and the

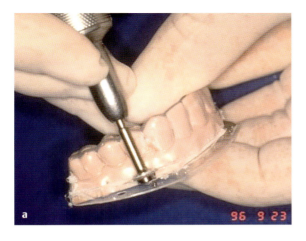 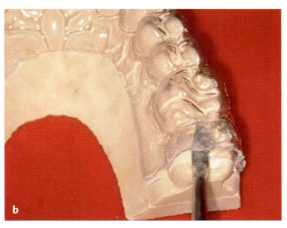

Fig. 15.**18** **Establishing the U-shaped outline.**
a A trimming disk, in a low-speed handpiece, is used to form the outline of the appliance on the cast. The borders of the appliance should be 2.0–3.0 mm onto the facial and lingual gingiva.
b The plastic is cut away from the distal of the terminal molar and, working from posterior to anterior, the appliance can be levered from the cast.

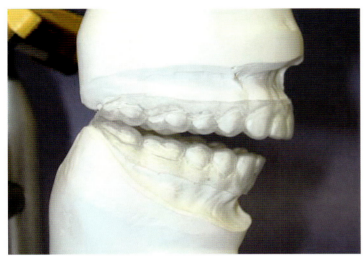

Fig. 15.**19** There is disproportionate anterior bite opening due to a thickness of plastic between the terminal molars.

cast. The removal process is initiated in the posterior and continued anteriorly until the appliance can be lifted from the cast (Fig. 15.**18b**).

The borders of the full-arch appliance are established with curved Mayo scissors so that it extends 2.3 mm onto the facial and lingual gingiva except for the lingual of the lower incisor area. As with the canine-to-canine plastic retainer, the appliance should extend as far as possible in the mandibular lingual area without impinging on the lingual frenum, usually about 5.0 mm. This reduces tongue awareness of the plastic edge.

Schedules of wear and care of the appliance are essentially the same as those described for canine-to-canine appliances: in most cases, full time for two days and then at night only (LaBoda et al. 1995; Alexander 1977; Lindauer and Schoff 1998).

Equilibration is strongly recommended after placement of full-arch Essix plastic retainers because any thickness of plastic covering the terminal molars closer to the hinge axis of the mandible will induce a proportionately larger opening in the incisor area because the anterior teeth are further away from the hinge axis (Sheridan et al. 2001) (Fig. 15.**19**).

The equilibration technique is as follows:
1. When the appliance is seated, identify the posterior interferences with articulating tape between the seated appliance and the opposing dentition when the patient taps the teeth together in centric relation (Fig. 15.**20a**).
2. Using a bur or scalpel, reduce excessive contact points, as indicated by the articulating tape, until reasonably balanced bilateral centric contact is established. Since the thermoformed plastic covering the buccal section teeth is so thin (< 0.5 mm), it is more practical to remove all the plastic at the interference point rather than trying to reduce it incrementally a few thousandths of an inch at a time (Fig. 15.**20b**). The perforation of the appliance does not affect the structural integrity of Essix C+ plastic.

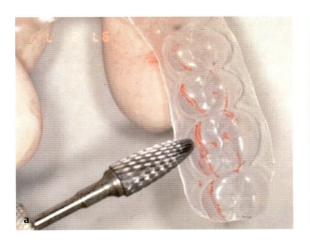 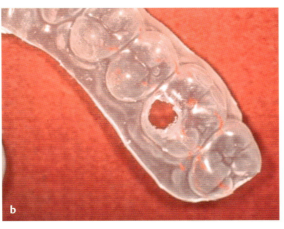

Fig. 15.**20** **Equilibration technique.**
a Articulating tape will reveal the interferences in centric relation. These can be removed with an appropriate bur in a handpiece. This procedure will significantly reduce the anterior open bite induced by the plastic covering the molars.
b The area-identified hyperocclusion that has been reduced. Since the plastic is less than 0.5 mm thick, it is advisable to cut the plastic completely away in the excessive contact area rather than just the surface area.

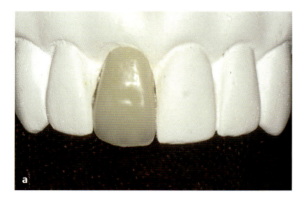
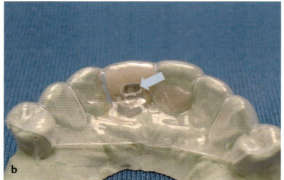

Fig. 15.21 **Construction of an Essix retainer/bridge.**
a A pontic of correct color and size is fitted to the edentulous area on the cast. It should be tacked to the cast with a material, such as acrylic or stone, that will not melt during thermoforming.
b A deep groove cut into the lingual of the pontic to mechanically lock it into the thermoformed plastic appliance.

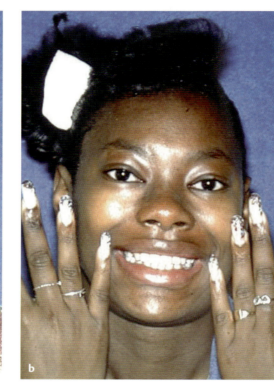

Fig. 15.22 **Esthetics of the Essix bridge.**
a The patient's esthetic pretreatment facial presentation, obviously compromised due to missing anterior teeth.
b Patient's esthetic posttreatment facial presentation has been demonstrably improved with the Essix bridge in place.

Replacement of Missing Teeth with an Essix Retainer/Temporary Prosthesis

Occasionally it may be necessary to place pontics in an Essix retainer because teeth are congenitally missing or lost through trauma. The conventional method is to place a pontic in a Hawley-type framework. However, these appliances, often called "flippers," are bulky, unstable, and marginally esthetic. Conversely, exceptionally esthetic and stable temporary bridges can be fabricated quickly and inexpensively from 0.040 in. Essix type C+ plastic, which is rugged and abrasion resistant, and can withstand the demands of function (GAC International Inc. Central Islip, NY).

The construction of an Essix retainer/bridge is as follows:
1. To replace a missing incisor, obtain a working cast and fit an appropriate pontic to the cast (Fig. 15.21 a).
2. Cut a wide and deep mesiodistal groove into the lingual surface of the pontic (Fig. 15.21 b). When the plastic sheet is thermoformed over the cast, it will conform to this trench and mechanically lock the pontic into the plastic.
3. After applying separating medium to the edentulous area of the cast, tack the pontic in place with quick-cure acrylic or light-cured composite gel (Fig. 15.21 b). Do not use wax because it would melt when hot plastic sheet material was thermoformed over it.
4. Thermoform abrasive-resistant 0.040 in. Essix type C+ plastic over the cast and, as with other thermoformed Essix appliances, immediately enforce the retentive undercuts gingival to contact points with a blunt-tipped instrument and use a refrigerant spray to cool the plastic quickly to room temperature as depicted in Fig. 15.12 h.
5. When the appliance is removed from the cast, trim it to canine-to-canine or full-arch form as previously described for fabrication of the canine-to-canine retainer.

The patient will wear the Essix bridge during the day for obvious esthetic reasons, so the conventional at-night-only retention schedule is reversed. The Essix retainer/prosthesis is not to be worn while sleeping. This allows the supporting tissues a nocturnal period of an appliance-free physiologically normal oral envi-

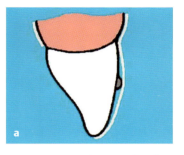 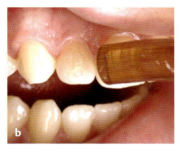 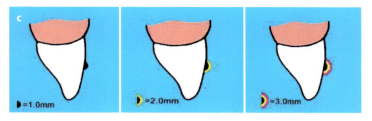 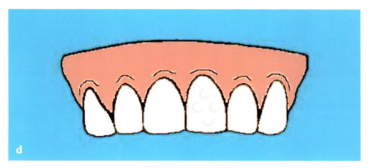

Fig. 15.**23** **Mounding to induce force.**
a The force against the tooth is generated by the resilient plastic pressing against the composite mound on the enamel surface.
b A mound of bonding composite, 1.0 mm thick, is placed on the enamel surface and light-cured. This mound is not noticeable.
c The thickness of the mound can be periodically increased for additional tooth movement at subsequent office visits.
d The type of movement depends on the position of the bonded mound on the crown. Placed incisally, it will induce tipping; placed gingivally, more bodily movement; placed distally, movement about a mesial vertical axis; and placed mesially, movement about a distal vertical axis.

ronment. Also, the patient should be instructed on how to remove the mechanically locked pontic for cleaning, if necessary. As with any plastic appliance, it should be cleaned with a toothbrush and water but not with toothpaste because the abrasives in toothpaste will eventually ruin the reflective qualities of the appliance and compromise its esthetic qualities.

The before and after portraits in Figure 15.**22** demonstrate the esthetic qualities of an Essix bridge.

Dual-Purpose Removable Retainers for Minor Tooth Moving and Stability

Occasionally appliances are necessary to realign anterior teeth that have had minor relapse and, when aligned, to hold them in their new positions. This is usually required when patients have ignored their initial retention directives or when late crowding has occurred after the patient has been relieved of a retention schedule. In these situations, the most convenient appliance would be one that can move teeth and subsequently serve as a retainer. This type of appliance is dynamic in one sense, because it will move teeth, and a retainer in another, since it will hold the teeth in their new positions. The crowding involved in these retreatment cases is usually minor and will nearly always require interproximal reduction to create space for resolution of the crowding. If moderate-to-severe crowding has occurred, fixed appliances are a better treatment option.

There are three basic forms of dynamic/retention appliances:
1. Clear plastic appliances, usually canine-to-canine, commonly called Essix appliances, that do not involve setting up teeth on a cast and can be modified during treatment.
2. Overlay plastic devices, commonly known as positioners, that require resetting the teeth on a cast.
3. Spring retainers constructed of wire and plastic.

Clear Plastic (Essix) Corrective Retainers

A clear plastic canine-to-canine retainer can be modified to align teeth that have slightly shifted from their orthodontically finished position (Sheridan 1994a). The modified clear plastic retainer is indicated when the patient or clinician does not relish another round of fixed appliances or treatment with an esthetically obvious wire-and-plastic appliance. Unlike other corrective retainers, Essix retainers do not involve setting up teeth in ideal positions on the working cast. They have other specific advantages:
1. Force application can be applied precisely.
2. The appliance is practically invisible, and patient acceptance is usually enthusiastic.
3. Tooth movement is rapid and precise, and can be accomplished in increments during sequential visits.
4. Fabrication is a fraction of the cost of conventional removable tooth-moving appliances.

Teeth can be moved when there is appropriate force, space, and time. With a modified Essix retainer, the force and space are incorporated into the appliance by the clinician. The patient must provide the time by wearing the appliance as directed – that is full time, with the exception of eating and cleaning, until the desired tooth movement has occurred; then at night only when it is being utilized as a retainer. Also, it is best to use a plastic that can induce a stronger force and more positive resiliency than Essix C+ retainer plastic. Essix 1.0 mm "A" plastic is recommended for this purpose.

Mounding to Induce Force

Force can be induced in the appliance by utilizing the inherent resilience of the Essix "A" plastic as it presses against an object that interferes with its resting state (Fig. 15.**23a**). That object is a 1.0 mm mound of composite placed on the enamel surface with an conventional acid-etch technique and subsequently light-cured or time-cured (Fig. 15.**23b**). The mound can be sequentially

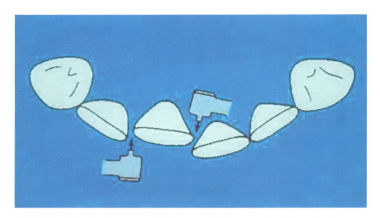

Fig. 15.24 Creating interproximal space with interproximal stripping is necessary to relieve the crowding without expansion of the arches or the extraction of teeth.

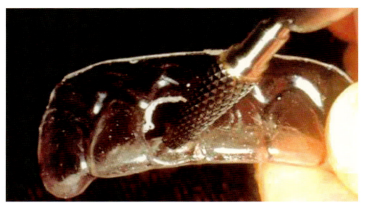

Fig. 15.25 A window, to provide space for the target tooth to move into, is cut into the plastic with an acrylic trimming bur.

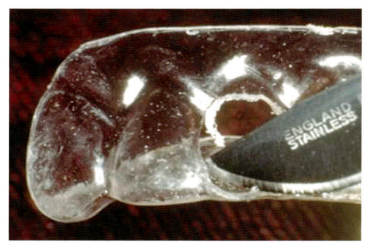

Fig. 15.26 The rough margins of the window, caused by the trimming bur, can be made smooth by trimming the borders of the window with a scalpel.

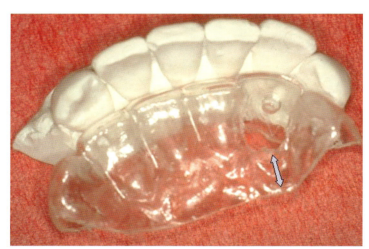

Fig. 15.27 An adequate border of plastic (arrow) should be present for strength and resiliency.

built up at subsequent visits to induce progressive tooth movement throughout the course of treatment (Fig. 15.23c). Since the force is induced by the composite mound on the enamel surface, not by resetting teeth, the initial appliance is not altered. Therefore, a series of appliances is rarely, if ever, necessary.

The composite mound, bonded to the enamel surface, can induce a variety of biomechanical forces: placed incisally, more tipping; placed gingivally, more bodily movement; placed distally, movement about a mesial vertical axis; and placed mesially, movement about a distal vertical axis (Fig. 15.23d).

Space is another requirement for aligning crowded teeth, and it is usually needed proximally, facially, or lingually. Interproximal clearance is obtained by judicious stripping with an abrasive strip or an air-turbine handpiece (Sheridan 1985) (Fig. 15.24). Space for facial or lingual movement is obtained by cutting a window into the plastic appliance. This is accomplished by using a plastic trimming bur turning at slow speed (Fig. 15.25). The resultant border of the window will have a frayed texture. This rough margin can be made smooth by finishing the borders of the window with a scalpel (Fig. 15.26). Since tooth movement must be unimpeded,

particular attention must be given to the size of the window. It is best to err on the side of a bigger, rather than a smaller, window. A 2.0–4.0 mm gingival border of plastic should remain after cutting the window to ensure the strength and resiliency of the appliance (Fig. 15.27). Tongue irritation may develop from the edges of the lingual window because there is a tendency for patients to explore the window with the tongue. Supplying the patient with bracket wax to wipe into the window will alleviate that aggravation.

Another method of creating space is to block out the cast to create space for the target tooth to move into by placing a thickness of acrylic or light-cured composite on the surface of the target tooth proportional to the amount of projected tooth movement (Fig. 15.28). This will cause a space for tooth movement between the tooth and the plastic in the thermoformed appliance. If the patient presents with average overbite and overjet, however, there may be interference on the plastic bulge caused by the plastic adaptation over the blockout material when placed on the lingual of upper incisors or the facial of lower incisors.

Removable Retainers 325

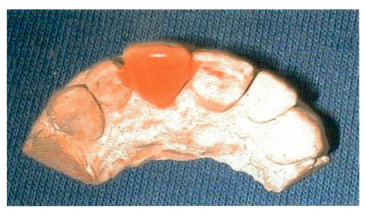

Fig. 15.**28** **Acrylic placed on the cast will provide the space necessary for the tooth to move into in the thermoformed appliance.** However, this may cause interference with the bite if placed on the lingual of the upper incisors or the facial of the lower incisors.

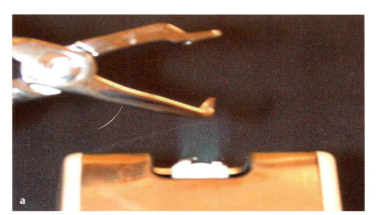

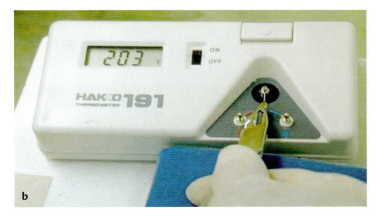

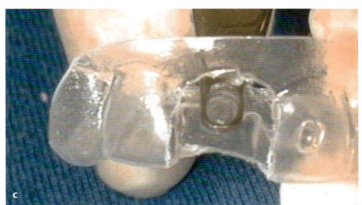

Fig. 15.**29** **Using thermoforming pliers to induce force.**

a Heating the tips of Hilliard thermoforming pliers will ensure that they will induce appropriate force into the thermoformed plastic.

b The correct range of thermoforming temperatures can be determined by the digital readout on a HAK<0 digital thermometer.

c Hilliard thermopliers will create a force-inducing projection within the plastic appliance that will ultimately move the tooth in the desired direction.

Using Thermoforming Pliers to Induce Force

An alternative method of incorporating tooth-moving force within the plastic appliance is using the thermoforming pliers to efficiently and rapidly induce a tooth-moving force into an Essix plastic appliance. These pliers allow the clinician to move teeth and to tighten an Essix appliance for a better fit with an uncomplicated chairside procedure. Unlike the composite mounding technique, these pliers induce a force-inducing bump directly into the Essix plastic appliance. The technique is deceptively simple:

1. The bulb-tip of the pliers is heated to a temperature that thermoforms Essix plastic (Fig. 15.**29a**).
2. Thermoforming temperature (about 93 °C [200 °F] for Essix "A" plastic) is determined by a readout on a HAK < O digital thermometer (Fig. 15.**29b**).
3. The pliers are placed where the force-inducing bump is indicated. When the handles of the pliers are slowly squeezed together, a sturdy tooth-moving projection will be developed in the Essix appliance (Fig. 15.**29c**).

When this modified appliance is seated on the patient's teeth, the thermoformed bump will exert pressure on the target tooth. It

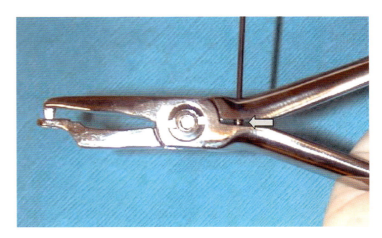

Fig. 15.**30** The size of the force-inducing projection can be increased on sequential office visits by adjusting the hex screw in the handle (arrow).

can be reenforced, in 1.0 mm increments, at subsequent appointments to effect additional tooth movement without the fabrication of an additional appliance. Adjustments for increasing the size of the force-inducing bump are made by adjusting the hex screw in the handle of the appliance (Fig. 15.**30**).

Clinical Case Examples

The following clinical case reports demonstrate the type of tooth movement that an activated Essix appliance can typically accomplish.

Case 1. A middle-aged woman presented with malaligned mandibular incisors (Fig. 15.31a). Buccal section intercuspation was acceptable. She had previous orthodontic treatment and was reluctant to go through another round of fixed appliances.

The case required interproximal incisor stripping and 3 mm of labial lateral movement on both lateral incisors. Three composite mound applications, the initial and two additional 1.0 mm buildups, created the force necessary for appropriate alignment. When tooth movement was complete with a single appliance (Fig. 15.31b), the appliance was employed as a retainer to be used at night only. The patient was seen every two weeks. Treatment time was five months, and chair time was minimal, involving impressions, placing the appliance, and sequential mounding. The patient was delighted with the esthetic (invisible) feature of the appliance.

Case 2. This case involving a middle aged man is typical of a patient who was concerned with the lower right lateral incisor that had relapsed slightly from its finished position (Fig. 15.32a). A 1.0 mm composite mound was placed on the facial of the lateral incisor and the Essix appliance was placed after a window, to provide space for the tooth to move into, was cut out on the lingual. The patient was given bracket wax to place over the lingual window to compensate for any tendency of the edges of the lingual window to irritate the tongue. The appliance was placed, and the patient returned two weeks later for reinforcement of the initial mound with another 1.0 mm layer of composite. The lateral was in acceptable alignment at the next appointment (Fig. 15.32b), and the patient was told to use the appliance as a retainer to be worn at night only.

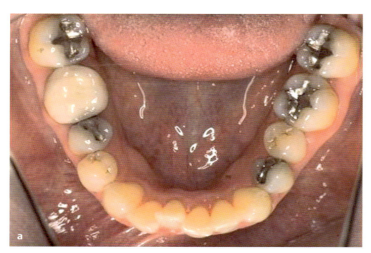
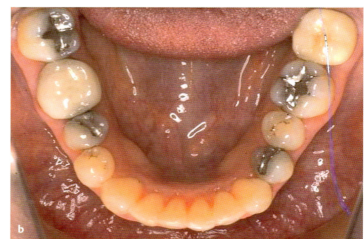

Fig. 15.**31** Case 1. A middle-aged woman presenting with malaligned mandibular incisors.

a The pretreatment incisor crowding of the mandibular central incisor that requires interproximal reduction to gain space for the tooth to move into.

b Posttreatment corrected incisor alignment. The patient was seen every two weeks. Treatment time was five months.

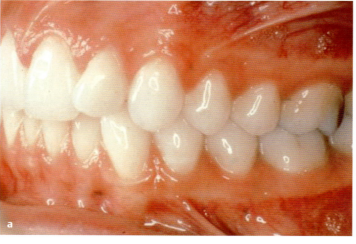
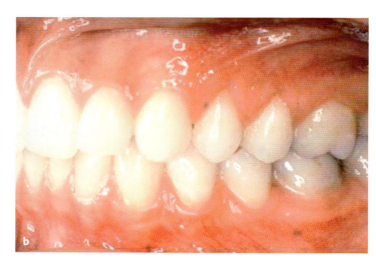

Fig. 15.**32** Case 2. A middle aged man's lower right lateral incisor had relapsed slightly from its finished position.

a The left lateral incisor had relapsed from its previously corrected alignment, and the patient did not want to go through another round of fixed appliances to have it corrected.

b The lateral incisor was brought into excellent alignment. Tooth movement was accomplished with two sequentially placed force-inducing composite mounds on the target tooth. The treatment was complete within two visits that were two weeks apart.

Overlay Full-Arch Plastic Devices (Positioners)

A positioner is a plastic device that is most effective in altering tooth positions when it is placed immediately upon removal of the fixed orthodontic appliance (Fig. 15.**33a**). Normally, it is fabricated by removing the archwires 4–6 weeks before the planned removal of the fixed appliance, taking impressions of both arches, taking a registration bite of occlusal relationships, and resetting the teeth in the laboratory to induce the minor changes to effect the desired movement (Fig. 15.**33b,c**). All teeth should be included in the positioner to prevent supereruption of those teeth not contained within the appliance. As part of the laboratory procedure, bands and brackets are trimmed away, and any band space is closed. The positioner is then fabricated by forming either a hard rubber or soft plastic material, usually 2.5–3.5 mm thick, that conforms to the laboratory setup, thereby producing a device from resilient plastic material that can move teeth into their desired positions.

Use of a tooth positioner, rather than performing final positioning with archwires and fixed appliances, has three advantages: (1) When completing an orthodontic case, it can alter minor tooth positional discrepancies and, therefore, allow the fixed appliance to be removed more quickly; (2) it can alter minimal occlusal relationships, for example, correcting a bite that has slipped one or two millimeters from its desired position; and (3) if the gingiva is swollen, the massaging action of the positioner overlying the tissue will quickly return it to normal proportions.

The disadvantage of a positioner is that it requires considerable laboratory time to construct, since the teeth have to be manually reset prior to constructing the appliance. Also, it is advisable to mount the case on a fully adjustable articulator due to the thickness of the interocclusal material that will alter the hinge axis relationship of the mandible. Also, a positioner tends to increase overbite more than the settling induced with vertical elastics and, therefore, may be contraindicated in cases that initially present with a deep bite. This disadvantage becomes an advantage if a positioner is used on a patient with minimal overbite in the finished case. Additionally, positioners do not hold corrected minor rotations well and, since they are removable appliances, cooperation with the schedule of wear is, of course, essential.

Spring Retainers

The indication for constructing a spring retainer is usually to correct some minor relapse of the anterior teeth from their finished position. This wire-and-plastic appliance is nearly always used after interproximal stripping has been done to create enough space to provide the room required to align the relapsed teeth without expansion, usually 1–3 mm. The fabrication of the spring retainer, which should be undertaken after creating enough interproximal space to resolve the crowding, involves taking an impression, pouring the cast, sectioning selected teeth from the cast, and, as with positioners, resetting the teeth on the cast to acceptable positions (Fig. 15.**34a**). The wire and plastic appliance should then be constructed from this configuration (Fig. 15.**34b**).

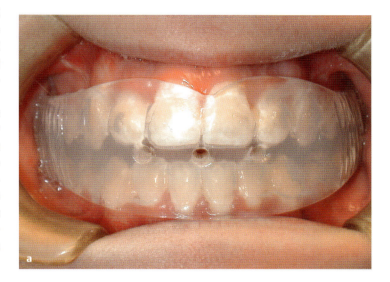

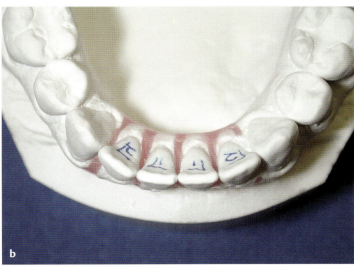

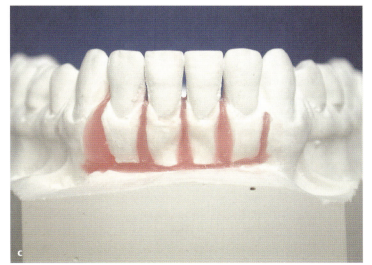

Fig. 15.**33** **Overlay full-arch devices.**
a The full-arch plastic positioner covers all teeth from terminal molar to terminal molar in both arches.
b The occlusal view of the teeth that have been repositioned on the working cast in the laboratory.
c The facial view of the teeth that have been repositioned on the working cast in the laboratory.

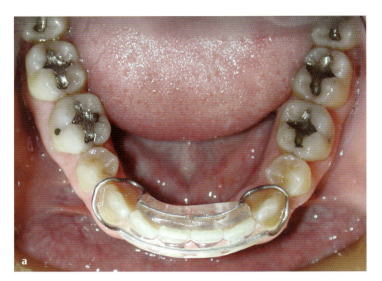 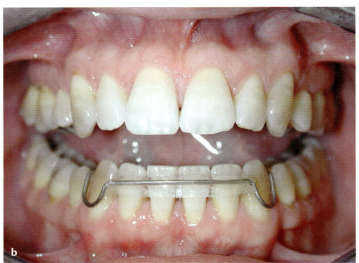

Fig. 15.**34** **Spring retainers.**

a The occlusal view of the spring retainer repositioning the right lateral incisor.

b Facial view of the spring retainer with the labial bow and clear acrylic pad.

Once the incisors are aligned, the dynamic phase of the spring retainer is complete and the appliance can still be worn as a conventional retainer to maintain the correction.

Fixed Bonded and Cemented Retainers

Fixed orthodontic retention is normally used in situations where arch instability is anticipated due to the relapse potential of certain corrected orthodontic results or when the patient's cooperation with removable appliances is questionable.

The usual indications for fixed retention are:
- Stabilization of the tooth positions of the finished case, especially until growth is essentially complete
- Holding space closed
- Holding space open: maintaining bridge or implant space
- Keeping extraction spaces closed in adults

The Canine-to-Canine Fixed Bonded Retainer

The bonded canine-to-canine retainer has all but replaced the banded-canine-and-soldered-lingual-wire variety because of the esthetic drawbacks of the bands on the canines and the creation of band space when these appliances are removed. Bonded canine-to-canine retainers are used most commonly in the lower arch to hold the anterior teeth in their posttreatment position until the cessation of the active growth period. They are, in the main, physiologically acceptable because they hold the esthetic presence of the anterior teeth while allowing the buccal section teeth to adapt to stress, diet, lifestyle, and aging.

The obvious disadvantage of bonded retainers is that, with the appliance in place, it is more difficult to clean the interdental areas. Additionally, when used on the upper anterior teeth, they can cause interference with the opposing dentition.

Direct Bonding of the Canine-to-Canine Retainer

The canine-to-canine retainer can be bonded only to the canines (by-passing the lateral and central incisors) with a relatively heavy stainless-steel wire and canine pads that have been sandblasted on the ends for a more tenacious bond (Fig. 15.**35a**). However, most clinicians prefer to use a lighter braided or twisted wire to allow some physiological movement within the periodontal ligament, to include all the incisors in the bonding sequence for additional appliance stability, and to prevent movement or rotation of the incisors to the labial (Fig. 15.**35b**). In extraction cases, especially in the adult patient, it may be judicious to extend the canine-to-canine wire to incorporate the terminal bicuspids (Fig. 15.**35c**). This precaution will prevent the extraction space from reopening. The formed canine-to-canine retainer wire can held be in place with interproximal floss or wire ligatures (Fig. 15.**35d**), and then directly bonded to the lingual surfaces of the anterior teeth after they have been treated with an appropriate acid-etch technique.

Indirect Bonding of the Canine-to-Canine Retainer

To save chair time and probably get more accurate placement of the bonded canine-to-canine retainer, many clinicians find that it is more efficient to bond the wire with an indirect technique like the one described below:

1. Form the wire on a canine-to-canine working cast, tack it to the teeth with a bonding composite, and cure the composite after a separating medium has been applied to the lingual surfaces of the canines and incisors on the cast (Fig. 15.**36a**).
2. The transfer tray should be constructed of transparent mouthguard plastic (2–3.0 mm thick in sheet form) that has been thermoformed over the cast and lingual wire (Fig. 15.**36b**).
3. Remove the tray from the working cast and clean the bases of the bonding composite (the side facing the enamel) with a cotton swab and water, and dry (Fig. 15.**36c**).
4. After appropriate acid-etch protocols have been completed, apply a thin film of bonding composite to each base, and place the transfer tray over the teeth. After curing time, remove the transfer tray, and check the interproximal areas to ensure that they are free of composite bonding material. Due to the transparency of the tray plastic, the bonding composite can be light cured.

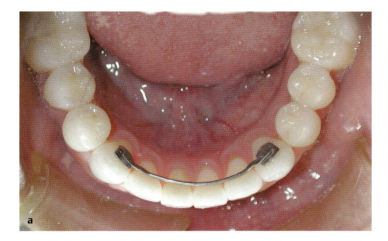
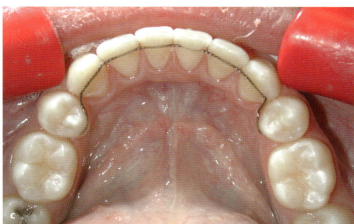
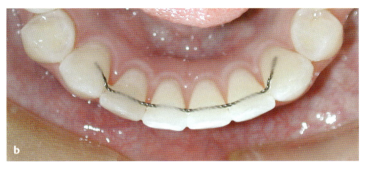
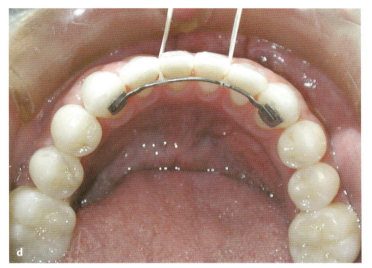

Fig. 15.**35** Direct bonding of the canine-to-canine retainer.
a The canine-to-canine fixed retainer bonded only to the canines.
b All the incisors are bonded to the canine-to-canine wire. The flexible braided wire allows physiological movement within the periodontal ligament and, therefore, will prevent labial or rotational incisor movement.
c Including the terminal bicuspids (bridging the extraction site) will prevent the extraction spaces from reopening.
d Holding the canine-to-canine wire in place with dental floss will stabilize it until it can be bonded to the lingual of the incisors.

Holding a Space Closed with a Fixed Retainer

A fixed permanent or semipermanent fixed retainer is indicated after space closure when stability is not predictable. This is relevant when a maxillary midline diastema has been closed during treatment because it is so prone to opening, even after frenectomy and since the reopened space is in the center of the smile, that it is particularly aggravating to the patient (Edward 1993). Accordingly, very long-term retention of the resolved diastema is nearly always indicated. The most reliable method of doing this is by holding the teeth on each side of the closed space together with a sectional bonded retainer constructed from a flexible wire to allow some slight physiological movement within the periodontal membrane during function (Fig. 15.**37**).

The wire can be fabricated using a working cast as a template. It can be attached to the teeth directly or indirectly as described in the previous section (canine-to-canine fabrication). Since most of these appliances are made for maxillary midline diastemas, it is essential that they do not interfere with the opposing incisors in centric occlusion. Therefore, assuming normal overbite and overjet in the finished case, the wire is bonded more cervically and usually gingival to the cingulum crest. That being the case, it is imperative that the patient be instructed on the use of a floss-threading device to clean the area gingival to the bonded wire.

Holding a Space Open with a Fixed Retainer

In certain cases it is essential to hold spaces open at a constant dimension until an appropriate more permanent prosthesis can be fabricated. This has become more pertinent since the use of osseointegrating implants has become popular in replacing teeth that are congenitally missing or lost through trauma (Moskowitz et al. 1997). The maintenance of space can and should be relatively short-term if an implant or bridge is to be placed in an adult. It may be long-term if the patient is an adolescent because implants, and occasionally bridges, are not indicated until the patient has completely finished the growing, usually age 18 years in females and 21 years in males. The maintenance of an anterior space due to a missing tooth usually involves the incorporation of a pontic into the fixed appliance. The maintenance of a posterior space usually does not.

The space for a posterior tooth can be maintained with a fixed appliance with a wire and bonded composite appliance, but a pontic is usually not necessary. A sturdier wire such as a 0.018 in. × 022 in. edgewise can be bonded to the border teeth. It should be bent so that the wire in the edentulous area is gingival to the occlusal plane to minimize the possibility of distortion during function (Fig. 15.**38a**). Usually small, shallow preparations are cut into the proximal enamel of the border teeth for better retention of the wire and to keep the terminal ends of the wire level

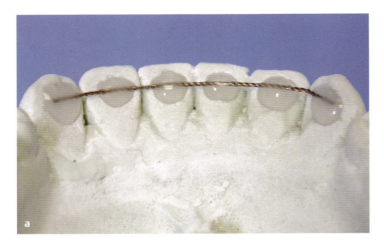

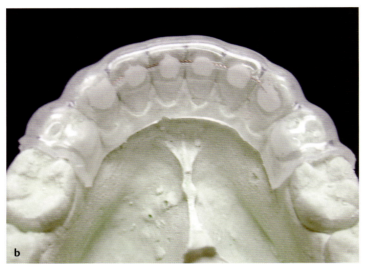

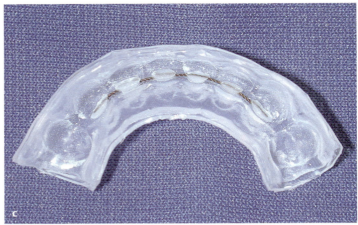

Fig. 15.**36** **Indirect bonding of the canine-to-canine retainer.**
a Tacking the formed wire to the cast with composite assures accurate placement prior to thermoforming plastic over the cast.
b The carrier material is thermoformed over the working cast. Since the material is transparent, light-curing of the composite is possible.
c The bracket bases can be cleaned with a wet cotton swab and then dried with compressed air. This step is required to ensure an uncontaminated composite surface.

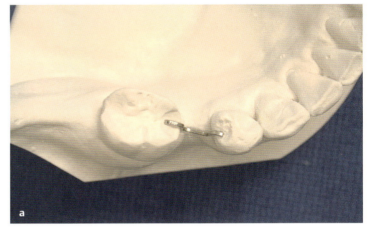

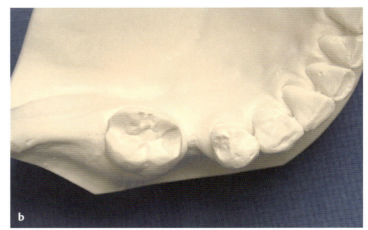

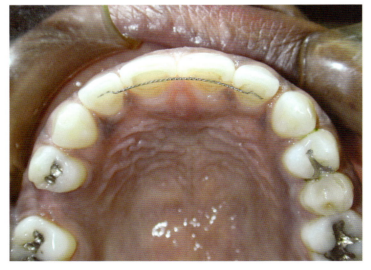

Fig. 15.**37** Retaining the diastema closure with a flexible, and lingually placed, bonded wire prevents the strong relapse tendency of any diastema closure.

Fig. 15.**38** **Maintaining space for a posterior tooth.**
a This wire design spans the posterior edentulous space and prevents the wire from being distorted by occlusal forces.
b The terminal ends of the wire on the border teeth are flush with the marginal ridges due to the shallow preparation cut into enamel.

with the marginal ridges, thereby preventing interference with the bite (Fig. 15.**38b**). This appliance also makes an excellent space maintainer for young patients who have prematurely lost a deciduous second molar.

References

Alexander RG. Retention: a practical approach to that critical last step to stability. Clin Impressions. 1977; 6: 3.

Behrents, RG. A treatise on the continuum of growth in the aging craniofacial skeleton. Ann Arbor MI: University of Michigan Center for Human Growth and Development; 1984.

Blake M, Bibby K. Retention and stability: a review of the literature. Am J Orthod Dentofacial Orthop. 1998; 114: 299–306.

Edward JG. Soft tissue surgery to alleviate orthodontic relapse. Dent Clin N Am. 1993; 37: 205–225.

LaBoda M, Sheridan J, Weinburg R. The feasibility of open bite with an Essix retainer. [Thesis]. Baton Rouge LA: Louisiana State University Department of Orthodontics; 1995.

Lindauer SJ, Schoff R. A comparison of Essix and Hawley retainers. J Clin Orthod. 1998; 32 (2): 95–97.

Little R, Reidel R, Artun J. An evaluation of changes in mandibular anterior alignment from 10 to 20 years postretention. Am J Orthod Dentofacial Orthop. 1998; 93: 423–428.

Moskowitz EM, Sheridan JJ, Celenza F, Tovilo K, Munoz A. Essix appliances: provisional anterior prosthesis for pre and post implant patients. New York State Dent J. 1997 (April): 32–35.

Proffit WR. Equilibrium theory revisited. Angle Orthod. 1978; 48: 175–186.

Reitan K. Principals of retention and avoidance of posttreatment relapse. Am J Orthod. 1969; 55: 776–790.

Sheridan JJ. Air-rotor stripping. J Clin Orthod. 1985; 19: 1.

Sheridan JJ. Essix appliances: minor tooth movement with divots and windows. J Clin Orthod. 1994a; 28 (11): 659–663.

Sheridan JJ. Essix technology for the fabrication of temporary bridges. J Clin Orthod. 1994b; 28 (8): 482–486.

Sheridan JJ, LeDoux W, McMinn R. Essix retainers: fabrication and supervision for permanent retention. J Clin Orthod. 1993; 27 (1): 37–45.

Sheridan JJ, et al. Demineralization and bite alteration from full-coverage plastic appliances. J Clin Orthod. 2001; 35 (7): 444–448.

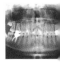

16 Treatment Planning for Mandibular Distraction Osteogenesis

Jason B. Cope

In recent years, a number of experimental and clinical investigations have demonstrated that gradual mechanical traction of bone segments at a craniofacial osteotomy site generates new bone parallel to the direction of traction (Samchukov et al. 1998a, 2001; Cope et al. 1999b). This phenomenon, known as distraction osteogenesis, has opened up new possibilities in the correction of craniofacial deformities by orthodontists and maxillofacial surgeons. Specifically, the process is initiated when incremental traction is applied to the reparative callus that joins the divided bone segments and continues as long as this tissue is stretched. The traction generates tension within the callus and stimulates new bone formation parallel to the vector of distraction.

Importantly, distraction forces applied to bone also create tension in the surrounding soft tissues, initiating a sequence of adaptive changes termed distraction histogenesis (Samchukov et al. 1998a, 2001). Under the influence of tensional stress produced by gradual bony distraction, active histogenesis occurs in different tissues, including periosteum, mucosa, muscle, and neurovascular tissue (Samchukov et al. 1998a, 2001). These adaptive changes in the soft tissues may allow larger skeletal movements while minimizing the potential relapse seen in large acute orthopedic corrections (Cope et al. 1999b).

Clinically, distraction osteogenesis consists of five sequential periods: (1) osteotomy, (2) latency, (3) distraction, (4) consolidation, and (5) remodeling (Samchukov et al. 2001). After the bone is surgically separated into two or more segments, the latency period begins. This is the duration from bone division to the onset of traction and represents the time allowed for reparative callus formation. The distraction period follows and is the time when gradual traction is applied and new bone, or distraction regenerate, is formed. After traction forces are discontinued, the consolidation period commences and lasts until mineralization of the regenerate bone is complete. At that time, the distraction device is removed and unrestrained functional loading begins. From the time of device removal up to a year later, the regenerate bone is continuously remodeled (Samchukov et al. 2001).

The application of distraction osteogenesis to the craniofacial skeleton has the potential to greatly enhance our ability to treat both complex and routine surgical patients. Although osteodistraction has gained widespread use in the maxillofacial region over the last few years, most reports and meetings have focused on the application of distraction to significant craniofacial deformities and syndromic patients, with few clinicians using the technique for the surgical-orthodontic procedures commonly seen in private practice. This chapter demonstrates the use of osteodistraction for treating two types of mandibular deficiencies – (1) a large sagittal deficiency that might normally be corrected in private practice with a bilateral sagittal split ramus osteotomy followed by immediate mandibular advancement, and (2) a large transverse deficiency that might normally be corrected by various extraction patterns. Further, this demonstrates that the use of distraction osteogenesis on these types of cases does not preclude obtaining high-quality facial esthetics and an ideal functionally-based occlusion, i.e., a bilateral mutually protected occlusion (maximum intercuspation having canine guidance in lateral excursion and incisal guidance in protrusion with the condyle located in a centrically related position).

Clinical Case Studies

Mandibular Lengthening

Case Study 16.1

History

This young male patient, 15 years 9 months old, presented with the chief complaint of "I don't like the way my front teeth stick out" (see Figs. 16.1.**1–11**). His maturational status was established as 16 years 0 months based on cross-referencing with Todd's *Atlas of Skeletal Maturation* (Todd 1937).

Predistraction Orthodontics

Treatment Plan

Widen the maxilla with rapid palatal expansion. Once expansion is achieved, stabilize the maxilla with an 0.036 in. stainless-steel (SS) transpalatal arch. Band the maxillary and mandibular first and second molars; bond the remaining teeth with 0.018 in. straight wire (Roth) appliance. Slenderize maxillary and mandibular anterior teeth and close spaces. Level, align, and coordinate maxillary and mandibular arches. Extract the third molars three to six months prior to surgery. Advance the mandible via distraction osteogenesis, then finish and detail the occlusion.

Treatment Progress

After the arches were coordinated, presurgical progress records were taken. The records included (1) intraoral and extraoral photographs (Figs. 16.1.**12–17**); (2) two sets of mounted and one set of unmounted study models; (3) lateral (Fig. 16.1.**18**), lateral oblique, posteroanterior (PA), and submentovertex (SMV) cephalometric and panoramic radiographs; and (4) a computed tomographic (CT) scan of the maxilla and mandible for production of a stereolithographic model (Medical Modeling, Denver, CO, USA). These records were used to formulate the distraction treatment plan-predicted movements (Figs. 16.1.**19–24**) (Table 16.**2**), including device fabrication and orientation (Figs. 16.1.**25–29**), surgical technique (Figs. 16.1.**30–32**), and distraction protocol.

Distraction Treatment Planning

It is critical to extensively plan treatment in preparation for osteodistraction. There are several reasons for the importance of this. The first is that relatively few clinicians have experience with the technique. Secondly, the distraction process is dynamic in nature, which is atypical for most surgeons. To explain, most surgical techniques rely on diagnosis and treatment planning based on a static presurgical position and a static postsurgical position. At the time of surgery, the surgeon osteotomizes the bone in its presurgical position, moves it to its postsurgical position, then rigidly fixes it in place using plates and screws. Because distraction regenerate formation occurs over a period of weeks to months, clinicians have the opportunity to modify the biological process.

Orthodontists are trained to essentially re-diagnose a case at every appointment, subsequently making mid-treatment corrections if necessary. Therefore, it is important for both the surgeon and orthodontist to be involved with presurgical distraction treatment planning. Figures 16.1.**19–32** illustrate our particular method of treatment planning and surgical technique.

Distraction Protocol

Latency

During the seven-day latency period, the patient was monitored on the third and seventh days. Postoperative swelling on the third day was similar to that seen following impacted third molar removal. The patient reported that analgesics were only required for three days postoperatively and that his throat was more sore (from the endotracheal tube) than was his mandible (from the osteotomy). In addition, varying degrees of paresthesia were present in the soft tissue overlying the chin and lips (Table 16.**3**). On the third day, the distraction splint was delivered and adjusted to the current occlusal scheme. In addition, light Class II elastics (Guerrero and Bell 1999) (¼ in., 4 oz) were worn from the mandibular first premolars to the maxillary canines. The patient was instructed to wear both the splint and elastics 24 hours per day.

Distraction

When the patient returned on the seventh day, he had only worn elastics 12 hours a day due to miscommunication. Minimal facial swelling was present and maximum opening was 23 mm. Minor erythema was present in the buccal mucosa overlying the anterior aspect of the distraction screw, so an acrylic shield was made to protect the cheek. The patient was instructed to activate the devices using an Allen wrench for 270° or 0.45 mm twice per day (total of 0.9 mm per day).

On the fourth day of distraction, maximum opening was 28 mm, and protrusive/excursive movements were 4 mm. The patient reported no pain upon device activation. He did, however, note sporadic "electric shocks" on his chin, indicating that sensation was returning. At this point, it appeared that the mandible had moved anteriorly more than half the necessary distance to correct the deficiency (6 out of approximately 10 mm) (Fig. 16.1.**33**). However, the mandible should have only moved forward 3.15 mm (seven activations) at this point. The patient demonstrated that he knew exactly how to activate the device. Mandibular manipulation revealed that the patient was posturing the mandible forward. Since the splint had been made to mimic ideal function through the full distraction distance and no premature contacts were detected, it was concluded that the elastics were causing the mandibular posture. At this point, the elastics were changed from a Class II to a very slight Class III vector for three days, to overcome muscle splinting.

By the eighth day of distraction, maximum opening was 34 mm, and protrusive/excursive movements were 5 mm. Mandibular posturing was resolved, and the mandible was in the anticipated position. The patient did report minor discomfort when wearing the Class III elastics, so they were changed to anterior and posterior vertical box elastics (¼ in., 6 oz). The patient was reminded what the final mandibular position should look like based on incisor overjet and overbite relationships and instructed to call if he thought device activation should stop before his next appointment.

On the eleventh day of distraction, maximum opening was 35 mm, and protrusive/excursive movements were 5 mm. The mandibular position was almost ideal, but the midlines were not coincident, so the devices were differentially activated to obtain coincident midlines and idealize the mandibular position.

Consolidation

Distraction was complete on the 11th day (Figs. 16.1.**34–40**) and the patient was monitored weekly for the next two weeks. During this time, the regenerate increased in radiodensity as seen on the panoramic radiograph (Fig. 16.1.**41**). On the seventh day of consolidation, maximum opening was 38 mm, and protrusive/excursive movements were 5 mm. The overbite and overjet relationships were good. Due to lack of complete curve of Spee leveling presurgically, occlusal contacts in the premolar region were not ideal, so box elastics were continued. Minor repositioning bends were placed in both archwires to idealize the final tooth positions. On the 14th day of consolidation, functional movements remained constant, and additional repositioning bends were placed in both archwires. By the 28th day of consolidation, substantial mineralization of the regenerate was evident. Functional movements remained the same, and the patient reported considerable sensitivity return in the soft tissues of the anterior mandible. The functional occlusion looked good, and elastic wear was tapered to nighttime only. On the 39th day of consolidation, the patient presented with swelling of the left mandibular angle. No purulence was noted in the area, either extraorally or intraorally where the devices passed transmucosally. The patient was placed on 150 mg of clindamycin four times a day for 10 days. After three days, the swelling had resolved, and no further sequelae were observed. The distraction devices were removed under local anesthesia on the 49th day of consolidation and one screw from each bone plate was replaced for long-term follow-up via cephalometric superimposition.

Remodeling (Postdistraction Orthodontics)

Artistic finishing procedures and final occlusal detailing were initiated one week after the distraction devices were removed. The archwires were cut distal to the canines, and posterior vertical elastics (¾ in., 2 oz) and an anterior box elastic (¼ in., 6 oz) were worn 24 hours a day for two weeks, at which time they were worn for an additional week at night time only.

Retention

All appliances were removed at this time, and a maxillary Hawley and a mandibular bonded canine-to-canine retainer were placed (Figs. 16.1.**42–49**). The maxillary retainer was worn 24 hours a day for three months, at which time retainer wear tapered to nighttime only. The mandibular retainer will remain in place indefinitely. Some have voiced concern that distraction might not be stable; however, no evidence of skeletal relapse was seen two years after appliance removal (Figs. 16.1.**50–58**).

Final Evaluation

The desired treatment objectives, i.e., ideal facial esthetics with a bilateral mutually protected occlusion and a healthy periodontium, were accomplished. Several issues should be discussed, however, when considering distraction osteogenesis versus traditional orthognathic surgery. These include (1) the direction of movement, (2) neurosensory issues, (3) stability/relapse potential, and (4) clinical management during the distraction process.

Concerning the direction of bone movement, three primary factors influence the final position of the distal bone segment – intrinsic factors (muscle forces, occlusal forces, vascular supply), extrinsic factors (device material properties), and distraction device orientation (vector) (Cope et al. 2000). Taken together, these factors determine both the final position of the bone segment as well as the path it takes during distraction. The occlusal splint worn during latency and distraction had several functions. First, since the occlusion changes daily during distraction, the splint provided a relatively constant and stable occlusion, which protected against nocturnal bruxing and/or mandibular posturing, both of which would be deleterious. Bruxing could introduce undesirable forces on the mandible, possibly leading to strains within the regenerate that are not favorable for osteogenesis (Cope et al. 2000) Mandibular posturing may confuse clinical judgment during decisions on how much distraction device activation is necessary. In addition, the occlusal splint increased the vertical dimension of occlusion, thereby minimizing the amount of mandibular closing during the period when the regenerate was not completely mineralized. The suprahyoid muscles, in turn, could not generate as much downward and backward tension at the anterior mandible, minimizing the potential production of shear stresses within the regenerate and the possibility of an anterior open bite (Cope et al. 2000).

Two potentially misleading points that may be inferred from the cranial base superimpositions should be clarified (Fig. 16.1.**59**). Although it appears that the lower lip moved backward after distraction, this was not the case. Actually, the lower lip was everted by the anterior aspect of the distraction device, and after device removal, the lip returned to its normal position. It also appears that a slight open bite developed during lengthening. This was not the case, however. A splint was worn during distraction and the rigid distraction device was oriented parallel to the maxillary occlusal plane, both of which minimize or eliminate this potential problem. More importantly, both cephalometric and articulator prediction methods accurately indicated that the lower anterior facial height would increase during distraction, not as a result of bite opening but rather as a result of lack of complete presurgical curve of Spee leveling and as a result of the final occlusal relationship with the maxillary occlusal plane. At the completion of distraction, the overbite was approximately 1 mm. By the end of consolidation, this relationship had increased to 2.5 mm, almost entirely as a result of controlled tipping/retraction and relative extrusion of the maxillary incisors by 1 mm and 2 mm, respectively. Slight anterosuperior rotation of the posterior aspect of the distal segment also occurred. Both of these occurrences probably resulted from anterior and posterior box elastic wear during distraction and consolidation. Importantly, an increase in lower anterior face height was desired to minimize the dished facial appearance (due to a prominent pogonion) that was present prior to treatment. It was anticipated that normal growth of the maxilla would continue in a downward and forward direction, which may have been enhanced by rapid palatal expansion. In addition, the mandibular plane was opened by curve of Spee leveling to increase the lower anterior facial height.

The patient reported that neurosensory perception was never completely lost. It is suspected that any sensory deficit was due to mental nerve manipulation during dissection for inferior bone plate placement. By the fourth day of distraction, the patient reported approximately 20% of presurgical sensation. Interestingly, sensation began to return during distraction, up to 45%, rather than decrease as might be anticipated (Table 16.3). This is in concurrence with Makarov and colleagues (1998), who reported that neurosensory loss was usually related to surgical procedures themselves rather than to bone segment distraction. Importantly, when the device was removed and the mental nerve was again subjected to manipulation during dissection, the patient experienced a transient hyperesthesia, followed by a decrease in soft-tissue sensation. By the time of appliance removal, neurosensory perception had returned to 100% and 70% of pretreatment values on the right and left sides, respectively. Considering these facts, it may be prudent to use either a bone-borne device with the anterior bone plate fixed posteriorly enough to avoid mental nerve dissection/exposure or to use a hybrid device with a tooth-borne component on the distal segment. Another sensory-related concern is the potential for pain during distraction. This is rarely a problem, however, and this patient reported that he felt no pain during distraction. In fact, he remembered more discomfort associated with palatal expansion than with distraction device activation.

Osteodistraction stimulates adaptive changes in the surrounding soft tissues referred to as distraction histogenesis (Samchukov et al. 1998a, 2001). This process may facilitate larger skeletal movements and minimize the potential for relapse (Cope et al. 1999b). Although not directly related to relapse, one particular area of concern in this case was the use of Class II elastics during distraction as suggested by Guerrero and Bell (1999) for "unloading" of the condyles. After eight days of light Class II elastic wear, the patient appeared to have been distracted about 3 mm more than should have been the case. This was eventually found to be caused by mandibular posturing as a result of Class II elastic wear, which should not have been unexpected considering the number of patients undergoing orthodontic treatment only who posture their mandible during and after Class II elastic wear. It is therefore suggested that particular attention be placed on elastic vectors. Elastics with vertical vectors, rather than Class II vectors, should be worn during latency, distraction, and consolidation. TMJ pain during distraction suggests either the presence of subclinical signs prior to treatment, in which case osteodistraction should have been precluded from the outset, or that improper device orientation has unfavorably loaded the joints. The use of Class II elastics during distraction may, in fact, cause undetected anterior mandibular posturing, which may lead to apparent relapse as these patients are studied long-term. For example, once distraction is stopped prior to complete skeletal deficiency resolution, the regenerate will go on to fully mineralize. If the incomplete skeletal correction is later detected, a second surgical procedure would be required. If it is not detected, however, and these patients continue to function after orthodontic treatment, they may undergo apparent relapse (mandibular repositioning) due to premature distraction cessation, rather than to true skeletal relapse.

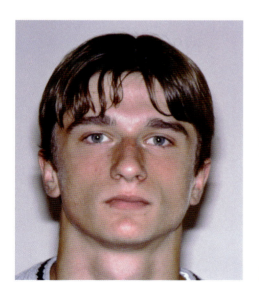

Fig. 16.1.**1** **Pretreatment frontal facial view.**

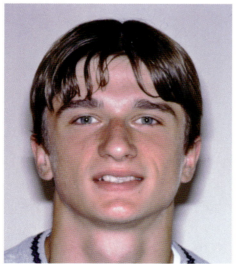

Fig. 16.1.**2** **Pretreatment frontal facial view smiling.** At maximum smile, 4 mm of maxillary central incisor was visible.

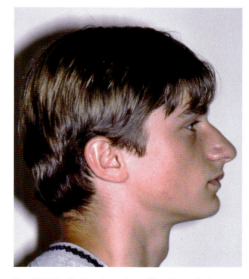

Fig. 16.1.**3** **Pretreatment profile.** The soft tissue profile was convex overall, with a retrusive mandibular profile and a moderate mentolabial sulcus. The nasal and chin projections were prominent, which minimized the facial convexity, camouflaged the true maxillomandibular discrepancy, and created a dished appearance. The upper lip was slightly procumbent, and the lower lip was slightly retrusive.

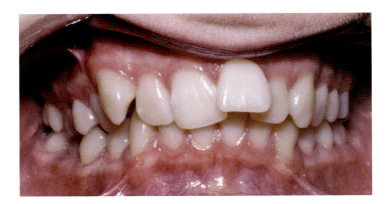

Fig. 16.1.4 **Pretreatment anterior view.** The frontal and lateral occlusal cants were level and the curve of Spee was 3 mm. The maxillary and mandibular dental midlines were coincident with each other and with the facial midline. The maxillary incisors were relatively upright except for the left central incisor, which was flared and blocked-out to the facial.

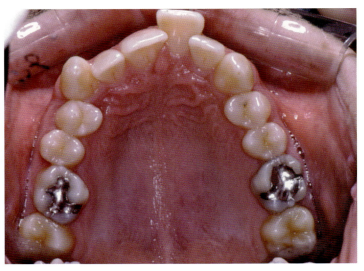

Fig. 16.1.5 **Pretreatment maxillary occlusal view.** The maxillary arch was V-shaped and constricted anteriorly with 8 mm of crowding, based on occlusogram analysis. The maxilla was also narrow posteriorly when the mandible was postured forward into a Class I position.

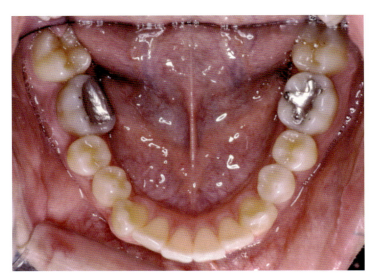

Fig. 16.1.6 **Pretreatment mandibular occlusal view.** The mandibular incisors were flared and the mandibular arch was V-shaped with 3 mm of crowding.

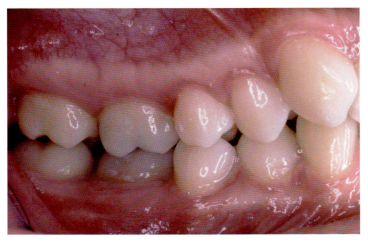

Fig. 16.1.7 **Pretreatment right buccal view.** The patient presented in the permanent dentition with a Class II molar and canine relationship.

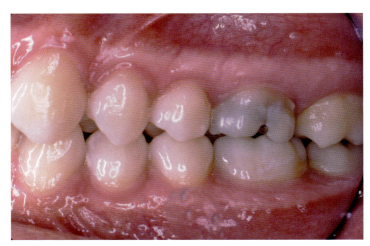

Fig. 16.1.8 **Pretreatment left buccal view.**

Table 16.1 Cephalometric Summary.

Cephalometric Area of Study	Cephalometric Measurements	Pretreatment (Norm)	Presurgery (Norm)	Postdistraction (Norm)	Posttreatment (Norm)
Maxilla to cranial base	S–N–A	84.8° (80.9)	84.1° (81.4)	84.5° (81.4)	84.0° (81.4)
	N–A/FH	89.9° (90.0)	88.8° (90.0)	90.1° (90.0)	89.4° (90.0)
Mandible to cranial base	S–N–B	79.8° (77.6)	78.4° (78.2)	81.5° (78.2)	82.2° (78.2)
	N–Pg/FH	87.8° (82.9)	86.6° (82.5)	88.4° (82.5)	88.8° (82.5)
Maxillo-mandibular relations	A–N–B	5.0° (3.3)	5.7° (3.2)	3.0° (3.2)	1.8° (3.2)
	A–B/OP	9.4 mm (−1.2)	9.4 mm (−1.2)	2.7 mm (−1.2)	0.8 mm (−1.2)
Vertical relations	N–ANS	57.1 mm (52.8)	58.3 mm (53.4)	58.8 mm (53.4)	58.5 mm (53.4)
	ANS–Me	59.9 mm (68.7)	61.5 mm (71.2)	64.8 mm (71.2)	64.8 mm (71.2)
	Go–Me/FH	16.2° (28.5)	17.0° (28.7)	20.1° (28.7)	20.5° (28.7)
	S–Gn/FH	57.8° (63.1)	58.5° (63.5)	57.8° (63.5)	57.0° (63.5)
Maxillary and mandibular incisor position	U1/S–N	119.7° (103.0)	114.5° (105.2)	110.4° (105.2)	110.4° (105.2)
	U1/N–A	34.8° (22.1)	30.5° (23.8)	25.8° (23.8)	26.4° (23.8)
	U1/A–Pg	9.1 mm (3.5)	7.7 mm (3.5)	6.0 mm (3.5)	6.0 mm (3.5)
	L1/Go–Me	99.3° (95.9)	88.6° (95.9)	100.4° (95.9)	94.8° (95.9)
	L1/N–B	23.1° (25.3)	11.0° (26.4)	29.2° (26.4)	24.3° (26.4)
	L1/A–Pg	−1.1 mm (1.8)	−6.8 mm (2.7)	3.6 mm (2.7)	2.5 mm (2.7)
	U1/L1	117.0° (129.2)	132.9° (126.6)	121.9° (126.6)	127.5° (126.6)
Soft tissue	Gl′–Sn–Pg′	22.9° (6.7)	21.7° (6.7)	17.7° (6.7)	17.8° (6.7)
	Nasolabial	115.1° (110.8)	116.7° (110.8)	109.2° (110.8)	116.7° (110.8)
	Ls(pSn–Pg′)	2.8 mm (2.6)	1.9 mm (2.3)	2.5 mm (2.3)	1.2 mm (2.3)
	Li(pSn–Pg′)	0.7 mm (2.1)	−2.4 mm (2.3)	2.2 mm (2.3)	−0.1 mm (2.3)
Other	N–A–Pg	4.6° (3.9)	4.9° (3.9)	3.6° (3.9)	1.4° (3.9)
	N–S/OP	3.8° (14.3)	5.9° (12.9)	9.2° (12.9)	9.5° (12.9)

Note: Norms based on Michigan Growth Study (Riolo et al. 1974) (age and sex matched).

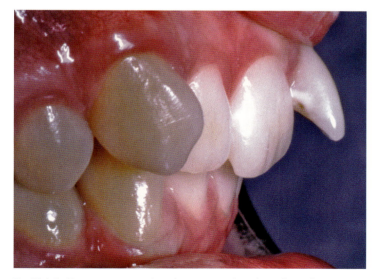

Fig. 16.1.9 **Pretreatment overjet.** The overjet and overbite relationships were 7 mm and 5 mm (70%), respectively.

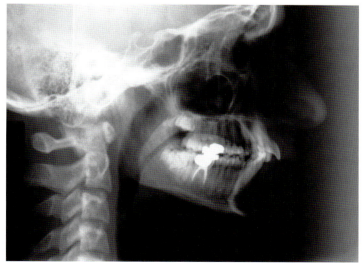

Fig. 16.1.10 **Pretreatment lateral cephalometric radiograph.** All anteroposterior skeletal measurements indicated a Class II skeletal deepbite relationship (Table 16.1). Both the maxilla and mandible were large and positioned slightly forward relative to the cranial base. However, the maxilla was slightly further forward. Pogonion was also prominent. A mandibular plane angle of 16.2°, a decreased Y-axis (57.8 °), and a lower anterior facial height 9 mm less than normal suggested a horizontal growth pattern.

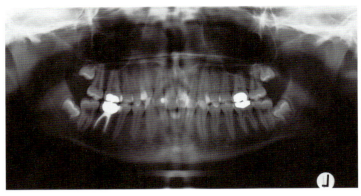

Fig. 16.1.**11** **Pretreatment panoramic radiograph.** Based on the panoramic (Coutinho et al. 1993) and the hand-wrist (Todd 1937) radiographs the patient was on the down slope of his growth curve and future growth was expected to be minimal.

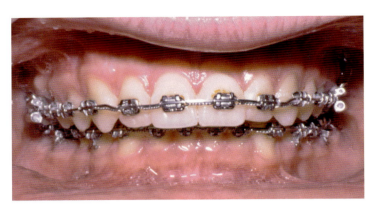

Fig. 16.1.**12** **Presurgery anterior view.**

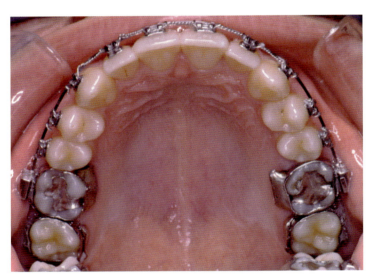

Fig. 16.1.**13** **Presurgery maxillary occlusal view.**

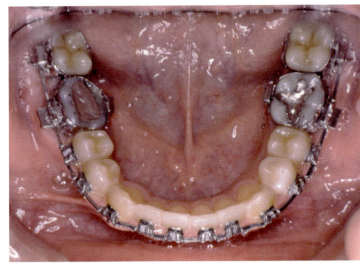

Fig. 16.1.**14** **Presurgery mandibular occlusal view.**

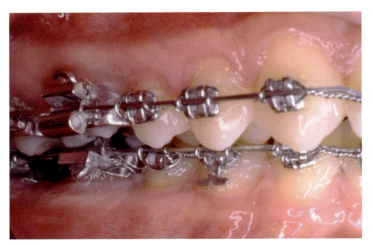

Fig. 16.1.**15** **Presurgery right buccal view.**

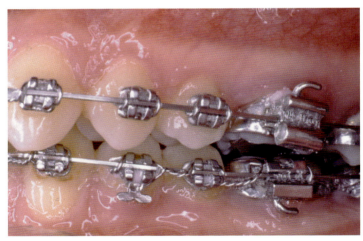

Fig. 16.1.**16** **Presurgery left buccal view.**

Table 16.2 Distraction Prediction Data (Mandibular Lengthening). In order to ensure that every possible detail was accounted for during predistraction treatment planning, four different methods of prediction were used to analyze bone segment movement during distraction. Taken together, the prediction data suggested that the mandible would come forward about 10 mm with a slight increase in the mandibular plane angle and lower anterior face height. Importantly, the anterior movement with the occlusogram was not as great as with the other methods, plus no vertical prediction was possible. This was most probably due to the inability of the two dimensional occlusogram to accurately represent the vertical dimension, i.e., the remaining mandibular curve of Spee.

Prediction Method	Anteroposterior (mm)		Vertical (mm)
	Right Side	Left Side	
Occlusogram	6.5	7	N/A
Cephalometric 4 mm vertical	11 mm superior margin		4
	9.5 mm inferior margin		
Model repositioning instrument	9.5		5
Mandibular position variator	9	10	5

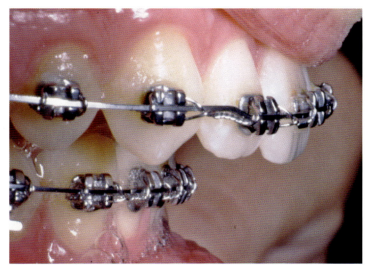

Fig. 16.1.**17** **Presurgery overjet.**

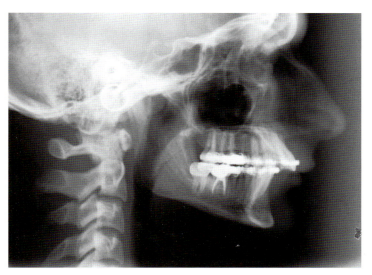

Fig. 16.1.**18** **Presurgery lateral cephalometric radiograph.**

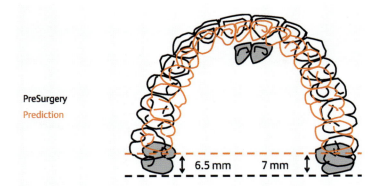

Fig. 16.1.**19** **For occlusogram analysis, the maxillary and mandibular occlusal surfaces of the presurgical models were photocopied, then traced on acetate film.** The tracings were superimposed and slid across one another until the desired final occlusal scheme was obtained, then anteroposterior measurements were recorded. This method indicated that the left and right sides would come forward 7 mm and 6.5 mm, respectively. As this occurred, the midline moved to the right 1 mm.

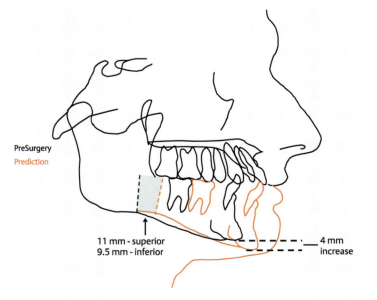

Fig. 16.1.**20** **For cephalometric analysis, the distal segment was moved until the final overjet and overbite were ideal.** For this tracing, the superior and inferior anterior osteotomy margins moved 11 mm and 9.5 mm anteriorly, respectively, and the lower anterior face height increased by 4 mm. This suggested that the distal segment would rotate slightly downward as distraction proceeded.

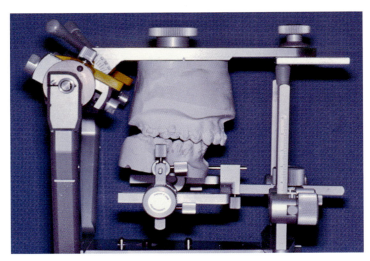

Fig. 16.1.**21** **The SAM Model Repositioning Instrument (Great Lakes Orthodontics, Tonawanda, NY) allows unmounted presurgical mandibular cast repositioning in three dimensions without cutting or sectioning the model.** Movements can then be measured in millimeters and referenced to the original cast position.

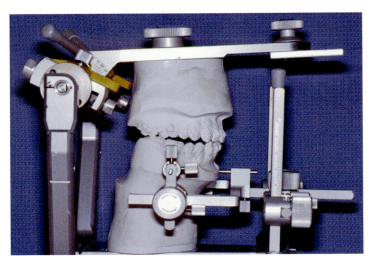

Fig. 16.1.**22** **For this case, vertical measurements were recorded for the left posterior, the right posterior, and anterior regions.** The anteroposterior movement was also recorded. This method indicated that the vertical left posterior dimension would not change, but the right posterior would increase 1 mm. The anterior vertical dimension increased by 5 mm during mock distraction and the model moved anteriorly 9.5 mm. This suggested that the mandibular plane would open during distraction, but that an ideal overjet relationship would be achieved.

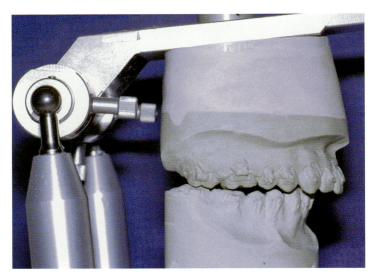

Fig. 16.1.**23** **The SAM Mandibular Position Variator is designed for repositioning the condylar elements during splint fabrication.** Each condylar element has two gears (one each in the X and Y planes), which are calibrated in millimeters such that when activated in either the X or Y plane, the maxillary model moves either posterior or superior, respectively. This gives a corresponding representation of anterior or inferior mandibular movement. For distraction, one set of mounted presurgical models was transferred from a SAM 3 articulator to the variator.

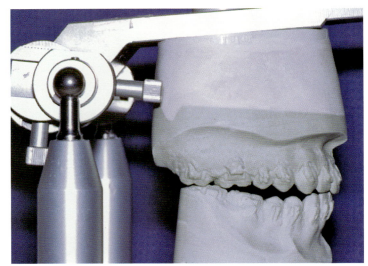

Fig. 16.1.**24** **The gears were activated to move the mandibular model into its desired final position.** This method indicated that the right and left mandibular sides would move anteriorly by 9 mm and 10 mm, respectively. Interestingly, by the end of mock distraction, the incisal guide pin was 5 mm off of the incisal table. Again, this indicated that as distraction proceeded, the mandible would rotate downward until the desired overjet was achieved. In the final position, there was again an openbite in the buccal segments.

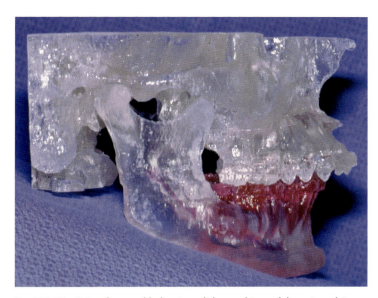

Fig. 16.1.**25** **Using the mandibular stereolithographic model as a template, a polyvinyl siloxane impression was taken and poured in dental stone to create a working model.** This model was then used to fabricate the bilateral distraction devices along the predetermined vector of distraction. Note that the model is differentially colored to highlight the mandibular nerve and tooth roots.

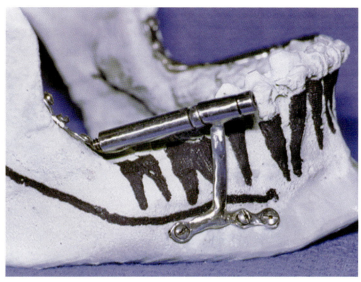

Fig. 16.1.**26** **Lateral view of the working model.** 2.0 mm stainless steel bone plates (KLS Martin, Jacksonville, FL) were adapted and fixed to the anterior aspect of the ascending ramus and the inferior cortex in the molar/premolar region using surgical screws. The bilateral distraction screws were cut to the appropriate length, oriented parallel to both the maxillary occlusal plane (Samchukov et al. 1998c) and the sagittal axis of distraction (Samchukov et al. 1998b) and soldered to the bone plates. The distraction screws were threaded (4/40") such that every 360° revolution advanced the distal mandibular segment 0.6 mm. The devices were removed from the models, tested for strength and range of activation, and polished. They were then transferred to the stereolithographic model, and screw lengths were determined for each hole in the bone plates. All materials were then sterilized and prepared for surgery. Note that the device is oriented parallel to maxillary occlusal plane.

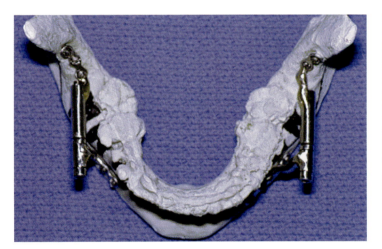

Fig. 16.1.**27** **Occlusal view of the working model.** Note that the devices are oriented parallel to each other and to the sagittal axis of distraction.

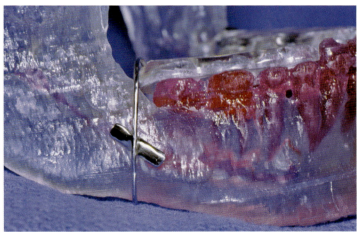

Fig. 16.1.**28** **In order to presurgically determine the location of the osteotomy and to minimize the potential of inferior alveolar nerve damage during surgery, a surgical template was fabricated for use during surgery.** Briefly, a sectional occlusal splint for each side of the mandible was fabricated on a mandibular model. An 0.036" SS wire was embedded into the occlusal surface of the acrylic so that the wire extended from the distal of the 2nd molar and out over the lateral surface of the mandible. The splint was then transferred to the stereolithographic model where the "osteotomy guide" wire was ideally adapted to the lateral surface of the mandible extending down to the inferior cortex, thereby representing the osteotomy line. Next, three 0.036" SS wires (nerve marker) were soldered to the osteotomy guide wire directly over and parallel to the inferior alveolar nerve. The surgical templates were then sterilized and prepared for surgery.

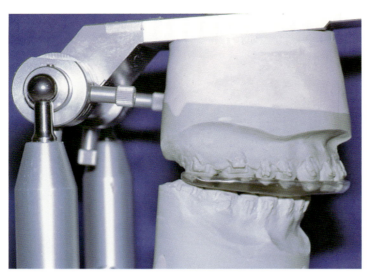

Fig. 16.1.**29** **Using the variator, a maxillary occlusal splint was constructed to minimize occlusal changes during distraction.** The splint was made to the presurgical mandibular position, then the occlusal surface was relined as the mandible was "distracted" forward on the variator.

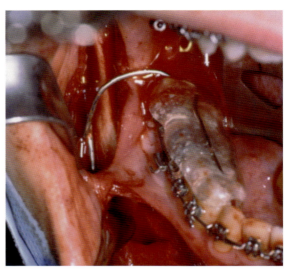

Fig. 16.1.**30** **All procedures were performed under general anesthesia with nasoendotracheal intubation.** The soft tissue incision was similar to that made during a standard sagittal split ramus osteotomy. The first incision was initiated halfway up the anterior border of the ramus and extended approximately 2.5 cm anteroinferiorly into the buccal vestibule lateral to the 2nd molar. The tissues were dissected through the mucosa and periosteum to the bone. Subperiosteal dissection continued in the retromolar region up the anterior border of the ramus to release the tendinous fibers of the temporalis muscle insertion. A second incision was then made in the buccal vestibule lateral and inferior to the molars/premolars. After the mental nerve was identified and dissected, subperiosteal reflection was completed inferior to the nerve.

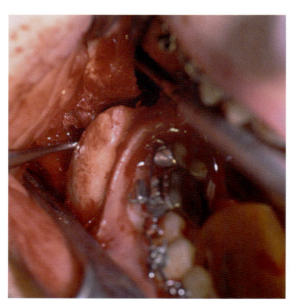

Fig. 16.1.**31** **The distraction device was positioned so that the posterior bone plate fit the anatomy of the anterior ascending ramus and the anterior plate fit the anatomy of the inferior cortex of the corpus.** Holes were drilled into the mandible using the bone plates as templates, then the device was removed. The surgical template was positioned on the occlusal surfaces of the right posterior teeth and a reciprocating saw was used to osteotomize the mandible. The osteotomy began in the retromolar region approximately 5 mm distal to the 2nd molar, and continued inferiorly along the osteotomy guide wire to the superior aspect of the inferior alveolar nerve marker. The saw blade was then repositioned at the inferior cortex, where the osteotomy continued superiorly to the inferior aspect of the inferior alveolar nerve marker. The saw blade and surgical guide were then removed, and the osteotomy was completed by gently torquing an osteotome between the bone segments, taking care not to impinge the inferior alveolar nerve.

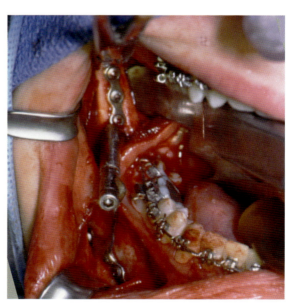

Fig. 16.1.**32** **After completing the osteotomy, the distraction device was repositioned and fixed using the previously measured screws.** The tissues were reapproximated and sutured in layers using 3–0 and 4–0 chromic gut sutures. A similar procedure was then performed on the contralateral side. At the end of surgery, anterior and posterior vertical box elastics (¼ in., 6 oz) were worn in order to restrict mandibular movement during the early postoperative (latency) period. The total surgery time was approximately one-and-a-half hours. The patient tolerated the procedure well and, after an hour of recovery, was conscious, cooperative, and discharged home. He was instructed to maintain a liquid diet for the seven-day latency period, followed by a soft diet during distraction and the first week of consolidation.

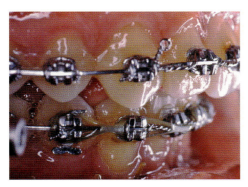

Fig. 16.1.**33** **Four-day interdistraction lateral overjet.**
Note the minimal overjet relative to presurgery photo (Fig. 16.1.**17**).

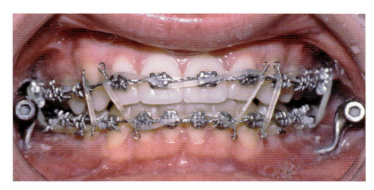

Fig. 16.1.**34** **Postdistraction anterior view.**

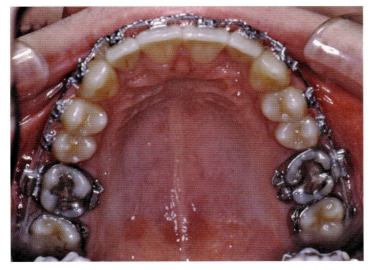

Fig. 16.1.**35** **Postdistraction maxillary occlusal view.**

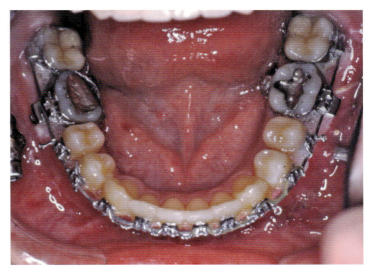

Fig. 16.1.**36** **Postdistraction mandibular occlusal view.**

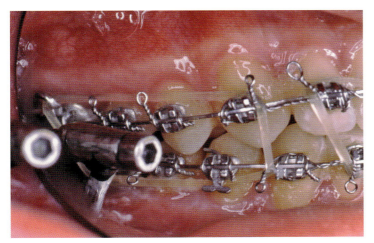

Fig. 16.1.**37** **Postdistraction right buccal view.**

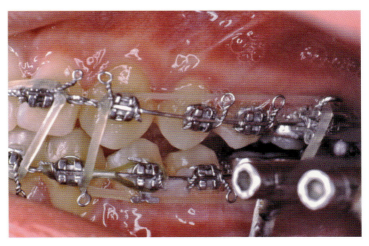

Fig. 16.1.**38** **Postdistraction left buccal view.**

344 Treatment Planning for Mandibular Distraction Osteogenesis

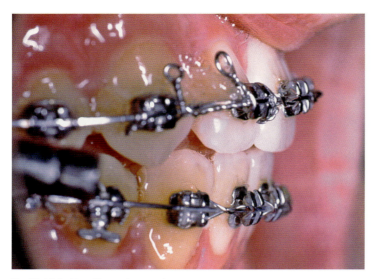

Fig. 16.1.**39** Postdistraction overjet.

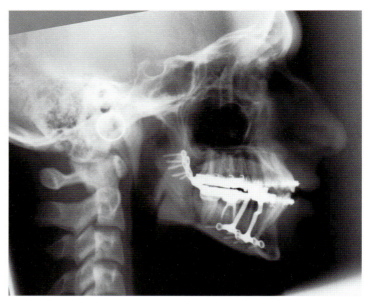

Fig. 16.1.**40** Postdistraction lateral cephalometric radiograph.

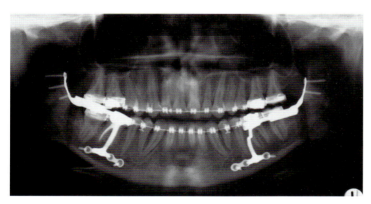

Fig. 16.1.**41** Postdistraction panoramic radiograph.

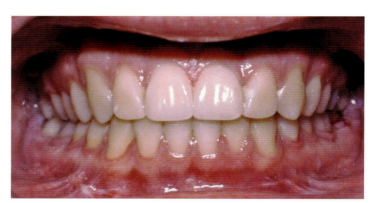

Fig. 16.1.**42** Posttreatment anterior view.

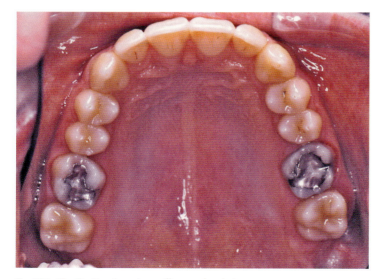

Fig. 16.1.**43** Posttreatment maxillary occlusal view.

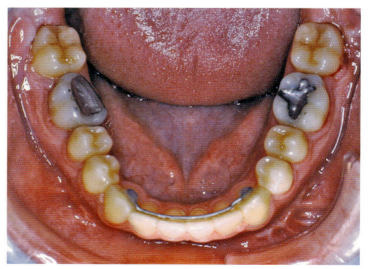

Fig. 16.1.**44** Posttreatment mandibular occlusal view.

Clinical Case Studies

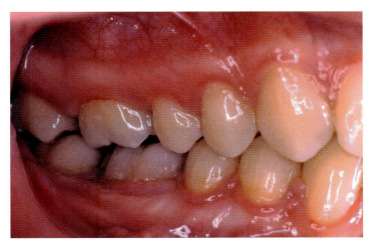

Fig. 16.1.**45** Posttreatment right buccal view.

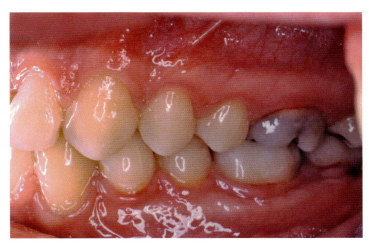

Fig. 16.1.**46** Posttreatment left buccal view.

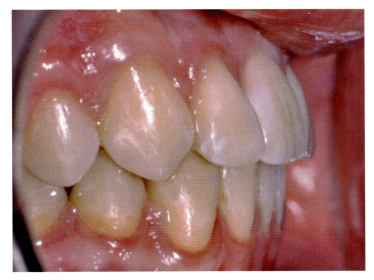

Fig. 16.1.**47** Posttreatment overjet.

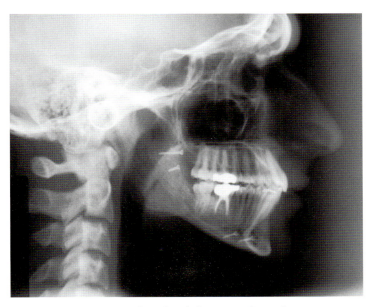

Fig. 16.1.**48** Posttreatment lateral cephalometric radiograph.

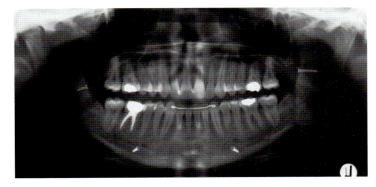

Fig. 16.1.**49** Posttreatment panoramic radiograph.

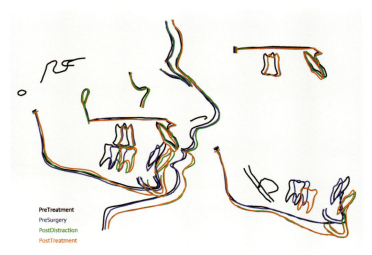

Fig. 16.1.**50** Cephalometric superimpositions.

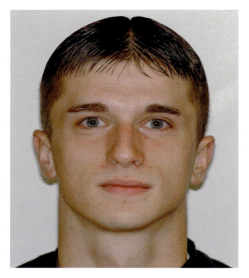

Fig. 16.1.**51** Two-year posttreatment frontal facial view.

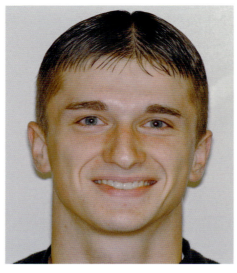

Fig. 16.1.**52** Two-year posttreatment frontal facial view, smiling.

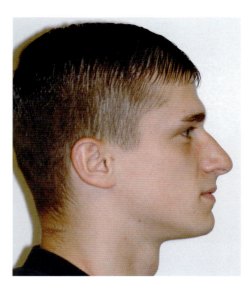

Fig. 16.1.**53** Two-year posttreatment profile.

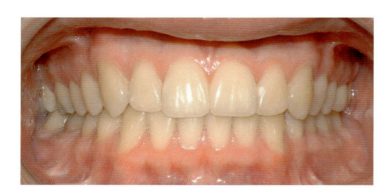

Fig. 16.1.**54** Two-year posttreatment anterior view. Note that the midline has shifted slightly.

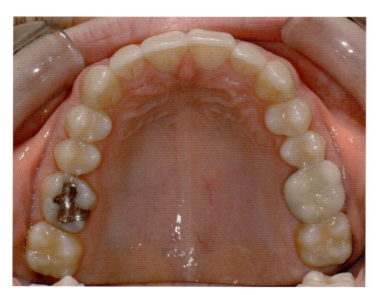

Fig. 16.1.**55** Two-year posttreatment maxillary occlusal view. Note that the maxillary left lateral incisor moved palatally slightly.

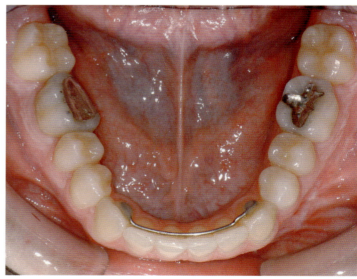

Fig. 16.1.**56** Two-year posttreatment mandibular occlusal view.

Clinical Case Studies

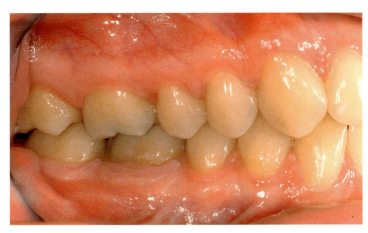

Fig. 16.1.**57** Two-year posttreatment right buccal view.

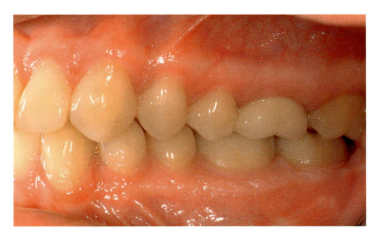

Fig. 16.1.**58** Two-year posttreatment left buccal view.

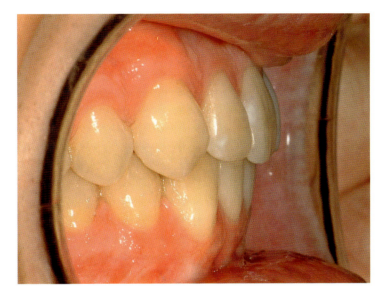

Fig. 16.1.**59** Two-year posttreatment overjet.

Table 16.**3** Functional and Neurological Data.

Time Point	Functional Movements (mm)				Lip and Chin Soft Tissue (%)	
	Opening	Protrusion	Right Lateral	Left Lateral	Right	Left
Pretreatment	54	8	8	7	100	100
Latency day 3	15	4	4	4	5	10
Distraction day 4	28	4	4	4	20	20
Distraction day 8	34	5	5	5	30	30
Distraction day 11	35	5	5	5	40	45
Consolidation day 14	38	5	5	5	50	50
Consolidation day 49	40	5	5	5	70	70
Remodeling day 7	32	4	4	4	0	0
Remodeling day 21	38	5	5	5	70	50
Posttreatment day 0	45	6	6	6	100	70
Posttreatment month 21	53	7	8	8	100	100

Mandibular Widening

Case Study 16.2

History

This young male patient, 16 years 5 months old, presented with a chief complaint of "I want my teeth straightened" (Figs. 16.2.**1–10**).

Predistraction Orthodontics

Treatment Plan

Band the maxillary first and second molars; bond the remaining maxillary teeth with a 0.022 in. straight wire (Roth) appliance. Level, align, and idealize the maxillary arch. About six months prior to mandibular osteotomy, correct the root position of the mandibular left canine such that the root is distal to the osteotomy site (Figs. 16.2.**11, 12**). Widen the mandible via distraction osteogenesis, followed by movement of the mandibular anterior teeth to the left in order to fit the right lateral incisor into the arch. Then coordinate the arches, and finish and detail the occlusion.

Treatment Progress

After the maxillary arch was idealized, presurgical progress records were taken. The records included (1) intraoral and extraoral photographs (Figs. 16.2.**13–17**); (2) two sets of mounted and one set of unmounted models; and (3) lateral (Fig. 16.2.**18**), lateral oblique, posteroanterior (PA), and submentovertex (SMV) cephalometric and panoramic (Fig. 16.2.**19**) radiographs. These records were used to formulate the distraction treatment plan predicted movements (Figs. 16.2.**20–23**) (Table 16.**4**), including device orientation, device fabrication (Figs. 16.2.**24–26**), surgical technique (Fig. 16.2.**27**), and distraction protocol.

Distraction Protocol

Latency

During the seven-day latency period, the patient was monitored on the third and seventh days (Fig. 16.2.**28**). Postoperative swelling on the third day was similar to that seen following genioplasty. The patient reported that analgesics were only required for two days postoperatively. On the third day, the distraction splint was delivered and adjusted to the current occlusal scheme (Fig. 16.2.**29**). In addition, anterior and posterior vertical box elastics (¼ in., 6oz) were worn. The patient was instructed to wear both the splint and elastics 24 hours per day during distraction.

Distraction

When the patient returned on the seventh day, he was instructed to activate the devices using an RPE key 0.5 mm twice per day (total of 1.0 mm per day). The patient reported minor discomfort upon device activation. On the 11th day of distraction, the approximate amount of space was 10 mm, so distraction was stopped.

Consolidation

Distraction was complete on the eleventh day (Figs. 16.2.**30, 31**), and the patient was monitored weekly for the next two weeks. During this time, the regenerate increased in radiodensity. After two months of consolidation, tooth movement of the mandibular anterior teeth into the distraction regenerate was slowly begun. After three months of consolidation, the distraction device was removed by the orthodontist without need for anesthesia. A month later, the regenerate bone had completely mineralized (Figs. 16.2.**32, 33**). Tooth movement in the mandibular anterior region progressed normally (Figs. 16.2.**34–38**). Upon completion of treatment, all mandibular anterior teeth fit nicely into the arch. A bilateral mutually protected occlusion with a healthy periodontium was achieved (Figs. 16.2.**39–43**).

Final Evaluation

Unlike mandibular anteroposterior distraction, transverse distraction required substantially more postdistraction orthodontics. This was due to the fact that it took more time to fit the blocked-out tooth into the arch. Even then, it has taken substantial time to correct the root position of this particular tooth.

Clinical Case Studies

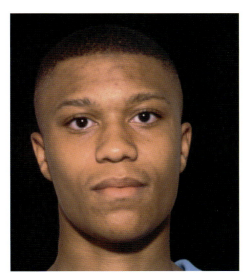

Fig. 16.2.**1** Pretreatment frontal facial view.

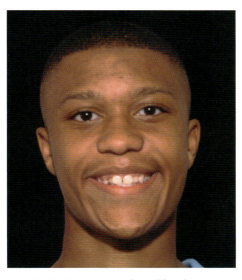

Fig. 16.2.**2** Pretreatment frontal facial view, smiling. At maximum smile, the entire clinical crown of the maxillary central incisor as well as 2 mm of gingival display was visible.

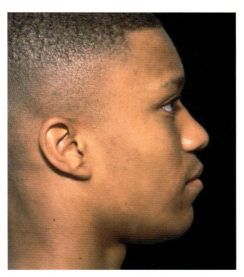

Fig. 16.2.**3** Pretreatment profile. The soft tissue profile was convex overall, primarily due to maxillomandiublar dentoalveolar protrusion.

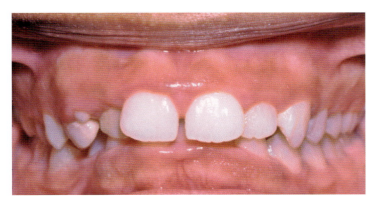

Fig. 16.2.**4** Pretreatment anterior view. The frontal and lateral occlusal cants were level, and the curve of Spee was deep with 100% overbite.

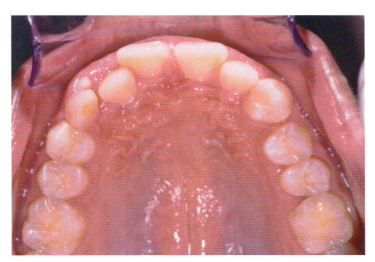

Fig. 16.2.**5** Pretreatment maxillary occlusal view. The maxillary arch was U-shaped and constricted anteriorly (relative to the mandibular) with 4 mm of crowding, based on occlusogram analysis. Both lateral incisors were blocked out of the arch to the lingual.

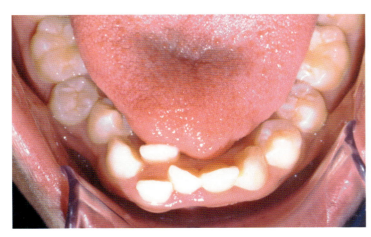

Fig. 16.2.**6** Pretreatment mandibular occlusal view. The mandibular arch was more V-shaped with 10 mm of crowding. The right lateral incisor and 2nd premolars were completely and partially blocked out of the arch to the lingual, respectively.

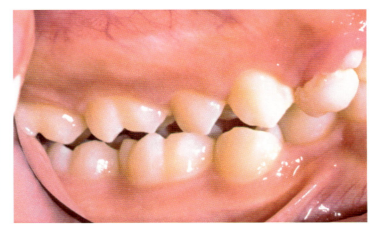

Fig. 16.2.**7** Pretreatment right buccal view. The patient presented in the permanent dentition with a Class I molar and canine relationship.

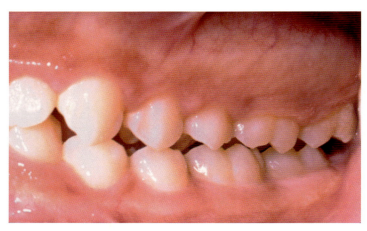

Fig. 16.2.**8** **Pretreatment left buccal view.**

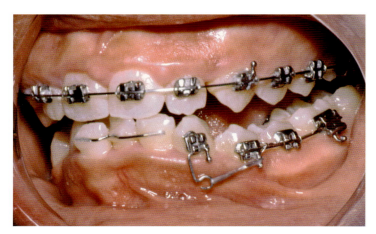

Fig. 16.2.**11** **Predistraction left buccal oblique view.** The mandibular incisors (right central to the left lateral) were bonded together as a unit. The mandibular left buccal segment (left canine to 1st molar) were bonded with brackets. A power arm was placed on both the buccal and lingual of the canine to distalize the root out of the eventual osteotomy site.

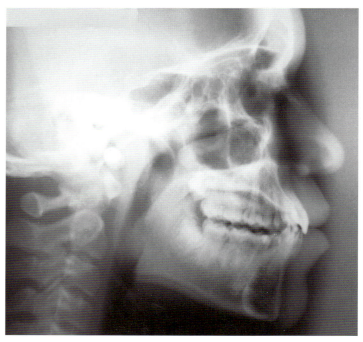

Fig. 16.2.**9** **Pretreatment lateral cephalometric radiograph.** All anteroposterior skeletal measurements indicated a Class I skeletal deepbite relationship. Both the maxilla and mandible were large and positioned slightly forward relative to the cranial base.

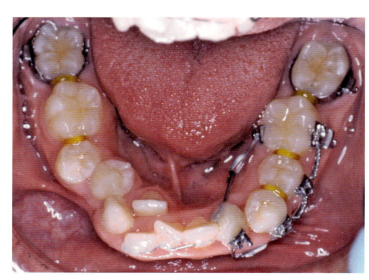

Fig. 16.2.**12** **Predistraction mandibular occlusal view.**

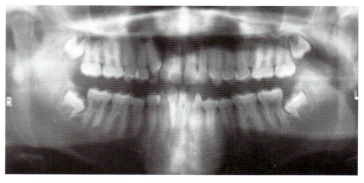

Fig. 16.2.**10** **Pretreatment panoramic radiograph.**

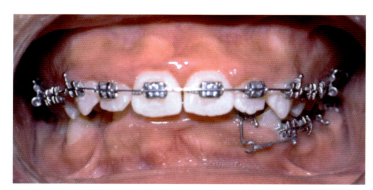

Fig. 16.2.**13** **Presurgery anterior view.**

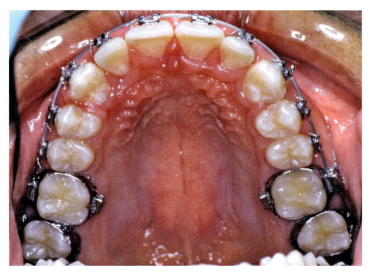

Fig. 16.2.**14** Presurgery maxillary occlusal view.

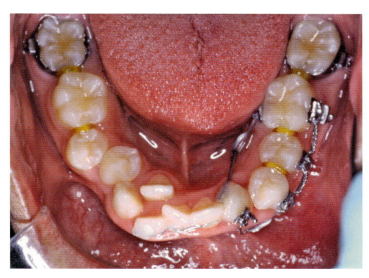

Fig. 16.2.**15** Presurgery mandibular occlusal view.

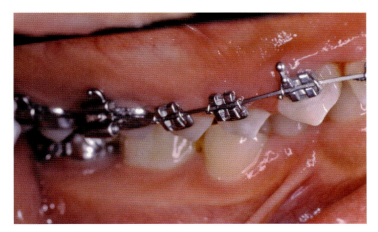

Fig. 16.2.**16** Presurgery right buccal view.

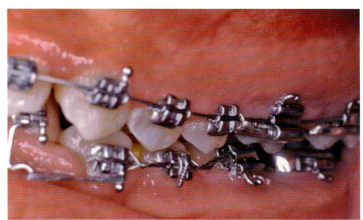

Fig. 16.2.**17** Presurgery left buccal view.

Table 16.**4** Distraction Prediction Data (Mandibular Widening). As the mandibular cast was "distracted" transversely, measurements were recorded using a Boley gage between the cusp tips of one side of the mandible with their contralateral counterparts.

Tooth	0–5 mm	5–10 mm	0–10 mm
LL2–LL3	5.0	5.1	10.1
3 Cusp tips	5.1	4.5	9.6
4 Distal cusps	3.0	5.5	8.5
5 Mesiolingual cusps	5.0	3.5	8.5
5 Distolingual cusps	4.6	3.5	8.1
6 Mesiolingual cusps	4.0	3.8	7.8
6 Distolingual cusps	2.0	5.0	7.0
7 Mesiolingual cusps	3.6	2.3	5.9
7 Distolingual cusps	2.1	2.8	4.9

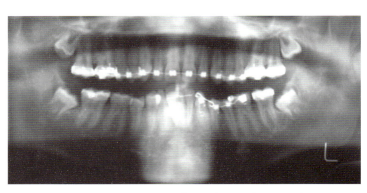

Fig. 16.2.**19** **Presurgery panoramic radiograph.** Note that as much space as possible was opened between the roots of the mandibular left lateral incisor and the canine.

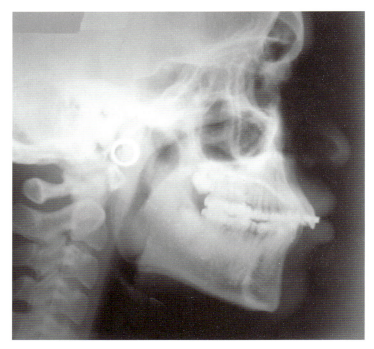

Fig. 16.2.**18** **Presurgery lateral cephalometric radiograph.**

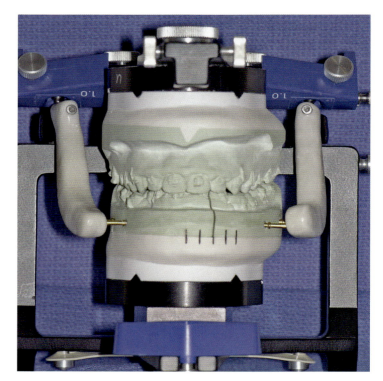

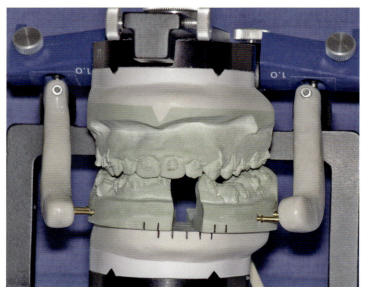

Fig. 16.2.**21** **Distraction prediction with articulator instruments.** CHRI after 10 mm of distraction. Note that the mandibular cast, and consequently the mandibular anterior teeth, move forward relative to the maxillary during transverse distraction.

Fig. 16.2.**20** **Distraction prediction with articulator instruments.** Panadent Articulator with custom components of the Condylar Housing Rotation Instrument (CHRI). Using principles of restorative dentistry, the mandibular cast was attached to the lower mounting of the articulator using Pindex pins (Coltene Whaledent). The maxillary cast was then mounted the mandibular cast. The mandibular cast was then sectioned at the planned osteotomy, then marked at every 5 mm increment. A rotational element was then fabricated such that both halves of the mandibular cast could be rotated about the condylar elements, thereby simulating mandibular symphyseal distraction. The mandibular cast was then "distracted", and measurements recorded between the cusp tips of one side of the mandible with their contralateral counterparts (Table 16.**4**). Importantly, the data indicated that as distraction proceeded anteriorly, increased width of the posterior teeth would also occur. This was not anticipated during pretreatment orthodontics, consequently the maxillary arch was too narrow. When this was realized, the maxillary archwire was expanded to compensate for the apparent width discrepancy.

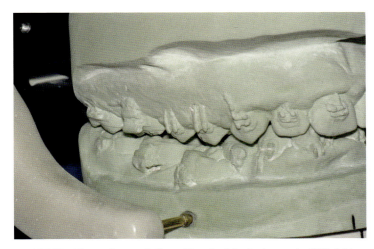

Fig. 16.2.**22** **Distraction prediction with articulator instruments.** CHRI right buccal.

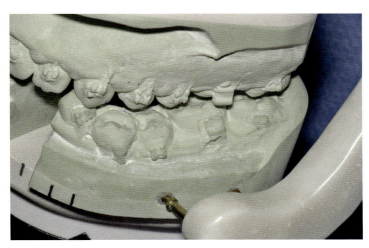

Fig. 16.2.**23** **Distraction prediction with articulator instruments.** CHRI left buccal. Note the crossbite created by mandibular distraction.

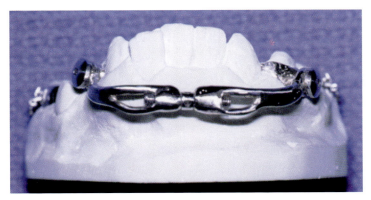

Fig. 16.2.**24** **Anterior view of custom distraction device.** The device was made from 3 components: 1) a Compact RPE (Ormco Corp, Glendora, CA) attached to 2) scrap parts of a Cantilever Bite Jumper appliance (Ormco Corp, Glendora, CA), which were soldered to 3) standard orthodontic bands. The Compact RPE was threaded such that every 360° revolution widened the mandible 1.0 mm. The devices were removed from the models, tested for strength and range of activation, and polished. All materials were then sterilized and prepared for surgery.

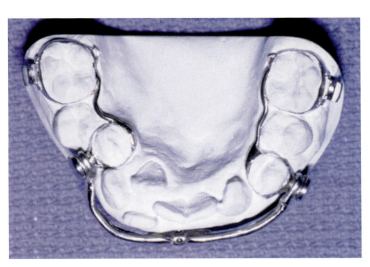

Fig. 16.2.**25** **Occlusal view of distraction device.**

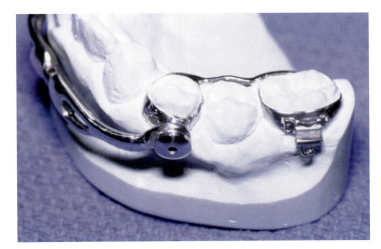

Fig. 16.2.**26** **Lateral view of distraction device.**

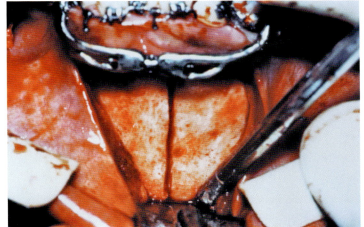

Fig. 16.2.**27** **Osteotomy completion.** All procedures were performed under intravenous conscious sedation with local anesthesia. The approach was identical to that made during a standard genioplasty: a transoral labial vestibular incision sharply dividing the mentalis muscles, sharp dissection through mucosa and periosteum to bone, and subperiosteal dissection exposing the entire anterior mandible, inferior border and mental nerves. Anteriorly, the mucogingival tissues were retracted with a modified interdental retractor and the roots of the incisor teeth were identified. Interdental osteotomies were begun with a fine rotary osteotome and copious saline irrigation through the lateral cortex only. A thin reciprocating saw continued the osteotomy through the inferior border and medial cortex. Fine spatula osteotomes were used from the alveolar crest inferiorly along the interdental osteotomy through the medial cortex to ensure complete separation of the bony segments.

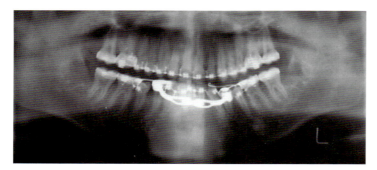

Fig. 16.2.**28** Postoperative panoramic radiograph.

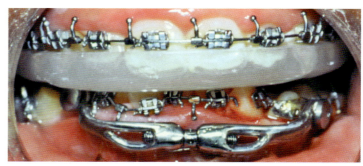

Fig. 16.2.**29** **Postoperative photo of distraction device and occlusal splint.** Using the Sam variator, a maxillary occlusal splint was constructed to minimize occlusal changes during distraction. The splint was made to the presurgical mandibular position, then the occlusal surface was relined as necessary during mandibular distraction.

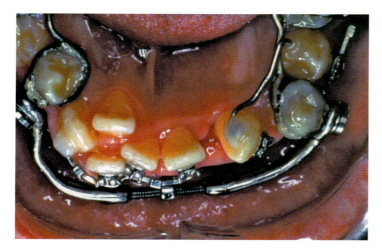

Fig. 16.2.**30** **Immediately postdistraction mandibular occlusal view.** Note the migration of mandibular left lateral incisor and canine toward each other into the distraction site as a result of the principal dentoalveolar and gingival fibers stretched in response to distraction forces (Cope et al. 1999a)

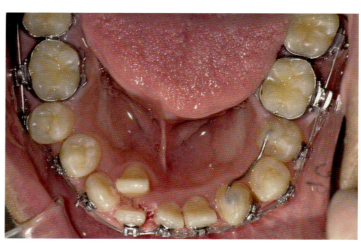

Fig. 16.2.**32** **Four-month postdistraction mandibular occlusal view.** Note that the mandibular anterior teeth are slowly being moved to the left.

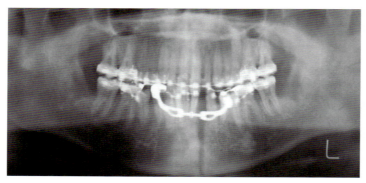

Fig. 16.2.**31** **Immediately postdistraction panoramic radiograph.**

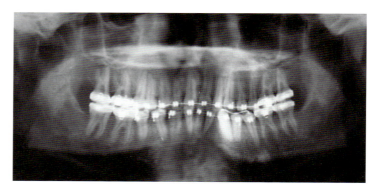

Fig. 16.2.**33** **Four-month postdistraction panoramic radiograph.** Note that the distraction regenerate has completely mineralized.

Clinical Case Studies

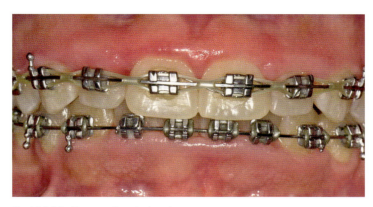

Fig. 16.2.**34** Ten-month anterior view.

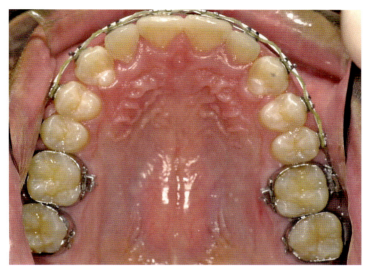

Fig. 16.2.**35** Ten-month maxillary occlusal view.

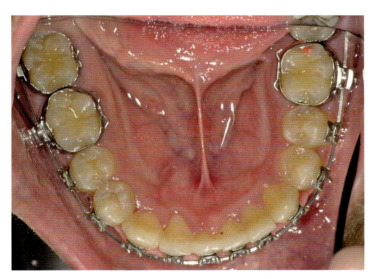

Fig. 16.2.**36** **Ten-month mandibular occlusal view.** Note that the mandibular right lateral incisor is in the arch; labial root torque is being used to move the root anteriorly.

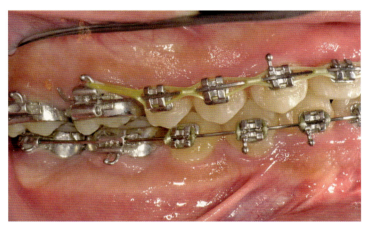

Fig. 16.2.**37** Ten-month right buccal view.

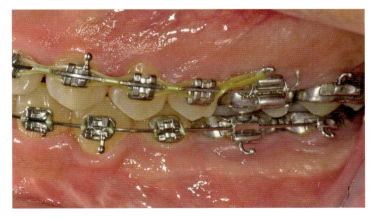

Fig. 16.2.**38** Ten-month left buccal view.

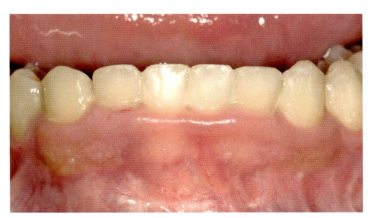

Fig. 16.2.**39** Posttreatment mandibular anterior view.

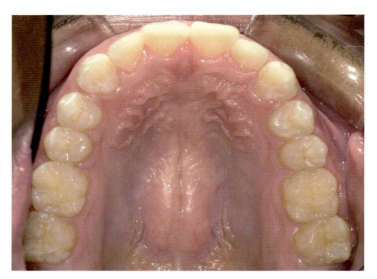

Fig. 16.2.**40** Posttreatment maxillary occlusal view.

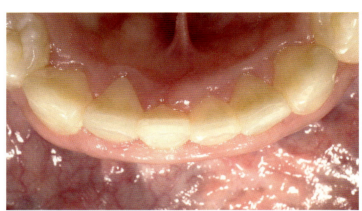

Fig. 16.2.**41** Posttreatment mandibular anterior occlusal view.

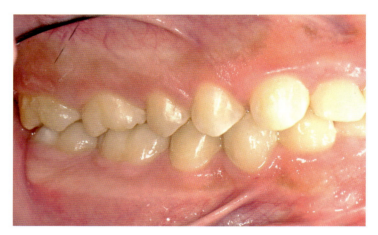

Fig. 16.2.**42** Posttreatment right buccal view.

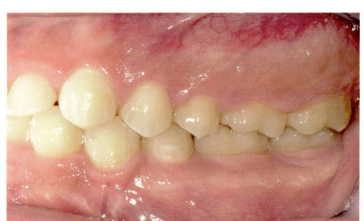

Fig. 16.2.**43** Posttreatment left buccal view.

Summary

Since the distraction process is dynamic and occurs over an approximately three-month period, it is extremely important for these cases to be simultaneously monitored by both the orthodontist and the oral surgeon. This is still a relatively young procedure, and the specifics of each clinician's role have yet to be clearly defined. In general, however, the orthodontist's role is that of initial skeletal deficiency diagnosis; surgical referral; presurgical orthodontic leveling, aligning, and arch coordination; distraction treatment planning for device selection and orientation; interdistraction distal segment and occlusal control via interarch elastics; determining the end point of distraction; and postdistraction orthodontic finishing procedures. The surgeon's role is that of distraction treatment planning for device selection and orientation; surgical management of osteotomy and device placement; postoperative monitoring; determining the end point of consolidation; and device removal. Although these duties are more or less the responsibility of a specific clinician, it is really a combined effort, and considerable time should be spent reaching collective decisions.

Finally, osteodistraction is a dynamic process that occurs over several days to several weeks. This may seem foreign to clinicians who are accustomed to osteotomies followed by immediate bony movement. Initially, it makes treatment planning more difficult, as well. Even when considering this and the fact that distraction devices must remain in place for approximately three months, osteodistraction still provides several advantages over traditional methods of orthognathic correction. Distraction osteogenesis allows the orthodontist, who has an intimate understanding of the occlusal goals and who will finish the occlusion after distraction is complete, to have more control over the final position of the mandible. This should also provide more consistent results since the final mandibular position will be determined with the patient sitting in a chair with little or no swelling and comfortable enough to undergo mandibular manipulation as opposed to lying intraoperatively in a supine position with perioral swelling and unable to undergo manipulation.

References

Cope JB, Harper RP, Samchukov ML. Experimental tooth movement through regenerate alveolar bone: a pilot study. Am J Orthod Dentofacial Orthop. 1999a; 116 (5): 501–505.

Cope JB, Samchukov ML, Cherkashin AM. Mandibular distraction osteogenesis: a historical perspective and future directions. Am J Orthod Dentofacial Orthop. 1999b; 115 (4): 448–460.

Cope JB, Yamashita J, Healy S, Dechow PC, Harper RP. Force level and strain patterns during bilateral mandibular osteodistraction. J Oral Maxillofac Surg. 2000; 58: 171–178.

Coutinho S, Buschang PH, Miranda F. Relationships between mandibular canine calcification stages and skeletal maturity. Am J Orthod. 1993; 104 (3): 262–268.

Guerrero CA, Bell WH. Intraoral distraction osteogenesis: maxillary and mandibular lengthening. Atlas Oral Maxillofac Surg Clin N Am. 1999; 7 (1): 111–151.

Makarov MR, Harper RP, Cope JB, Samchukov ML. Evaluation of inferior alveolar nerve function during distraction osteogenesis. J Oral Maxillofac Surg. 1998; 56: 1417–1423.

Riolo ML, Moyers RE, McNamara JA, Hunter WS. An atlas of craniofacial growth: cephalometric standards from the University School Growth Study, the University of Michigan. Ann Arbor MI: Center for Human Growth and Development, University of Michigan; 1974.

Samchukov ML, Cherkashin AM, Cope JB. Distraction osteogenesis: origins and evolution. In: McNamara JA, Trotman CA, eds. Distraction osteogenesis and tissue engineering. Ann Arbor, MI: Center for Human Growth and Development, University of Michigan; 1998a: 1–36.

Samchukov ML, Cope JB, Cherkashin AM. The effect of sagittal orientation of the distractor on the biomechanics of mandibular lengthening. J Oral Maxillofac Surg. 1998b; 57 (10): 1214–1222.

Samchukov ML, Cope JB, Harper RP, Ross JD. Biomechanical considerations for mandibular lengthening and widening by gradual distraction using a computer model. J Oral Maxillofac Surg. 1998c; 56 (1): 51–59.

Samchukov ML, Cope JB, Cherkashin AM. Biological foundation of new bone formation under the influence of tension stress. In: Samchukov ML, Cope JB, Cherkashin AM, eds. Craniofacial distraction osteogenesis. St. Louis MO: Mosby-Year Book; 2001: 21–36.

Todd TW. Atlas of skeletal maturation. St. Louis MO: CV Mosby; 1937.

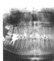

Index

A

abrasive disks for enamel stripping 294
absent teeth, congenitally
 see congenitally missing teeth
acrylic
 of activator, trimming or grinding 87–89
 of occlusal bite blocks
  in maxillary expansion 161
  with twin blocks 104
activator therapy 73, 90
 construction bites *see* construction bites
 dentoalveolar effects 87–88
 failures 87
 forces 75–76
 indications 78
 lower incisor area 88–89
 mode of action 76
 preconditions for success 87
Adams clasp
 functional magnetic system 130
 twin blocks 105
age
 goals of treatment related to 8
 jaw growth related to *see* growth
 maxillary expansion effects related to 167–168
aims of treatment *see* goals
air cooling for grinding of teeth 290
air-rotor stripping 292
airway patency, upper, evaluation 27–28
Alexander Discipline 235–260
 arch form 238–239
 bracket selection and prescription 235–238
 case studies 240–259
 evidence-based studies 260
 in maxilla 239
 treatment mechanics 239
Align technology 276, 277, 278, 282, 283, 284, 285
aligners *see* Invisalign
alveolar dehiscence and fenestration with maxillary expansion 175, 176
alveolar nerve, inferior, minimizing damage in mandibular distraction osteogenesis 341
anchorage
 bionator 93
 dental 261
 edgewise appliances 36
 in extraction site/space closure 205–221, 227
  finishing procedures 220–221, 221
  glossary of notation and abbreviations 205
  group A 210–213, 219, 221
  group B 129, 205–208, 221
  group C 214–219, 219, 221
  maximum anchorage mechanics, case study 240–249
  segmented arch approach 227
 functional magnetic system 130
 skeletal *see* miniscrews; palatal implants; skeletal anchorage

vestibular screen 70; *see also* fixation
Andresen and Häupl activator 75
Angle, Edward Hartley 35
 "Old Glory" skull in textbook of 13
 serial extraction 33
angulations
 Alexander Discipline 235, 237
 buccopalatal, of posterior teeth, causes 156
anterior biteplane in Hawley retainer 314
anterior teeth (tooth segments)
 common presentations following space closure 230
 controlled tipping in group A anchorage control 211–212
 crossbite correction 3
 open-bite, management with twin blocks 107
 retraction 227, 229
anticurvature bends in group C anchorage control 219
apnea, obstructive sleep, rapid maxillary expansion 174–175
appliances
 edgewise *see* edgewise appliances
 factors affecting early use 24
 functional *see* functional orthodontics
 lingual *see* lingual appliances
 maxillary expansion 30
 removable *see* removable appliances
 retention *see* retention
 in serial extraction followed by 34–36
 twin block *see* twin blocks
arch (and archform), dental
 in Alexander Discipline 238–239
 center of resistance of upper arch (C_{Res}) in group A anchorage control 210
 lateral expansion 286
 length deficiency problems, activators and 83–84
 maxillary, presentation with 29
 sagittal expansion 286
 in screening therapy, expansion 73
 in twin block treatment, case studies
  after treatment 110, 117
  before treatment 108, 115
 see also full-arch plastic retainers; segment arch mechanics
archwires (in anchorage control)
 Alexander Discipline 240
  case study of extraction treatment 240, 242, 243, 244, 245, 246
  case study of nonextraction wk 250, 252, 253, 254, 255, 256
 in extraction therapy 220
articulator instruments, distraction prediction with 352–353
a-siloxane *see* vinyl polysiloxane
asymmetric space closure in extraction therapy 219
attachments, Invisalign System 280–282
auto-blocking self-expanders 164
AutoBite 276

B

ball-shaped miniscrew head 266
Balthers bionator *see* bionator
band cement, temporary fixation of twin blocks 105
behavioural patterns 23
bicuspids *see* premolars
bimaxillary crowding, enamel stripping 297–302, 305–307
bimaxillary protrusion of teeth, extraction case 240–249
bionator (of Balthers) 75, 90–94
 anchorage 93
 indications 94
 principles 90–92
 in slow maxillary expansion 166
 trimming 93
 types 92–93
bite registration
 with functional magnetic systems 130
 with twin blocks for deep overbite 102
 see also construction bites; occlusal bite blocks; open-bite; overbite
biteplane, anterior, in Hawley retainer 314
Bolton analysis 22
bonded maxillary expanders 160, 161
bonded retainers 328–331
bone
 anchorage *see* miniscrews; palatal implants; skeletal (bone) anchorage
 remodelling *see* remodelling
brachyfacial patients, interarch compression spring effects on dentition 188
brackets
 Alexander Discipline
  case study of extraction treatment 240, 242, 244
  case study of nonextraction treatment 250, 252, 253
  selection and prescription 235–238
 Edgewise *see* Edgewise appliances
 in rapid maxillary expansion in conjunction with treatment of sagittal maxillary deficiency 169, 172, 173
breathing (respiration)
 abnormal modes 27–28
 construction bites and 77
 vestibular screen with holes for 71–72
buccal occlusion with interarch compression springs 184, 189, 190, 191, 192, 193, 196, 197, 198, 199, 203
buccal segment in group C anchorage, uprighting 217–219
buccinator loops (with standard bionator) 92
buccopalatal angulation of posterior teeth, causes 156
bumper (screening appliances) 73
Burstone CJ and segment arch mechanics 222

Index

C

camouflage 14
canine
   impaction, enamel stripping 305
   intrusion by segmented spring 225, 227
   maxillary, in Alexander Discipline 239
   retraction in Alexander Discipline 240, 243
   root correction 231–232
canine-to-canine Essix retainer 318
   corrective 323–325
   fabrication 318
   modified 323
canine-to-canine fixed bonded retainer 328
caries predisposition with stripping 296
casts (dental)
   construction bite 70
   with Hawley retainer 314–318
   with implants 274
     in miniscrew insertion 270
caudal direction, growth rotation in 15
causation (etiology) 1
cement, temporary fixation of twin blocks 105
cemented retainers 328–331
center of resistance (C_{Res}) of upper arch in group A anchorage control 210
cephalometry 1, 7–8
   in Alexander Discipline
     after treatment 248, 258
     before treatment 242, 252
   construction bites 77–78
   in functional magnetic system treatment, case studies before/after treatment 138, 143, 148, 152
   interarch compression spring space closure of congenitally missing bicuspids 195
   in interceptive treatment 25, 29
     serial extraction and mechanotherapy after treatment 40, 41, 48, 50, 56, 58, 59, 60, 65
     serial extraction and mechanotherapy before treatment 38, 39, 44, 45, 54, 55, 65
   in mandibular distraction osteogenesis 337, 339, 345
     post-treatment 334, 337
     pre-treatment 337
   in twin block treatment, case studies before/after treatment 110, 113, 117, 119
     poor results 122, 125
cervical facebow see facebow
Charles H. Tweed International Foundation for Orthodontic Research and Education 34
clasps
   functional magnetic system 129, 130
   Hawley retainer 313
   twin blocks 105
class I malocclusion
   Alexander Discipline 240
   enamel stripping 297–300
   full-arch plastic retainers 320
   interarch compression springs 179, 180
   serial extraction 34
class II bionator (standard bionator) 92
class II elastics see elastics
class II malocclusion
   activators and construction bites 84, 86
   Alexander Discipline 250–259
   camouflage 14
   enamel stripping, case studies 303–304, 306–307
   functional jaw orthopedics 94–99
   functional magnetic system treatment, case studies 141–154

interarch compression springs 179, 180, 181, 188, 192–193
   non-compliant patients 190
   treatment planning 192–193
interceptive treatment 25
   serial extraction and mechanotherapy 62
lower lip shield 71
rapid maxillary expansion 169
twin blocks, case studies 108–122
class III bionator 93
class III elastics see elastics
class III interarch compression springs 182, 184, 197, 198, 198–200
class III malocclusion
   progression 12
   rapid maxillary expansion 169
clear plastic retainers 314–318
   corrective 323–325
ClinCheck 277, 280, 281, 283
coils, maxillary expanders with 163–164
cold-cure acrylic (of occlusal bite blocks) 104
composite, temporary fixation of twin blocks 105
compression spring, interarch see interarch compression spring
computer programs and analysis 9–12
   in interceptive treatment 24–25
computerized tomography 9–10, 20
Condylar Housing Rotation Instrument (CHRI) 352, 353
cone-beam CT 20
cone-beam volumetric tomography 20
congenitally missing teeth 19
   Alexander Discipline 250, 251
   fixed retainers with 329
   interarch compression spring space closure 195–197
   removable full-arch plastic retainers 322
conically-shaped miniscrew body 267
consolidation period in mandibular distraction osteogenesis 332
   in mandibular lengthening 334
   in mandibular widening 348
construction bites 69, 76–87
   execution 78
   high 78, 79
   low 78, 79
   rules for two variations of 78
   in twin block treatment 104
   types 78
convergent rotation 15
cooling for grinding of teeth 290
co-operation, patient
   with headgear
     in extraction site closure with group A anchorage control 210–211
     non-provision of 211–212
   in maxillary expansion 159
corrective clear plastic retainers 323–325
cost–benefit–risk ratio 2
Cranial Facial Analysis with Difficulty, case studies of serial extraction and mechanotherapy
   after treatment 41, 48, 50, 57, 59, 61
   before treatment 39, 45, 55
cross-shaped miniscrew slots 267
crossbite 28
   anterior, correction 3
   posterior, causes 155–156
   severity, indicating transverse maxillary deficiency 156
   surgically-assisted maxillary expansion 174
crowding
   bimaxillary, enamel stripping 297–302, 305–307

edgewise treatment 66
mandibular, interarch compression springs 198, 199
mild, treatment decisions 11
screening therapy 73
Crozat appliance 278
cylindrically-shaped miniscrew body 267

D

Damon low-friction brackets, Eureka Springs with 189
deband records in anchorage control in extraction therapy 220–221
deciduous dentition, screening therapy 73
deep overbite
   activators and 83
   bite registration with 102
   intrusion arches in correction of 222–225
   twin blocks in management of 106
Delaire mask, rapid maxillary expansion in conjunction with 169, 170, 171
dental floss, space availability checking in Invisalign System 283–284
dentin, risk in grinding toward and into 90, 289
dentition see tooth
dentoalveolar effects of activators 87–88
dentoalveolar overbite and activators 83
diagnosis, therapeutic 1–17
diamond burs for enamel stripping 292, 293, 294
diastema, maxillary midline 21–22
   closed with fixed retainer 329
digital technology 23
direct bonding of canine-to-canine retainers 328
distal movement of teeth, skeletal anchorage 262
distraction osteogenesis, mandibular 332–357
   for lengthening (case study) 337–348
   for widening (case study) 348–355
diverging rotation 15
dolichofacial patients
   interarch compression springs 202
     effects on dentition 188
   mandibular advancement surgery following 1st premolar removal 203
double-helix spring
   in group A anchorage control 212–213
   in group C anchorage control 217–219
   in root correction 230, 232
driftodontics, Alexander Discipline 239
dual-purpose removable retainers 323
dynamic diagnosis 1
dynamic forces, activator therapy 76
dynamic/retention appliances 323
dysfunction, soft tissues and 4
dysplasia, skeletal, functional jaw orthopedics 75
dysplastic relationship (skeletal and neuromuscular components) 14

E

early treatment see interceptive orthodontics
ectopic eruption 20
edgewise appliances/brackets 35–36
   case studies 37–61
     with Edgewise brackets 190
     following functional magnetic system treatment 137, 143–145, 148–149, 153
elastic(s)
   class II 179, 180, 181
     in Alexander Discipline 250, 254
     in orthognathic surgery 202

elastic(s) class III
  in Alexander Discipline 240, 244, 245
  in group C anchorage 215, 216–217
  finishing 240, 246
elastic clasps, functional magnetic system 129, 130
Elliot separator 294
enamel
  mesiodistal reduction *see* stripping
  polishing, instruments 291, 292–294
equilibration, technique with full-arch plastic retainers 321
eruption 20–21
  ectopic 20
  failure (unerupted teeth) 19, 20
Essix clear plastic retainers 314–318
  case example 326
  corrective 323–325
ethylene vinyl acetate (EVA) system 292
etiology 1
Eureka Springs 184, 185, 188
  with Damon low-friction brackets 189
  in orthognathic surgery 202
  with removable appliances 201
EVA system 292
evidence-based diagnosis 15–16
evidence-based studies of Alexander Discipline 260
expansion appliances, maxillary 30
extraction
  in Alexander Discipline, case study 240–249
  anchorage control in site/space closure *see* anchorage
  incisor *see* incisor
  Invisalign treatment combined with 287
  premolars *see* premolars
  serial *see* serial extraction
extrusion of teeth
  activator trimming 87
  Invisalign System 285
  skeletal anchorage 262

F

facebow in Alexander Discipline 239
  case study of extraction treatment 240, 243, 250, 252
  case study of nonextraction treatment 251
facial appearance (balance, harmony, profile etc.)
  with Alexander Discipline
    after treatment 241, 247, 249, 257, 259
    before treatment 241, 257
  with functional magnetic systems
    after treatment 140, 145, 149, 153
    before treatment 138, 141, 146, 150, 153
    during treatment 139
  with Invisalign System, Align technology's request for photographs of 279
  with mandibular lengthening (by osteodistraction)
    after treatment 346
    before treatment 335
  with mandibular widening (by osteo-distraction), before treatment 349
  with serial extraction and mechanotherapy 35
    case studies after treatment 39, 42, 47, 49, 51, 52, 56, 58, 59, 61, 64
    case studies before treatment 37, 43, 53, 64
  with twin blocks
    case studies after treatment 108, 111, 112, 117, 119, 120, 123, 124, 125
    case studies before treatment 108, 111, 112, 114, 118, 120, 123

finishing elastics 240, 246
finishing procedures in anchorage control in extraction therapy 220–221, 221
finite element method 9–12
fixation of twin blocks, temporary 105–107
  see also anchorage
fixed maxillary expanders 160–164, 175, 176
fixed retainers 328–331
flossing for space availability checking in Invisalign System 283–284
forces
  with Alexander Discipline 235, 260
    case study 240
  with clear plastic corrective retainers, inducing 323–325
  with functional therapy 68
    with activators 75–76
    application 68
    elimination 68, 69–74
  with interarch compression spring 179–182
  with maxillary expanders 164
  with segmental arch springs 222, 224, 225
forecasting *see* prediction
Forsus spring 185, 186, 188
Fränkel appliance 95
  in slow maxillary expansion 166
full-arch plastic devices, overlay *see* positioners
full-arch plastic retainers 320–321
function, soft tissues and 4
functional orthodontics (and appliances) 68–94
  magnetic system *see* magnetic system
  principles 68
  twin blocks (for mandibular advancement) *see* twin blocks
functional orthopedics 68, 75, 94–99
functional shift in transverse maxillary deficiency 157

G

gingiva (mucosa)
  in enamel stripping
    maintaining normal papillae 295–296
    regaining lost papillae 296
  eruption impeded by 20
  miniscrew insertion through (using punch instrument for perforation) 268
gingival neck of miniscrew 267
goals/aims/objectives of treatment 8, 13–15
  age-related 8
  in interceptive guidance of occlusion 24–25
  with vestibular screen 69
Graber, Tom 127
grinding of teeth (technique), risks 289–290
growth (jaw – mandible and maxilla) 155
  activator therapy and forces of 76
  age-related changes 2, 3, 8
    puberty 99–100
  extremes 25
  mean annual mandibular, appliances enhancing extent of 24
  proprioceptive stimulus 101
  rotation (in treatment) 15
guidance (tooth)
  with activators 87
  of occlusion, interceptive 33–67

H

"H" activator 78, 79, 80
  construction bites for 78

Haas expander 160, 161, 167, 168
habits 23
handpiece, enamel stripping 294–295
Häupl K 68
  see also Andresen and Häupl activator
Hawley retainers 221, 313–314, 322
  in mandibular distraction osteogenesis 334
headgear
  Alexander Discipline in class I bi-maxillary protrusion extraction case 240, 244
  in extraction site closure with group A anchorage control, patient co-operation 210–211
  Reverse (Delaire mask), rapid maxillary expansion in conjunction with 169, 170, 171
  screening appliances 73
healing, miniscrews 266
heat-cured acrylic (of occlusal bite blocks) 104
Herbst appliance compared with interarch compression springs 184
histiogenesis, distraction 335
Howe pliers in trial activation of titanium T-loop retraction springs 208
hyoid triangle 27
Hyrax expander 160, 161, 167

I

imaging (radiology) 9
  3D 9, 20
  miniscrew insertion site 270–271
  of transverse maxillary deficiency 156–157
  see also specific modalities
impaction
  canine, enamel stripping 305
  molar 21
    skeletal anchorage 262, 264
implants 261–275
impressions
  for Hawley retainer 314–315
  for Invisalign System 282–283
incisors
  in activator therapy 88–89
    extrusion of 87
    intrusion of 87
    lower 88–89
    protrusion of 87, 88
    retrusion of 87, 88
    upper 89
  in Alexander Discipline 239
    missing 250, 251
  congenitally missing right central, interarch compression spring space closure 196–197
  intrusion (in deep overbite correction) 222, 223, 224
    and retrusion 226
  mandibular *see* mandible
  maxillary central, overlapping, enamel stripping 303–304
  recontouring 293
  root correction 231–232
indications (for treatment) 2
  activator therapy 78
  bionator therapy 94
  fixed retainers 328
  full-arch plastic retainers 320–322
  Invisalign System treatment 285–287
    combined with extraction therapy 287–288
  screening therapy 73
  skeletal orthodontic anchorage 262
indices (in objectifying of treatment) 2
indirect bonding of canine-to-canine retainers 328–331

inferior alveolar nerve damage in mandibular distraction osteogenesis, minimizing 341
interarch compression springs 179–204
    case studies 189–203
    dentition and the effects of 188
    description and comparisons of various appliances 184–185
    disadvantages 204
    forces/moments/analyses 179–182
    relapse following rapid tooth movement utilizing 200–201
interceptive (early/preventive/prophylactic) orthodontics 18–32
    occlusion 19–20, 33–67
interdental stripping *see* stripping
intrusion (of teeth)
    activator trimming 87
    deep overbite correction by 222–225
    in implantology 274
        skeletal anchorage 262, 263
    Invisalign System 285
Invisalign (aligner) System 276–288
    attachments 280–282
    clinical approach 278–280
    clinical aspects 283–285
    impression-taking 282–283
    indications 285–286
    principles 276–277

J

Jasper jumper compared with interarch compression springs 184
jaw
    functional orthopedics 68, 75, 94–99
    growth *see* growth
    see also mandible; maxilla
jumpers compared with interarch compression springs 184

K

Kesling's positioner 276
kinesiographic recording 4, 5
Kjellgren B 33
Körbitz, narrow slipper analogy of 95

L

labial bow (lip bar) 79
    class II (standard) bionator 92
    class III bionator 93
    Hawley retainer 313, 314
    open-bite bionator 93
labial fold and vestibular screens 69
latency period in mandibular distraction osteogenesis 332
    mandibular lengthening 333
    mandibular widening 348
lateral expansion of dental arch 286
light maxillary expansion 167
lingual appliances 278
    arches 232
lip
    lower
        in mandibular lengthening (by osteodistraction) 334
        shield 71
        twin block for class II malocclusion regarding 114

seal 4, 5
    with functional magnetic system 137, 140, 150, 153
    vestibular screen and 70
    see also entries under labial
lip bar *see* labial bow
loading, implant 274
    miniscrew 265, 269, 270, 271, 272
loading areas, bionator 93
loss of teeth, early 20
low-friction Damon brackets, Eureka Springs with 189

M

machine insertion of miniscrews 269
Magnetic Expansion Device 167
magnetic resonance imaging 9
magnetic system, functional (FMS) 127–154
    case studies 137–154
    design 128
    fabrication 130
    mechanism of functional correction 132–136
    modus operandi 131
malfunction, soft tissues and 4
malocclusion
    activators 83
    class I, serial extraction 34
    class II/III *see* class II malocclusion; class III malocclusion
    twin blocks in correction of *see* twin blocks
mandible
    in Alexander Discipline
        archwires 240, 244, 250, 254, 255, 256
        brackets 240, 244, 250, 253
        treatment mechanics 239
    construction bite for markedly forward positioning of 78, 79
    construction bite with opening of 84–86
    construction bite with retrusion or posterior positioning of 78, 84–86
    construction bite for slightly forward (anterior) positioning of 78, 79
    construction bite without forward positioning of 83
    crowding, interarch compression springs 198, 199
    distraction osteogenesis *see* distraction osteogenesis
    functional advancement
        with magnetic system 130
        with twin blocks *see* twin blocks
    growth *see* growth
    incisors
        Essix appliance with misaligned 326
        Invisalign treatment combined with extraction 287
        stripping vs extraction of a 296
    molar impaction 21
    patient advancing, in prediction of response to functional advancement 101–102
    rest position *see* rest
    retainers, in distraction osteogenesis 334
    retrognathism
        activator therapy 89
        functional magnetic system, case studies 137–145
        functional orthopedics 95–97
        serial extraction and mechanotherapy, case study 43, 44
    retrusion *see* retrusion

surgical advancement following 1st premolar extraction 203
see also jaw
maxilla
    in Alexander Discipline
        archwires 240, 242, 250, 252–256
        brackets 240, 242, 250, 252
        treatment mechanics 239
    anatomy 155
    expansion *see* maxillary expansion
    growth *see* growth
    incisors, overlapping central, enamel stripping 303–304
    narrow dental arch, presentation with 29
    narrow slipper analogy of Körbitz 95
    prognathic *see* prognathic maxilla
    retainers, in mandibular distraction osteogenesis 334
    retrognathism, case study of serial extraction and mechanotherapy 43, 44
    sagittal deficiency, case study of rapid maxillary expansion in conjunction with treatment of 169–174
    transverse deficiency 155
        diagnosis 155–157
    see also bimaxillary crowding; bimaxillary protrusion; jaw
maxillary expansion 30, 155–178
    age and effects of 167–168
    early 155–178
        case studies 169–174
    forces 164
    late 174
    rapid *see* rapid palatal expansion
    rate, and its dental and skeletal effects 166–167
    retention and stability 175
    side-effects 175, 176
    surgically-assisted 174, 276
    timing 157–158
    types of expanders 160–164
maxillary midline diastema *see* diastema
maxillomandibular transverse differential, assessment 157
maxillomandibular width differential, assessment 157
mechanical separator in enamel stripping 294
mechanotherapy 31
    serial extraction followed by *see* serial extraction
Merrifield, Levern 35
mesial movement of teeth, skeletal anchorage 262
mesial out-rotation of molar 232, 233
mesiodistal enamel reduction *see* stripping
micrognathia (small mandible), functional orthopedics 95
midcourse changes in treatment 1, 11
midline diastema, maxillary *see* diastema
Mills, Christine 107
miniscrews 262, 263, 270, 270–272
    considerations in use of 265–270
    disadvantages 272
    insertion, instruments for 268–269
    for palatal implants 272
    removal 265, 271
    requirements for anchorage with 265
Minne Expander 163, 167
missing teeth
    congenitally *see* congenitally missing teeth
    dental implants as replacements 274
    fixed retainers with 329
    removable full-arch plastic retainers with 322

mixed dentition, screening therapy 73
molars
    extrusion
        activators and 87
        skeletal anchorage 263
    impaction *see* impaction
    intrusions 274
        activators and 87
        in implantology 262, 274
    mandibular 1st, in Alexander Discipline 239
    maxillary 1st, class II interarch compression springs and forces on 182
    rotation 232
    "tip-back" 225, 232, 234
    tipped, skeletal anchorage for uprighting of 262
moments
    interarch compression spring 179–182
    segmental arch spring 222
Moorrees CFA 33, 34
mounding to induce force with clear plastic corrective retainers 323–324
mouth breathing (oral respiration) 27–28
    vestibular screens and 71–73
mucosa, gingival *see* gingiva
multibanded-multibracket appliance 34–35, 62
muscle contractions, activator therapy and forces of 76

N

narrow slipper analogy of Körbitz 95
nerve damage in mandibular distraction osteogenesis, minimizing 341
neuromuscular structures 4
    dysplastic relationship of skeletal and 14
    eliminating dysfunction 4, 5
neurosensory deficits in mandibular distraction osteogenesis 335
nickel–titanium (NiTi) wires
    interarch compression springs 199
    maxillary expansion 164
nocturnal enuresis, rapid maxillary expansion 175
noncompliant class II patients, interarch compression springs 190

O

objectives of treatment *see* goals
obstructive sleep apnea, rapid maxillary expansion 174–175
occlusal bite blocks (of twin blocks) 104
occlusion
    buccal, with interarch compression springs 184, 189, 190, 191, 192, 193, 196, 197, 198, 199, 203
    positions
        interceptive treatment for 19–20, 33–67
        mandibular manipulation for 5
    see also malocclusion
"Old Glory" skull 13
open-bite (malocclusive)
    activators and 83
    twin blocks in management of 106
        anterior teeth 107
open-bite bionator 92–93
oral breathing *see* mouth breathing
Ortho-Strips system 292

orthognathic mandible with prognathic maxilla, functional orthopedics 97
orthognathic surgery, interarch compression springs in 202
orthopedic vs surgically-assisted maxillary expansion 174
orthopedics, functional 68, 75, 94–99
oscillating handpiece, enamel stripping 294–295
osseointegration, concept/principle of 261, 266
osteodistraction *see* distraction osteogenesis
osteotomy in mandibular distraction osteogenesis 332
    mandibular lengthening 333, 341, 342
    mandibular widening 348, 350, 353
overbite
    activators and 83
    Alexander Discipline, case studies 240, 241, 250, 251
    brackets (on expanders) increasing and securing 169, 172, 173
    deep *see* deep overbite
    interarch compression springs 198, 199
overjet
    Alexander Discipline, case studies 241, 250, 251
    bite registration (for twin block treatment) 102
    in mandibular distraction osteogenesis
        inter-treatment 343
        post-treatment 334, 344, 345, 347
        pre-treatment 337
overlay full-arch plastic devices *see* positioners

P

palatal bar
    class II (standard) bionator 92
    class IIL bionator 93
    open-bite bionator 93
palatal expansion, rapid *see* rapid palatal expansion
palatal implants 272–273
palatal vault
    miniscrew insertion on 271
    morphology indicating skeletal deficiency 156
Panadent Articulator 352
patient co-operation *see* co-operation
perforated plastic trays for impression-taking for Invisalign System 283
periodontium (periodontal tissue)
    assessment 7–8
    in enamel stripping
        pretreatment breakdown 308–311
        risk of accelerated breakdown 296
photographs
    diagnostic 27
    Invisalign (aligner) System 278
    intraoral 276
    see also facial appearance
pilot drill for self-tapping miniscrews 267, 268
pin and tube system for maxillary expanders 163–164
planning of treatment
    interarch compression springs for class II malocclusion 192–193
    mandibular distraction osteogenesis
        for lengthening 333
        for widening 348
plastic(s), thermoforming *see* thermoforming devices
plastic positioning devices *see* positioners

plastic retainers 314–318, 323
    clear *see* clear plastic retainers
    full-arch 320–321
plastic trays, perforated, for impression-taking for Invisalign System 283
platform of miniscrew 267
pliers, thermoforming 325
    corrective clear plastic retainers 325
    splint aligners 276
polishing of enamel, instruments 291, 292–294
polyurethane, aligners made from 277
polyvinyl siloxane *see* vinyl polysiloxane
positioners (overlay full arch plastic devices) 327
    Kesling's 276
posterior teeth (tooth segments)
    anchorage 225
    buccopalatal angulation, causes 156
    common presentations following space closure 230
    crossbite, causes 155–156
    sliding 4
postural rest *see* rest
prediction (forecasting) 11–12
    mandibular osteodistraction
        in lengthening 339
        in widening 351, 352, 353
premolars (bicuspids)
    congenitally missing, interarch compression spring space closure 195–196
    extraction
        following functional magnetic system treatment 137, 140
        Invisalign treatment combined with 287
        mandibular advancement surgery following, of 1st premolars 203
        plastic retainer holding extraction site closed 318
    recontouring 293
pressure machines for thermoforming plastic 316
preventive orthodontics *see* interceptive orthodontics
profile *see* facial appearance
prognathic maxilla
    with orthognathic mandible, functional orthopedics 97
    with retrognathic mandible, functional magnetic system 141–145
progressive activation of twin blocks 102
prophylactic orthodontics *see* interceptive orthodontics
proprioceptive stimulus growth 101
prosthetic implants 261–275
protrusion of teeth
    activator trimming and 87, 88
    bimaxillary, extraction case 240–249
Proxoshape set 292
pubertal growth spurts 99–100
punch instrument for miniscrew insertion 268

Q

Quad-helix (of Ricketts) 163
    case study 150, 151
    in maxillary expansion 161, 164, 167

R

radiography
    miniscrew insertion site 271
    transverse maxillary deficiency 156–157

radiology see imaging and specific modalities
rapid palatal (maxillary) expansion (RME; RPE) 28, 29–30, 155, 167
   in conjunction with treatment of sagittal maxillary deficiency, case study 169–174
   in obstructive sleep apnea 174–175
recontouring by stripping see stripping
records
   deband, in anchorage control in extraction therapy 220–221
   essential diagnostic 1–2
remodelling, bone
   with mandibular distraction osteogenesis 332
     in mandibular lengthening 334
   with miniscrews 266
removable appliances
   interarch compression springs with 201
   maxillary expanders 160
   retainers see retention
reproximation chart with Invisalign System 280
reshaping by stripping see stripping
respiration, abnormal modes of 27–28
rest (postural)
   mandibular manipulation for 4, 5
   registration of position at 4
retention (and retainers) 313–331
   in Alexander Discipline 239
   fixed retainers 328–331
   Hawley-type appliance see Hawley retainers
   in mandibular distraction osteogenesis 334
   in maxillary expansion 175
   miniscrew 266
   removable retainers 313–328
     case examples 326–327
retraction
   in Alexander Discipline 240, 243
   in deep overbite correction, intrusion and 225
   see also titanium T-loop retraction springs
retrognathism
   functional appliances 89, 90
     limited response to mandibular advancement with twin blocks 120
   mandibular see mandible
   maxillary, case study of serial extraction and mechanotherapy 43, 44
retrusion
   incisors in activator therapy, trimming and 87, 88
   mandibular
     in activator therapy, construction bite with 78, 84–86
     functional magnetic system treatment 150–155
     twin block treatment 101, 102, 114, 118, 120, 123, 126
reverse curve of Spee, mandibular archwire with 250, 254
Reverse Headgear (Delaire mask), rapid maxillary expansion in conjunction with 169, 170, 171
reversed bionator 93
rhinomanometry 28
rhythmic forces, activator therapy 76
Ricketts RM
   quad-helix of see quad-helix
   Rocky Mountain analysis 11, 29
root
   correction (following space closure)
     retraction en-mass in group A anchorage control 212
     in segmented spring mechanics 231–232
   resorption with maxillary expanders 175, 176
rotating handpiece, enamel stripping 294–295
rotation (in treatment) 15

Invisalign System 285–286
molar 232
wings for, Alexander Discipline 235
Roux hypothesis 68

S

sagittal expansion of dental arch 286
sagittal maxillary deficiency, case study of rapid maxillary expansion in conjunction with treatment of 169–174
sagittal plane (with activators)
   movements of posterior teeth 90
   trimming for sagittal control 87–88
SAM Mandibular Position Variator 340, 341
screening therapy 68, 69–73
   indications 73
screw(s), maxillary expanders with 160–161, 176
   see also miniscrews
screw advancement system, twin blocks 103
screwdriver (miniscrew)
   for insertion 268–269
   for removal 271
segment arch mechanics (springs) 222–234
   root correction closure 231–232
   space closure 227
self-drilling miniscrews 267
self-expanders (maxillary) 164
self-tapping miniscrews 267
semi-rapid maxillary expansion 167
sensory deficits in mandibular distraction osteogenesis 335
serial extraction followed by mechanotherapy 33–67
   case studies 37–66
shape (tooth) abnormalities 22–23
size (tooth) abnormalities 22–23
skeletal (bone) anchorage 261–262
skeletal dysplasia, functional jaw orthopedics 75
skeletal effects of maxillary expansion 166–167
skeletal vs dental discrepancy in timing of maxillary expansion 159
sleep apnea, obstructive, rapid maxillary expansion 174–175
sliding movements 4
slots, miniscrew 267
slow maxillary expansion 166, 175, 176
soft tissues
   activator therapy and stretching of 76
   and function 4
   in mandibular distraction osteogenesis 335
space
   availability checking in Invisalign System 283–284
   creation, with corrective clear plastic retainers 324
   held close
     with fixed retainer 329
     with removable retainer 320
   held open with fixed retainer 329–331
space closure
   anchorage control see anchorage
   congenitally missing teeth 195–197
   extracted teeth
     asymmetric 219
     interarch compression spring, incisors 196–197
     segment arch mechanics 227
Spee, mandibular archwire with reverse curve of 250, 254
splint aligners see Invisalign System

spring(s) see double-helix spring; interarch compression spring; segment arch mechanics; titanium T-loop retraction spring
spring retainers 327–328
static forces, activator therapy 76
steel (surgical) miniscrews 265–266
stepwise advancement, twin blocks 103
stripping, interdental (mesiodistal enamel reduction) 289–312
   adverse effects 296
   amount of enamel removal 290–291
   case studies 297–311
   gingiva in see gingiva
   instruments 291–294
   optimal technique 294–295
   risks in grinding teeth 289–290
study models with construction bites 77
supernumerary teeth 19
surgical steel miniscrews 265–266
surgically-assisted maxillary expansion 174, 176

T

T-loop springs see titanium T-loop retraction springs
teeth (dentition and single tooth)
   activators regarding movements of 90
     trimming of 87–88
   anterior see anterior teeth
   distal or mesial movement, indicating skeletal anchorage 262
   eruption see eruption
   extraction see extraction
   extrusion see extrusion
   grinding (technique), risks 289–290
   guidance see guidance
   impaction 21
   interarch compression spring effects on 188
   intrusion see intrusion
   loss, early 20
   maxillary expansion effects on 166–167
   missing see missing teeth
   posterior see posterior teeth
   rapid movement utilizing interarch compression springs, relapse following 200–201
   screening therapy with mixed and deciduous dentition 73
   size and shape abnormalities 22–23
   supernumerary 19
   see also specific teeth
temporary anchorage devices 262
   dental implants as 273–274
temporary fixation of twin blocks 105–107
therapeutic diagnosis 1–17
thermoforming devices (with plastics)
   pliers see pliers
   for retainer fabrication 316–318, 318
     full-arch retainers 320
thread of miniscrew 267
three-dimensional imaging 9, 20
timing of treatment 11, 12
"tip-back", molar 225, 232, 234
tipping, controlled
   in group A anchorage 211–212
   in group C anchorage 215
titanium miniscrews 265, 266
titanium T-loop retraction springs (TTLRS) 219, 221, 227
   in group A anchorage control 210, 211
   in group B anchorage control 206, 219
     fabrication and preactivation 207
     trial activation 208

titanium T-loop retraction springs (TTLRS)
   in group C anchorage control   214–215, 215, 216, 216–217
      intraoral reactivation   216–217
tongue
   bionators and the   90–91
   shield, in vestibular screen   70, 71
   see also lingual appliances
tooth *see* teeth
ToothShaper software   276
torques, Alexander Discipline   235, 237
Total Space Analysis (TSA) and TSA Difficulty, case studies of serial extraction and mechanotherapy   37, 38, 43, 44, 53
traction, extraoral   24, 25
   see also distraction osteogenesis
transfer trays for canine-to-canine fixed bonded retainers   328
transgingival (transmucosal) portion of miniscrew   267
transpalatal arches   232
transverse maxillary deficiency *see* maxilla
trays
   for impression-taking for Invisalign System   283
   transfer, for canine-to-canine fixed bonded retainers   328
Treat software   280, 284
triangular clasps, functional magnetic system   130
trimming
   activator   87–88
   bionator   93

tungsten carbide (TC) burs for enamel stripping   292, 294
Tuverson technique for mesiodistal enamel reduction   291, 292
   modified   292
Tweed, Charles H   34, 35
Tweed–Merrifield Edgewise Appliance   35–36
   case studies   37–61
twin blocks   101–126
   activation   102, 103
   active phase of treatment   105
   case selection   101–102
   case studies   108–125
      poor/limited responses   120–125
   clinical management   105–107
   construction   104
   design   104
   support phase of treatment   105
Twin Force   185, 187, 188

U

U-shape of full-arch plastic retainers   320
ultrasound, 3D   9
unerupted teeth   19, 20

V

"V" activator   78, 79, 81
   construction bite for   78

vacuum machines for thermoforming plastic   316, 318
vertical plane/dimension
   with activators
      problems relating to   83–86
      trimming for vertical control   87
   in deep overbite correction   102
vestibular screen   69–70
   goals of treatment with   69
video imaging   11, 12
vinyl polysiloxane (polyvinyl siloxane; a-siloxane)
   for impression-taking
      Hawley retainer   315
      Invisalign System   282
virtual models (Invisalign System)   276, 277
Vitallium miniscrews   265

W

water cooling for grinding of teeth   290
wedge (wooden) in enamel stripping   294
wiggle analysis in case studies of serial extraction and mechanotherapy
   after treatment   41, 49, 51, 57, 59, 61
   before treatment   40, 46, 56
wings, rotational, Alexander Discipline   235
wooden wedge in enamel stripping   294

X

X-rays radiography *see* radiography